LAYAYOGA

LAYAYOGA

The Definitive Guide to the Chakras and Kundalini

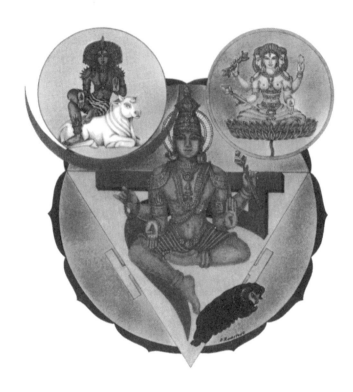

Shyam Sundar Goswami

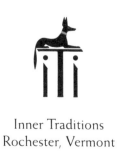

Inner Traditions
Rochester, Vermont

Inner Traditions International
One Park Street
Rochester, Vermont 05767
www.InnerTraditions.com

Library of Congress Cataloging-in-Publication Data

Goswami, Shyam Sundar.
    Layayoga : the definitive guide to the chakras and
kundalini / Shyam Sundar Goswami.
       p.   cm.
    Originally published: Boston : Routledge & Kegan Paul, 1980.
    Includes index.
    ISBN 978-0-89281-766-5
    1. Yoga, Laya. 2. Chakras. 3. Kundalini. I. Title.
BL1238.56.L38G67   1999
294.5'436—dc21   99-10266
                              CIP

Printed and bound in India by Replika Press Pvt. Ltd.

10 9 8 7 6

To Wani
Goddess of Words

'uttishthata jagrata prapya waran nibodhata'
                    —Kathopanishad, 1. 3. 14

Arise, awake and seek a teacher;
First know 'Who art Thou'.

This Upanishadic saying reverberates in
the Greek maxim

'Γνῶθι   σεαυτόν'

engraved in the temple of Apollo at Delphi.

Contents

Expounded by Shiwa; The Chakra
System as Expounded by Bhairawi; As
Explained by Rishi Narada; As Explained
by Mahidhara; As Explained by
Brahmananda; As Explained by
Jñanananda; As Explained by Lakshmana
Deshikendra; As Explained by
Brahmananda Giri)

1 Muladhara (Terminology, Position,
Description, Explanation) – 2 Swadhi-
shthana (Terminology, Position, Descrip-
tion, Explanation) – 3 Manipura
(Terminology, Position, Description,
Explanation) – 4 Hrit (Terminology,
Position, Description, Explanation) –5
Anahata (Terminology, Position,
Description, Explanation) – 6 Wishuddha
(Terminology, Position, Description,
Explanation) – 7 Talu (Terminology,
Position, Description, Explanation) – 8
Ajña (Terminology, Position, Description,
Explanation)

Ajña System – 9 Manas (Terminology,
Position, Description, Explanation) – 10
Indu (Terminology, Position, Description,
Explanation) – 11 Nirwana (Terminology,
Position, Description, Explanation) –
Sahasrara System – 12 Guru
(Terminology, Position, Description,
Explanation) – 13 Sahasrara
(Terminology, Position, Description,
Explanation) – The Chakra Table

The Vertebral Column – The Cranial
Cavity – The Spinal Cord – The Filum
Terminale – The Central Canal – The
Brain – The Medulla Oblongata – The
Pons – The Midbrain – The Interbrain –

Contents

Illustrations

Foreword to the Second Edition

by Georg Feuerstein, Ph.D.
Founder-Director of the Yoga Research Center
and author of *The Shambhala Encyclopedia of Yoga*

This unique volume focuses on one of the most recondite aspects of Tantra: the esoteric process by which the ordinary human body is transmuted into a "divine body" *(divya-deha)*. In such a body, every cell is suffused with consciousness, and it is endowed with extraordinary capacities *(siddhi)*.

At the heart of Tantra is Kundaliniyoga, and at the core of Kundaliniyoga is Layayoga. Tantra, or Tantrism, is a spiritual tradition that crystallized in the opening centuries of the first millennium C.E. and reached its zenith around 1000 C.E. It represents a remarkable synthesis and understands itself as the teaching for the present age of darkness *(kali-yuga)*. Among its central tenets is the notion that the body is not, as taught by more ascetical schools, an obstacle on the path to enlightenment. Rather, it is a manifestation of the ultimate Reality and hence must be fully integrated into one's spiritual aspirations. The early Tantric adepts *(siddha)* developed an approach that is body-positive and epitomized in the concept of "body cultivation," or *kaya-sadhana,* which in due course led to the creation of Hathayoga with its many purificatory practices *(sadhana),* postures *(asana),* and techniques of breath control *(pranayama).*

The purpose of these practices is not merely to acquire physical fitness and mental health, but primarily to awaken the body's dormant psychospiritual power called kundalini-shakti. When this power, which is a form of conscious energy, is fully aroused it begins to transform the body. It leads to the ecstatic realization of one's true identity as the pure, universal consciousness *(cit),* and it also progressively renders the body transparent to that supreme consciousness.

This alchemical process of transmutation of the very constituents of the body is the domain of Layayoga. Laya refers to the absorption of the elements *(tattva)* constituting the body, which occurs when the kundalini power rises from the psychoenergetic center *(cakra)* at the base of the spine toward the center at the crown of the head. In its ascent along the spinal axis, it must pierce a series of psychoenergetic centers, each of which relates to specific psychosomatic functions and also anatomical structures. As it passes through each center, the kundalini absorbs each center's elements and correlated function. This induces a deepening state of mental concentration and conscious lucidity, but at the same time decreases physical animation. Thus the outside observer would notice a drastic decrease in metabolism and spontaneous suspension of breathing. In a way, the ascent of the kundalini amounts to a consciously undergone death process.

If the yogin remains long enough in this state of suspended animation, the body simply dies. But this is not the intended outcome of Tantra. Rather, the successful practitioner of Tantrayoga must next skillfully guide the kundalini from the crown center back to its home at the base of the spine. This restores all the bodily functions, yet brings a new element into play: the gradual suffusion of the body with consciousness. For the Tantric adept, enlightenment is nothing unless it includes the body. Thus the delicate process of Layayoga is designed to bring enlightenment down to earth, into the body—a quite literally breathtaking adventure.

Shyam Sundar Goswami, who was an adept of Layayoga, sifted through no fewer than 282 Sanskrit texts to gather all the relevant information about the process of absorption *(laya-krama)* into one volume. This book is a testimony to his spiritual stature and tremendous scholarship, but also to the yogic heritage of India. Nowhere else on earth can one find such profound knowledge about esoteric anatomy and the subtle energetic work

necessary to achieve full enlightenment.

I hope this volume will help correct prevalent, especially New Age, misconceptions about the cakras and nadis. The information locked away in the Sanskrit scriptures and presented here comprehensively for the first time is based on actual yogic experimentation and realization, which makes Shyam Sundar Goswami's compilation an extremely valuable gift to genuine Yoga practitioners. I would like to commend the publisher for reissuing this book, which has been out of print for many years.

Foreword

It has been expounded in the wedamantra: 'yogeyoge tawastarang wajewaje hawamahe. sakhaya indramutaye' (—Rigweda-sanghita, 1. 30.7). That is, with our hearts attuned, we worship with deepest love Indra (Supreme Power-Consciousness) so as to be able to practise samprajñata yoga (with all its parts successfully, by removing all obstacles that distract the mind), and then (by developing supreme unaffectedness) asamprajñata yoga.

This worship is ishwarapranidhana, that is, concentration in deepest love for God. Love-concentration causes samadhi. Patañjali has also said: 'ishwarapranidhanad wa' (samadhi is also attained by love-concentration on God) (—Yogasutra, 1.23) and 'samadhisiddhi rishwarapranidhanat' (the accomplishment of samadhi is effected by love-concentration on God) (—ibid., 2.45).

There are Oupanishada explanations of the Waidika 'yogeyoge'. It has been stated: 'yogena yogo jñatawyo yogo yogat prawardhate' (—Soubhagyalakshmyupanishad, 2.1). That is, yoga is to be known by yoga, and yoga develops from yoga. This means that the attainment of asamprajñata yoga is accomplished by samprajñata yoga; asamprajñata yoga develops from samprajñata yoga. Again, 'yogena yogang sangrodhya . . . ' (—ibid., 2.12). That is, controlling yoga by yoga. This means that samprajñata yoga is controlled by asamprajñata yoga. In other words, samprajñata samadhi is transformed into asamprajñata samadhi when control develops to its highest degree.

The nonappearance of the absorbed writtis (linawritti) is the limit of control (—Adhyatmopanishad, 42). At this stage, natural mental absorption, leading to mind-transcendent state, occurs (—Akshyupanishad, 2.3).

Yoga means samadhi. So it has been stated: 'sa gha no yoga a bhuwat . . . ' (—Rigweda-sanghita, 1.5.3), that is, the yogi is established in yoga. Here, yoga is samadhi.

Waidika 'yogakshemah' (—Maitrayani-sanghita, 3.12.6; Shuklayajurweda-sanghita, 22.22; Taittiriya-sanghita, 7.5.18) means the preservation of samadhi. It has been stated that yoga is the attainment of that which is otherwise unobtainable. What is that thing? It is that which is beyond the senses and mind. It is Brahman (Supreme Consciousness). The attainment of Brahman is not possible without recourse to samadhi (—Nrisinghatapinyupanishad, Part 2,6.4; Atmopanishad, 4; Annapurnopanishad, 4.62; Trishikhibrahmanopanishad, Mantra Section, 161-2; etc.). All this indicates that yoga is samadhi. The word kshema means preservation. So 'yogakshema' is the preservation of samadhi. This is why it has been stated: 'yogang prapadye kshemang cha kshemang prapadye yogang cha' (—Atharwaweda-sanghita, 9.8.2). That is, I may attain yoga (samadhi) and kshema (preservation) and kshema and yoga. The attainment of samadhi and its preservation is the aim of the practice of yoga.

Yoga is hidden in the wedamantra (—Rigweda-sanghita, 10.114.9) as bijas which are its original form. The bijas are four: 'yang', 'ung', 'gang', and 'ah'. Again, 'yang' is composed of two bijas, 'ing' and 'ang'. When the powers locked in the bijas are roused and harnessed, the nada-bindu factor is absorbed into the bija aspect, and then the bijas, being arranged in order, constitute the shrouta word 'yogah', which in that form, as well as in its complex spiritual forms, occurs frequently in the Sanghitas of the Weda.

The two matrika-letters ing and ang represent agni (fire) and soma (moon), or pingala and ida. Pingala and ida cause respiratory motions which are based on yang bija. When yang is roused, respiration is suspended because of the absorption of pingala and ida in the sushumna, and as a result kumbhaka is effected. At this stage, the yang-force is transformed into yama (control). The emergence of yama occurs in three stages: physical control in relaxation in asana, vital control in kumbhaka, and sensory control in pratyahara. At the pratyahara stage, the bija ung is roused and radiates udana force, by which concentration develops in three stages in the mental field: dharana, dhyana and samprajñata samadhi. At the samadhi stage, yama (control) becomes sangyama (super-control).

In samprajñata samadhi, the bija gang is roused as concentration-knowledge-light (prajñaloka). Associated with gang is wisarga (ah); it is represented by the sign:. Wisarga is Kundalini. Kundalini is roused in samadhi and illuminates the whole superconcentrated mind by her splendour. Then, Kundalini absorbs super-consciousness by her absorptive power to effect a mind-transcendent stage in which samprajñata samadhi is transformed into asamprajñata sama-dhi. Finally, Kundalini herself is absorbed into and united as one with Parama Shiwa—Supreme Consciousness. This supreme absorptive yoga is layayoga. Rigweda calls it the attainment of the state of Indra in yoga (—Rigweda-sanghita, 4.24.4).

There is a clear indication of the layayogic absorptive process in the Atharwaweda-sanghita, 9.8.2. It has been stated there 'ashtawingshani

shiwani shagmani sahayogang bhajanta me', that is, all the cosmic principles together become beneficial and pleasant when they are devoted to yoga. This means that the cosmic principles, after being roused from the absorptive state of yoga, become propitious. This yoga is absorptive concentration. It is layayoga.

The nature of layayoga has been expounded in the following mantra:

'jyotishmantang ketumantang
trichakrang sukhang rathang
sushadang bhuriwaram.
chitramagha yasya yoge 'dhijajñe
tang wang huwe ati riktang pibadhyai'
(—Rigweda-sanghita, 8.58.3)

That is, ordinarily, this luminous and living force is latent in the body with its three sheaths (matter-life-mind), and is capable of becoming quiescent. When, by absorptive concentration, this highest, splendorous, and omnipotent power is in union with Supreme Consciousness, a 'deathless substance' (amrita) starts to flow. It is then necessary, by purificatory and vitalizing exercises, to prepare both body and mind for the utilization of this substance. This splendorous power is Kundalini.

This is Waidika layayoga. Its successful practice and accomplishment can be achieved only under the direct instruction of a teacher (guru).

In this book, Waidika layayoga and its Tantrika and Pouranika interpretations are clearly and elaborately elucidated. The author is a renowned teacher of yoga, whose work is based not only on his lifelong study and practice of yoga, but also on direct instruction by advanced layayogis. The book will prove especially useful to all serious readers who feel the need for attaining mental control and concentration in their every-day life.

Calcutta   Acharyya Karunamoya Saraswati

Preface

This book aims to present layayoga authentically and elaborately. For this purpose it was necessary to investigate and study the immense number of ancient documents of the rishis who expounded yoga.

The present work is essentially based on the Rigweda-sanghita, containing 10,589 mantras; 179 Upanishads; 67 Tantras having over 10,000 pages which contain innumerable verses, and 9 Tantrika manuscripts having 386 pages; 23 Puranas, containing 451,000 verses; the 100,000-verse Mahabharata of Wyasa, which includes the Bhagawadgita; the 29,000-verse Yogawashishtha-Ramayana of Walmiki; and Yoga-darshana of Patañjali, containing 195 aphorisms.

From these sources, 4,122 mantras and verses have been quoted in this work. The mantras and verses had to be translated. They contain 1, 2, 3 or 4 lines each. All this was necessary in order to find out—rather rediscover—the original form of this yoga—the form which was given by the rishis of ancient India, who were the exponents of yoga. The rishis introduced a system of technical terms to interpret the hidden meaning and various processes of yoga to their pupils. It is our purpose to paint a genuine picture of layayoga—layayoga as it was known and practised in ancient India.

With regard to the English translation of the Sanskrit texts cited in this work, I wish to say that an attempt has been made to give, in many cases, the secret and yogic meanings in preference to the literary translations. However, in each case, a complete reference has been given which includes the title of the book or manuscript, number of the mantras and verses whenever possible, chapters, etc. This may be helpful to research students of yoga. The edition and the author's or editor's name have been given in the bibliography. For explanation of transliteration of Sanskrit terms the reader is referred to the Note on Pronunciation at the end of the book (p. 328).

Moreover, it was absolutely necessary to have the guidance of competent and well-experienced layayoga gurus for the right understanding of the Sanskrit texts and a practical knowledge of the various processes of layayoga. This has been specially utilized in the part dealing with Concentration Practices (Part 3 of this book), and to which my guru's contribution is the greatest. My own personal experiences also have been helpful.

An important question may be raised in connection with this study: What is the significance of layayoga and its utility in our lives? The whole book gives the answer. Still it can be added here, that a serious student, determined to make experiments by undergoing the layayoga practices, will discover the tremendous power of thought and concentration which usually remains hidden. Concentration becomes so real and forceful that at a certain stage it rouses a latent power which is at zero level in our ordinary state of existence; now, he is in contact with that power which becomes the gigantic power-reality in his life. This power no longer exists in imagination, but becomes such a powerful force that it is able to alter the vital functioning of the body to a state of suspension, and transmute mental consciousness into a mind-transcendent form; and, in the ordinary state of existence, it causes perfect vital functioning, and makes the mind forceful, constructive, attentive and tranquil. All this means that an unknown aspect of our existence begins to manifest itself on the surface stratum of our lives which illuminates our mind from within, and vitalizes our body through an established vital control. This unsuspected power has been termed Kundalini, and layayoga has demonstrated the possibility of rousing it. Layayoga has also shown that these practices can be successfully carried out without abandoning the 'world-path'. Many accomplished layayogis are examples of this.

Kundali-power operates in the chakra-system. There is no possibility of tracing the chakras in the nervous system or any other part of the body. They are not material but dynamic graphs of power operations. This does not mean that they are fictitious. There is a definite relation between the chakras and certain vertebro-cranial points. These points in the medulla spinalis and the brain are also related to certain points on the surface of the body. The nervous points can be determined approximately through the surface points. The nervous points are closely related to certain positions where the replicas of the chakras appear in deep thought-concentration and certain physical effects are also produced. This is the first time that an interrelation between the chakra-system and the cerebrospinal system has been demonstrated on a scientific basis.

Owing to the failure in understanding the principles of yoga, there have been many misconceptions and illusions about the chakras, and especially about Kundalini. As for example, the theosophical interpretation of them. To start with, the theosophists acquired their knowledge of Kundalini and the chakras from the Sanskrit works dealing with the subject. But then the original accounts were distorted, either on purpose or due to a lack of understanding, which needs, first, the technical knowledge, and second, the guru's direct instructions. Here is an example: C.W. Leadbeater (Lead-

beater, C.W., *The Chakras*, The Theosophical Publishing House, Adyar, Madras 20, India, 1952, p. 20) says that the crown chakra (that is, the sahasrara), described in Indian books as thousand-petalled, which is really not very far from the truth, has 960 radiations (i.e., petals) of its primary force in the outer circle. This means that the sahasrara has only 960 petals instead of 1,000. This indicates a complete lack of understanding of the organization of the sahasrara. The sahasrara is the expansion of the pranic bindu which is in a supremely concentrated state when prana becomes patent and causes an emission of 50 power-units, and each of these units becomes potentized 20 times to manifest its full creativity. This means $50 \times 20 = 1,000$, and so, the sahasrara has exactly 1,000 petals, neither less nor more.

One cannot have anything against a personal or a group experience, but when such recently acquired experiences are presented to challenge the age-old yogic experiences, which have been verified by the yogis from time immemorial, it becomes like a 'frog in a well challenging a frog of the ocean'.

There is another important point which I want to make clear. It has been stated (Arundale, G.S., *Kundalini*, The Theosophical Publishing House, Adyar, Madras, India, 1947, p. 17) that there is a danger of sexual stimulation in relation to the rousing of Kundalini. The yogic experiences are quite the contrary. The rousing is indispensably associated with the fully controlled sex urge. It has also been stated (Leadbeater, C.W., *The Chakras*, The Theosophical Publishing House, Adyar, Madras, India, 1952, p. 64) that there are dangers in rousing Kundalini prematurely. Under certain conditions, Kundalini may be roused automatically, without the knowledge of the person concerned. But this does no harm. A practitioner cannot rouse Kundalini if he is not prepared for it. In fact, there is no such thing as prematurely rousing Kundalini, and there is no danger when Kundalini is roused.

It has also been supposed that Kundaliniyoga is materialistic yoga. Is there any such thing as materialistic yoga? Ramakrishna says that real spiritual knowledge cannot arise if Kundalini is not roused. Is he mistaken? Wama says that without the awakening of Kundalini, liberation is not possible. Is he wrong? Tailanga has stated that the rousing of Kundalini leads to yoga. Shankaracharya himself was an accomplished yogi in Kundaliniyoga. Arawinda has called Kundalini the divine force. Did all these spiritual leaders and yoga masters follow materialistic yoga? We understand that Kundalini is the spiritual dynamism which remains latent when coiled, but becomes real in life when it is roused. The real spiritualization of human life occurs through dynamic Kundalini.

The author does not claim that this work is a complete exposition of layayoga. It cannot be so, because many layayoga manuscripts appear to have been lost during the course of time. It may be that there are manuscripts dealing with layayoga lying in the private libraries of yogic scholars in India, and one day they may become generally accessible.

The author is also quite conscious of the limitations of his knowledge, capacity and time. The only remedy is if an advanced layayogi, who possesses more extensive material, undertakes to make a complete work on layayoga.

Last, the author hopes that the present work may inspire women and men all over the world to introduce concentration, as an indispensable practice, into their lives.

Stockholm   Shyam Sundar Goswami

Acknowledgments

First, I wish to thank the great authority on the Wed*a*, Acharyya Karunamoya Saraswati, Calcutta, for his kindness to write a foreword to this work.

The Plates II and 28 are photographs of my pupil Mrs Karin Schalander, Stockholm; Plate III is reproduced with the permission of Acharyya Karunamoya Saraswati himself; Plates 1-26 have been made under my guidance, by my pupil Mrs Dea Ramstedt, Stockholm, and Plate 27 by Mrs Ramstedt and Dr Ulf Jansson, Stockholm. The Plates II and 28 have been taken by Mr Leif Persson, Gräsmark, Sweden.

I wish to thank them all.

Shyam Sundar Goswami

My Initiation into Layayoga

'Layayoga has assumed an intermediate position between hathayoga and rajayoga. The most complicated processes of hathayogic pranayama and the very advanced and difficult rajayogic processes of concentration have been simplified in layayoga. The essence of mantrayoga has also been introduced in layayoga. So it is a most practical form of yoga suited to nearly all persons desiring to develop concentration'— said my Master after my initiation.

It had not been an easy matter for me to penetrate deeply into the subject of layayoga and understand its fundamental principles. Even prolonged study was not enough. I felt the necessity of having instructions directly from a master of layayoga. It seemed absolutely imperative to learn many unknown aspects of this yoga and its various hidden practices from a guru.

The first meeting with my Master occurred in this way. One day a friend of mine came and asked me whether I would be interested in seeing a great yogi who happened to be in Calcutta. I was rather surprised—such a yogi in such a noisy city! When I expressed my thoughts to my friend, he said: 'A yogi can be in the forests of the Himalaya or in a big city; a real yogi is as unconcerned with his own environment as he is with himself.' I realized that what he had said was true. I accepted his invitation and accompanied him.

We entered a spacious clean room. A dignified middle-aged man was sitting on a couch and a number of men—I presumed them to be his disciples—sat on a carpet on the floor. My friend immediately bowed his head to the yogi's feet and received his blessing. I followed my friend's example, who then introduced me to the yogi. He received me in a very kindly manner. He asked us to sit down. This was in the evening. However, I did not ask about anything. I only looked at him continuously. I sensed in him a very serene, internally joyous, and kindly person, and also that his inner being was all purity and full of power. I had never had such an experience before in connection with anyone.

The thought came to me: What makes a man like this. Was it a sign of awakened spirituality? What mode of life does he lead? I resolved to investigate all these things. The first meeting ended in this way. I spent some hours there. My friend and I bowed to his feet and said good-bye to him. The Master left Calcutta after some days.

When he returned to Calcutta next year I visited him more often, almost every day. I wanted to know more about him in my own way. So one day I asked: 'Is it necessary to accept God as the ultimate reality?' Other disciples who were there appeared to be amazed at my question. Perhaps they thought that the question indicated atheistic tendencies. Smiling, the Master replied: 'It is not a question of necessity; you can neither accept nor reject it. This is the position.'

His statement was not clear to me. I pondered over it again and again. Many thoughts came into my mind: Does the Master want to avoid the subject? If so, why? My thoughts were continuing in this way when the Master suddenly interrupted them by saying: 'It is not that the subject needs to be avoided.' I stared at him. Did he read my thoughts? The Master continued: 'It is avoided in a life that is not spiritually illuminated. Mere intellection is inadequate for the purpose.'

I said: 'If our intelligence and our thoughts and our reason are unable to find God, then He cannot be found, and, consequently, there will always be speculation.'

Master: 'For you, the senses and intelligence are the only criterions—the only instruments for acquiring knowledge. You are normally endowed with them and have learnt how to use them. You have no other means. But the Supreme God is beyond intelligence, and the senses cannot reach Him. This is why the senso-intellectual means are inadequate.'

I said: 'When we have no other means than the senses and intelligence for the acquisition of knowledge, how can we know God?'

Master: 'The senses and intelligence are only partially suited even for knowing the external world, and that is their limit.'

I said: 'Partially suited?'

Master: 'Yes. The senses have limitations. First of all, the power of the senses varies in different species and also in different individuals of the same species. The differences in power may also be due to age, the state of health, heredity and other factors. Even supposing that a normal, healthy young person has very good sensory powers, they are still limited. There are three fundamental limits in relation to sensory objects—minute objects, concealed objects, and far distant objects. If the normal senses are unable to overcome these barriers, then it is quite possible that they do not perceive certain objects at all.'

I said: 'But the range of the senses can be enhanced by the use of sensitive instruments.'

Master: 'That is true. But the material instruments, however refined they may be, are still material. They cannot reach what is beyond the material. There is no possibility of "seeing" the mind with the help of these instruments. Even a most sensitive instrument has its limits, which it cannot surpass. The three sensory barriers can be modified by the use of appropriate instruments, but the limitation is still there.

'Therefore, the knowledge acquired through the normal senses is limited; and the enhanced sensory power due to the use of sensitive apparatus is also limited, and, consequently, imperfect. How can you acquire perfect knowledge of a reality which is perfect through imperfect sensory means?'

I said: 'The imperfections of our senses are made up for, at least to a great extent, by intelligence if it is highly developed. This is the reason why it is necessary to utilize our senses together with our intelligence so as to know the world.'

Master: 'We must not forget that our intelligence is also limited.'

I continued: 'According to the degree of development, the power of intelligence varies. But human intelligence has reached very far. It has discovered many hidden laws of nature, and created things that are almost unbelievable. It has altered the face of our earth. It has revolutionized our thoughts and mode of living and has tremendously increased our knowledge.'

Master: 'All this is true. But still that very highly developed intelligence of ours has failed to know God. God has not been found in the various forms of energy that are active around us; or in inert matter; or in molecules, atoms and elementary particles; or in radiation; or in the earth or in the atmosphere. Our intelligence has tried to explore matter in every possible way, and found nothing else but matter-energy and energy-matter. Are not all these indicative of its limitations? Even our intelligence in the so-called scientific field has failed to know mind, and scientific attempts are being made to demonstrate that mind is an unknown form of matter, or that it derives from matter; an attempt is being made to restrict the mind to the cranium.'

I said: 'But the philosopher's intelligence appears to have sensed that there is something which is beyond matter. Even the human mind is considered to be too small. There has been talk of a cosmic mind or greater intelligence, and also of God. Anyhow, everything appears to be uncertain, speculative. What can we do?'

Master: 'So long as the highest spiritual

truth is left to the judgment of those who think that what is obtained through human intelligence aided by instruments is the real truth, and anything else is not truth but superstition and nonsense; so long as God is sought for in terms of philosophic thought and reasoning alone, He will appear to be far way from us.'

I said: 'In that case, even religion does not help us very much. The priests have worshipped God ritualistically for hundreds of years in the temples, but how many of them have known God. The One-God conception has been the ideal of many who go to the churches for the absolution of their sins and to be in contact with God; but they hear only words—empty words, and come back with that. Those who join in the mass prayers in the mosques, tell us the same story. How many of them have real love for humanity? All these things show the failure of religion.'

Master: 'We have to go deep to understand the role of religion in human life. First of all, the *rishi*s of ancient India have declared that Dharma—you may call it religion if you like—is perpetual. It is not made by man but remains as an intrinsic part of the cosmic world and in the lives of all beings—eternally. It is the grand support of the universe and all beings. It is Brahman—God who sustains everything. Therefore, the awakening of God within us and seeing God in the universe is religion.'

I said: 'How can religion be perpetual when a particular religion originates from a spiritual leader? And in all such religions there are great diversities. One says God is one; the other says God is many. One thinks God is without form, while the other thinks God has forms. One is of the opinion that love for God is the means, while others consider that divine wisdom leads to God. There are also prayers, ritualistic worship and many other means. Where does the solution lie?'

Master: 'First of all, you have to understand that religion in its real spiritual form cannot be created by a man. Religion is the natural spiritual principle, divine in character, which operates along with the principle of "cosmosity" in which the original creativity is manifested. It is the spiritual aspect of the Supreme Power which is all God. Therefore, it is perpetually existing without any interruption. Consequently, it cannot be man-made. The *rishi*s did not make any religion, but explained different aspects of religion which are always in existence. Neither did any "incarnation" found any individual religion, but expounded and strengthened religion which is eternally existing.'

I said: 'But what about Buddhism, Christianity or Islam? Were they not founded by men?'

Master: 'Long time after K*rishna* left our earth, Gout*ama* Buddha came to this world. He can be considered as the first spiritual leader in India whose name has been associated with the introduction of Buddhism. Buddha revived yoga by his own example—yoga which had become corrupted and abused by that time. In his life, he showed how to reach the final stage of spiritual yoga. He showed how, by making our consciousness void—free from all mundaneness, we could realize directly the ultimate reality where everything else is non-being. This is nirwa*na*.'

I said: 'What about Jesus Christ? About Mohammad?'

Master: 'Jesus Christ was a great spiritual leader in Western Asia at that time and is regarded as an incarnation. He manifested his spirituality in that high degree, where his consciousness, raised above all worldliness, and in a state of concentratedness which contained God alone, became godly, and finally, the divine consciousness was reabsorbed in God. It was possible for his intimate disciples, who realized God in Christ and in themselves, to develop Christianity, through which, being spiritually inspired, they wanted to give the essence of spiritual truth to man for his salvation.

'Mohammad also realized God within, in concentration, and wished to communicate the spiritual truth to man.'

I said: 'If such great spiritual persons as Buddha, Christ and Mohammad are the founders of the great religions, why are they not effective?'

Master: 'So long as the spiritual currents flow in a religion or in one of its forms or doctrines by the tremendous spiritual impetus of a great religious leader, religion remains alive and,

3

consequently, becomes fruitful. But as soon as spirituality ebbs, religion becomes mere words without life.

'When the spiritual force imparted by Buddha in his doctrine began to be diminished as time passed distortion and corruption came, and spirituality was replaced by the dead words of theory. At a certain time Shankara, who realized Brahman in samadhi, was able to destroy the Buddhistic doctrine of lifeless words as then preached by the followers of Buddha, and to establish the Oupanishada One-and-All Brahman doctrine. This was possible because of his great spiritual power combined with the extraordinary brilliance of his intellect. But when Shankara's spirituality began to ebb in his followers in later times, the Brahman doctrine likewise assumed wordiness without spiritual life. In this condition it was unable to stand against the bhakti doctrine of the great bhakti-yogi Chaitanya, who was immersed in the deepest love of God, both in concentration and in daily life.

'A religion or a doctrine when not strengthened by spirituality, cannot meet the spiritual needs of man. But even when a religion deteriorates through the withered spirituality of its adherents, there will always be some silent spiritual persons who uphold that faith or religion—the real yogis, otherwise the religion would become extinct. This is true of all religions.'

Now I recollected the three great silent yogis: a Buddhist yogi who attained a very high level in samadhi; the well-known Christian yogi, Saint John of the Cross, from whose heart intense love ascended towards God in deep concentration; and a great Muslim yogi, Abdul Gafur, who was endowed with great spiritual power.

I said: 'It seems strange that God is not reflected in the unusually brilliant intelligence of a genius; the scientists do not know God; the philosophers only speculate about God; and God appears to remain hidden even to most followers of religion. Why is God very far away from us! Is religion superfluous for man living in the modern world?'

Master: 'God is far away when the "sight" is submerged in the materiality of our existence; it cannot go beyond the sensory boundary; and hence God is so far away that he is not seen at all.

'God is very far and also very near. When God is "seen" within, he is ever present in our consciousness; the contact is never lost. When God is seen within, he is also seen without; and he is also seen in what is beyond both within and without. God is within and also outside and is what is neither within nor outside. No one can say "It is this, it is not that". It is an infinite ocean of Being and Consciousness.

'And also God cannot be denied. To deny God means to accept the permanent limitation of our beingness. In our being also lies the substance of infinity which becomes illumined in the Beingness of God. God is our being in its supreme stratum.'

I was highly impressed by the profundity of the Master's knowledge; and not merely that, I began to feel a real spiritual foundation upon which his knowledge was based. I began to appreciate that something deep and powerful was utilizing his intellect as an avenue for the outward expression of inner truth. I was proud of my learning and I devoted fifteen or sixteen hours a day to my studies. My pride began to be demolished; my arguments began to fail. However, I put one more question, and that was the last of its kind.

I asked: 'Why is this "cosmosity" which is the root of all our sufferings?'

Master: 'It can as well be said that because of the "cosmosity" we are given a chance to enjoy so much.'

'Why has the universe been manifested? Who can answer that, and if it is answered, who can understand it? When human power cannot produce it, when human intelligence cannot penetrate into it, how can that question, as such, be helpful. Human intelligence is too small to solve the mystery of the appearance of the universe. But there is the possibility of the human mind being in a state in which the image of the universe is not recorded, and the mind is in tune with something which is neither material nor mental, but the non-material-nonmental reality. In this reality there is no trace of the universe, of mind or of matter. Its realization is both mental and nonmental. The mind of our everyday life, which perceives the world, desires, feels pleasures and pains, thinks and wills, is not all, but only one aspect of our being, represented by I-consciousness around which is whirling the sensory world. Again, the mind in its other aspect completely closes its doors to the world and does not desire, think, and will, but realizes the Supreme Reality which is all, and besides which there is nothing else. Ultimately this unitary experience merges into a beingness which is itself the beingness of Supreme Consciousness.

'The Infinite Power Principle is the being of the Infinite Supreme Consciousness. In its purely power aspect, that is, power isolated from Supreme Consciousness, it is no longer infinite as it is no longer the being of the Infinite Consciousness. Thus it is as if a finite section of the infinite being in which the Infinite Consciousness appears as a finite being. This finiteness in infinity is the phenomenon of the mental and material universe. The universe is real when the Infinite Consciousness is veiled, but unreal when the finite being is no being as is "seen" in the Supreme Being.

'The finite being manifesting as the I-consciousness is nil at the infinite point, but this nothingness appears to be something when the supremeness of the Being is veiled. In other words, a phenomenon of Godlessness, which is in reality a nonbeing, emerges as a being. But there is a possibility of arousing spirituality amidst mundaneness, which leads to liberation. Spirituality is the awakening of Godliness in consciousness. So spirituality is not something engrafted into man; it is in the highest aspect of his nature, through which man can manifest his God-being, which is his own being in its supreme aspect. Without spirituality man is a hopelessly restricted being moving aimlessly, with his lust and greed, in the mundane ocean.

'Religion is the means to the spiritual realization of God. Without this realization, religion is mere words, or an order of no value. That is dead religion. Real life comes to religion through yoga. Yoga is the intrinsic part of religion. Without yoga religion is no religion; without yoga religion is lifeless. All the great spiritual leaders and many of the adherents of a religion have made yoga the basic spiritual practice.

'The natural transformation of sense-consciousness, which is perceptive in character, and in which uncontrolled thoughts are constantly arising—and these thoughts are often tinged with unrestrained and unspiritual affectiveness—into a nonoscillatory concentrated form, in which is held what is spiritual and divine—is yoga. Yoga is the highest order of the human mind. And still in its supreme aspect, yoga is the supreme spirituality in which beingness is only of God. There is nothing else, all is God.'

The Master stopped. It was very late at night. So I bowed to him and left with a 'heart' full of deep thoughts.

I began to ponder over what the Master had said in our long discourse. Many thoughts came to my mind. What is this life! We find that living is associated with desiring, willing, thinking and emoting. These activities usually have two modes of expression. In one, we see that man desires and experiences pleasure in enjoyment and also suffers pain and sorrow. In pleasure-seeking, he does not hesitate to commit excesses. He becomes sensual and greedy. We all see that, in spite of his sexual, alimentary and other excesses, he is able to manifest his other qualities. He thinks brilliantly and constructively. He becomes an educationist, scientist, artist, and philosopher.

But do we find in him spirituality as a mode of being in his life? Does he not live without God? Many people may talk of God and religion, but mostly it is mere talk. Of course, there are a limited number of people who think of religion seriously, who search for God sincerely, and are moral and spiritual by nature. Therefore, it is possible for man to manifest his spiritual qualities despite his sensuality, greed, and all excesses.

Is it possible to make spirituality a living factor in life when there is so much strong worldly desire for the satisfaction of which the whole being is involved? If we are advised to renounce all worldliness, it would be impossible to achieve, because of our supreme attachment to sensory objects; if we are asked to reject sexual and other pleasures, it will not work, because they are as deeply ingrained in us as if they were parts of our organism.

Does initiation help? This thought came into

my mind. Is it not necessary to be spiritually prepared? Am I really qualified for it? I also thought the opposite. Will not initiation release spiritual qualities in my nature? It may be that a certain degree of preparedness is necessary for a pupil; but will not initiation itself sow the spiritual seeds in him? This is how my thoughts continued for some months.

One day the friend who first introduced me to the Master came to my house and told me: 'The Master has fixed the date of your initiation which will take place outside Calcutta in a lonely place; so be ready for it.' I was very surprised to hear this news. The thought came into my mind: 'Has the Master seen something in me of which I am unconscious myself?' I do not know. I could not speak for some time. My friend smiled and said: 'Everything will be all right.' He was himself an initiate.

However, my initiation took place on the date fixed. In initiation, the guru gives to a faithful and serious disciple a specific m*a*ntr*a*. The m*a*ntr*a* is a great aid to concentration. Initiation was rather sudden in my case. I also heard from our mother (the Master's wife) that the Master's initiation also happened suddenly and that in connection with it a miracle occurred.

The Master began to feel spiritual thirst when he was young. Day by day it grew more and more intense and ultimately it drew him to a great Tantrik*a* and l*a*y*a*yog*a* master, Bholanath*a*. He told my Master: 'Your spiritual aspiration will be consummated through the Tantrik*a* form of yoga.' Then he gave some instructions to the Master and asked him to come back after a few months.

The Master went back home and started to carry out the instructions given him. He then began to feel a very great desire for initiation, and this continued to increase. He became restless, and one day he ran to the Tantrik*a* yog*i* Bholanath*a*.

The guru said: 'It is just the time for your initiation. I will perform it to-day. Go and take your bath.' After doing this the Master returned to his guru. Then the guru said to him: 'Now you have to bring the bilw*a* leaves (Aegle Marmelos—wood-apple) for worship and

oblation. The leaves should be new and not spotted or torn.' Then he pointed to a bilw*a* tree situated at a little distance from the place, and said: 'That tree is very big, and good leaves are only on a thick branch which is very high. It may even be impossible for you to reach the branch with a long bamboo pole. You need not worry. Go and stand under the branch calmly and the branch will come down to you by itself. Do not be afraid: go!' The Master was very much surprised to hear this. However, he went there and saw the enormous bilw*a* tree. He also found the huge branch bearing good leaves, but it was so high that he could not reach it even with a very long pole. Then he stood under it calmly. After a while the Master saw that the immensely thick branch was bending slowly downward and it came down so much that it was possible for the Master to take some leaves with his hands. He came back with the leaves. The guru initiated him, and also taught him more spiritual practices. At that time the Master was about nineteen years old.

After my initiation the Master instructed me in the first stage of concentration according to l*a*y*a*yoga. He said: 'Concentration should be practised every day and regularly. The morning is the best time for it. Concentration may be divided into two parts: preliminary and regular. As soon as you get up, sit on the bed in a yog*a* posture, facing towards the north and concentrate on a white divine form, as advised, in the white twelve-petalled lotus just above the head. Then think that the *amrita*—the immortal life-substance—is flowing from the divine form by which you have been completely bathed; then think that "I have been energized and immortalized by *amrita*; I have no disease, no senility, no death, no sorrow" Think deeply, make your thinking vital. The regular concentration can be done either after this, or after your bath, which should be taken after the evacuation of the bowels and oral cleansing. Better do this part of the concentration after your bath.'

One day the Master talked about the purification of the body. He said: 'The purification of the body is an intrinsic factor in concentration. We know that food, water and air are absolutely necessary for maintaining life in the body. The functioning of the life-energy in relation to the body causes two phenomena: keeping the body alive and making the mind perform its sensory functions.

'The life-energy is composed of two factors— one is fundamental and the other is secondary. The fundamental factor is involved in exhibiting developmental functions which maintain growth, development, vitality, and bodily health. The secondary factor is concerned with the reproduction of the species, the sexual function. Associated with the functioning of the life-energy in the body is the manifestation of sense-consciousness. In other words, the mind is manifesting its sensory functions in relation to the developmental and sexual functions.

'The developmental and sexual energy— each has two principles, activation and restraint. But the activation factor is more powerful and predominant in a living body; and, as the mind is closely linked to the living body it is manifesting its sensory functions along with the developmental and sexual functions. Through its sensory functions the mind is cooperating with the living body in its functions.

'In sensory functions, the control factor of the mind is recessive, very weak. This is why the multiformity of the mind is associated with the living body at its common level. The sensory mind is utilizing its intelligence mainly in creating uncontrolled thoughts, and its will is restricted merely to the phenomenon of conation. The sensory mind, through its conative function, is playing a dominant role in the living body, and exercising its influence directly on the muscles, and indirectly on the internal organic functions.

'The conative functions of the mind are principally five. They are: (1) speech, (2) prehension, (3) locomotion, (4) excretion, and (5) reproduction. The developmental function is helped by the sensory mind through prehension and locomotion which directly influence the muscular system, and through it the organic system. The mind is directly helping the organic system by the process of excretion. The mind is playing a great role in sexual function through its involvement in the process of reproduction.

However, on the one side, the sensory mind is aiding the developmental and sexual functions, and on the other side, it is utilizing these functions to serve its own purposes.

'The main object of the sensory functions of the mind is to experience pleasure in enjoyment by establishing a direct sensory contact with a sense object. Without this sensory contact enjoyment is incomplete, pleasure is partial. One cannot get full satisfaction by merely thinking of food, it must be tasted. The full sexual enjoyment is not possible by sexual thoughts alone; it requires sensory contact with the object.

'The pleasure-pattern, which is an intrinsic mode of the mind, excites it to experience pleasure often to a degree which causes excesses, and consequently sexual functions are carried on beyond a normal point. The pleasure-pattern which is based on pleasure impressions acquired through previous experiences, develops as affection in the sense-consciousness, which causes desires. Desires excite three phenomena in the mind: the rousing of strong passion, volition and conation, and uncontrolled thoughts. The pleasure-desires drive the mind to establish sense connection with the objects in order to experience great satisfaction by enjoying them again and again, and to an increasing extent. In this way the excesses are committed willingly and with great pleasure.

'So the mind manifests its sensory functions to give a material shape to its pleasure-desires to fulfil the enjoyment of the "I", and, in this enjoyment, there is a sensory relation with an appropriate object in the material field. The constant penetration of the sense objects, as images, into the sense-consciousness causes an oscillatory state in which the intellective and volitive aspects of the mind also take part. The pleasure-pattern, which is the basis of the sensory mind, creates a pleasure-loving tendency and the mind exhibits it in thoughts, feelings and actions. In the mind all sensory images, all thoughts, all feelings and the impressions of all actions are recorded, and that makes it multifarious. It is a state of anti-concentration.

'Deconcentration is the mode adopted by the sensory mind. It is mainly due to the recessiveness of the control factor of the mind. Unless the control factor is awakened, it is not possible to transform the oscillatory consciousness into a state of concentratedness. In *yoga*, the process of *yama* (control) has been prescribed for this purpose. The *yama* process consists of eight stages, and the power of control develops stage by stage, and at the final stage control reaches its highest limit and becomes supercontrol leading to *samadhi*.

'The control of the sensory mind is impossible, unless not only the sense-consciousness itself, with its thoughts, feelings, and volitions, but also the body, which is used by it as its apparatus, and the sense objects are taken in consideration. This means that a state common to the mind, body and objects, and anti-oscillatory in character, is established. According to *yoga*, it is a state of purity, in which the mind, the body, and the sense objects undergo purification.

'The sensory phenomenon is in the nature of thought-word form. Unless it is changed into a form in which the control factor, that is almost dormant, is awakened, real concentration is not possible. The thought-word form of the mind is neutralized step by step by a process of purification effected by the introduction of suprasound power in word-form, that is *mantra*. The word-form of *mantra* does not create thoughts in the mind, but it neutralizes the sensory mind when the power residing in it is awakened, and develops the power of control. So *mantra* develops *yama* (control) by effecting a purification of the mind.

'But as the sensory mind is in relation to the body and sense objects, they also should be purified by *mantra*. The sense objects in effect are parts of the mind. The purification of the mind is not complete without the purification of the sense objects. A purified mind will be polluted by contact with the sense objects when they are not purified. This means that purification, only at the mental point, does not work satisfactorily. Even the purified mind in relation with the sense objects manifests pleasure-pain feelings and the control power becomes ineffective. But it will be different when the purified mind comes in contact with the purified objects. In the purified objects the pleasure-giving factor begins to be more and

more submerged, so the control influence of the purified mind is not hindered when the mind comes in contact with a purified object.

'Similarly, the body, which is the instrument of the sensory mind, should be purified for the right functioning of the purified mind. The control factor of the purified mind cannot be aroused fully when the mind utilizes an impure coarse apparatus. The impurified sense objects stimulate the sensory aspect of the mind and thus an anti-concentration state is created in sense-consciousness. The impure body becomes a hindrance to concentration by facilitating the sensory functions of the mind. Therefore, the purification of the mind, the body and the sense objects should be achieved simultaneously.

'There is a difference between the ordinary purification and the refinement by *mantra*, that is, the *mantra* purification. For health, it is necessary to eat pure food. Pure food helps the developmental function of the body. But the enjoyment factor in relation to food will remain the same. To control this, the *mantra* purification is absolutely necessary. But the ordinary purification is far from worthless, rather it is very necessary, because the *mantra* purification works most satisfactorily in pure foods.

'The general purification of the body is effected by taking pure and well-balanced food, drinking pure water, breathing pure air, maintaining vigorous circulation by appropriate exercise, internal cleansing, baths, and sleep, rest and relaxation. Such a body maintains its developmental function at a high level. But, even such a purified and vitalized body has not been purified enough to be utilized as an apparatus by the mind, purified by *mantra*, for the manifestation of its spiritual qualities. This indicates that the body also needs *mantra* purification.

'The *mantra* purification of the body is done by the use of food and water purified by *mantra*, by the practice of the purificatory breathing process, and by the *mantra* nyasa (touching) process. The purificatory breathing process is very important. A specific pranayamic breathing, in conjunction with *mantra*, causes an internal deep purification of the life-force and the body. When the body is purified in this manner, the mental control and concentration work without much interruption and more effectively. But the purificatory breathing process and nyasa do not work in a satisfactory manner unless the body undergoes general purification. So the ordinary purification of the body is also important and it is closely connected with the mantra purification.

'The body is externally cleansed by bathing. But when the baths are taken in conjunction with mantra the purificatory effects will be increased. The internal cleansing as prescribed in hathayoga causes internal purification of the body and this is very important. In addition to it, clean water purified by mantra is used for deep internal purification.

'There is a process, called achamana (water-sipping) in which water purified by mantra is drunk for deep internal purification. The process consists of the following: first hollow the right palm by making a shape like a cow's ear in which the forefinger, middle finger and ring finger are conjoined, and the little finger and the thumb are free; now place a very small quantity of clean water in the hollow; purify the water by mantra and drink it. The drinking should be done three times. Every morning it should be done. The quantity of water should be so small that it does not add to the contents of the stomach but is immediately absorbed.

'There is another process called *aghamarshana* (pharyngonasal deep purification). The essential part of it is as follows: a handful of clean water purified by mantra should be drawn through the left nostril and then, after washing away the internal impurities, the water should be expelled through the right nostril. It is a difficult process.'

I asked: 'The subject appears extremely complex: where should one start?'

The Master replied: 'The method of concentration consists of three fundamental parts: purification of body and mind by mantra, purification of the sense objects by mantra, and concentration practice.

'The purification of body and mind is effected by the right application of purificatory pranayamic breathing, comprising the processes of drying, burning, renovating and strengthening with mantra. This creates a favourable condition for concentration.

'Second, the sense objects should be purified by mantra. This creates a state in which the control factor of the mind works in relation to the purified objects without being ineffective. Experience teaches us that, in the beginning, we have to start with those objects which are related to the alimentary and sexual functions. Most of the abuses and excesses come through these channels, and man experiences greatest pleasure in relation to them. Man has not selected only those foods which make the body vital, strong and healthy. He has included in his diet many foods which may be unnecessary; he prepares many dishes mainly for their palatability, and eats in excess of his need for enjoyment. Similarly, clean water is enough for health and quenching thirst. But man has introduced alcoholic drinks for creating an artificial exhilaration which goes very well with other excesses.

'The pleasure-feeling rises to its highest point in sexual gratification which is often carried to excess. It is of no use merely to say "control this passion". Behind the passion lies the strongest force—we call it sexual energy—which is an intrinsic part of the life-force and with which is associated the perpetuation of the human race. It is not easy to "kill" or suppress sexual passion. To absent oneself from the object of sexual attraction or to apply artificial control does not work. If the control is to be successful, it should be developed normally and in relation to sexual objects. As the sensory mind normally tends to establish a sensory relation with the sexual objects because of the influence of its pleasure-desires, and, as, under this condition, there are experiences of greatest pleasure, all these should be accepted as a fact and control should start here. Control should be natural, not artificial and ineffective.

'The normal control power begins to develop when the body-mind purification by mantra is accomplished. This is the first requisite. As the sensory mind flows naturally and constantly towards the sense objects, no premature attempt should be made to withdraw the mind from the objects, but the connection should be made through mantra. The control power of the mind develops through mantra. Foods and drinks should be purified by mantra. The sensory relation with the sex objects should also be made through mantra. In this manner, the control power over sexual passion will develop step by step, not by withdrawal, but through contact, and at a certain point the sexual passion will normally disappear.

'Last—the concentration practice. Concentration is holding in consciousness an image which occupies the whole conscious field, and there is no stain or dark spot, and the holding is continuous, not interrupted, and not replaced by anything else. Concentration is only possible when consciousness is uniform in character and, consequently, one-pointed. But the sense-consciousness which is our consciousness in everyday life is oscillatory; in it undulations are constantly going on, owing to the sensory projections and senso-mental radiations to consciousness. This is an unsuitable state for concentration. The students of yoga know this. Some sort of mental focusing can be attained by much effort in such a state, but it is extremely difficult to develop real, natural and deep concentration on such a substratum.

'Our position is this. For the practice of concentration we need nonundulatory consciousness as the background. But our consciousness is undulatory, so how can we concentrate successfully? This is the greatest problem. Theoretically, concentration itself can transform the oscillatory consciousness to a state of uniformity. But the difficulty is that concentration does not go well in a diversified consciousness.

'Hathayoga solves this problem by controlling the sensory projections and senso-mental radiations by making the body-apparatus sensorially inoperative by kumbhaka. But this is a very difficult method. In rajayoga this problem does not arise. The rajayoga process of concentration starts when a student is already established in concentration. Rajayoga aims at purifying consciousness to the highest degree and transforming it in the state of samprajñata samadhi (superconscious concentration) which will be effortless and the normal mode of the mind. The final goal of rajayoga is to get this super-purified and super-

illuminated consciousness absorbed completely into Supreme Consciousness in asamprajñata samadhi (non-mens concentration). Layayoga achieves this goal by arousing Kundalini (the spiritual aspect of the Supreme Power) and gets all the cosmic principles absorbed into it. But the awakening of Kundalini requires deep concentration. So a modified method, termed bhutashuddhi, has been introduced to develop concentration.

'Mantrayoga presents a unique method which is extremely helpful for making concentration deep, real and normal. This method has also been adopted in layayoga. The method consists of the following factors:

'First, the consciousness is moulded into the mantra-form through the mental transformation of the waikhari (gross, sensory) sounds of the mantra. By the mantra-practice, the mantra-form will gradually be changed to living mantra when consciousness is in a state of concentratedness. Then, ultimately from the living mantra, living God, in an appropriate form, emerges, and concentration now becomes deep, real and automatic. The living God in form is called Ishtadewata, that is God who appears in a form from the mantra-sound by his will.

'In order to make the mantra-work successful, it may be necessary to apply certain specific processes which are as follows: (1) Achamana; (2) Kaminitattwa; (3) Mantrashikha; (4) Mantrachaitanya; (5) Mantrarthabhawana; (6) Nidrabhanga; (7) Kulluka; (8) Mahasetu; (9) Setu; (10) Mukhashodhana; (11) Karashodhana; (12) Yonimudra; (13) Pranatattwa; (14) Pranayoga; (15) Dipani; (16) Ashouchabhanga; (17) Utkilana; (18) Drishtisetu; (19) Special dhyana; and (20) Kamakaladhyana.

'These processes are highly technical and are executed with appropriate mantras and with concentration. They should be learned from a guru.

'It is not an easy thing to make Ishtadewata appear from the mantra. It is also not an easy thing to make the mantra living. So long as it is not possible to achieve this, an easier means has been adopted in mantrayoga for the development of concentration. It is this: a replica of Ishtadewata as an object of concentration is made.

For this purpose, a gross image from some suitable material is made. This image is not an imaginary representation of I*shta*dewata, but a close copy of the real form. It is a tangible form easy for the sense-consciousness to hold. It is not idolatry. This is a wrong term, only used by those who are ignorant of the subject.

'By seeing the gross image of I*shta*dewata again and again, a clear picture is formed in the sense-consciousness. The gross image is made life-like by m*a*ntr*a*, and in certain cases quite living, and then it begins to be steady in the consciousness, and gradually fills the whole consciousness, and no other objects penetrate consciousness. Now concentration becomes very deep. This state can only be reached when the body and mind are purified by m*a*ntr*a*, and the life-impartation to the image is done by m*a*ntr*a*. In this manner, concentration becomes real and deep.

'I*shta*dewata is God in form. The form arises from the living m*a*ntr*a* and is created by God himself. So it is not imaginary. God appears in form, otherwise the mind will not be able to receive it. It is absolutely necessary to have a form which can be held in consciousness in concentration.

'There is also mental worship which helps to establish concentration. In the m*u*ladhar*a* chakra, I*shta*dewata is worshipped with the smell principle; in the swadhi*shth*ana centre, with the taste principle; in the m*a*nipur*a* centre, with the sight principle; in the anaha*ta* centre, with the touch principle; in the wishuddh*a* centre, with the sound principle; in the h*ri*t chakra, with all the five principles; and in som*a* chakra, with spiritual qualities. Then a student is able to hold in his consciousness the pure luminous form of I*shta*dewata in concentration.

'Thereafter, concentration develops into samadhi in which the most subtle form of I*shta*dewata is held naturally in superconsciousness. This is the last stage of form. Then comes the realm of formlessness. Here, I*shta*dewata is without form; he is now the Supreme God. This is the stage of *asamprajñata* samadhi.'

Now I had a better opportunity, because of our intimate relation, to observe the mode of life the Master was leading, his actions in every-day life. I learned from his teachings as well as from his life. I found that y*a*ma and niy*a*ma were fully established in him. Truthfulness was the cornerstone of his life. He did not touch any thing which was acquired in an immoral way. He was content, and, usually, he remained absorbed in himself and silent, even when there were people around him. He had superpowers, but he rarely used them.

The Master observed br*a*hmacharya (sexual control) up to the age of twenty-eight years. During this period, he led a continent life for eight years while with his wife. Thereafter, he had children. Then he devoted himself to perfect the process of Adamantine Control.

I have learnt from his teachings and life that premature continence does not help in controlling the sex urge. Sexual excesses are also enervating. To be away from the sex objects also does not help. Senseless sexual gratification decreases power. Sexual efficiency demands control while alone as well as in contact.

Sexual efficiency is closely related to physical vigour, mental creativity and concentration. It should be developed by appropriate means. Its component parts are: (1) sexual passivity while alone and also together; (2) sexual creativity at will; (3) sexual purity; (4) adamantine control.

On one occasion, the Master talked about the four great systems of yog*a*. He said: 'There are four great systems of yog*a*: m*a*ntr*a*yog*a*, layayog*a*, h*a*thayog*a* and rajayog*a*. Each has its own characteristic feature, each has its specific practices. Each aims at the attainment of samprajñata yog*a*, and through it asamprajñata yog*a*. This is the final form.

'M*a*ntr*a*yog*a* is that form of yog*a*, in which word-thought forms, associated with the multiform consciousness, are transformed into supraword form, that is m*a*ntr*a*. M*a*ntr*a* effects the concentrated form of consciousness which leads to samadhi.

'M*a*ntr*a* is the suprasound power in word form. When the m*a*ntr*a* is rightly worked upon, it becomes a living power from which arises the living I*shta*dewata—God in form. Now concentration becomes very deep.

'L*a*yayog*a* is that form of yog*a* in which

concentration is developed through the absorption of all cosmic principles, leading ultimately to samadhi.

'Hathayoga is that form of yoga in which dynamic livingness, with which is associated the oscillatory form of consciousness, is transformed by the pranayamic process into a passive form of existence which effects concentratedness of the consciousness, leading to samadhi.

'By the pranayamic breath-control, a non-respiratory state is gradually developed in which a natural cessation of respiration occurs. This is called kewala kumbhaka. In kewala kumbhaka concentration becomes the normal mode of consciousness.

'The control of the inspiratory and expiratory acts is done by sahita pranayama. An internal purification is necessary for making the pranayama work. For this purpose, internal cleansing, purificatory diet and control exercise are instructed in hathayoga. By the pranayamic process, the body begins to be refined normally, all the vital activities are normalized and brought to a new level and normal health is established. This super-purification is called nadishuddhi.

'At this state, health, vitality, absence of unpleasant body odours, wholesome breath, appearance of a pleasing, slightly fragrant smell, cheerfulness and calmness and concentratedness of the mind—all these arise.

'Rajayoga is that form of yoga in which concentration is developed to non-mens concentration—asamprajnata samadhi which is rajayoga—the highest form of yoga.'

I have seen the Master in a state of samadhi. He usually assumed the corpse posture (shawasana) in which he lay on a bed with his face upward, and arms by his sides. The body remained completely motionless, without breathing, without pulse, and, apparently, without signs of sense activities. In this death-like condition he would stay for long periods.

He also used to go into very deep concentration in a sitting posture. It was his common practice to sit outside in the sun with a newspaper, supporting his elbows on a small stool, placed in front of him, as if he were reading. He might perhaps read the paper for a short time, but very soon he became still and his eyes closed. He remained in this position for hours. Shouting often could not make any impression on him. Many times it was necessary to awaken him for his lunch by shaking him vigorously. After being aroused, when he first opened his eyes, his look appeared meaningless, as if he was not of this world. After some time, he came back to his worldly self.

One day I asked the Master: 'Is the mind unconscious and dark while the body remains death-like in samadhi?'

The Master replied: 'No. The mind is super-conscious and super-illumined.'

S. G.

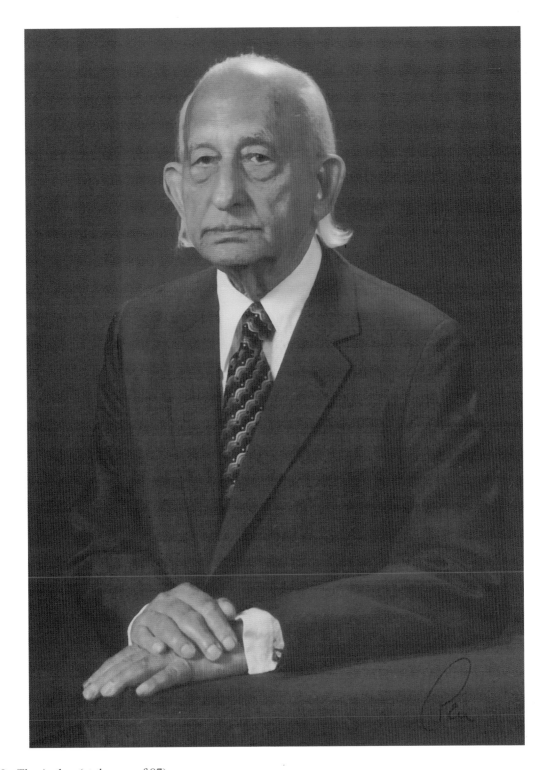

I   The Author (at the age of 87)

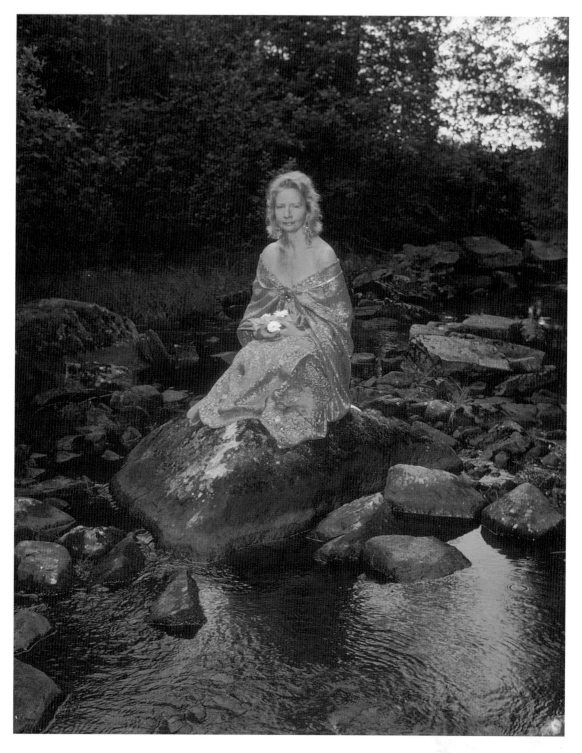

II   Wani

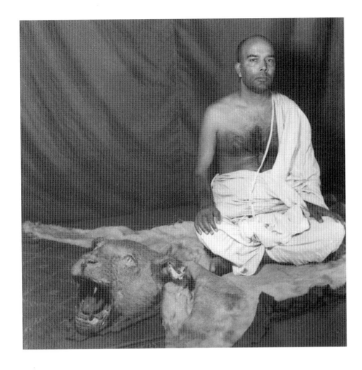

III   Acharyya Karunamoya Saraswati

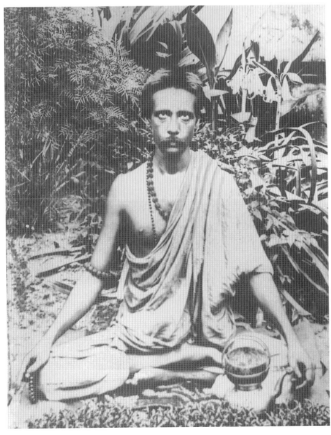

IV   Master: Sreemat Dwijapada Raya

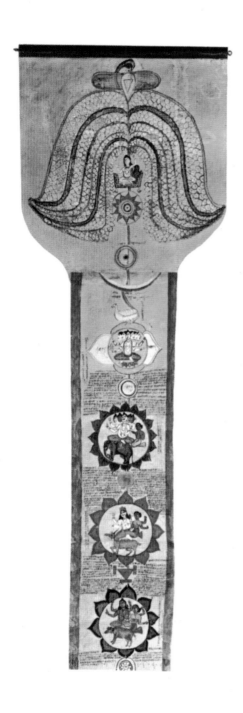
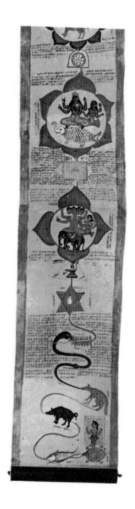

V   An Ancient Picture of the Chakra System (belonging to the Author's library)

Introduction

It is the discovery made by yoga that mind is the repository of prodigious power—mental dynamism—which manifests itself when mental consciousness is transmuted into a concentric form. It is the process of centralization of consciousness when it is reduced to a 'point'. This means that consciousness enters the bindu state. Bindu is a state in which power is at maximum concentration. When mental consciousness is in the bindu state, diversified mental powers are collected and highly concentrated as mental dynamism. The greater the concentration of power, the less are the dimensions, but the more increased the potency. Bindu—the power point—is a natural and indispensable condition associated with power in its operation. Bindu occurs both in the mental and material fields. The atom is the bindu of matter; the nucleus the bindu of a protoplasmic cell; and samādhi consciousness the bindu of the mind.

The reduction of the diversification of mental consciousness is the process of concentration leading to the bindu stage. The inner nature of the mind is to tend towards bindu, though it is rather unobservable when mind exhibits its multiform functions. At this state, the higher mental-energy system remains almost dormant; but it is fully activated in concentration. Even in diversified mental states, towards-the-bindu-motion operates fragmentarily. An example is the function of attention in relation to physical sensory perception and intellection. Physical sensory perception and associated intellection are due to the limiting influence on the mind.

Pragmatically, it is important and indispensable for determining the individual's position in the world around him and to see the world in a practical manner. But it is not the whole picture of the mind, it is only a fragment. It is a great mistake to think that the whole mind is what is represented by perception, intellection and will at the physical sensory level. One may even go so far as to assume that the mind is identical with the brain. The brain is important when, and as long as, mind exhibits physical consciousness. But when mind in its supramental aspect functions as superconsciousness the brain is not important to it; the brain then, practically remains a passive non-mental apparatus.

Principles of Chakra

The ancient yogic interpretation of mind and concentration is fundamentally based on the chakra organization and its function. Kundalini is indispensably connected with it. Kundalini is vitally connected with the chakra system and the whole body system as their static background. Kundalini also plays a most important role in the spiritualization of mind and the development of absorptive concentration. The chakras indicate the levels of spiritual consciousness and of absorptive concentration. The chakra system is actually a system of subtle power operations around some centralized force. The chakra is a natural dynamic graph, exposing the exact picture of the constituent powers operating in it.

Chakras as Myth

There is a viewpoint according to which the chakras are not real but imaginary. It is essentially based on the evidence that the chakras are seen neither when dissecting the body nor on its microscopic examination. This indicates that the chakras are beyond the range of both normal sight and extended sight. In other words, they are beyond our physical senses both normal and instrumentalized. But this does not prove their nonexistence.

Sensory perception is a sense-section by which only a segment of the whole is mentalized. Physical sense has four fundamental limitations, namely, size, obscurity, distance and time. This limited sensory power can be enhanced to a certain extent by the use of sensitive instruments. First of all, what we see with our eyes in the body are bones, muscles, blood vessels, nerves, organs, etc., which form the gross aspect of the body. When a bone is covered by muscles, or an organ is enclosed in its cavity, we do not see them, we only see the outer covering. This is the limitation by obscurity. So the gross structure of the body can be partially seen by the sense of sight. It is a very superficial observation of the body, a larger part of which remains hidden. For the observation of the minute structure of the body, it is absolutely necessary to magnify the small objects. For this purpose a powerful microscope is used. It is now possible to study the ultrastructure of the cells through the electron microscope. This has disclosed the molecular constituents of the living organisms. At the molecular level, the chakras are not seen.

Does the molecular study of the living organisms reveal its whole organization? Is that all, what we see by means of the microscope? The molecular structure is based on atoms, and the atoms are built up of what are known as elementary particles. So we find that there are two levels above the molecular level: atomic and subatomic. We have also been able to see atoms, but not elementary particles. They are so minute that they are not observable even with the most powerful instrument. They are inferred. However, the chakras are not seen at the atomic and subatomic levels. Are they inferred? Before an answer is given, we want to discuss another viewpoint about the chakras.

Anatomical Interpretation of Chakras and Nadis

There are viewpoints according to which the chakras are nerve plexuses, and the nadis are nerves or blood vessels. Dr Bamandas Basu[1] has expressed the opinion that a more accurate description of the nervous system has been given in the Tantras than in the medical works of the ancient Hindus. The Tantrika nomenclature has been regarded as anatomical terms, and an attempt has been made to explain them accordingly.

According to Professor Brajendranath Seal,[2] the adhara (muladhara) chakra is the sacro-coccygeal plexus; the swadhishthana chakra is the sacral plexus; the manipuraka (manipura chakra) is the lumbar plexus; the anahata chakra is the cardiac plexus; the bharatisthana (wishuddha chakra) is the junction of the spinal cord with the medulla oblongata; the lalana chakra lies opposite to the uvula, and is supposed to be concerned with the production of ego-altruistic sentiments and affections; the ajña chakra belongs to the sensory-motor tract, and the afferent nerves to the periphery rise from this chakra; the manas chakra is the sensorium, and receives the afferent nerves of the special senses; the soma (indu) chakra is a sixteen-lobed ganglion in the cerebrum above the sensorium; it is the seat of the altruistic sentiments and volitional control; and the sahasrara chakra is the upper cerebrum with its lobes and convolutions.

The anatomical interpretation of the chakras is basically wrong. First of all, an accurate knowledge of both the chakra system and

Western anatomy is required to correlate them. Usually, even a good Sanskrit scholar does not possess all the necessary information on the chakras, and so he is not in a position to make a comparison between the two systems. On the other hand, a Tantrika yogi is generally not well versed in modern anatomy and physiology, and is therefore unable to correlate them. (The form 'yogi' has been preferred to 'yogin', and is used throughout in this book.) The yogi utilizes the knowledge of the chakras in his yoga practices; and to do this no anatomical knowledge of the chakras is really necessary. But a person who has a knowledge of anatomy and physiology as well as a correct understanding of the chakras, and utilizes his knowledge of the chakras in his yoga practice, finds that there cannot be any real identification of the chakras with the nerve plexuses. But this lack of identification does not interfere with his yoga practice. The yogis have been continuing their practices in this way from time immemorial, the teaching being imparted by the gurus to their disciples, who also become proficient in time. The yogis, in absorptive concentration, when the outer world and along with it their own bodies are completely forgotten, experience a new inner world in each chakra. To them the chakras are inner power phenomena; they are vivid and 'seen'. It will not serve any purpose of theirs to identify the chakras with the nerve plexuses.

This study has been undertaken not so much to understand this yoga better, but to find out whether the Tantrika terms can be used to name some physical organs or structures having no clear-cut names in the ancient Indian books on anatomy. Firstly, the main reason for this shortcoming is not due to a lack of knowledge, because even in what we have, we find that they had great anatomical and physiological knowledge, but because most of the works on the subject have been lost. Secondly, if we think that the Tantrika terms are merely anatomical terms, then they lose their essential character and specificality. But, first, we have to see whether or not this identity is possible.

Professor Seal has identified the muladhara, swadhishthana, manipura and anahata chakras with the coccygeal, sacral, lumbar and cardiac plexuses respectively. This identification is based on a lack of the right knowledge of the real locations of these chakras. The chakras are in the sushumna, and the sushumna is inside the vertebral column. These nerve plexuses are situated outside the vertebral column. So there cannot be any identification. Professor Seal says that the bharatisthana (wishuddha chakra) is the junction of the spinal cord with the medulla oblongata. The upper end of the spinal cord is continuous with the medulla oblongata. The upper border of the spinal cord is at the level of the foramen magnum. It is the upper border of the atlas vertebra. He appears to indicate that the point where the upper end of the spinal cord and the lower end of the medulla oblongata meet is the bharatisthana, that is, the wishuddha chakra. Actually, this description does not name the chakra, but merely gives its location. He has also stated that 'This also comprises the laryngeal and pharyngeal plexus'. If he means that these two plexuses are included in the wishuddha chakra, then it must be pointed out that these two are the nerve plexuses; the laryngeal plexus is situated on the external surface of the inferior constrictor muscle of the pharynx, and the pharyngeal plexus, called plexus pharyngeus ascendens, lies on the ascending pharyngeal artery in the wall of the pharynx. In that case, the wishuddha chakra would have to extend to the outside of the vertebral column. If the chakra were stripped of the plexuses and pushed upward into the medulla oblongata, it could be made a nerve centre there. The medulla oblongata has a number of centres which include the respiratory and the vasomotor centres. However, in that case the functional identification should be made.

There is still another difficulty. The wishuddha at the medullary level may clash with the lalana (talu) chakra. He has not identified the lalana with any specific anatomical structure, but only says that it is 'supposed to be the tract affected in the production of ego-altruistic sentiments and affections'. According to him the lalana lies opposite the uvula. This means that the lalana is situated in the palatine region, above which is the ajña and below which is the wishuddha. The palatine region roughly corresponds to the medulla oblongata. It has been clearly stated that the wishuddha is situated in the neck region which corresponds approximately to the middle of the cervical vertebrae.

Professor Seal says that the sensory-motor tract comprises the ajña and manas chakras. This statement is not clear. Moreover, he says that the manas chakra is the sensorium. Seal also asserts that it is the sensory tract at the base of the brain. According to him the manas chakra receives the sensory nerves of the special senses, coming from the periphery. The sensorium generally is any nerve centrum; broadly speaking, it is the sensory apparatus of the body as a whole. It is the seat of sensation. More clearly, it can be said that the manas chakra is the seat of perception. But in what part of the brain is it actually situated? Seal has, of course, roughly indicated that it is at the base of the brain.

There are a number of events that take place during the centripetal passage of nervous impulses from the periphery to the brain, namely, stimulation of the receptors, transmutation of the stimuli into nerve impulses, conduction of sensory impulses to the neurons in the brain, and neuronal transmission and projection on the sensory areas of the cerebral cortex. The whole chain of events is physicochemical, not psychical, in character. Recently, it has been postulated that the cerebral cortex is a way station from which sensory impulses are finally relayed to what has been termed centrencephalic system consisting of the mesencephalon, diencephalon and part of telencephalon. It has no clear-cut anatomical boundary, but, functionally, forms an integrated unit. It appears that both the cerebral cortex and the higher brain stem serve as the neuronal background for sense consciousness. However, it is here that a superphysicochemical event occurs, following or accompanying the nervous events. We can place the manas chakra somewhere in the higher brain stem.

If the manas chakra is identified with a particular area or centre of the higher brain

stem, then the chakra itself cannot be regarded as the seat of consciousness. There is no possibility of finding consciousness in the brain substance. We cannot detect the mentative energy factor in the chemical and electrical energy systems of the brain. We cannot say that the neural activity itself produces consciousness, as it is not known how the change occurs. The findings that lesions in the higher brain stem cause the loss of consciousness do not indicate that consciousness permeates through the brain. The brain stimulation activates the subconscious mechanism which relays impulses to the mind, and as a result consciousness is evoked. Consciousness, which is nonspatial in character, cannot be located in the three-dimensional brain.

It has also been postulated that an intense dynamic neuronal activity, different from the low level activity of sleep, elicits an interaction between brain and mind, and under this condition perception occurs. How is this dynamic brain activity caused? The sensory impulses are not the cause, because they also come into the brain during sleep when no consciousness is evoked. The cause appears to be intrinsic. The specific dynamic brain activity can be explained as the neural counterpart of subconscious activity, roused subconsciously to receive sensory messages. The unconscious neural mechanism is, so to speak, bridged by the subconscious mechanism to consciousness. The brain-mind interaction indicates that mind is an entity lying extraencephalically, but when a relation between it and the brain is established, the brain exhibits specific dynamic activity, and is evoked subconsciously. Consequently, it is a mistake to regard a chakra as a nerve plexus or a brain centre or substance. If it is possible to demonstrate that the chakras are the different levels of consciousness and the subtle dynamic graphs, then, it will at once be clear that the brain is only a gross outline of the inner power operation.

Professor Seal states that the ajña chakra is the centre of command over movements. Hence, it is a motor centre. The motor centres are in the cerebral cortex. But, according to some current notions, the motor impulse originates somewhere in the higher brain stem and is radiated to the cerebral cortex. In that case, the ajña is situated below the manas in the higher brain stem. The external location-point is the space between the eyebrows, which corresponds roughly to the caudal part of the third ventricle of the brain.

Seal maintains that the soma (indu) chakra is a sixteen-lobed ganglion comprising the centres in the middle of the cerebrum, above the sensorium; it is the seat of the altruistic sentiments and volitional control. These qualities are mental and cannot be a function of any brain centre. It may be that the physical counterpart of the mental functioning is a certain brain centre or area located in the telencephalon. He identifies the sahasrara chakra with the cerebral cortex. This is a mistake. The sahasrara is not in the sushumna, but is situated extra-cranially. It is more correct to say that the convoluted surface of the cerebral hemispheres is the material replication of the subtle nirwana chakra, which has 100 petals.

The well-known author of the Aryashastra-pradipa,[3] a scholastic work on ancient Hindu religion and thought, and a great sanskritist, has identified the muladhara, swadhishthana, manipuraka and anahata chakras with the ganglion impar or coccygeal plexus, hypogastric or pelvic plexus, solar or epigastric plexus, and cardiac plexus respectively. It is astonishing that he has also made the same mistake. The coccygeal plexus is connected with the ganglion impar, situated at the union of the two sympathetic trunks at their caudal ends. The other plexuses are sympathetic. However, these plexuses are situated outside the vertebral column, whereas the chakras are in the sushumna, which is inside the vertebral column. So these chakras cannot be identified with the nervous plexuses.

The identification has been carried out still farther. Purnananda Brahmachari[4] has identified the sahasradala lotus (sahasrara chakra) with the telencephalon; dwadashadala lotus (guru chakra) with the diencephalon; chandramandala (moon-circle), amakala and nirwana-kala with the upper part of the corpus callosum; samana (samani) and unmana (unmani) with the middle part of the corpus callosum; nirodhini (nirodhika) and wyapika with the lower part of the corpus callosum; and mahanada with the fornix. He also says that the seat of bindu is in the pineal gland (body) and that of the ajña in the pituitary body.

It has already been mentioned that the sahasrara is an extracranial chakra, so it cannot be identified with the telencephalon. As the dwadashadala (guru chakra) is a part of the sahasrara, and, consequently, is situated extra-cranially, it cannot be identified with the diencephalon. The chandramandala, amakala and nirwanakala are inside the sahasrara, hence, they cannot be identified with the upper part of the corpus callosum. Samani and unmani are two forms of subtle power roused in deep concentration, when dhyana is about to be transformed into samadhi. Therefore, they cannot be identified with the material brain structure. Nirodhika and wyapika are also power-forms operating at the lower level, and cannot be identified with the brain structures. Mahanada is the power-station where pranic motion almost stops in deep concentration. It is situated between the nirwana chakra above, and the indu chakra below. Its corresponding physical point is in the corpus callosum. Consequently, it cannot be identified with the fornix. Similarly, it is a fallacy to make bindu and ajña identical with the pineal and pituitary bodies respectively.

Dr Vasant G. Rele[5] has identified the muladhara chakra with the pelvic (inferior hypogastric) plexus. Similarly, the swadhishthana has been identified with the hypogastric (superior) plexus; the manipura chakra with the plexus of the coeliac-axis (coeliac plexus); the anahata chakra with the cardiac plexus; the wishuddha chakra with the pharyngeal plexus; the taluka (talu) chakra with the cavernous plexus; and the ajña chakra with the naso-ciliary extension of the cavernous plexus. We have already noted that this identification is baseless. First, the chakras are situated within the vertebral column, whereas these nervous plexuses are lying outside it, and, consequently, there cannot be any identification between them. Second, the chakras are subtle force-centres, but the nervous plexuses are gross structures. It cannot be demonstrated that the powers residing in the chakras are also in the nerve plexuses. By concentration and pranayama, these latent powers lying in the chakras can be roused; but these processes have no such effects on the nervous plexuses. So the correspondences can neither be ascertained scientifically nor are they in agreement with the technical description of the chakras.

Moreover, Dr Rele has identified the shaktis (powers) residing in the chakras with the efferent impulses exercising an inhibitory influence generated through the subsidiary nerve centres in the spinal cord. The shaktis are conscious powers; they act directly on any physical organs, and unlike the nervous impulses they never act unconsciously. They control the chakra organizations, and the yogis arouse them to develop their concentration to the dhyana level to be able to do dhyana on the deities situated in the chakras. The chakras are also the centres of pranic forces and specific sense principles. An alteration in the functions of the body can be made by pranayama and concentration. The nervous impulses are physico-chemical phenomena whereas the shaktis are subtle and conscious.

Swami Wiwekananda[6] has vaguely stated that the different plexuses having their centres in the spinal canal can stand for the lotuses. The chakras cannot be explained physiologically as they are subtle centres, and the nervous plexuses are gross structures. Swami Sachchidananda Saraswati[7] presents this in a more sensible way. He says that the nervous plexuses are not the chakras, but they are the gross indicators of the inner regions where the chakras are. According to him, the ganglion impar or the coccygeal plexus is the indicator of the muladhara chakra; the hypogastric plexus, solar plexus, cardiac plexus, carotid plexus (plexus caroticus internus), and cavernous plexus are the indicators of swadhishthana, manipura, anahata, wishuddha and ajña chakras respectively. But this is also misleading. The better method to determine the locations of the chakras has been presented in Section 12 of this book.

Arawinda[8] says that the centres (chakras) are in the subtle body, not in the physical body; but as the subtle body is interfused with the gross body, there is a certain correspondence between the chakras and certain centres in the physical body. So the real nature of the chakras has been disclosed by him.

Dr Gananath Sen[9] has used the terms ida and pingala to mean the two sympathetic chains of ganglia, and the sushumna for the spinal cord. He has named the spinal cord sushumnakanda, and the medulla oblongata sushumnashirshaka. Dr Rele[10] has also identified the ida pingala nadis with the two gangliated sympathetic trunks, one on each side of the vertebral column, and the sushumna nadi with the spinal cord. Professor Brajendranath Seal[11] has identified the ida and pingala with the left and right gangliated sympathetic trunks, but the sushumna nadi with the central canal of the spinal cord. According to Purnananda Brahmachari[12] the sushumna is the spinal cord and brahmarandhra (brahma nadi) is identical with the central canal.

Wiwekananda[13] says that the ida and pingala are the sensory and motor fibres in the spinal cord through which the afferent and efferent currents travel. So the sensory and motor impulses in the spinal cord have been identified with the ida and pingala nadis respectively. About the sushumna, he says that it is a hollow canal, running centrally through the spinal cord, and the canal is continuous within the fine fibre which starts at the end of the spinal cord and goes downward to the lower end, situated near the sacral plexus. This fibre is clearly the filum terminale. From this description it appears that he has identified the sushumna with the central canal within which there is no nerve matter, but it contains the cerebrospinal fluid. According to him, the mind is able to send messages without any wire (that is, without passing through the nerves), and this is done when the yogi makes the current pass through the sushumna.

Now, let us first consider whether we are justified in identifying the sushumna with the spinal cord. First, the sushumna nadi has been described as extremely subtle and spiralled; but the spinal cord is a gross nervous structure, measuring in width at the level of the cervical enlargement 13-14 mm, of the lumbosacral enlargement 11-13 mm, and of the thoracic portion about 10 mm. Consequently there cannot be any identification between the two. Second, the sushumna nadi arises from the nadi centre called kanda-mula, lying just below the muladhara chakra, which corresponds approximately to the point below the inferior end of the filum terminale. It ascends through the filum terminale, central canal, fourth ventricle, cerebral aqueduct, third ventricle, telencephalon medium, anterior commissure, fornix, septum pellucidum, corpus callosum and longitudinal fissure, to reach the central point of the cerebral cortex. On the other hand, the spinal cord extends from the lower border of the first lumbar vertebra, or the upper border of the second lumbar vertebra to the upper border of the atlas, and ends in the lower part of the medulla oblongata at the level of the foramen magnum. From this it is clear that the sushumna cannot be identified with the spinal cord.

There is another important point which needs our attention. Inside the sushumna are three more nadis. Within the sushumna is wajra, within the wajra is the chitrini and within the chitrini is the brahma nadi. If the sushumna is the spinal cord, how are these three nadis to be explained? Can the wajra, chitrini and brahma nadis stand for the white matter, grey matter and central canal respectively; or, should these three nadis be identified with the meninges, white matter and grey matter? The meninges also consist of three layers, dura mater, arachnoid mater and pia mater. Here we really do not know what to think. The nadi can stand for the white or grey matter. But it cannot be identified with either the meninges or the central canal, neither of which are composed of nervous tissue.

Dr Gananath Sen[14] has exclusively used the word nadi to signify nerves. He also says that probably the Greek word neuron (a nerve) is derived from the Sanskrit word nadi. Professor Brajendranath Seal[15] appears to have the same opinion. Dr Rele[16] also has the same opinion. He says: 'Wayu-nadis, i.e., nerves of impulse.' He has clearly identified wayu with nervous impulse.

The Greek word neuron means sinew, cord, and nerve. Now this word is used to mean a nerve cell with its axonal and dendritic processes, and it is considered to be the structural unit of the nervous system. The word nerve has many meanings. But from the medical viewpoint, a nerve is a tubular elongated structure consisting of bundles of nerve fibres or axons of nerve cells, which convey impulses, and a connective tissue sheath, called epineurium, which encloses these bundles. The word nerve may also mean energy, force, vitality.

Now, let us consider the meaning of the word nadi. Nadi has been derived from 'nada' (or nala) to mean motion or regulated motion. In other words, nadi is energy in motion, or activated energy. When the energy in motion is vehicled in a material structure, nadi is a nerve. Otherwise, nadi is 'wireless' force-motion. The word wayu has been derived from 'wa' to mean motion, that is, energy in motion. So the word wayu can stand for nadi. There is another word in Sanskrit—'snayu' which has been used for nerves. According to Dr Gananath Sen[17] this is a mistake. He maintains that the meaning of the word snayu is fibrous tissues generally, and ligaments particularly. But it appears that the word 'snawa' has been used in the Atharwawedasanghita to signify very slender threadlike structures. Can they not be nerves?

Now, let us come to our point. We are not justified in using the word 'nadi' exclusively for the nerve. In yoga, the term nadi has been used in a technical sense. The nadi-chakra or nadi organization is not the nervous system. In the nervous system, energy is propagated through the medium of the nerves, and the energy itself appears to be electrical in nature, functioning on the physico-chemical basis. This 'wired' energy is restricted in its functions. There is another aspect of the energy which is free from this material bondage. This means that its function is not restricted by the nerves, and, consequently, it is conducted in a 'wireless' manner to produce deep effects. This energy works in a supramaterial field having unbounded potency, and it also glides into matter to reinforce the nervous energy. This field is subtle, and the energy is subtle. The word 'subtle' (sukshma) has been used technically to indicate what is not material. It is Patañjali's third form of matter (bhuta). This subtle aspect of energy has been termed prana wayu which operates without nerves. This non-nervous operation is, therefore, only pranic force-motion lines of direction, technically termed nadis. To avoid confusion and make the nadis distinct from the nerves, it has also been termed yoga nadi. It is now also clear why we cannot identify wayu with nervous impulse. A nervous impulse is a wave of negative electrical force based on the chemical energy system. Its activities are limited by the nerves. Wayu is the patent form of latent prana—the basic energy. Wayu is in constant motion and creates subtle lines of direction, called nadis.

Arawinda[18] states that the pranic energy is directed through a system of numerous channels, called nadi,—the subtle nervous organization of the psychic body. The nadis, or the system of nadis, have been described as the subtle nervous organization of the psychic body. The nervous organization he mentions here is not the gross nervous system. It is the 'subtle' nervous system, and this is clear by his using the word 'subtle' nervous organization. We already know the meaning of the word subtle. To avoid confusion we would prefer to use 'the nadi organization' instead of the subtle nervous organization. But the nadi organization is not only of the psychic body, but essentially of the pranic body (pranamaya kosha); on the one side, the pranic body extends to the material body (annamaya kosha), and on the other, to the mental body. The 'channels' mentioned here are not actually some tubular substance, but the subtle lines of direction caused by the pranic energy.

Now we come to the nadis ida and pingala. The origin of the ida and pingala is the same as of the sushumna. But they extend beyond the vertebral column and ascend to reach the ajña chakra, about the level of the caudal part of the third ventricle of the brain, where they are united with the sushumna. The ida and pingala are also subtle nadis, otherwise there cannot be any union with the sushumna. Though, anatomically the two gangliated sympathetic trunks extend from the base of the skull to the coccyx, they are too gross to be identified with the subtle ida and pingala. The functions of the ida and pingala are not those of the sympathetic nervous system. The ida and pingala have also been identified with the sensory and motor impulses in the spinal cord. This cannot be, because they are not the gross nerve fibres carrying nervous impulses. They are subtle nadis which are themselves force-motion lines, conveying pranic forces to the mind and body. Moreover, they are not within the vertebral column, but outside it.

Here it is not a question of deciding whether the ancient Indian medicine has presented sound anatomical and physiological knowledge; and it is unnecessary to explain here the Waidika and Tantrika chakra system and Kundalini in terms of modern anatomy and physiology. To do so means to limit the energy-confining only to the physical field, ignoring its supramaterial manifestation. As physiology is understood today, we cannot go farther than the molecular level. Even this does not explain the whole matter. It will be very helpful if we remember what Arawinda[19] has said: 'I am afraid the attempt to apply scientific analogies to spiritual or yogic things leads more often to confusion than to anything else—just as it creates confusion if thrust upon philosophy also.'

Enough has been said to indicate that neither can the chakras be identified with the nervous plexuses, nor the nadis with the nerves.

Yogic Exposition of the Chakras

There are no indications of the chakras either in the gross aspect of the body or at the molecular and atomic levels. Are we then forced to conclude that the chakras belong to the realm of nonentities? Another important question is linked with the answer given to this question, namely, is the modern scientific conception of matter the borderland of our knowledge? At one level matter is seen in its gross form, and at another level it is constituted of minute particles and energy. Here we find the conversion of matter into energy, and energy into matter. This may explain how the materiality of matter is maintained, but it is not enough to account for the manifestation of life in matter and the connection of mind with the brain. We cannot escape by saying simply that protoplasm is the living matter and mind is the function of the brain.

The elementary particles are very minute; they are so small that they are not seen even with the help of the most sensitive instruments. But they still have mass; and theoretically it is possible to reduce mass step by step to a point where there is no longer any mass. According to Kanada, this is the stage of anu—a non-magnitudinous point. The nearest approach to anu is seen in the neutrino, which has no mass, no charge and a very slight interaction with matter. This indicates that there is a possibility of energy becoming free from the bondage of the particles in a graduated manner. In this transition period, certain particles may pass into the stage of anu where they are only energy—energy without any material form and free from matter-bondage. This is subtle energy. Where does it go? It does not return to the material field, as it cannot function there; it is not destroyed; then it must have a field of operation. This has been termed by the yogis the subtle power-field.

The yogis explain this in the following manner. The decentralized subtle forces, technically termed mahabhutas (metamatter) pass to a level, called subtle elliptical body (kanda-mula), where they are equalized to form an undifferentiated metamatter force. At this point, metamatter force tends towards grossness and materialization on a descending scale, and finally, it is transformed into material energy which operates in the material field. Material energy undergoes fragmentation. It is the process of transformation of energy, first, into just a trace of minute matter-fragments which, at a certain stage on a descending scale, appear as elementary particles, and second, into atoms and molecules, and finally into gross matter. At the gross level, matter exhibits specific sense qualities, derived from

five forms of tanon (tanmatra) associated with metamatter forces, which react on the physical senses. On the other hand, when energy becomes free from particles at the energy level of matter, a part of it may break the bondage of matter, due to the activation of the latent metamatter force, the outer expression of which is material energy, and becomes transformed into metamatter force to function in the subtle power-field. Hence, matter does not end at the level of the elementary particles, but is continuous with metamatter in the subtle power-field. The yogic explanation gives an answer to Hoyle's statement that matter comes from nowhere. This nowhere is the subtle metamatter field which is beyond all observations, even with the aid of the most sensitive instruments.

The yogis say that pranic dynamism releases three forms of energy which give rise to the three phenomena: laghiman (rarefaction), animan (subtilization), and mahiman (magnification), which cause the emergence of life force, mind, and matter respectively. The supremely concentrated prana as bindu (power-point) becomes expanded and active at a certain 'critical' moment, and is expressed as radiant dynamism. Radiant dynamism is transformed into petaline dynamism consisting of the centrally situated massive mental consciousness, around which is the circular pranic force-motion, and surrounding it is a petaline formation of an extraordinary character. The whole organization has been technically termed the sahasrara chakra. Below the sahasrara, the three basic forms of pranic energy coalesce to form a central power-flow, termed the sushumna. The sushumna retains the threefold nature of pranic energy, and so there are three power-flows in it. The outer flow is the sushumna itself; internal to it is the wajra-flow; and the third, which is inside the wajra, is the chitrini-flow.

The sushumna power-flow exhibits two fundamental characters: vertical force-motion, expressed as centrifugal and centripetal force-motion lines, and spiral force-motion. The chitrini energy tends to be centralized in a circular form at certain points throughout its course, due to the influence of the spiral force-motion. The centralized circular power follows the pattern of the *sahasrara* and presents three aspects: a central pericarpial formation, a circular force-motion around it, and a peripheral petaline formation. The whole circular organization is called *chakra*. There are nine main *chakras* in the *chitrini*, namely *nirwana*, *indu*, *manas*, *ajña*, *wishuddha*, *anahata*, *manipura*, *swadhishthana* and *muladhara*.

Thus, the *chakras* are in the subtle power-field which comprises the mental and meta-matter realms. Is this yogic explanation based on pure inference? No, the *chakras* are 'seen' with the 'mental eye'. This requires an explanation.

Perception is the process of receiving and being conscious of an object. Perception has several strata. At its lower stratum, physical sense apparatus is involved in perception and there is the awareness of a sense quality in a modified form. There are five main sense qualities: smell, taste, sight, touch and sound. These qualities are an aspect of matter. The awareness of the sensory form of matter occurs in consciousness. This indicates that sense qualities are outside the boundary of consciousness, and they are to be brought into consciousness by some appropriate means. This implies that there is a distance factor. Moreover, the penetration of sensory forms into consciousness and their recognition are based on the principle of selection and rejection. If the distance and selection-rejection principle were not operating, then all sense qualities would be the simultaneous content of consciousness.

There are five classes of receptors, each endowed with the power of receiving only a particular form of sense quality. After the sense qualities are received by the receptors, sensory paths are created from the receptors, first through the sensory nerves and then through the neuronal connections in the brain, to the cerebral cortex, and thence to an area of the higher brain stem. Nothing more is known about sensory path in its nervous aspect, and there is no further trace of it in the brain. This has resulted in too much speculation. For instance, that the end point of the sensory path is in a certain area of the brain which is in connection with consciousness. But this connection does not necessari-

ly indicate that this particular brain area itself is the seat of consciousness. It may mean that the area is in some way connected with consciousness; and when this area is damaged or removed, the connection is cut off. If this brain area is the seat of consciousness then is consciousness distinct from brain, or is it identical with the brain, that is, brain = consciousness?

But, actually, consciousness has not been traced to that area or any other part of the brain. The sensory path which has been created is observable up to the brain; it is observable because it is a physicochemical process. But how the physicochemical process in that brain area causes the appearance of consciousness is not known. How the metamorphosis of physicochemical energy into consciousness occurs has not been explained. How physicochemical events in the brain suddenly occur as psychic events cannot be explained. Consequently, it is not easy to make mind = brain.

There may be another possibility. Psychical events may accompany or immediately follow the physicochemical events in the brain. If this is accepted, then it will mean that brain and consciousness are not identical, but are two separate entities, and their interconnection is experienced in a particular brain area. To explain this, it has been postulated that certain specific dynamic actions of the brain, in which certain areas of the cerebral cortex and the higher brain stem are involved, are the essential conditions for the relation between the brain and consciousness. How the specific dynamic actions, which are physicochemical in nature, can establish a relation with consciousness which lies beyond the brain itself, is neither known nor explained.

Molecular, atomic, and subatomic activities are all disconnected from consciousness, and are not a fact in consciousness. It is certainly a suggestion that a relation is established between brain and consciousness when the former exhibits specific dynamic actions. If we accept consciousness as something which is neither a physicochemical phenomenon nor explainable in terms of matter, then we think of consciousness as something which is outside the sphere of chemical and electrical energy, something which is neither bound by nor composed of molecules, atoms and elementary particles. In that case, the brain-consciousness relation is deeper and more complex.

There is an important query regarding the specific dynamic action of the brain. How is it caused? If we say that neural-neuronal, centripetal conductions are the cause, then we have to accept that this brain state is continuous, without any interruption, because these conductions are continuous. It has not been demonstrated that there is some controlling mechanism in the brain to exercise control over these conductions. In that case, how is sleep-unconsciousness produced? The specific dynamic actions certainly disappear during sleep. What makes them disappear? Here is a clear indication that the specific dynamic action of the brain, if there is any, is not caused by neural-neuronal conductions, but by something else which operates from outside the brain.

Now, let us consider two important factors: distance and sensory capacity. Taste and touch operate in direct contact with the receptors in the tongue and skin respectively. The distance factor operates in smell, sight and sound. This means that the receptors and sense-objects are not situated in direct contact with each other, but are separated by a certain distance. The distance varies, but there are certain upper and lower limits of perception, beyond which no perception takes place. Between the upper and lower limits sensory capacity varies in different species and also in the same species. Apart from distance, there is another factor, size or magnitude of the sense-objects. If the size of an object diminishes below a certain point, it is not perceptible. Here, the sense capacity also varies in both different species and the same species. There is still another factor. If a sense-object remains within the range of the right distance, and its size is also suitable for perception, then there will be no perception if it is obscured. As an example, if a certain object is placed inside a closed box situated within the range of vision, then only the box will be seen, not the object inside the box. That object has been obscured by the box, which the eyes cannot see through. Other examples are: bones covered by muscles, brain covered by the skull, etc.

The time factor is also operative in perception. Events which occurred in the past are only remembered, but not 'seen'. Only present events are perceived directly. There is no direct knowledge of future events.

All this indicates that sensory capacity is not a fixed thing, but relative, variable, conditional and temporal. The sense qualities themselves are also variable. If this is so, we can postulate that there is a possibility of ultimately attaining a perfect and absolute sense capacity; and that the most subtle sensory forms may exist. Can this be actually demonstrated?

Let us say that normal sensory capacity is X. Now, the question is whether we can perceive sense-qualities beyond X or not. Our experience is that by using appropriate instruments we can perceive those sense-qualities which are imperceptible at X. The instrumental observations indicate that the barriers of distance, size and obscurity have been overcome to a considerable extent, and that certain details and factors which are never seen at X have become visible. Symbolically we may call this instrumentalized, extended sense capacity Y. This shows that the sensory capacity can be increased beyond the normal limit by instrumental aid. But future events are not revealed by these instruments.

Now, the question is whether X can be extended to Z without Y. Z stands for supra-normal sensory capacity. It has also gradations. Its existence has been demonstrated by the yogis. Yogic experiences may be divided into three categories. First, there is an extension of the normal limit of power without any instrumentation. This may be called extended, normal sensory capacity, XA. Those yogis who have been established in pranayama are able to exhibit XA. As, for example: there is a tree in front of us at a distance when the normal eyes can see its trunk, branches and leaves, but not in greater details. If a swarm of ants moves upward on the surface of the trunk, the ants will not be seen from that distance by the normal eyes. But a yogi can see them very clearly. This has been demonstrated. In a similar manner smell and sound are experienced.

Second, there can emerge an uncommon and new pattern of sense-qualities which is never experienced by normal sensory power. This specific sense capacity may be called XB. A yogi has the capacity XB. He experiences supersmell, supersight and supersound.

The following are instances in my own experience. I was in a sitting position on my seat in a very dark room on a dark night, fully awake but calm. There was no notion of seeing or hearing anything uncommon. I spent about an hour like this. Then, suddenly I saw a beautiful light of vermilion colour, by which the whole room was lit up. I got up amazed and looked at the light for some minutes. The light was very beautiful, cool and localized, and the room was beautifully illuminated. I went outside to see if anything had happened there, but found nothing. I hastened into the room and saw that the light was still glittering. After 10 minutes or so, the light gradually became dim and finally disappeared. The room was again dark. I saw this light with my eyes, which were neither closed nor covered. In my judgment it was a superlight.

The other experience was that: I happened to be in a place where a room was given me to sleep in, which had on the wall a beautiful picture of Sri Chaitanya, the great bhaktiyoga master. One dark night, the room being also very dark, I was in a sitting attitude, calm, but awake. When about 30 minutes had passed, I suddenly saw, to my great surprise, that very bright yellow rays were radiating from the body of Chaitanya in the picture. The whole picture was beautifully illuminated, and even part of the room was lit up. Before this occurrence, I had not thought at all of the picture. I was fully awake at the time. The light phenomenon continued for about 4 or 5 minutes. In those days I was able to see clearly and minutely things in deep darkness, without the help of light.

Third, there are real supranormal sensory perceptions, Z perception, in which the barriers of distance, size, obscurity and time are completely overcome. A yogi can perceive a happening occurring far away from him and barriered by mountains, buildings, etc. He can correctly foretell future events. All this has been demonstrated.

So the position is this. The gross aspect of matter presents sense-qualities in a form which may be termed sensory form 1. It is perceived by normal sensory capacity (X-capacity). The range of normal sensory capacity can be increased to a degree when the perception of sense-qualities lying beyond the normal sensory limit occurs. The sense-qualities do not change at this stage, but are barriered, which is overcome by extended, normal sensory capacity (XA-capacity).

We also find that the pattern of the sense-qualities perceived by normal sensory capacity and extended, normal sensory capacity is associated with a new, or an altered form of sense-qualities, which is only perceived by specific sensory capacity (XB-capacity). Above all these is the sensory form 2 which is perceived by instrumentalized, extended sensory capacity (Y-capacity). Thereafter, there is a gap in the perception of sense-qualities at the subatomic level. There are no records of any sensory experience at this stage known to me. But theoretically there is no reason why this should be impossible.

The supranormal sensory experience develops after the specific sensory experience. In this experience, sensory form 1 is perceived. But sensory form 1 is concealed by the barriers of distance, size, obscurity and time. In this perception, these barriers are overcome by developing supranormal sensory capacity (Z-capacity).

What is the mechanism which is brought into play in the above forms of perception? In normal sensory perception, the receptors are stimulated, and sensory nervous paths are created which join the appropriate brain areas. In extended, normal sensory perception, specific sensory perception, and instrumentalized sensory perception, the same receptor-brain nervous paths are used. But in supranormal sensory perception, the nervous paths are not used, because the receptors cannot be stimulated by sensory form 1, which is obscured by the barriers of distance, size, obscurity and time. In that case, how does this form of perception take place? It indicates that the 'wired' nervous paths are too gross for this kind of perception; and since this perception is a fact, there must be some subtle 'wireless' conduction-system for this purpose. These nonnervous, subtle conduction-lines are technically termed na*di*-paths. When the pranic forces are roused and become more concentrated by pra*n*ayama and concentration, they can be made so sensitive that they receive the vibrations, motions, or radiations of the sense-qualities even when these are obscured. The end-points of pranic forces in the head and skin of the body receive the refined sensory vibrations and transmit them to the ch*a*kras, from where the sense-qualities are transmitted to the subconscious mind in the ajña ch*a*kra. Precognition is only affected by the subconscious mind. The subconscious mind is also able to receive directly all sense-qualities when it is sensitized by pra*n*ayama and concentration.

Supranormal perception indicates the existence of subtle na*di*-paths. It also shows that consciousness is outside the boundary of the brain. Most people are unable to utilize these paths, because their powers in this direction are undeveloped. The neural-neuronal paths of conduction, occurring in common sensory perception, stop at certain points in the brain. These are the end points of the gross, brain paths. The sensory qualities conveyed by sensory conduction are released from the nervous envelopment at these brain points and are received and conveyed by pranic forces to the na*di*-field, and then to the subconscious mechanism, from where they are radiated to consciousness. It appears that brain dynamism is an aspect of pranic dynamism, and mental dynamism extends through pranic dynamism to the brain.

The sensory forms are a series of graduated forms. On the lower scale the sensory forms are gross, and as they ascend the scale they become more and more minute. Sensory capacity also changes and becomes increasingly powerful in the perception of more minute sense forms. Our normal sensory capacity can be extended to perceive not only sense-qualities lying beyond the normal but also a new type of sense-qualities. Minute sensory forms, existing in the internal form of matter as molecules and atoms are perceived by the electron microscope. But sensory forms existing at the subatomic levels

are so minute that they cannot even be perceived by the use of the electron microscope. This does not indicate that the sensory forms are non-existent here. The sensory forms continue from the atomic-subatomic level and extend to the subtle metamatter state.

At the metamatter stage, sensory forms are subtle and exist as subtle smell, taste, sight, touch and sound, isolated from each other. They are the fundamental aspects of meta-matter. The m*a*habh*u*tas are reducible to the most concentrated forces called t*a*nmatras. At the t*a*nmatra level, sensory forms are the subtlest, and these are the perfect and final forms. Beyond this point, there are no sensory forms. It is the borderland of sense-form. For the perception of these subtle phenomena, it requires perfect 'nose', 'tongue', 'eye', 'skin' and 'ear'. This means that it is the final and most perfect sensory experience which can only be achieved by yogic 'mental eye'. It is the superconscious perception, and consciousness elevated to the concentration level is the only apparatus for its attainment. This perception has two levels: dhyana-perception and samadhi-perception. The former develops into the latter.

Dhyana is that state of consciousness in which the body becomes completely motionless like a mountain; the senses of smell, taste, sight, touch and sound become inoperative, and, consequently, the outer world is no longer the content of consciousness; consciousness remains unaffected by intellective functions and thoughts; such consciousness, thus being empty, coils to a point in which all its power is in full concentration. In this state, concentration exhibits the power of holding only one object fully. When such a concentrated consciousness is exposed to an object, it penetrates into the deeper aspects of the object and gets its inner subtle power-graph properly imaged in consciousness, and the image is fully illuminated because the revealing quality of consciousness is now maximally roused; then consciousness expands to a certain degree for the magnification of the image of the power-graph which, finally, is transferred to highly rarefied thought. In this way, a perfect and complete knowledge of the unknown and the subtle aspect of an object is attained. Samadhi is the full extension of dhyana when the perception is absolute and automatic. The chakras have been 'seen' in this manner.

Is the mental 'vision' of subtle phenomena a fact? Are the subtle phenomena real? Our answer is, that the chakras are subtle, but not imaginary. Each chakra contains specific power phenomena which can be made to manifest physically by appropriate means. This fact clearly indicates that the chakras exist and their powers can be made to manifest themselves on the physical plane. Let us take the muladhara chakra as an example. The power apana residing there can be roused, controlled, and made to exhibit a strong upward motion by dhyana and pranayama. When this upward apana motion is most forceful, the physical body rises off the ground and begins to levitate by itself without any mechanical aid. There is no form of energy operating in the body which is able to do this. Consequently, it definitely manifests the existence of the chakra, the pranic power and its influence on the body.

There are other forms of power in the chakras, and they can also be roused by dhyana. Dhyana in the muladhara develops natural health and strength of the body and intellective power, and prolongs life. Dhyana in the swadhishthana chakra develops a diseaseless and vital body and intellectual power. Dhyana in the manipura chakra develops the natural immunity of the body, the attainment of long life, and the release of certain uncommon powers. Dhyana in the anahata chakra develops an inner beauty, and makes the body highly attractive; there is also an intellectual development above normal and an acquisition of uncommon sensory powers. Dhyana in the wishuddha chakra develops a body adamantine in hardness and strength, and absorptive mental concentration. All these phenomena indicate that the chakra powers can be made to manifest in the body.

Experiences of the Yogis

Kundaliniyoga forms a highly important part of the yoga practices; and it has been practised
26

by the yogi gurus and their disciples from time immemorial in India. This is indicated by the fact that the great yogi Shankaracharya,[20] who became famous by expounding the monistic doctrine of Brahman in his well-known commentary, 'Sharirakabhashya', on the Brahmasutra (Wedanta-darshana) of Wyasa, had experience in this yoga, and gave an account of this in two of his unique works, Ananda Lahari (Wave of Bliss) and Yogatarawali. In the Ananda Lahari, the essence of Shankara's direct experience in Kundaliniyoga is presented. The Ananda Lahari is considered to be such an important document that there are now known to be thirty-six commentaries on it. The work is an elaboration of the principles of this yoga contained in the Subhagodaya, a stotra by the celebrated Goudapada. It indicates that Goudapada himself practised Kundaliniyoga, and presented certain principles of this yoga in the Subhagodaya. Goudapada, who was almost certainly taught this yoga by his guru Shuka, the son of the famous Krishna Dwaipayana Wyasa, was expected to teach it to his disciple, the famous yogi Gowindapada, and Shankara must have obtained his knowledge of it from the latter. This shows the great antiquity of Kundaliniyoga.

Shankara has clearly stated what happens in Kundaliniyoga when Kundalini, being roused, passes through the brahma nadi and pierces all the chakras and reaches the sahasrara to be in union with Parama Shiwa; and then returns again to the muladhara. He says[21]: Having pierced all the principles (situated in the chakras) —'earth' in the muladhara, 'water' in the swadhishthana, 'fire' in the manipura, 'air' in the heart (that is, anahata), 'void' (akasha) above it (that is, wishuddha), mind (manas) between the eyebrows (that is, ajña), and having thus passed through the kulapatha (that is, the path through which Kulakundalini, or Kundali-power, passes; it is the brahma nadi which starts from the muladhara and terminates in the nirwana chakra where the sushumna also terminates), you (Mother Kundalini) are in union (in mind-transcendent concentration) with your husband (Parama Shiwa) in the secret aspect of the sahasrara chakra (that is, the all-absorbing path leading to infinity; it is beyond the sahasrara, and consists of Bindu, Nada, Shiwa-Shakti, Sakala Shiwa, and then Parama Shiwa where the union in yoga occurs). The life-essence flows like a stream from your feet ('feet' symbolizes union in yoga) by which the whole body is sprinkled; and then you again return to your own abode, and in doing so, you cause the chakras to become manifest. There (in the muladhara) you assume your own form, like a coiled serpent (that is, $3\frac{1}{2}$ coils around Swayambhu-linga), and sleep (become latent in samadhi) in the cavity of the kulakunda (the triangle in the muladhara).

Shankara has also mentioned the names of the following chakras in the Ananda Lahari: muladhara in verse 41, swadhishthana in verse 39, manipura in verse 40, wishuddha in verse 37, and ajña in verse 36. There is no clear mention of the anahata chakra, but in verse 38, the word sangwit-kamala (knowledge-lotus) occurs, and it has been interpreted as referring to anahata chakra. But Shankara has clearly used the word anahata in verses 3 and 9 of the Yogatarawali.

Shankara has disclosed the contraction process which is a part of the mantra process in rousing Kundalini in Kundaliniyoga. The contraction process comprises locks (bandhas) in conjunction with pranayama.

Shankara says that by the application of the anal-lock (mulabandha), navel-lock (uddinabandha = uddiyanabandha) and neck (or chin)-lock (jalandharabandha) (in conjunction with sahita kumbhaka) Kundalini is roused and enters into the sushumna (that is, the brahma nadi lying within the sushumna). Moreover, he states that sahita kumbhaka, practised in conjunction with anal-, navel-, and chin-locks, finally develops into kewala kumbhaka (automatic breath-suspension)[22].

Tailanga Swami[23], the great yoga master, has also mentioned the contraction process. He says[24]: By the application of the contraction process (consisting of different locks) the door of Kundalini should be opened, and the passage leading to liberation (that is, the chitrini nadi in which the chakras are strung) should be pierced (by Kundalini). This yoga (that is, Kundaliniyoga) should be practised after hearing the Wedanta (that is, purifying the mind by hearing and thinking of Brahman).

The well-known Tantrika yogi Ramaprasada[25] has recounted his experiences of Kundaliniyoga in some of the spiritual songs (Padawali) he composed. He relates[26] that the muladhara contains 4 petals in which are situated the 'earth' principle and Power Dakini, and here lies Kundalini in $3\frac{1}{2}$ coils round Shiwa (Swayambhu-linga); the swadhishthana has 6 petals where the deities Wishnu and Waruna, and Power Rakini reside; the manipura has 10 petals and a triangular region containing the bija of Wahni, and Power Lakini resides here; the anahata has 12 petals and a hexagonal region in the pericarp containing the wayu-bija; there resides Power Kamini (Kakini); the sixteen-petalled lotus wishuddha contains vowels (the first 16 matrika-letters) and there the Deity Wishnu is seated on naga (the celebrated serpent) or on an elephant, and Power Shakini; the dwidala (the two-petalled, that is, ajña) is situated in the space between the eyebrows; on its petals are the matrika-letters 'hang' and 'kshang'; there is situated chandra-bija ('thang'), from which nectar oozes; here are also Shiwa-linga (Itara-linga), a circle and a triangle; it is the seat of the mind. This is the clear picture of the chakras. Ramaprasada also states[26] that Kulakundalini is in the muladhara; she is also in the sahasrara and the chintamani-pura (hrit chakra); concentration (on chakras, deities, etc.) is to be done in the interior of the body according to the instructions of the guru: there is Brahma, and four other deities; Dakini and five other Powers; the lord of elephants (gajendra), makara, ram, black antelope and the second elephant, the realization of these occurs when there is automatic breath-suspension (in deep concentration). Ramaprasada's own chosen place for concentration is the hrit chakra (Padawali, Nos 126, 142, 161); his own experience is that Kundalini is in the muladhara as well as in the sahasrara (No 107); he says that there are four Shiwas residing in the muladhara, swadhishthana, throat-region (wishuddha) and the eyebrow space (ajña) (No 104); Srinatha (Supreme Shiwa) is in the thousand-petalled lotus (No 104); a yogi always does concentration on Kundalini in form in the muladhara and sahasrara (No 156).

All these statements indicate that he had full knowledge of the chakras and realized Kundalini and the chakras directly in yoga.

Ramakrishna[27], the great yogi, spiritual teacher and prophet, has expressed his own experiences of Kundalini and the chakras[28]. He 'saw' how Kundalini, being roused, ascends through the sushumna (in fact, through the brahma nadi), and as Kundalini enters into a chakra, the chakra turns its face upward and 'blooms'. He saw that the roused Kundalini passes from the muladhara to the swadhishthana and then to the manipura and the other chakras, and finally, to the sahasrara. He says that the chakra system is like a plant with branches and flowers all made of wax, but actually they are in the nature of life-force (chinmaya). He speaks of one of his experiences, when he saw that a youthful person resembling himself, had entered the sushumna and made each chakra turn upward and open by a 'deep contact' with the tongue, one after another, from the bottom to the top. In this manner, he saw that the muladhara, swadhishthana, manipura, anahata, wishuddha, ajña and sahasrara had turned their heads upward and bloomed.

Ramakrishna has described the movements of Kundalini as supreme-force (mahawayu) motions. He experienced five forms of motion leading to samadhi: ant-like, frog-like, monkey-like, bird-like and snake-like; when these motions reach the sahasrara, samadhi is attained. In deep thought, he perceived Kundalini. He says that real spiritual knowledge does not arise if Kundalini is asleep, and when Kundalini passes through the different chakras, various spiritual experiences occur. According to him, Primordial Supreme Power (Adyashakti) resides in all beings (in the muladhara) as Kulakundalini, sleeping like a coiled serpent.

The celebrated Wama[29], generally known as Wama Kshepa, an accomplished Tantrika yogi, had direct perception of Kundalini and the chakras. He says[30] that the first practice in yoga for the initiated Tantrikas is the rousing of Kundalini. This yoga process is very ancient and highly scientific. In Kundaliniyoga, the practitioner experiences how Kundali-power is working in different chakras and what is happening there. There are specific experiences, associated with blissfulness, in each chakra, when Kundalini passes through it. These experiences are characteristic of the Tantrika method. In other religions there must also be some means of arousing Kundalini, otherwise it is impossible to proceed beyond the lower mental plane. Kundalini may be automatically roused in intense love, intense happiness, intense sorrow, intense pain and intense fear. But she may again return to a dormant state. This is why the guru's guidance is so important.

From his own experiences in Kundaliniyoga, my guru has said that Kundali-power becomes dynamic in the muladhara by intense thought-concentration in combination with the mantras, pranayama and bandhas, and passes upwards through the brahma nadi, by piercing chakra after chakra, and finally reaching the sahasrara. When Kundalini reaches a chakra, the head of the chakra turns upward and the whole contents of the chakra—mahabhuta, tanmatra, Deity, Power, everything—first becomes fully illuminated by the light from Kundalini, and then are absorbed into Kundalini. When Kundalini is roused, real concentration starts, and as she goes upward, it deepens more and more. Thought-concentration of the bhutashuddhi process becomes transformed into real concentration through roused Kundalini. When thought-concentration on Kundalini becomes most intense, the chakras automatically appear in consciousness. This is the indication that Kundalini is about to be roused.

My guru has said that after the union of Kundalini with Parama Shiwa in thought-concentration in bhutashuddhi, Shiwa-Shakti should then be transformed into Ishtadewata, and is to be brought first to the sahasrara, and then to the hrit chakra, where concentration should be done. Thought-concentration on Ishtadewata is a very efficient means of transforming thought-concentration into real concentration. It is a great help in making bhutashuddhi more effective and preparing the practitioner for the practice of Kundaliniyoga.

It appears that thought-concentration on Shiwa-Shakti in form, as Ishtadewata, is also an ancient practice and part of bhutashuddhi, though usually omitted; and this is indicated in Shaṅkara's Ananda Lahari, Verse 8.

Kundalini

Kundalini has been called Kundali-shakti (-power), that is, power in coil. The basic word is kunda or kundala meaning what is spiral or in coil. The term Kundalini or Kundali has been used in yoga in a technical sense, and can be called the spiraliform power, or energy. So Kundalini may be called 'spiraline'. We will elaborate the technical meaning of it later.

Kundalini has been called Spirit-fire, Serpent-fire, Serpent-power, Serpentine Power, Annular Power, Cosmic Electricity, and so on. This does not help very much in understanding the real nature of Kundali-power.

On the physical plane, all energy appears as chemical, mechanical and electrical. Can we find any trace of Kundali-energy in muscular, nervous, glandular, respiratory, cardiac, alimentary and eliminative functions of the body, in cellular activities, at the atomic and subatomic levels? Is it possible to find this energy playing a part in the mental field, in perception, intellection and affectivity?

Kundali-energy cannot be identified with the energy operating in the body at all its levels, or with the tissues and structures of the body. The energy functioning in the body is physico-chemical in nature; it is derived from food, and when food is not supplied, it comes from the tissues of the body. So this energy is actually food-tissue energy. Food is converted into energy and tissues in the body on the one side, and on the other, the tissues are converted into energy to maintain the more vital parts of the body, as in inanition. If Kundalini is identified with the chemical energy, then it is also the tissues of the body. Such a gross transformation of Kundalini is contradictory to its real nature.

Is it possible to identify Kundalini with special forms of energy in the body? As, for example, muscular energy? Here, also the same objection arises. Muscular energy is essentially chemical energy derived from food. Food also becomes a part of muscle. The energy is involved in muscular contraction. Contraction is initiated by motor nervous impulses. The nervous control is not purely a nervous factor; with it the chemical factor is also involved, because at the nerve endings acetylcholine is also released.

Muscular contraction causes muscular movements. A large part of skeletal, muscular movements is carried out automatically, and it is said that they are controlled by the spinal cord and the lower brain. In everyday life we execute innumerable movements in this way. But also a very large part of skeletal muscular movements is done by volition. Over and above those willed actions which are indispensably necessary in our daily life we can execute movements for muscular growth and development. By systematic application of physical culture, an extraordinary muscular growth can be attained, and strength, speed and endurance can be developed to a very high degree. These are isotonic muscular work. But skeletal muscle can be made to exhibit a very powerful isometric contraction, which enables an expert to support on his chest a weight of 5 tons, and on his throat $\frac{1}{2}$ a ton. This isotonic and isometric muscular work is of a conscious type. This great muscular power also depends on food. Thus, in fact, food energy is the basic part without which the body will collapse. Food, combined with muscle training, causes the development of such muscular power. We find that there is really no scope here for Kundalini.

But there are instances which indicate that there is also a possibility of attaining unusual muscular power without specific muscular training and 'athletic' diet. The author knows a number of hatha yogis who have demonstrated extraordinary strength and endurance. Their bodies are not of the athletic type, but graceful. How has this been possible? We cannot introduce Kundalini here, as the basic energy part is still chemical. The question is whether 'will' can do so, and if it can, whether Kundalini is involved in it.

By the application of will on skeletal muscle, a particular muscle or a particular group of muscles can be isolated and controlled; different degrees of contraction can be attained; contraction can be made hard as stone; controlled movements of the diaphragm, control of sphincter muscles, and full relaxation of muscles are achieved. This voluntary control[31] can be developed to an extent when it is possible to attain the following: the passing of the fluid contents through the alimentary canal, urethral suction of fluid and air, voluntary ejaculatory control and very powerful voluntary vaginal contraction.

It is generally thought that this muscular control indicates mental influence on muscles. But it is not so simple. Mind cannot be in contact with the muscle. The brain and mind are bridged by nadi and subconscious mechanisms. The will, being patterned into a definite thought and purpose, develops as conation. This is the extreme mental border. Thereafter, conative impulses are generated and pass in an unconscious form the bridge mechanism and are finally transferred to an appropriate brain area. Then they take the usual course— the motor impulses to the muscles. This 'will' is not effective without the help of the nerve force. Such a weak will cannot be the seat of Kundalini, and as the will is associated with chemical energy for its final effectiveness, it cannot be identified with Kundalini; and without Kundalini the will, combined with nerve force, can do extraordinary things in the body.

What about extraordinary muscular strength demonstrated by the hatha yogis without physical culture? The yogis are able to concentrate pranic force by pranayama and to direct it through the nervous mechanism to the skeletal muscles. We shall come to this factor later.

Can Kundalini-energy be identified with nerve energy? The energy system operating in the nervous system is not different from the other systems of the body. Basically, it is physicochemical, but the metabolism in the brain is slight in comparison with other parts of the body. This is why the brain is extremely resistant to the effects of inanition. Though its loss of mass is very slight, there is still some loss, which indicates its dependence on chemical energy. The electrical power, exhibited especially in nerve impulses, functions on the basis of chemical energy, and not without it. Nerve impulses are intrinsically associated with the nerve structure. The electrical phenomena in the nerves may be a replication of the particles-energy system at the atomic level. Here too, the energy is unconscious in nature, and is associated with extremely minute matter and these are interchangeable. So Kundalini cannot be identified with the brain or any nerve structure or nerve energy.

Dr Rele[32] has identified Kundalini with the right vagus nerve. This means first, that Kundalini is a nerve impulse limited to the right vagus nerve and secondly that it is physicochemical energy.

The vagus nerve, which is the most widely distributed of the cranial nerves, passes from the medulla oblongata through the neck and thorax into the abdomen. It is a mixed nerve, containing essentially three groups of nerve fibres: branchiomotor, efferent parasympathetic and afferent. If Kundalini is the vagus, or the right vagus, is Kundalini then identified with all three groups or only one, possibly parasympathetic? In any case, Kundalini appears to be fragmented and materialized. Moreover, its power becomes very limited. The parasympathetic portion of the vagus exerts an inhibitory influence on the heart, coronary arteries and bronchi, but accelerates the activities of the smooth muscles of the alimentary canal. On the other hand, the sympathetic stimulation produces just the opposite effects. Then, for the efficient functioning of these organs, both the harmonious parasympathetic and sympathetic activities are absolutely necessary. By making Kundalini the vagus nerve, its power has been very much restricted, and it is made to depend upon the sympathetic functioning in a state of normal health. This Kundalini cannot exercise full control over these organs alone. First, the limitation on Kundalini comes by making it the nerve force which is physicochemical in nature; and second, it has been more restricted by making Kundalini the right vagus nerve. Is it this material Kundalini that the yogis strive to realize in deep concentration? Is the yogi's Kundalini so fragmented and limited? Is Kundalini a chemical phenomenon?

Perhaps, the identification can be explained in a different manner. Kundali-energy may reside in the vagus nerve (or the right vagus) ordinarily in a latent form when the normal nerve function goes on; but when it is roused by some processes, it exercises control over the vagus nerve when the ordinary nervous function is transformed into an extraordinary control power by which the heart is completely stopped and a prolonged breath-suspension occurs; and all these things are done voluntarily. Under ordinary conditions, our will does not act directly on the autonomic nervous system; however, it can be stimulated electrically. The exhibition of this unusual control power may be explained in two ways: Kundali-energy, when roused, exhibits this control and at the same time it becomes reflected on the mind, and this results in its becoming a conscious phenomenon; or, the will is directly infused by Kundali-energy when it is able to cause such an extraordinary control power. However, it appears that Kundali-energy is different from the nervous energy which is linked to the nerve structure and is physico-chemical and unconscious in nature. Kundali-energy either functions directly through the will or it works independently and at the same time influences the mind to become involved in it. If Kundalini is not nervous energy, then it is unnecessary to make it the vagus, or right vagus, nerve. Kundalini is also different from will-power, because the ability of the will to control the autonomic nervous system and the involuntary organs is due to Kundalini.

Even this explanation of Kundalini does not reveal its real nature. It is also our assumption that Kundali-power is involved in the control of the autonomic nervous system. Yogis have demonstrated that this control can be achieved by pranayama and concentration. In pranic and mental control Kundalini is indirectly involved. But in the conscious application of the control power over the autonomic nervous system and involuntary organs, Kundalini is not involved. Rather, when Kundalini is roused, an absorption of pranic forces occurs stage by stage, and as a consequence basal metabolism is progressively decreased. So there is no point in making Kundalini the right vagus nerve.

It is a fallacy to think that the sleeping Kundalini resides in the solar plexus. Kundalini does not lie in a gross nervous plexus, as it has been called by the yogis supremely subtle. The yogis say that Kundalini is situated in a coiled form in the subtle muladhara, lying within the vertebral column. The solar plexus is outside the vertebral column. The roused Kundalini rises upward and pierces all the chakras which are subtle power-centres lying inside the vertebral column. These chakras cannot be identified with the gross nervous plexuses lying outside the vertebral column. So, Kundalini neither resides in the solar plexus nor passes through the nervous plexuses.

Nature of Kundali-energy

Up to now we have said what Kundalini is not. This neti-neti (not this—not this) deliberation is very helpful in understanding the real nature of Kundalini. It can be prefaced with a brief consideration of the energy-system operating in the body, even at the risk of some repetition.

The characteristic of the living body is to exhibit activities, viz., cellular, nervous, glandular and muscular, which are associated with livingness. The energy which supports these activities is derived from the tissue-substances (carbohydrates, fats and proteins) by catabolic process. On the other hand, the decay of the tissue-substances is prevented by the anabolic utilization of food. This energy release is a chemical process. This energy-cum-tissue is material in character, and perhaps it may be sufficient to explain physical activities. But really it is not very simple. The phenomenon of consciousness is intermingled with the physical activities. Of course, in most of the vital activities of the body consciousness is not involved. But conscious actions are also an integral part of the bodily functions. Perception, intellection, thought, attention and willing are not possible without consciousness. But in the body, only physicochemical events are observable in perception. How consciousness is evoked or linked with the unconscious physicochemical process is not known. We cannot say that consciousness is located in a certain area of the brain and is 'ignited' by the neuronal conduction, because the same process does not cause consciousness to appear in sleep. The observed fact that the damage of a certain brain-spot produces unconsciousness, may not really indicate that it is the seat of consciousness. It may mean a lack of interaction or an effacement of the material replication of consciousness. That the whole nervous paths and brain are not utilized in the subconscious (generally known as extra-sensory) mode of perception (which definitely occurs), clearly shows that consciousness is beyond the brain.

If this is so, then there must be some form of energy which is not based on the physicochemical system of the body, but is operative in its super-physical character. This subtle energy-system is the 'wireless' system which operates without being vehicled by the nerves. Technically, it is called the nadi system. The 'wired' or the nervous system is an extension of the 'wireless' or the nadi system into the material field.

In the nadi-field, dynamic prana energy is in constant motion. What is the static counterpart of dynamic prana? Take an atom for example. It is the composite of two forms of energy: energy in motion and energy in static form, called the nucleus. If we regard nadi-chakra (-field) as similar to an atom, then prana is its electrons, but what is its nucleus? This is the first time we are compelled to enquire what is the static form of energy as the background of the dynamic prana.

We find that there are three states of pranic operation: a control influence exercised on pranic forces, pranic concentration, and pranic latency, that is, a state of suspension or near-suspension of prana. Under the control influence, pranic energy functions powerfully and harmoniously, and the force-motions take right directions. These effects are shown both in the body and mind. The body becomes purified, healthy, vigorous and diseaseless, the mind becomes clear, forceful and better controlled. This is in itself a great achievement in one's life. The method consists in developing a 'sushumnitc'

force-motion to act successfully on the static force which must have been polarized with dynamic prana. We experience a transference of control element to the active pranic energy, and it is due to the static source, because there are no other sources. This process is technically termed nadishuddhi—normalization of pranic activities. This fact also indicates that dynamic prana functions both in the body and in the mind. It regulates in a specific manner the functions of the body.

Pranic concentration is the transformation of the diversified pranic activities to a highly concentrated state when pranic potency is increased to an extraordinary degree. An example of the increased pranic potency is to levitate the body. This fact also indicates that pranic forces can operate in the body directly.

Thirdly, a state of pranic latency or suspended animation is produced when pranic energy is absorbed, step by step, into an unknown power. So we find that an influence of an unknown power is completely hidden from our observation and its presence unsuspected under ordinary conditions of life, whereas under certain unusual circumstances it is exercised on pranic dynamism, and ultimately there is a possibility of a complete withdrawal of pranic functions. This unknown power has been called in yoga Kundalini. Ordinarily, it is latent, but under certain special conditions, it becomes patent.

What is the real nature of Kundalini? It has been argued that energy polarizes itself as static and dynamic, and the dynamic form is the pranic force, and its static support is Kundalini. Can we trace this relation between prana and Kundalini? The sum total of the activities in which the body, the life-force and the mind are involved is the dynamic aspect of our existence, and the whole phenomenon may be called pranic dynamism. This is observable. But can prana function alone, without a static background? In its normal functioning there is no indication of what is the static aspect of prana. But if there is the polarization of energy, the dynamic form must have a static form, and consequently, prana must have its static form. This static form has been considered as Kundalini.

That there is an intimate relation of Kundalini

with prana is indicated specially in pranic concentration and suspended animation. These two phenomena definitely show the influence of Kundalini on prana. In a state of normal pranic function, no relation between them is observable. It is because prana functions by its own power, and these energy-functions are supported by static Kundalini silently. But there are instances when Kundalini acts on prana, and this active influence of Kundalini changes the character of the normal function of prana. In this case, Kundalini is expected to be dynamic, at least partially. Then what would be the static support of the dynamic Kundalini?

The active influence of Kundalini on prana can be explained by assuming that it is due to an emanation of force from Kundalini which itself remains static, or partly static. But when prana is absorbed by Kundalini, does it still remain static?

The following are the signs of gradual pranic absorption: first, a motionless body; second, the decrease of metabolism lower than basal metabolism; third, stoppage of vital functions of the body; fourth, inoperation of the sensory system. It appears that pranic absorption is associated with a corresponding change in Kundalini, from its static to its dynamic form. The experiences of the yogis support this. The yogis experience directly that Kundalini is roused in the muladhara centre and passes upward through the brahma nadi, piercing all the chakras, to the sahasrara. This means that static Kundalini becomes dynamic in Kundalini-yoga, and exhibits motion—the Kundali-force motion. Consequently, Kundalini leaves the muladhara and goes to the sahasrara.

Some objections have been raised against the actual rousing and passing of Kundalini from the muladhara to the sahasrara. The muladhara has been considered as the static pole in relation to the whole organism. In the muladhara, Kundalini as static power maintains the dynamic form of energy which is the sum total of the activities of the living organism. So Kundalini cannot be made dynamic, it always remains static in the muladhara. The rising of Kundalini has been interpreted as sending forth an emanation or ejection in the likeness of Kundalini which passes through the various chakras and become united with Mahakundalini in the sahasrara, and in this process the coiled Kundalini does not actually move from the muladhara. It has been further stated that if Kundalini leaves the muladhara and goes upward, then it means that Kundalini ceases to be Kundalini. In this case, dynamic Kundali-power will enhance the vital vigour instead of causing the suspension of animation. And so it has been concluded that, ordinarily, prana is diffused over the whole organism, and the pranic dynamism is supported by static Kundalini in the muladhara; in Kundaliniyoga, prana becomes converged, and this is also supported by static Kundalini in the muladhara.

The theory of the nonascent of Kundalini and Kundalini-emanation has been specially advanced by Professor Pramathanatha Mukhopadhyaya[33]. Wiwekananda[34] has clearly said that Kundalini, the coiled-up energy, can be roused and made active and consciously made to pass upward through the sushumna when it acts upon centre after centre. He further says that the rousing of Kundalini is the only means of attaining divine wisdom; and when it passes from centre to centre, layer after layer of the mind opens up. He also admits that a minute portion of Kundalini energy can, as a small current, be set free and may pass through the sushumna. However, according to Wiwekananda, the rousing of Kundalini and its passing through the chakras are facts, and are intimately associated with the lighting up of the dormant layers of the mind; but, under certain conditions, some currents from Kundalini may pass through the sushumna.

Arawinda[35] recognizes the actual passing of Kundalini to sahasrara, and also an ejection from Kundalini as the ascending current going up to the sahasrara. He also says that a mere ejection from Kundalini cannot cause a radical change. In other words, the full release of spiritual force and the growth of superconsciousness are linked to the rousing of Kundalini and its ascent through the chakras.

It is not necessary to assume that all along the muladhara is the permanent static centre. The muladhara has been evolved last, after all other chakras came into being. Pranic dynamism in the form of prananation (pranic radiation) has caused the emergence of the chakras. Before the formation of the muladhara, pranic dynamism started to operate. In that case, its static polarity could not be static Kundalini in the muladhara, but some other static power centred somewhere. The yogis say that it was the $3\frac{1}{2}$-coiled Kundalini, residing in the sahasrara, which was the static support of pranic dynamism at the beginning; and after the emergence of the muladhara, the $3\frac{1}{2}$-coiled Kulakundalini became the static support of the dynamic prana whose activities now have been more diffused and diversified to maintain animation in the gross body. Also there is 8-coiled Kundalini lying throughout the sushumna with 1 coil in each chakra.

So the rousing of Kundalini in the muladhara and its ascent will not cause the total collapse of the living organism. The rousing of Kundalini is the dynamization of Kulakundalini. This will not cause an excess of pranic force, because the ascent of Kundalini is associated with the withdrawal of prana, causing the suspension (to a varying degree) of animation. When Kulakundalini is roused, it becomes uncoiled without being non-Kundalini, and its dynamization causes the absorption of prana, and its motion becomes uninterrupted and highly concentrated. It is not necessary to interpret the ascending Kundalini as the dynamic counterpart of the static Kundalini in the muladhara. Kundalini is actually dynamized, and only when this prodigious power is fully and wholly roused, does the whole power, in concentration and motion, transform the mind in the sahasrara into a supermind—a mind in samadhi. When Kulakundalini is dynamized, the muladhara ceases to be a static centre, and Kundalini in $3\frac{1}{2}$ coils in the sahasrara becomes the static support. This is not to deny that under certain circumstances the static Kulakundalini sends forth emanations to exercise its control influence on prana.

When Kulakundalini becomes dynamic, Kundalini in the sahasrara becomes the static support. The eight-coiled Kundalini is absorbed, step by step, into Kulakundalini when it passes through the different chakras, thus strengthening the Kulakundalini-motions. When Kulakundalini reaches the sahasrara, it becomes united as one with the sahasrara Kundalini, and the whole Kundalini becomes dynamic, and its static support is Kundalini lying beyond the sahasrara and extending from the Supreme Bindu to Sakala Shiwa. Again, when the united Kundalini as Nirwana (all absorbing) power enters into the beyond-sahasrara-Kundalini, it (Kundalini beyond the sahasrara) becomes dynamic and the static support is Parama Shiwa—Supreme Consciousness. Kundalini is finally absorbed into Supreme Consciousness.

These Kundalinis—Kundalini in the muladhara, the eight-coiled Kundalini in the other chakras, Kundalini in the sahasrara, and Kundalini beyond sahasrara—are not different entities, but the different aspects of the same Kundalini. Dynamization of Kundalini takes place step by step. The dynamization is essentially the unfoldment of spiritual consciousness and associated yoga power stage by stage.

Prana is the dynamic counterpart of the coiled Kundalini. Prana is the energy-whole which creates mind, life and matter. The yantra—the real dynamic graph of the pranic operation—is the chakra system. The chakras and associated nadis form the nadi organization. Only a part of pranic energy is at play in the body and mind, which is required for the maintenance of vitality and mentation according to one's capacity and possibility. The pranic function at the common level is an unconscious radiation of pranic energy from the chakras into the body, and that aspect of the mind which is functionally connected with the brain. The chakras are the reservoirs of prodigious powers, which are ordinarily latent. They can be unfolded by pranayama and concentration. These powers can manifest in the body as great vital, nervous and muscular strength, and in the mind as various unknown secret forces. They can also be manifested in the body in a wireless manner as superpowers. But still deeper, there is the coiled central force, remaining as static support of the central dynamism (prana) which maintains all dynamic expression of energies.

The uncoiling of the coiled central force is an

extraordinary occurrence in the human mind and body, in thoughts and actions. It is like a flood of splendorous divine force from which is being released a new form of consciousness which is not modified by what is called matter at all its levels, and is not dependent upon the mind which mentalizes consciousness. Because of the coiling, this latent central force is called Kundalini. But the meaning of coiling or Kundali is much deeper than its superficial significance, 'latency'. Kundalini is in $3\frac{1}{2}$ coils in the muladhara, in 8 coils, one coil in each of the eight chakras, in $3\frac{1}{2}$ coils in the sahasrara and in $3\frac{1}{2}$ coils beyond sahasrara. The first uncoiling of Kundalini takes place in the muladhara. Second, the uncoiling of the eight-coiled Kundalini, third the uncoiling of the sahasrara Kundalini, and finally Kundalini beyond sahasrara takes place. The uncoiling is the process of dynamization of Kundalini occurring in four stages. When Kundalini is uncoiled it becomes the sole dynamism. This dynamism reaches a stage of bodilessness and mindlessness and again becomes static in the form of infinite, whole supreme consciousness.

Kundalini as Kulakundalini is in $3\frac{1}{2}$ coils in the muladhara. The 3 coils indicate that Kundali-energy is latent in the material, nadi and mental fields, and the half coil shows that Kundalini is in a static form. One coil in each chakra indicates that the chakra is inactive and dark, and its powers remain unmanifested. Of the $3\frac{1}{2}$ coils in the sahasrara, the 3 coils indicate that Kundali-energy remains inoperative at the amakala, nirwanakala and nirwana shakti points. This means that samprajñata samadhi has not been developed, prakriti has not been absorbed, and Kundalini has not manifested all-absorbing power. The $\frac{1}{2}$ coil is indicative of its static state. Beyond the sahasrara, the first coil is at Para Bindu, the second coil is at Para Nada, the third coil is at Shiwa-Shakti, and the half coil is at Sakalashiwa. All this means that asamprajñata samadhi has not been attained.

But the significance of the coils goes further. The latency of Kundalini indicates that it is the static support of the prana as dynamism. The dynamic prana is the creative energy, supremely concentrated at the Bindu, and is about to be manifested. At a certain critical moment, the Bindu ejects its dynamic counterpart in the form of an expanded circle within which the pranic energy becomes more concentrated and assumes a triangular form from which power emanates. This triangle-imbedded circle is the first form of pranic-energy radiation in which lie three power components, technically termed 'a', 'u' and 'm' in coiled forms which constitute the radiant first mantra 'ong'. The coiled factor is the replication of Kundalini itself which is in $3\frac{1}{2}$ coils and the static support of prana. Prana exhibits the characteristic Kundali-coil in its motion which becomes spiral.

The pranic impulse consists of two principal factors which are exhibited in pranic motion. They are spiral and vertical. The spiral motion creates subtle dynamic graphs in the form of circles, called chakras; and the vertical motion causes the emergence of the sushumna field in which the chakras are systematically arranged. So the 'coil' is a fundamental factor which remains in static Kundalini as well as in dynamic prana. The coil is the actual potency which is released both in coiling and uncoiling.

When Kundalini begins to be uncoiled, the spiral pranic energy loses its dynamism and begins to be absorbed step by step into dynamic Kundalini. In this way, the chakras are absorbed into Kundalini. When Kundalini is in coils, pranic dynamism essentially manifests as pranic radiations through the sushumna as centrifugal and centripetal motions without any cessation; and its spiraline aspect goes to the pranic chakras and activates the centralized pranic forces. The pranic main currents and centralized pranic forces become more efficient functionally by nadi-shuddhi, when greater control influence is exercised on the body and mind.

But when Kundalini begins to be uncoiled, the central 'sushumnaite' prana currents begin to ebb and the centralized pranic forces are gradually withdrawn into the main pranic current. This is shown by the gradual decrease of the basal metabolism of the body and the cessation of the undulations of mental consciousness. The uncoiling of the $\frac{1}{2}$ coil causes Kundalini to enter into the brahma nadi. The uncoiling of the 3 coils produces control effects on the pranic forces, body and mind. The effects on the pranic forces are two: the absorption of the central pranic currents and the initiation of the Kundalini motion through the brahma nadi; and secondly, changing of the Kundalini motion to Kundalini radiation which causes the revitalization of the pranic forces and produces the nadishuddhi effects. The effects on the body are also two: first, the body undergoes a state of motionlessness in a natural manner, and second, the body functions healthfully and more efficiently, when it goes back to the ordinary state. The mental effects are also two: development of deep concentration and natural unfoldment of spiritual qualities. All this indicates the interrelation between Kundalini and prana.

When Kundalini is in coil, prana force exhibits its spiral motion by which the body is vitalized and mental dynamism operates. When Kundalini is uncoiled, the spiral energy of prana first becomes coil, and then is withdrawn into dynamic Kundalini. This causes the body to be naturally in a state of motionlessness and the slowing of the vital functioning. In this state the mind functions above the perceptive and intellective levels as real concentration. Before being really dynamic, Kundalini emits radiations through the sushumna. Under this condition, the mind becomes spiritual in nature, and an urge is felt to make and keep the body purified and vigorous.

Kundalini is roused consciously as in Kundaliniyoga, or unconsciously as in various religious and spiritual practices involving deep godly feeling. There are certain circumstances in life when Kundalini is also roused unconsciously. In intense fear of death as in severe diseases or some great danger; in deepest unbearable pain; or in intense happiness, an unconscious rousing of Kundalini may happen.

If sexual desire is conjoined with intense love for each other, then Kundalini may be roused unconsciously. When the heightened sexual force in deep love is under restraint in visual experiences or in close contacts, deep concentration at a certain point develops, which rouses Kundalini. But the sexual desire itself has no influence on Kundalini. When Kundalini is

roused, sexual desire is fully under control. The rousing of Kundalini is never connected with sexual indulgence. But when an intense mental depression is caused by excessive sexual enjoyment, Kundalini may be roused. But if this unconscious rousing is utilized spiritually, then this unconscious rousing becomes highly beneficial, otherwise, Kundalini goes back to 'sleep' again. On the other hand, highly intensified godly love (bhakti) in which there is no tinge of sexuality in any form, is a most powerful factor in rousing Kundalini.

In consciously rousing of Kundalini, it is felt and 'seen'. The passage of Kundalini through the different chakras is felt and seen. When the roused Kundalini passes through the chakras, they are at first fully illuminated, and then concentration becomes deeper, and finally they are absorbed into Kundalini. In this way, all principles located in the different chakras are absorbed step by step. Ultimately, a stage is reached when there is nothing but Kundalini in its subtlest, splendorous and mind-transcendently conscious form. The meaning of the subtlest is that Kundalini is subtler than anything else. In the material field, elementary particles are the minutest. But prana wayu is subtler than elementary particles. As prana wayu is absorbed into Kundalini, so the latter is subtler than the former. In a similar manner, the most refined mind is also absorbed into Kundalini, so it is subtler than mind. The subtler the power, the more forceful it is, and by its forcefulness it is able to absorb what is grosser than it. So, Kundalini cannot function in the material, vital and mental fields, but it tends to absorb them, to create a nonmaterial, nonvital and nonmental stratum where it is in full power and in illumination.

Kundalini is splendorous. Kundalini-'light' has three aspects: sunlike bright light by which subtle phenomena are illuminated and experienced in concentration; moonlike 'cool' light which deepens concentration; and firelike burning light which exhibits great absorption-power and develops absorptive concentration. Kundali-power is in the nature of illumination. It first illuminates appropriate objects and then they are absorbed into it. When everything is absorbed, Kundalini as Supreme and splendorous power remains, and this power is all consciousness. This is not mental consciousness, as mind is fully absorbed into it. It is mind-transcendent consciousness—Kundalini-consciousness. When mental consciousness operates in chitta, its material replica is found in the brain, and certain physical activities become conscious. Otherwise, nervous impulses, neuronal activities, organic and muscular actions, all are unconscious. The power that is capable of absorbing mind and radiates nonmental consciousness light is Kundalini. Kundalini in its fullest manifestation is supreme consciousness.

The Kundalini-emanations exercise a control influence on the body and mind, and as a result, the physical and mental activities are fully regulated and forceful. The roused Kundalini withdraws prana in stages. The first sign of pranic withdrawal is the natural establishment of asana in which an assumed body posture is held still, painless and effortless. Second, a gradual decrease of animation, which is accompanied by a decrease of metabolism below the basal metabolic level, a diminution of vital activities and a prolonged breath-suspension occur. This is the stage of pranayama. Third, a complete suspension of sensory functions occurs. This is pratyahara. Thereafter, the fully internalized consciousness undergoes the stages of dharana, dhyana and samprajñata samadhi. When Kundalini comes to the sahasrara, samprajñata samadhi takes place. Then Kundalini absorbs superconsciousness and its root, prakriti, and thus being in a mind-transcendent state, it remains alone in asamprajñata samadhi. Finally, Kundalini, in the final stage of asamprajñata samadhi, is entirely supreme consciousness, and its power aspect supports the infinite supreme beingness as real.

The roused Kundalini-energy is actually yama (control)-power which develops stage by stage as asana, pranayama, and pratyahara, and becomes sangyama (supercontrol) when dharana, dhyana and samprajñata samadhi are attained. Finally, sangyama is transformed into asamprajñata samadhi, the supreme control power. So Kundalini may be termed samadhi force, or yoga power. Arawinda[36] has aptly called

Kundalini yoga-shakti (-power). Yoga power actually operates in Kundalini-yoga.

After the union with Supreme Shiwa, Kundalini goes back to the muladhara, and in its descent, the chakras, their powers and divinities —all are restored. This recoiling process is essentially the spiritualization of consciousness which functions in everyday life. That is, it is a transference of spiritual reality, developed in concentrated consciousness, to sense-consciousness to be able to realize spiritual truth in our daily life. In the uncoiling and recoiling of Kundalini, the practitioner of Kundaliniyoga experiences the Divine in its formless aspect in supreme concentration as well as in form in post-concentration waking consciousness. So Arawinda[37] calls Kundalini a divine force.

Concentration

Concentration is not focused thought (bhawana) but is the process consisting of dharana, dhyana and samadhi. It does not come into being unless pratyahara is first established. In focussed thought, though mental efforts are made to centralize thought on a chosen object, yet it is often diversified; an automatic and uncontrollable penetration of other objective images occurs, and consequently the whole thought system is shaken.

Concentration is a mental process of reducing multiform consciousness to a point, termed bindu. The development of this mental power is dependent upon the transformation of the diversified pranic forces into a state of pranic concentration and withdrawal by which the vital and sensory functions become internalized. These are the processes of pranayama and pratyahara. Thereafter, and on the basis of pratyahara, pranic dynamism functions in the mind and rouses the slumbering mentative energy which expresses itself as dharana-power, the immensely strong power to hold the one-pointedness of consciousness in the form of only one object, for a sufficiently long time to be effective. This power grows step by step, and it is then possible to continuously maintain single-objectiveness of consciousness uninterruptedly and for a prolonged period of time. This produces very deep concentration; and from that deep concentration a 'mental light' comes into being which can be focussed on any object, inner or outer. This state of consciousness is called dhyana.

Prolonged and repeated dhyana deepens concentration so that it reaches the bindu state. This is the highest point of mental concentration in which consciousness is maximally concentrated to a point and the truth-exposing concentration-light shines forth. This is samprajñata samadhi. Ultimately, samprajñata samadhi consciousness is coiled into bodiless and mind-transcendent supreme consciousness in asamprajñata samadhi.

The general principles of concentration have been modified, specialized and elaborated in different systems of yoga to suit the particular needs of the practitioners. In the hathayoga method of concentration, an attempt has been made to obliterate the mental reaction effects from the brain by the pranic withdrawal by pranayama. It is necessary first to elevate pranayamic breathing to the nadishuddhi level for this purpose. For the effectiveness of the nadishuddhi pranayama, the body needs to be purified and vitalized by the practice of posture exercise, internal cleansing and right diet.

In rajayoga, centralized thought, combined with spiritual reflection, is applied for the attainment of pratyahara. The intensified thought causes pranic withdrawal and sensory control. Thereafter, the dharana power is roused and gradually dhyana and samadhi are attained.

In mantrayoga, concentration is attained by the use of mantra. Mantra is an aspect of Kundalini, and it is in sound-form. So mantra is actually Kundalini in mantra form. The mantra sound cannot be heard by the physical ear. The replication of mantra on the physical plane is the lettered waikhari sound which is audible. The waikhari mantra, in conjunction with pranayama and other special processes, is utilized, according to the direction of a guru, to enliven the mantra. In other words, it is the rousing of Kundalini in mantra form. When the mantra-Kundalini is roused, it exhibits its absorptive and control powers by which, step by step, the control of prana and the senses is attained. The influence of the outer objects on the mind is neutralized by the mantra power. Consequently, it is a great help in the attainment of pratyahara and self-control.

Then mantra-Kundalini is transformed into Ishtadewata—the metamorphosis of subtle Kundalini through the mantra power into an appropriate divine form. At this stage, dharana and dhyana are attained. After this, Ishtadewata is again transformed into subtle Kundalini when samprajñata samadhi is attained. Finally, Kundalini absorbs the mind and all other things and remains alone, and is then absorbed into Supreme Consciousness in asamprajñata samadhi.

In Kundaliniyoga, which is the fundamental part of layayoga, concentration is attained through the roused Kundalini. So in this yoga, the rousing of Kundalini is the essential process. This rousing is only possible in the muladhara chakra. Focussed thought is the main factor of the rousing process. The intensified thought, in conjunction with pranayamic breathing, mantras and bandhas, becomes so forceful that ultimately it makes static Kundalini dynamic. If the centralized thought is imbibed with intense godly love, thought power is much enhanced. The roused Kundalini exhibits higher control power by which dharana, dhyana and samadhi are attained.

Notes

1 Sarkar, Professor Benoy Kumar, *Hindu Achievements in Exact Science*, Longmans, Green, London, 1918, p. 59.
2 Seal, Brajendranath, MA, PhD, *The Positive Sciences of the Ancient Hindus*, Moti Lal Banarsi Dass, Delhi, 1958, pp. 219–21.
3 *Manawatattwa, by the author of the Aryashastrapradipa*, N.C. Mookerjee, Mahalakshmi Press, Barahanagar, 1901, p. 158.
4 Brahmachari, Purnananda, Sarala Yoga

Sadhana, a treatise in Bengali on yoga
Mitra Brothers, Calcutta, 1926, Preface,
p. 12.

5 Rele, Vasant G., FCPS, LM & S,
The Mysterious Kundalini, DB. Taraporevala
Sons, Bombay, 7th edn, 1928, pp. 23–7.

6 Wiwekananda (Vivekananda), Swami,
Raja-Yoga, Ramakrishna-Vivekananda
Centre of New York, Inc., New York,
1946.

7 Sachchidananda, Swami, Saraswati,
Gurupradipa, Shyambal Chakrabarti,
Calcutta, 2nd edn, 1930, pp. 225–6.

8 Aurobindo, Sri, *On Yoga II*, vol. 1, Sri
Aurobindo International University Centre,
Pondicherry, India, 1958, pp. 369, 373.

9 Sen, Gananath, Mahamahopadhyaya,
Kaviraj, M.A., L.M.S., Saraswati,
Pratyaksha- Shariram (Human Anatomy in
Sanskrit), 3rd edn, Kaviraj Charu Chandra
Bisharad, Kalpataru Ayurvedic Works,
Calcutta, 1924, Introduction, p. 14; Third
part, p. 3.

10 Rele, op. cit.

11 Seal, op. cit.

12 Brahmachari, op. cit.

13 Wiwekananda, op. cit.

14 Sen, op. cit.

15 Seal, op. cit

16 Rele, op. cit.

17 Sen, op. cit.

18 Aurobindo, Sri, *On Yoga I, The Synthesis
of Yoga*, Sri Aurobindo International
University Centre, Pondicherry, India,
1957, p. 611.

19 Aurobindo, Sri, *On Yoga II*, op. cit., vol.
2, p. 259.

20 Shankaracharya was born in the village of
Kaladi, in Kerala, South India. His date
has not been finally determined, but AD
788 has been generally accepted. But
according to an old register of the Gurus,
mentioned by Swami Sachchidananda in
his work entitled *Guru Pradipa*, op. cit., p. 3,
footnote, the latter was born in AD 130.

21 Shankaracharya, *Ananda Lahari*, Verses 9
and 10.

22 Shankaracharya, *Yogatarawali*, Verses 6
and 8.

23 Born in Holia, near Vizianagram, South
India, in 1608. He left his body in Waranasi
(Benares) in 1888.

24 Tailanga Swami, *Mahawakya-Ratnawali*,
1.13, 14, ed and trans. Umacharana
Mukhopadhyaya, Yogendranatha
Mukhopadhyaya, Calcutta, 1917.

25 Born in Halisahar (near Calcutta) in 1723.
He was a celebrated member, known as a
'gem' of the court of Maharaja Krishna
Chandra of Nadia (West Bengal, India).

26 Sena, Ramaprasada, 'Rampasad Sener
Granthabali', *Padawali*, Nos 215 and 216,
n.d., Basumati-Sahitya-Mandir, Calcutta.

27 Born in the village of Kamarpukur in
Hooghly district, West Bengal, India, on
18 February 1836.

28 (a) M(Mahendranath Gupta),
Shrishriramakrishnakathamrita, 5 vol, Anil
Gupta, Kathmrita Bhaban, Calcutta, India.
(b) Saradananda, Swami, *Shri-
shriramakrishnaleelaprasanga*, 2 vol, Swami
Atmabodhananda, Udbodhan Office,
Calcutta, India, 1957.

29 Wama (Wamacharana) was born in a
village named Atla in the Birbhum District,
West Bengal, India, in 1835.

30 Essentially based on Chattopadhyaya,
Pramode Kumar, *Tantrabhilaseer
Sadhusanga*, Part II, Mitra and Ghosh,
Calcutta, n.d.

31 Cf Shyam Sundar Goswami, *HATHA-
YOGA An advanced method of physical
education and concentration*, 2nd edn, L.N.
Fowler, London, 1963, pp. 104–6.

32 Rele, op. cit.

33 Avalon, Arthur (Sir John Woodroffe), *The
Serpent Power*, 5th edn, Ganesh, Madras,
1953, pp. 297–313.

34 Wiwekananda, op. cit.

35 In Aurobindo, *On Yoga II*, vol. 2, op. cit.

36. *Ibid.*

37. *Ibid.*

PART 1

FUNDAMENTALS
OF
LAYAYOGA

CHAPTER 1
Layayoga
and
Ashtangayoga

Layayoga is one of the four great systems of yoga, the other three being mantrayoga, hathayoga and rajayoga. The Great Yogi Wishnu said to Brahma: 'Yoga is in many forms because of its different practices; of these, the main four are—mantrayoga, layayoga, hathayoga and rajayoga' (—Yogatattwopanishad, 19). It indicates the Waidika origin and the antiquity of layayoga.

The four great systems are the four forms of the original yoga termed Mahayoga—Supreme Yoga. Maheshwara said: 'Mahayoga is the fundamental yoga having four main forms—mantra, hatha, laya and raja yogas' (—Yogashikopanishad, 1. 129 – 130). So, layayoga is an elaboration of the fundamental yoga on a specific line to meet the spiritual needs of those disciples who are specially suited to it.

The eight practices, namely, yama (abstension), niyama (observance), asana (posture), pranayama (breath-control), pratyahara (sensory control), dharana (holding-concentration), dhyana (deep concentration) and samadhi (superconcentration), technically known as ashtangayoga (eightfold yoga), are the constituent elements of the general structure of mahayoga. Suta said: 'I am giving an exposition of mahayoga with its eight parts' (—Garudapurana, 1. 230.1). Consequently, layayoga as well as mantrayoga, hathayoga and rajayoga, each has eight parts. In other words, the basic pattern of layayoga consists of eight parts.

Layayoga has two fundamental forms—Waidika and Tantrika. Waidika yoga is the original form of yoga found in the Wedas in a concise version; it was explained by the rishis

(seers) in the Upanishads. Shiwa gave Waidika yoga a new character, and his explanations are collected in the Tantras. Consequently, it is called Tantrika yoga. In fact, the Tantrika yoga is not a different form of yoga but a modification of Waidika yoga. The various difficult processes of Waidika yoga were simplified and new processes incorporated, thus making it more adaptable to a larger number of persons.

So, the Tantrika form of layayoga came from Shiwa. It is also very ancient and is based on the Waidika form. It is said that Shiwa expounded twelve forms of yoga, namely, mantrayoga, hathayoga, bhaktiyoga, layayoga, kriyayoga, lakshyayoga, jñanayoga, uroyoga (rajayoga), wasanayoga, parayoga, amanaskayoga and sahajayoga. These are the Tantrika forms of yoga. Wishnu also said that yoga had many forms. Here Waidika yoga is indicated. So, both Waidika and Tantrika yoga have many forms. Of the many forms of yoga, mantra, hatha, laya and raja yogas are considered the foremost in the Waidika as well as in the Tantrika system. Ishwara said: 'There are four main forms of yoga—mantrayoga, hathayoga, layayoga and rajayoga' (—Shiwasanghita, 5.17). But before we proceed further, it is absolutely necessary to have a clear picture of the term yoga.

Yoga from the Mantra Viewpoint

The technical term 'yoga' belongs to those fundamental groups of letter-arrangements constituting word-formations which are unconnected with thought-language patterns, but arise from the sound-radiating power form called mantra. The mantra-form of yoga is 'Y–ang'–'U–ng'–'G–ang'–'Ah', which being modified, constitutes the shrouta word 'yogah' and then it assumes the language form 'yoga'.

The basic part of yoga is 'ya', which, at the mantra level, is 'Y-ang'. It is the centre of the concentrated energy in the form of control which is technically termed 'yama'. The yama (control)–energy is aroused and developed, by udana force, represented by 'U-ng', and becomes finally transformed into sangyama (supercontrol). At this stage, samadhi consciousness, represented by 'G-ang', develops and Kundali power is revealed. This is yoga.

Control

There are eight distinct stages of development of the control power. The great yogi Dattatreya said: 'I will explain to you the science of yoga having eight stages of practice' (—Darshanopanishad, 1.4). The great yoga master Ribhu also said: 'Yoga has eight stages of practice' (—Warahopanishad, 5.10). Ishwara said: 'Yoga consists of eight parts' (—Gandharwatantra, ch. 5, p. 25). Shiwa also said: 'Yoga consists of eight practices (—Wishwasaratantra, ch. 2, p. 11). So, both in Waidika yoga and Tantrika yoga the eight stages of practice have been accepted.

What is the nature of the control? It is a process by which an action or function, either of the body or the mind, is volitionally restrained with a view to reach a deeper aspect, which remains generally dormant, and bring into play a higher form of power and consciousness. An unknown inner power is released when the body is made quiescent by the control process, which keeps the body in an excellent state of health and vitality, either when the body is in motion or is immovable. The motionlessness of the body also exercises a great influence on the mind. In fact, it is an indispensable condition for the application of the control, directly and

effectively, to the mind. When the inner part of the mind is reached by control, the mind exhibits a trend toward tranquillity and shows better restraint when functioning at the sensory level. This control either causes an alteration in a common action or function to a desired pattern, or stops the action completely to bring about a state of motionlessness. To indicate the control the terms 'bandha', 'bandhana', 'rodha', 'nirodha', and 'nigraha' are used. There are other terms also.

The eight stages of control have technical names: yama (abstention), niyama (observance), asana (posture), pranayama (bio-energy-control or breath-control), pratyahara (sensory control), dharana (holding-concentration), dhyana (deep concentration) and samadhi (superconcentration). Atharwana said: 'The eight stages of yoga are abstention, observance, posture, bio-energy control, sensory control, holding-concentration, deep concentration and superconcentration' (—Shandilyopanishad, 1.2). These eight stages of control have also been accepted in Tantrika yoga. It is said: 'Abstention, observance, posture, bio-energy control, sensory control, holding-concentration, deep concentration and superconcentration are the eight parts of yoga' (—Tantrarajatantra, 27. 54–5).

First and Second Stages of Yama (Control)

The first two stages of control are yama and niyama. This yama (first stage of control) is the same word which stands for the original yama, that is control. The second yama (abstention) has been used in a technical and limited sense to indicate only the first stage of control. In niyama 'ni' has been prefixed to yama. 'Ni' indicates certainty. However, this strengthening of yama does not mean very much, as niyama has been used here in a restricted and technical sense, and stands for the second stage of control. It is more convenient to consider the first and the second stages of control together.

Abstention and observance constitute the

elementary regulation of thoughts, emotions and actions. But even these rudimentary control factors do not function in a satisfactory manner if the spiritual nature of man is completely dormant. In such a state, various unspiritual qualities arise and not only become so strong that a man forgets his innermost being almost completely, but also urge him to be externally minded. His unspiritual nature makes him passionately inclined to external objects he likes for enjoyment. Sensuality, greed, excesses and an inclination to softness are the predominant factors in his thought. Strong lustful desire and the feeling of satisfaction and pleasure in connection with it, and wickedness, pride, anger and the like make a man almost dead spiritually. He is completely disinclined to practise abstention and observance. He is unwilling and unable to abandon his mode of enjoyment because of his strong attachment to pleasure-giving objects.

Unless even a slight awakening of a man's divine nature takes place, it will not be possible for him to undertake the practice of abstention and observance. But how is this awakening possible, as he is antispiritual in nature? In a mode of life which is completely dedicated to excessive sexual gratification and other excesses, there cannot be only pleasures, but also sufferings, pain and sorrow. This is true not only in extreme cases, but in all other cases. Both pleasure and pain encircle our lives. In sensual pleasure, our spiritual nature sleeps, but in pain things change. In intense suffering, intense pain, intense sorrow, severe disease and fear of death the whole being is shaken, a deeper feeling awakens, a need for help from an unknown and invisible power is felt, some discernment is aroused. This is the right moment. Without waiting, just try to be in contact with that unknown and invisible being through prayer—deep and silent, and sincere prayer, with full belief and with full effort. This prayer is not asking for any material gain but for arousing the dormant spiritual nature. And at the same time try your best to be in contact with a saintly person. His understanding, his genuine sympathy, his kindness and his willingness to help will do you very much good. His mental purity and tranquillity, his

physical cleanliness and vitality, his emotional calmness and control will exert tremendous influence on you. And above all, his spiritual personality, his depth of inner knowledge and his very forceful and truthful expression—all these will be exceedingly helpful to you.

It is the moment when you should start a new life with a new programme. Your first programme is—ritualistic worship, spiritual study, ascesis and internal and external physical cleanliness. You are not expected at this stage to get your thoughts and emotions under your control. But you can control your actions very much by doing regularly the above four practices. Whatever happens do not stop but go on with them. Whatever thoughts, emotions and desires arise in your mind, without paying any attention to them, go on with the four practices. You will find that you are gaining in spiritual strength more and more and day by day. Then it will be your experience that you are manifesting a natural tendency to spiritual qualities, and have enough inner strength to do what is spiritual and not to do what is anti-spiritual. In this way, your spiritual endeavour will bring success.

That association with a saintly person is very helpful has been widely recognized. It is said: 'There are four door-keepers who are guarding the doors leading to liberation; they are control of the mind, reflection, contentment and the company of a spiritual person' (—M*a*hopani*sha*d, 4.2). The importance of worship is shown by the saying which runs thus: 'When the Supreme Spirit is directly known in concentration, all sins are destroyed, afflictions become attenuated and immortality is attained' (—Shwetashwataropani*sha*d, 1.11). Spiritual study plays an important role for a person who intends to lead a religious and virtuous life. It is said: 'The teacher instructs his pupils not to be inattentive to spiritual study' (—T*a*ittiriyopani*sha*d, 1.11.1). The importance of ascesis as an agent for the purification of the mind and as a necessity for the attainment of divine knowledge has been stressed. It is said: 'Ascesis, sensory control, spiritual actions, spiritual study and the like are the means of attaining the divine knowledge' (—Kenopani*sha*d, 4.8) About cleanliness it has been said: 'He who is endowed with spiritual

45

knowledge, established in concentration and purified by cleanliness, attains God' (Kathopanishad, 1.3.8).

In leading such a life, he will be able to develop enough power of control to practise regular abstention and observance. He should practise them volitionally in his thoughts, emotions and actions. These practices also develop his spiritual nature to such an extent that normally he will be able to manifest his spiritual qualities, at the right moment and in the right circumstances. The most important but most difficult practice is brahmacharya, that is, sexual control. Now it will be possible for him to practise it successfully. Sexual control is of two forms: complete and partial. The partial form is for married people. However, the complete form should first be practised for a sufficient length of time before undertaking the partial form.

Yama said to Nachiketa: 'I will explain briefly to you that truth for the attainment of which the spiritual students practise sexual control' (—Kathopanishad, 1.2.15). Once Sukesha, Satyakama and others—all were the sons of the rishis and devoted to God—went as pupils to the great spiritual teacher Pippalada to know about the Supreme Being. Pippalada said to them: 'All of you practise sexual control, and ascesis, and devotedness for a year and then come back; I will try to answer your questions' (—Prashnopanishad, 1.2). Here the importance of sexual control and ascesis for the right understanding of the highest spiritual knowledge has been clearly shown.

In regular abstention and observance, each consists of ten practices. Abstention consists of the following:

1 Ahingsa—Harmlessness; love for all
2 Satya—Truthfulness
3 Asteya—Non-theft
4 Brahmacharya—Sexual control
5 Daya—Mercy
6 Arjawa—Honesty
7 Kshama—Forgiveness
8 Dhriti—Firmness
9 Mitahara—Moderation in eating
10 Shoucha—Cleanliness

Observance contains the following practices:

1 Tapas—Ascesis
2 Santosha—Contentment
3 Astikya—Faith
4 Dana—Charity
5 Ishwara-pujana—Worship of God
6 Siddhanta-shrawana—Spiritual study
7 Hri—Modesty
8 Mati—Reflection
9 Japa—Mantra-practice
10 Wrata—Vow

These tenfold abstentions and tenfold observances were declared by the great yogi Dattatreya to his disciple Sangkriti (—Darshanopanishad, 1.6 and 2.1). So in the Waidika form of yoga ten practices constitute abstention and ten practices are also the constituents of observance. In the Tantrika form exactly the same number of practices constitute abstention and observance. Not only the same number but the same practices compose abstention and observance, with one exception. Vow, the tenth practice of observance has been replaced by homa (oblation) in the Tantrika form. Ishwara (Shiwa) expounded this tenfold abstention and observance to Dewi (—Gandharwatantra, ch. 5, p. 25).

The shortened forms of abstention and observance were also introduced. Agni said: 'Abstention consists of harmlessness, truthfulness, non-theft, sexual control and non-acquisitiveness, and observance contains cleanliness, contentment, ascesis, spiritual study and worship of God' (—Agnipurana, 372. 2-3). These shortened forms were also widely accepted.

Sexual control and cleanliness were elaborated in hathayoga. The Wajroli—adamantine control process—was developed from brahmacharya, and a system of internal baths (done without instrumental aid) from shoucha. Ascesis and diet also formed an important part of hathayoga. The mantra-practice was elaborated in mantrayoga. The worship of God was elaborated and developed into higher forms of concentration in layayoga and rajayoga. In rajayoga, the practice of asamprajñata samadhi (non-mens concentration) was specially developed.

Third Stage of Y*ama* (Control): As*ana*

Now we come to the third stage of control, that is as*ana*—posture. When 'yama' (control) is used in connection with the body, it usually takes the form 'ayama' to mean control. As for example, sh*arira* (body) + ayam*a* (control) form the term sh*arir*ayam*a* (body-control). The nature of control here is either to regulate the activities of the body to a desired pattern, or to stop all voluntary activities to make the body motionless. When regulated activities are desired the term 'wyayam*a*' is used. Here the prefix 'wi' indicates something specific. So wyayam*a* means the specific application of control to regulate the voluntary movements of the body to a desired pattern. Wyayam*a*, therefore, is a controlled movement system of the body. However, it has been generally used to mean physical education, and in a more restricted sense, muscular exercise.

When the stopping of all motions of the body is done in order to make the body motionless volitionally, as is required in yog*a*, by the application of control, a special technical term has been used in yog*a*. It is as*ana*, that is, posture. It is an arrangement or placement of the body to assume a particular position or posture. The posture may be of the static or dynamic type. But for the purpose of yog*a*, the posture is of the static type in which the body is maintained in a motionless state by a special arrangement of the limbs in an appropriate sitting position. When the body is made to assume such a motionless attitude in a sitting position it is called as*ina*, that is, in a state of sitting position by the special arrangement of the body and limbs. This special alignment of the body and limbs in a static posture is as*ana*, in which control is applied to stop all motions with a view to make the body motionless.

On the other hand, posture has been connected with the dynamic posture exercise in h*atha*yoga. Here, the body is made to undergo appropriate movements to assume a final posture, either in a sitting, standing or lying position. The original meaning of as*ina* has been extended, and the body now assumes many different as*anas*, through appropriate movements. However, in the word as*ana*, the term y*ama* in any form does not occur, but a new form as*a*, to mean a special arrangement of the body in a sitting posture, has been introduced in yog*a*. From as*a*, as*ana* has been formed.

The body should be cultured and made efficient and under control for spiritual development. It is said: 'May my body be efficient (for the attainment of spiritual knowledge)' (—T*aittiriy*opan*isha*d, 1.4.1). For the attainment of the highest spiritual stage both the body and the mind should be controlled. It is said: 'Only physical movements are not helpful, nor concentration alone is successful. He who knows how to practise physical control in combination with concentration, attains immortality' (—*I*shopan*isha*d, 9 and 11). Here is a clear indication that the body should be purified, vitalized and well-controlled by h*atha*yoga, and in that state of the body concentration will develop in a satisfactory manner. More clearly it is said: 'The yog*i* making his body as the lower piece of wood and the pr*anawa* (the first mantra) the upper piece of wood (used for kindling the fire), should do the churning which is in the form of concentration again and again until he realizes the Supreme Being' (—Shwetashw*ata*ropan*isha*d, 1.14). This means that in a purified body and with the help of the m*antra*, concentration develops to its highest limit and as a result God is revealed.

A yog*i* can attain such a purified and vitalized body that it is free from disease, senility, and is long-lived. It is said: 'When a yog*i* develops a highly purified body by yog*a*-fire, he becomes free from disease, his youth is prolonged and his life is extended; and the experience of super-smell, super-taste, super-sight, super-touch and super-sound occurs' (—Shwetashw*ata*ropan*isha*d, 2.12). So, it is possible to attain a yoga-fire body of super-purity.

The body should be trained to be in a state of motionlessness for a prolonged time without discomfort or pain. It is said: 'In s*amadhi* all senses cease to function and the body remains motionless like a piece of wood' (—Nadabindu-panishad, 3.3.2). The motionlessness of the body is developed by the practice of static posture. Moreover, by the practice of processes contained in hathayoga, not only the body is vitalized and controlled but also the mind is controlled and brightened.

The assumption of a folded-leg concentration posture is necessary for the practice of sensory control and concentration. As, for example: 'Once upon a time, the great yogi Mandawya, being desirous of withdrawing his senses into the manas-chakra—the subtle centre of the mind, assumed the lotus posture' (—Annapurnopani-shad, 3.3–4). That the static posture to be assumed for the practice of yoga should be a yogasana (concentration posture) has been stated: 'Assuming rightly a yoga posture, such as lotus posture, auspicious posture or happy posture, and facing towards the north' (—Amritanadopanishad, 18). The concentration postures when well mastered will be suitable for the practice of yoga. Aditya said: 'The three worlds are conquered by him who has mastered posture' (—Trishikhibrahman-opanishad, Mantra Section, 52). Dattatreya said: 'Assuming a yoga posture, one should always practise breath-control' (—Darshanop-anishad, 3.14).

When a posture is fully controlled, then it is to be assumed for concentration. Narayana said that there were two indications when the posture is fully controlled; the natural feeling of ease and comfort when a posture is assumed; and the ability to prolong the posture without discomfort (—Mandalabrahmanopani-shad, 1.1.5). There are also other indications when posture is mastered. It is said: 'Disease is eliminated by posture' (—Yogachudamanyup-anishad, 109). Also, 'All diseases of the body are destroyed by posture, even poisons are assimilated. Any one of the postures selected should be made comfortable, if it was not possi-ble for one to master all of them' (—Shandi-lyopanishad, 1.3.12–13), and 'The yogi being still in a posture (because of his mastery), well-controlled' (—Shandilyopanishad, 1.7.1).

In an impurified body, mind is usually rest-less. This is why Shiwa has said: 'How will it be possible to practise concentration without purifying the body? ... A purified body is full of vitality and is fit for concentration' (—Brihan-nilatantra, ch. 6, p. 41). The assumption of a concentration posture for spiritual practice requiring concentration is absolutely necessary. So it is stated: 'The mantra-practice, worship and other spiritual works should be done while assuming the lotus posture, auspicious posture, hero posture (wirasana) or other postures; otherwise there will be no success' (—Kularnawa, ch. 15, p. 74). Bhairawi said: 'I am explaining different postures to those who are desirous of attaining success in yoga. Without the assump-tion of an appropriate posture breath-control and other practices are not successful' (—Rudrayamala, Part 2, 23. 23). It is also said: 'By the practice of postures life is prolonged. ... For the purification of the body and for attaining success in yoga, posture is absolutely necessary' (—Rudrayamala, Part 2, 24. 38–39), and 'Posture helps to make the mind calm' (—Tantrarajatantra, 27, 59). 'By the practice of posture the body becomes disease-free, firm and efficient' (—Grahayamala, ch. 12, p. 85).

So, the importance of posture has been recog-nized in the Waidika as well as in the Tantrika form of yoga. It has been recognized that a purified and vitalized body is necessary for concentration; that posture plays an important role in making the body purer, healthful, youthful, efficient and long-lived; and also that a concentration posture is absolutely necessary for the practice of breath-control, sensory control and concentration; a posture should be fully controlled.

Posture has been fully elaborated in hathayoga. Innumerable postures were introduced and various scientific processes were developed in relation to postures (—Rudrayamala, Part 2, 24. 3). Many postures were also developed in Waidika yoga. So it is said that many postures were explained in the Weda (—Wishwasara-tantra, ch. 2, p. 11). In hathayoga, postures have been divided into three groups: dynamic posture exercise, static posture exercise, and concentra-tion postures. Dynamic posture exercise has been designed to exercise all the muscles of the body in conjunction with charana (contraction-control exercise). Static posture exercise trains the body to be still in different positions and develops vital endurance and the power of concentration. Concentration postures are for the practice of breath-control, mantra and concentration.

Fourth Stage of Yama (Control): Pranayama

The fourth stage of control is pranayama—breath-control. When 'yama' (control) is applied to control prana-wayus (different forms of bio-energy) the form 'ayama' is frequently used. The words nigraha, rodha and nirodha are also used to indicate control.

Pranayama is actually the process of controlling prana, the central bio-energy; and as this control is achieved through the process of the regulation of breath, it is usually called breath-control. It is said: 'He who is well-restrained in all his actions, should control bio-energy carefully through the breath-process; as a result of this the bio-energy becomes so rarefied as to increase the power of breath-suspension. Thereafter expiration should be made through the nostrils. This process makes the restless mind fit for concentration' (—Shwetashwataropanishad, 2.9). Here is a clear indication that the control of bio-energy is intrinsically associated with breathing. Furthermore, the rarefaction of the bio-energy causes a diminution of the internal organic activities to a very low level and this is helped by the decreased voluntary muscular activities in a static concentration posture. This physical state is an anti-oscillatory state of the mind. The rarefied bio-energy flow becomes very much less through the ida-pingala paths (the white and red energy lines), but is enhanced considerably through the sushumna path (the central energy line). This creates a state in which concentration becomes easy, prolonged and deep.

Ribhu, the exalted knower of Brahman, said: 'When the throbbing of all the bio-energies

ceases by the practice (of breath-control), the mind becomes non-mens, and what remains is the liberation' (—Annapurnopanishad, 2.33). When the bio-energy is rarefied by the practice of breath-control, it ceases to throb and becomes calm. This causes the mind to be free from oscillation.

A complete control of respiration is associated with that state of the mind which is beyond the perceptive, intellective, affective and volitive phenomena. It is said: 'The yogi will practise the absorption process in conjunction with the control of respiration and concentration; in this way when the respiration stops, the mind goes beyond the perceptive-intellective-affective states' (—Tripuratapinyupanishad, 5.10). By the process of breath-control respiration can be controlled to the point when it will automatically stop. It is the state of what is technically called kewala kumbhaka—automatic breath-suspension. At this stage the mind is also automatically in deep concentration. However, the breath-control should be regularly practised. It is stated: 'A student of yoga who is well-controlled in sleep and activities and lives on an abstemious diet, being in a lonely place with his mind without any thirst for wordly things and when the previous meal has been completely digested (that is on an empty stomach), should practise breath-control according to the process shown by his teacher' (—Soubhagyalakshmyupanishad, 2.2).

The importance of the control of the breath and the mind for the development of super-concentration has been fully recognized. It is said: 'The yogi should control the breath and the mind to accomplish superconcentration' (—Trishikhibrahmanopanishad, Mantra Section, 22). Breath-control, practised regularly, develops intelligence and the power of concentration. So, the great yogi Dattatreya said: 'The regular practice of breath-control develops intelligence. ... By breath-control that spiritual knowledge which leads to liberation arises (through super-concentration)' (—Darshanopanishad, 6.10–12).

Respiration is one of the intrinsic factors that causes the perceptive mind (chitta) to function, and hence the control of the mind is related to the control of respiration. It is stated: 'There are two causes which make the perceptive mind to oscillate; they are the latent impression of feeling (wasana) and respiration; if one is controlled, the other also becomes inoperative. Of these two, first respiration should be controlled' (—Yogakundalyupanishad, 1.1–2). The control of bio-energy means the control of respiration, as the former is inseparably associated with the latter, and through the latter the former control is achieved. So it is said: 'The control of prana is this: prana means physical respiration, and ayama means kumbhaka (breath-suspension)' (—Yogakundalyupanishad, 1.19).

The respiratory movements which are associated with the movement of air in the lungs, is a great factor in producing the oscillation of the mind. The diversification of the mind can be regulated by breath-control. It is stated: 'The respiratory movements cause the multiformity of the mind; when the former is motionless, the latter also becomes calm' (—Yogachudamanyupanishad, 89). It is also stated that the control of respiration causes both physical and mental development (—Warahopanishad, 5.46–49). Further, 'When the subtle energy line system (nadichakra) is purified by breath-control, done in a right manner, the bio-energy enters easily into the central energy line (sushumna) by bursting through its entrance and, as a result, the mind becomes absolutely calm' (—Shandilyopanishad, 1.7.9–10).

The process of breath-control consists of three acts: inspiring the atmospheric air into the lungs, expiring the air from the lungs, and the suspension of breath, either at the end of inspiration or of expiration. We have very ancient Waidika terms for the three respiratory acts, which are based on the Chandogyopanishad, 1.3.3. The word 'prana' is used to denote the action of expiring the air from the lungs. The actual process of expiring the air is 'prana' or 'pranana', that is, expiration. Similarly, the word 'apana' is used to denote the action of inspiring the air. The process of inspiring the air is 'apana' or 'apanana', that is, inspiration. The connection between the prana and apana is 'wyana'. This means that at the end of inspiration and at the beginning of expiration, or at the end of expiration and at the beginning of inspira-

tion, is the period in which the action of prana and apana has stopped. The cessation of prana or pranana (expiration) is 'aprana' (that is no expiration), and that of apana or apanana (inspiration) is 'anapana' (no inspiration). During the interval between the two processes there is neither inspiration nor expiration. This is wyana or 'wyanayana', that is, breath-suspension. So, we have the following terms:

Apana or Apanana	= Inspiration
Prana or Pranana	= Expiration
Wyana or Wyanayana	= Breath-suspension

The interval at the end of apana and before the commencement of prana is 'kumbhaka'. This is antah-kumbhaka (inspiratory breath-suspension). Again, the interval at the end of prana and before the commencement of apana is kumbhaka. This is bahya-kumbhaka (expiratory breath-suspension). Here, prana is expiration and apana is inspiration. These two terms are the same as older ones mentioned above. Here the term kumbhaka is used to denote breath-suspension, instead of wyana or wyanayana. This is based on the Muktikopanishad, 2,51–52.

Then we find that the term 'ruchira' was used synonymously with kumbhaka, that is, breath-suspension. And the terms 'rechaka' and 'puraka' for expiration and inspiration (—Amritanadopanishad, 9).

Pranayama (breath-control) has been defined as: 'Pranayama is that in which the Gayatri mantra, combined with seven wyahritis to which the pranawa ("Ong") is prefixed in each, and "shiras" (the last part of the mantra) are said mentally with controlled respiration' (—Amritanadopanishad, 10). This is the basic Waidika breath-control in which the measures of inspiration, breath-suspension and expiration are the same. The mantra used in this breath-control consists of about sixty units. This means that the duration of inspiration is sixty units of time, let us say 60 seconds. The time of breath-suspension and of expiration is also 60 seconds in each case.

The three respiratory acts have been explained as: 'The air should be expelled outside so as to make the lungs as if empty; this emptying is called expiration.

'When the air is inhaled like the sucking in of water through the stalk of a lotus, it is called inspiration.

'To be in a state when there is neither expiration nor inspiration and the body is completely motionless is called breath-suspension' (—Amritanadopanishad, 11–13).

So, during breath-suspension the body should be maintained absolutely motionless. In other words, breath-control should be practised when the static posture has been mastered.

The preliminary practices of breath-control, when a student of yoga assumes a sitting posture, are as follows: 'First a yoga posture should be assumed with the body erect, eyes non-moving, the upper teeth not touching the lower, the tongue retroverted (only in special cases), with chin-lock, the (right) hand on the nostrils to make breath-flow through a desired nostril, body motionless, and the mind at ease and concentrated, and then practise breath-control' (—Trishikhibrahmanopanishad, Mantra Section, 92–94).

The order of breath-control is as follows: 'First is expiration, then inspiration, then breath-suspension, and finally expiration; this is breath-control' (—Trishikhibrahmanopanishad, Mantra Section, 94–95). This means that the inspiratory part of breath-control should start after a preliminary expiration.

The actual breath-control process is as follows: 'First exhale the air from the lungs through the right nostril by closing left nostril with the fingers of the right hand; now inhale through the left nostril, counting 16, and then suspend the breath for 64 measures, and then exhale through the right nostril, counting 32. In this manner continue the process [both] in the inverse and [in] direct order' (—Trishikhibrahmanopanishad, Mantra Section, 95–98). Here, the relative measures of inspiration, suspension and expiration are 1–4–2. So the 1–1–1 measures are modified in this process.

It is clearly said that: 'Pranayama (breath-control) is composed of inspiration, breath-suspension and expiration. These three respiratory acts are in the form of "A", "U" and "M",

that is, pranawa, so the pranayama is of the nature of pranawa' (—Darshanopanishad, 6.1–2). Inspiration, breath-suspension and expiration are done in the following manner: 'Inspire through the left nostril slowly, counting 16 and at the same time doing the sound-process (japa) with "A" of the pranawa and with concentration; then suspend the breath for 64 measures and at the same time make the sound-process with "U" of the pranawa and with concentration; and, finally, expire the air slowly through the right nostril and at the same time count 32 and along with it make the sound-process with "M" of the pranawa and with concentration' (—Darshanopanishad, 6.3–6). So, the relative measures of inspiration, breath-suspension and expiration are 1–4–2, and the sound-process and concentration are added to the respiratory acts.

The breath-control process has two fundamental forms: sahita (inspiratory-expiratory-suspension) and kewala (noninspiratory-non-expiratory-suspension). The sahita is that form of breath-suspension which is done in conjunction with inspiration and expiration. The kewala is that form of breath-suspension in which there is no inspiration and no expiration, but only automatic breath-suspension. So it is said: 'Breath-suspension is of two kinds: sahita and kewala. Sahita should be practised until the yogi is able to do the kewala. Sahita breath-control includes suryabheda (right-nostril breath-control) ujjayi (both-nostrils breath-control), shitali (lingual breath-control) and bhastri (thoracico-short-quick breath-control)' (—Yogakundalyupanishad, 1.20–21).

During breath-control three forms of muscular control should be adopted. They are mulabandha (anal-lock), uddiyana (abdomino-retraction) and jalandhara (chin-lock). So it is said: 'During the four forms of breath-suspension, the three forms of control should be executed; they are anal-lock, abdomino-retraction and chin-lock' (—Yogakundalyupanishad, 1.40–41).

There are other measures in inspiration, breath-suspension and expiration. It is said: 'Breath-control is that in which the measure for inspiration is 12, for breath-suspension 16, and for expiration 10, along with the sound-process with "Ong". The measure in the elementary type is 12 (in inspiration), in the middle type 24, and in the highest type 36' (—Yogachudamanyupanishad, 103–104).

When breath-control is accomplished, certain signs appear. It is said: 'Thence the yogi's body becomes free from excessive fat and disease, eyes bright, countenance cheerful, sexual urge well-controlled and energy increased' (—Shandilyopanishad, 1.7.13:6).

So far we have talked about Waidika breath-control. Now, we shall consider the Tantrika form. It is said: 'Pranayama is that in which the breathing movements, due to the throbbing of the bio-energy, are controlled. During pranayama one becomes conscious of the divine power' (—Gayatritantra, 1.205).

By the control of breath the mind and the senses are spiritually purified. It is said: 'Breath-control is of many kinds. ... By breath-control the mind and the senses are purified' (—Kularnawa, ch. 15, p. 75). It is also said: 'The internal impurities are removed by breath-control. It is the best yoga practice. Without its help liberation is not possible. The yogis attain success through breath-control' (—Gandharwa tantra, ch. 10, p. 47). The throbbing of the bio-energy causes the oscillation of breath. By breath-control the throbbing of the bio-energy is controlled and the mind becomes calm. It is also said in the Gandharwatantra that the uncontrolled respiratory movements cause the mind to oscillate; when the breath is controlled, the mind becomes calm. Breath-control makes all forms of bio-energy calm. So it is said: 'The ten forms of bio-energy, such as prana, apana, etc. are made to stop their throbbing by breath-control' (Mundamalatantra, ch. 2, p. 3).

He who desires to control his breath should be moderate in eating, healthy, clean and sexually well-controlled. So it is said: 'One who is healthy and eats moderately can control breath and becomes a yogi. ... He who is clean and doing sexual control is able to control breath. Regular practice is absolutely necessary. Yoga is not possible without breath-control' (—Rudrayamala, Part 2, 17. 40–43).

In the Tantrika form the general terms for the three respiratory acts in breath-control—puraka (inspiration), kumbhaka (breath-suspension)

and rechaka (expiration), have been generally accepted. It is said: 'The inhalation of the atmospheric air into the lungs is termed puraka. The holding of the inspired air within, and without any inhalation or exhalation, is termed kumbhaka. Then the suspended breath should be expelled outside. This is termed rechaka' (—Phetkarinitantra, ch. 3, p. 4).

The process of breath-control and its measures are explained thus: 'Assuming the hero posture with the body erect, inspire the outer air through the left nostril for the measure of 16; then suspend the breath for the measure of 64, and thereafter exhale the air outside through the right nostril for the measure 32' (—Gandharwatantra, ch. 5, p. 25). Here the general measures—16–64–32—have been discussed. It is further stated: 'The measure for breath-suspension is four times the measure of inspiration, and the measure of expiration is half the measure of breath-suspension' (—Gandharwatantra, ch. 10, p. 47). So, the general measures are: 1–4–2. For the control of the nostrils during breath-control, it has been said: 'The thumb, ring, and little fingers should be used to control the nostrils, leaving the forefinger and the middle finger' (—Koulawalitantra, ch. 2, p. 6). About the forms of breath-control it is said: 'There are two forms of breath-control: one is with the mantra and concentration, which is called sagarbha, the other is without them and is called agarbha or wigarbha' (—Sharadatilaka, 25. 20–21). About the stages of breath-control, it is said: 'The early or first stage is that in which perspiration occurs due to the practice of breath-control. In the middle or second stage the body shakes (due to the arousing of inner power). In the highest or third stage the body levitates. The breath-control should be regularly practised until the third stage is reached' (—Sharadatilaka, 25. 21–22). It has been further stated: 'Breath-control consists of three stages: the highest, the middle and the first. At the highest stage, the body becomes light and levitates and the mind becomes calm. At the first stage perspiration is produced in the whole body, and at the second stage the body shakes. These signs appear after long practice. By regular practice the third stage is reached from

52

the first and through the second stage. The breath-control should be regularly practised in the morning and evening' (—Tantrarajatantra, 27.64–66).

The usual Tantrika terms for inspiration, suspension and expiration are puraka, kumbhaka and rechaka respectively. The terms ahara, dharana and apasara for inspiration, suspension and expiration respectively have also been used (—Tantrarajatantra, 27.67–68).

The usual measures in breath-control are 16–64–32, on the basis of 1–4–2. But the relative measures of 1–4–2 change according to the different forms and the nature of the mantras used. In one of the forms of breath-control, inspiration is done through the left nostril for the measure of 16 with the first 16 matrika-letters; then breath-suspension for the measure of 32 with the matrika-letters 32 from 'Ka' to 'Sa'; thereafter expiration through the right nostril for the measure of 16 using the letters from 'Ka' to 'Ta' (—Gayatritantra, 1.203–204). Here the relative measures are 16–32–16 at the ratio of 1–2–1, and the matrika-letters (sound-units) are used as mantra.

In another form, the 50 matrika-letters as mantra, said in regular order, with concentration together with initiation-mantra are used for inspiration; the 50 matrika-letters, first in the reverse order and then in the regular order with concentration and the initiation-mantra are used for breath-suspension; finally, the 50 matrika-letters in the reverse order with concentration and the initiation-mantra for expiration (—Kamadhenutantra, ch. 9, p. 10). The relative measures of inspiration-suspension-expiration are 50 + initiation mantra—10 + initiation mantra—50 + initiation mantra. This form of breath-control is for advanced pupils.

There is another Tantrika breath-control in which 'A' to 'Ksha'—the 50 matrika-letters—are used in inspiration, 'Ka' to 'Ma'—the 25 matrika-letters—are used in breath-suspension, and 'Ya' to 'Ksha'—the 9 matrika-letters—are used in expiration (—Wishwasaratantra, ch. 1, p. 10). It is a special breath-control in which the relative measures of inspiration, suspension and expiration are 50–25–9.

There is also a special breath-control process, called brahmamantra pranayama, in which a different technique has been used. Sadashiwa says: 'In this breath-control the brahmamantra (consisting of 7 matrika-letters) or only pranawa (Ong) should be used. Closing the left nostril with the middle and ring fingers of the right hand, inspire through the right nostril and at the same time do sound-process (japa) with brahmamantra or pranawa for 8 times; then closing the right nostril (the left nostril is already closed) with the thumb, suspend the breath for 32 measures with the mantra or pranawa; and finally, open the right nostril and expire through it slowly by counting the mantra or pranawa 16 times; in this manner inhale through the left nostril counting 8, suspend counting 32, and exhale through the left nostril counting 16; and again, inhale through the right nostril counting 8, suspend counting 32, and exhale through the right nostril counting 16. This is the brahmamantra pranayama' (—Mahanirwanatantra, 3.44–48). The measures of this breath-control are 8–32–16, the same ratio as 1–4–2. The characteristic feature of this breath-control is that the inspiration and expiration are done through the same nostril. In this respect it differs from both surya pranayama (right-nostril inspiratory breath-control) and chandra pranayama (left-nostril inspiratory breath-control).

The regular measures for inspiration, breath-suspension and expiration are 16–64–32. But one who is not able to use these measures should adopt lower measures. It is stated: 'He who is unable to use the measures of 16–64–32, should reduce them to 4–16–8; even one who is unable to use these reduced measures should use the measures of 1–4–2' (—Shaktanandatarangini, ch. 7, p. 16).

In the Tantrika form of breath-control, the three forms of special muscular control—chin-lock, abdomino-retraction and anal-lock, have also been introduced. It is stated: 'At the end of inspiration, chin-lock should be done. At the end of expiration, abdomino-retraction should be done, and during breath-suspension anal-lock, chin-lock and abdomino-retraction should be executed' (—Grahayamala, ch. 13, p. 102).

As in Waidika breath-control, Tantrika breath-control also has two fundamental forms: sahita and kewala. It is said: 'Breath-suspension is of two kinds: sahita and kewala. The sahita-suspension is that in which suspension is done with inspiration and expiration. The kewala-suspension is that in which suspension is automatic and effortless and where inspiration and expiration are completely absent' (—Grahaya-mala, ch. 13, p. 101).

It has been said: 'The body of a resolute yogi, who has mastered kewala-suspension, is as swift as the mind, and is diseaseless and without senility' (—Tripurasarasamuchchaya, ch. 3, p. 10).

About the signs which appear when the breath-control is accomplished, it is stated: 'The signs which appear after the perfection of breath-control are aroused internal powers, joy and satisfaction, purity of mind, calmness, bodily lightness, gracefulness and brightness' (—Tantrarajatantra, 27. 69). Further, 'When the breath-control is perfected, these signs appear: lightness of the body, cheerful countenance, brightness of the eyes, good digestion, internal purification and control, and joy' (—Grahaya-mala), ch. 13, p. 102).

Fifth Stage of Yama (Control): Pratyahara

Now we come to the fifth stage of control which is the control of the senses. The terms ayama, nigraha, rodha and nirodha are used for control. But in yoga, a special term 'Pratyahara' has been introduced for the control of the senses. This new term explains the nature of yama (control) involved in the control of the senses. The word pratyahara is derived from 'hri': to take away, to remove, to prevent, to disjoin, to withdraw, and to which 'prati' (= against) and 'a' are prefixed. So, the meaning of the term is to take away, remove or withdraw the senses from the objects, to prevent the senses from being in contact with the objects. The main point is that the nature of the control, in relation to the senses, is that which keeps the

senses from being in contact with the objects, that is, a process of abstraction or withdrawal. Therefore, the technical meaning of the word pratyahara is the sensory withdrawal, which can simply be termed sensory control.

It is said: 'The senses and the organs of action should be controlled in the manas (the sense-mind or the sixth sense), and the manas in the jñanatman (perceptive consciousness or mind)' (—Kathopanishad, 1. 3.13). Here the process of the actions of the senses and its control have been technically explained. The sensory impulse at the cerebral point is transformed into the udanic (pertaining to the udana—a form of bio-energy exhibiting upward radiation) radiation and is conducted to the sense-mind. The sense-mind is stimulated by the radiated udanic energy and creates and conducts manasa-radiation (highly rarefied subconscious radiation) to the perceptive consciousness where objective knowledge is formed. In the text two phases of control have been pointed out. During the first phase, the rousing of the sense-mind in response to the udanic radiation is controlled, and, as a result the sense-mind is neutralized. During the second phase, this neutralized sense-mind is withdrawn into the perceptive mind. This two-phased control process is technically termed pratyahara—sensory control. In the above text the word 'yama' has been used as a verb, meaning to control the senses. So, the term is 'indriya-yama' which stands for pratyahara.

A different technique of sensory control has also been expounded. It is stated: 'The senses should be controlled by the manas (will-mind) in the hrit (here, sense-mind)' (—Shweta-shwataropanishad, 2.8). This means that the transformed sensory impulse into udanic radia-tion should be neutralized in the sense-mind by will-mind, that is, before the creation of the sensory image in the perceptive consciousness. It can also be explained differently: 'By the concentrated mind the senses should be control-led in their particular seats in the chakras (subtle centres).' This process of sensory control has been specially adopted in layayoga. Here the term 'indriya sanniwesha' (sense control) has been used for sensory control in place of pratyahara. This form of sensory control has been more clearly expounded by the great yogi Mandawya in his own practice. It is stated: 'Once upon a time Muni Mandawya desired to withdraw his senses to the manas-chakra (a subtle centre which is the seat of sense-consciousness), and for that purpose he assumed the lotus posture with his eyes half-open and, stage by stage, disjoined his senses from the internal and external objects' (—Annapurnopanishad, 3. 3–4). The process described here consists of the withdrawal of the senses, from all objects, into the manas-chakra. It is a layayoga process. Here, a more direct term 'indriya sangharana', that is, sense-withdrawal, has been used for pratyahara.

There was an ancient form of yoga practice consisting of prana-apana sangyama, that is, breath-control, and the disjoining of the senses from their objects and other processes (—Kundikopanishad, 24–25). Here, the word 'sangshraya' in the verbal form and in the negative sense has been used. To denote negation it can be constructed as 'asangshraya' to mean disjoining.

About a special process of sensory control it has been stated: 'By the concentrated mind the senses should be withdrawn from their objects and the apana-energy should be drawn upwards into the abdominal region and held there' (—Trishikhibrahmanopanishad, Mantra Section, 115). It appears that the reverse apana-action is associated with the process of sense-withdrawal. Here, the term 'karana-samaharana' has been used to mean sense-withdrawal. However, the process of sensory control has been elaborated in this manner: 'On the eighteen vital points of the body, the mind should be concentrated, from one point to the other, with breath-suspension. This is sensory control. The eighteen points are: (1) big toe, (2) ankle, (3) calf, (4) thigh, (5) anus, (6) genitals, (7) heart, (8) abdominal region, (9) navel, (10) neck, (11) elbow, (12) root of the palate, (13) nose, (14) eye, (15) space between the eyebrows, (16) forehead, (17) knee, and (18) wrist' (—Trishikhibrahmanopanishad, Mantra Section, 129–133).

Dattatreya defined sensory control as: 'The senses naturally are in contact with the objects;

the withdrawal of the senses from the objects by the application of the power of control is termed sensory control' (Darshanopanishad, 7. 1–2). Here, the process involved in sensory control has been termed 'indriya aharana', that is sense-withdrawal, and this is to be effected by the well-developed power of control. The control process has been more fully described by Dattatreya. He says: 'According to the process of breath-control, breath should be suspended with concentration applied to the following points in succession: (1) root of the teeth, (2) neck, (3) chest, (4) navel region, (5) region of Kundali (coiled power), (6) muladhara (intra-coccygeal subtle centre), (7) hip, (8) thigh, (9) knee, (10) leg, and (11) big toe. This is called pratyahara by the ancient yogis who were masters of sensory control' (—Darshanopanishad, 7. 5–9). The processes involved in sensory control are two-fold: breath-suspension and holding the mind, that is, mental concentration, on certain vital points in the body in a particular manner and order. The concentration should be done along with breath-suspension. This is a very ancient method of sensory control.

Dattatreya expounded a higher process of sensory control in which mind is concentrated on the different subtle centres of the body. This is the layayoga method. He says: 'The yogi should assume the swastikasana (auspicious posture) and should be completely motionless; then he should inhale the atmospheric air and suspend the breath. During breath-suspension, the following points should be held in consciousness in succession: (1) feet, (2) muladhara (the intra-coccygeal subtle centre), (3) navel point (manipura—the intra-lumbar subtle centre), (4) heart point (anahata—the intra-thoracic subtle centre), (5) neck point (wishuddha—the intra-cervical subtle centre), (6) palatine point (talu—the intra-medullary subtle centre), (7) eyebrow point (ajña—the intra-cerebral subtle centre), (8) forehead point (manas and indu, which belong to the ajña system), and (9) head point (sahasrara—void centre)' (—Darshanopanishad, 7. 10–12).

In explaining sensory control, Narayana said: 'The control of the mind in respect of sensory objects is pratyahara' (—Mandalabrahman-

55

opanishad, 1.7). That is, the sense-mind should be so controlled as to cease all conduction to the perceptive consciousness. Here the term 'manas-nirodhana' (sense-mind control) has been used to explain the nature of the control.

It is said: 'The withdrawal of the senses from their objects, towards which they are naturally flowing, is called pratyahara' (—Yogachudamanyupanishad, 120). Here the word 'pratyaharana' (withdrawal) has been used to indicate the nature of the control, and from which the term 'pratyahara' originated. The great yogi Wishnu also said: 'It is evident that pratyahara is the process in which the yogi, being in kumbhaka, (breath-suspension) withdraws his senses from their objects' (Yogatattwopanishad, 68–69). Here also, the word 'pratyaharana' (withdrawal) has been used to explain the nature of the control. It is also stated that the control process is conjoined with breath-suspension.

Atharwana expounded five forms of sensory control to Shandilya. He said: 'The withdrawal of the senses from their objects by well-developed control-power is pratyahara; (the second form is) whatever sensory image shines forth in consciousness should be thought of as God, this is sensory control; (the third is) the abandonment of the fruits of all actions which are to be done everyday, this is sensory control; (the fourth is) the turning away from all objects, this is sensory control; (the fifth is) the holding (in consciousness) the eighteen vital points (of the body) in succession, this is sensory control. The vital points are: (1) foot, (2) big toe, (3) ankle, (4) leg, (5) knee, (6) thigh, (7) anus, (8) genitals, (9) navel, (10) heart, (11) neck, (12) larynx, (13) palate, (14) nostrils, (15) eyes, (16) the space between the eyebrows, (17) forehead, and (18) head. On these points the process of holding should be done on the ascending as well as on the descending scales' (—Shandilyopanishad, 8. 1–2).

All these are the Waidika sensory control. Now we come to the Tantrika sensory control. Shiwa said: 'The senses are constantly in contact with the objects; they should be withdrawn from their objects in a graduated manner' (—Niruttaratantra, ch. 4, p. 8). Ishwara defined

pratyahara as: 'The withdrawal of the senses from their respective objects, with which they are normally in contact, by well-developed control power is called pratyahara' (—Gandharwatantra, ch. 5, p. 25). It is said: 'The perceptive mind, because of the influence of desires, is in an oscillatory state; when the desires are controlled by pratyahara, it becomes concentrated on God' (—Rudrayamala, Part 2, 24. 137). Further, 'The perceptive mind is irresistible, firm, difficult to control and unwilling to obey; the withdrawal of it by the strength of control is called pratyahara. By pratyahara, the yogi becomes calm and is able to concentrate deeply and that leads to yoga' (Rudrayamala, Part 2, 27. 28–30).

A new and highly technical definition of sensory control is as follows: 'With the suspension of breath the mind should be concentrated on the muladhara centre and from there on all other subtle centres, step by step; this is pratyahara' (—Tantrarajatantra, 27.70). This is the form of sensory control which is specially adopted in layayoga.

The word 'yama' in the form of 'sangyama' has been used for the control of the senses. It is said: 'The sangyama (control) of the senses from their objects into the hrit centre by the will-mind is called pratyahara; this fifth process of control should be regularly practised by the yogi' (—Satwatatantra, 5.14). Sensory control has also been defined as: 'Even when the senses are in contact with the objects, the non-reception (in the sense-consciousness) of those (objects) is pratyahara' (—Paranandasutra, final section, 1. 42). Here, it is indicated that the sense-mind should be so controlled that it does not receive the dematerialized sensory impulses and, consequently, will not conduct sensomental impulses to consciousness.

Sixth, Seventh and Eighth Stages of Yama (Control): Dharana, Dhyana and Samadhi

The sixth, seventh and eighth stages of control are exercised in relation to the mind. In other words, the control of the mind is practised in three main steps, and each one has a technical name denoting the nature of the control. These names are Dharana, Dhyana and Samadhi, which will be explained.

1 Dharana (Holding-Concentration)

Dharana is the sixth stage of yama (control) and the first phase of mental control or concentration. Dharana is derived from 'dhri' meaning holding. Holding is a process of maintaining a particular form of consciousness without its transformation into another form. Therefore, holding is the process of concentration in which only one form of consciousness is maintained. This monoform consciousness is beyond perceptivity, intellectuality, affectivity, and volitionality.

Perception effects the oscillatory state of consciousness because of the constant sensomental radiations into it. The radiated energy in the conscious field is transformed into conscious forms or images which, in relation to the I-consciousness, are apprehended as what we call the external objects. According to the experiences in relation to the objects a conscious feeling of passion or aversion may be aroused. This is determined to a great extent by the desire-pattern which is based on pleasure-pain impressions, acquired before. The desire (kama) itself which is born of preformed impressions, when combined with the will-principle (manasyana) develops finally into conation (kriti). Conation may, or may not, be associated with affectivity.

On the other hand, intelligence plays an important role in perception. In a general way, it is a component part of apprehension. However, intellectuality becomes a predominant factor in certain types of apprehension. An apprehension can be so refined that higher and deep thinking and deliberation form its major part. Thinking and reasoning are the main functions of the intellective mind (buddhi).

Perception is the basis of consciousness at the sensory level. In this consciousness, not only perception, but also affection and volition and, to a certain extent, intellection are components. It is called the perceptive (sangjnana) field. When the intellective mind predominates in the perceptive field, clear thinking and sound reasoning become elements of consciousness. These are the functions of the intellective mind as mati (thought) and manana (reasoning). The intellective mind at a higher level, such as manisha (superintellect), exhibits a higher form of intelligence as deep thinking and deliberation. The intellect and superintellect modify the perceptive consciousness to a specific form called intellective consciousness (wijñana).

Both the perceptive and intellective forms of consciousness are multiform in character, though the latter is much more refined. The constituent elements of the perceptive consciousness are the knowledge-forms, principally of five varieties created by the five kinds of sensomental radiations in the conscious field. Each knowledge-form is a knowledge-unit which is termed writti (an imaged consciousness). By the appropriate combination of different knowledge-units a conscious pattern is formed which is associated with the phenomenon of the awareness of the objects. It is manifold in character and is constantly changing. Intelligence also radiates from the intellective aspect of the mind into the conscious field, and is manifested as conscious thoughts and intellectual creativity. When conscious thoughts are of a high order and intensive in character, consciousness assumes a new pattern called intellective consciousness, which is composed of thought-intelligence-units, also termed writtis.

At the sensory level the knowledge pattern is the awareness of sensory objects. Either the awareness, or the thought associated with it, is composed of knowledge and intelligence units so coalesced as to give a complete meaning. Each unit is a writti which is the knowledge minimum. Consciousness in the sensory or intellective field is maintained by the continuous arising of the writtis, one after another. It is like this, writti 1—pause—writti 2—pause— writti 3 and so on. The pause is so brief that it cannot be apprehended, and so there is an apparent continuity. A writti-chain creates a knowledge pattern of which a single writti may

57

manifest a knowledge of an object or the part of the knowledge of an object or objects. Therefore, our knowledge is a compound of writtis.

The writti-form of consciousness, the seat of which is either the perceptive or intellective field, has been termed 'sarwabhawatmabhawana' (—Annapurnopanishad, 1. 32)—the multifarious consciousness—manifesting manifold perception-thought phenomena. Unless the writtis are controlled, it is not possible to attain uniformity (samata) of consciousness. It is the background, or the actual state, of the concentratedness (ekagrata) of consciousness. This state should be developed from the state of deconcentration by the application of control.

The uniformity of consciousness is not an abnormal, unintelligent, unaffectionate and unillumined state. On the other hand, it is a supernormal, superintellective, superaffectionate and superilluminated state. So it has been called prajñana—superconsciousness. It is not based on perceptive-intellective knowledge phenomena, but on the dhi—concentrative mind which causes consciousness to assume the concentrative form. Superknowledge arises from concentration—not from perception and intellection. Superknowledge has two levels— inward and outward. At the outward level, superknowledge reveals the supermatter field, and thus the range of knowledge is increased to a very high degree. At the inward level, superknowledge manifests as spiritual light or divine knowledge.

In the intellective field, the concentrative mind manifests as attention (awadhana) and genius (pratibha). When the writtis flow in the conscious field, the specific function of the concentrative mind is almost hidden. Unless an appropriate condition in consciousness is created, concentration will not be possible. Concentration is essentially the development of that form of consciousness in which writtis cannot arise, and intellective, affective and volitive phenomena are not recorded, and the form itself does not change. A writti indicates a knowledge of an object or a part of the knowledge of an object. This is why writti 1 is not the same as writti 2, or writti 3. This shows the oscillatory character of the consciousness undergoing writtis. On the other hand, the consciousness in concentration shows that any point, measured by time, is that conscious form which is without manyness in character, but uniform. This is due to the influence of the concentrative mind.

In yoga, a unique method is introduced to raise our consciousness from the perceptive-intellective levels to the concentration level. The multifarious consciousness is intimately related to the body. The summation of all the activities of the body, which is indicated by the respiratory frequency and depth, may be regarded as an approximate index.

In normal, quiet breathing, the number of breaths is from 12–16 per minute. Let us take 16 respirations per minute in a resting state. Assume a cross-leg concentration posture as advocated in yoga. Then make your body completely motionless by passive conscious effort. When you have mastered the physical stillness, link your consciousness to the physical motionlessness. When this is controlled, any slight motion of the body, or even a tendency to movement will be recorded in your consciousness. However, by prolonged practice, a state of undisturbed consciousness, in conjunction with the motionlessness of the body, can be maintained for a desired period. This is posture control.

When the concentration posture is controlled in this manner and the mind made calm at the same time, the respiration rate of 16 per minute may decrease to 10, 8, or even less. This is due to the stillness of the body and calmness of the mind in which the suspension factor has been brought into play, which influences the respiratory rate. The respiratory rate of 16 per minute means that there are 16 inspirations and 16 expirations and a pause between them which is equal to zero. In other words—inspiration 16, expiration 16, and a pause between them; the pause = 0. If the pause 0 is raised to the inspiratory or expiratory value 16 and the inspiratory and expiratory values are reduced, then suspension will be a predominant factor in respiration. In yoga, the usual proportion has been fixed at the ratio of 1-4-2. If inspiration is 4, suspension will be 16, and expiration 8. If we make suspension equal to 64 seconds, then inspiration is 16 seconds, and expiration 32 seconds, that is, 4 counts inspiration in 16 seconds, suspension for 64 seconds, and 8 counts expiration in 32 seconds. Here, the value of 1 respiratory unit is 4 seconds. This is high R. unit. When a R. unit is reduced to 2 seconds, it is medium, a R. unit of 1 second is a low unit. In a grade using a low unit, the suspension is 16 seconds. In the medium grade, it is 32 seconds, and in the high grade 64 seconds. A student should start at the low grade and gradually proceed to the high grade.

The student should sit in a concentration posture and remain motionless and calm. Then he should practise breath-control in the following manner: inspire and concentrate on this in a passive way; then suspend and link the consciousness to the suspension and be conscious of that; and finally, expire with passive concentration. The counting of the number of units and the measure of each unit should be done consciously along with passive concentration. When the suspension is well-controlled, it will be easy and cause no disturbance.

After the suspension has been made easy by practice, matrika (supersound) units should be introduced in suspension. The 16 matrika-letters from 'Ang' to 'Ah' should be used in suspension. If the suspension is for 64 seconds, then each letter has the value of 4 seconds. This value is reduced to 2 seconds in suspension 32, and to 1 second in suspension 16. The increased or decreased time value is obtained by a slow or less slow mental sound-process essentially obtained by increasing or decreasing the nasal factor connected with each matrika-letter. During suspension, concentration should be made on the sound-process. The inspiration and expiration should be done with passive concentration and should be regulated by the respiratory units.

When the mental sound-process is fully established in suspension, the next step in practice is as follows: concentration should be done so deeply on the mental sound-process that the suspension time limit is totally forgotten. In this case, the suspension may be unconsciously prolonged or the expiration-inspiration is carried out unconsciously. Now, the 16 matrika-letters should be used in inspiration, suspension and expiration, thus making the ratio 1–1–1. When this is mastered, the 50 matrika-letters from 'Ang' to 'Kshang' should be used in inspiration-suspension-expiration as if one continuous act without any interruption in the mental sound-process at the junction between inspiration and suspension, suspension and expiration, and expiration and inspiration, and so on. In this manner, a monoform consciousness is created in which are held only the matrika-letters, flowing one after another but linked with one another by the nasal factor in mental sound-process, and the concentration is so deep that the respiratory phases do not break the concentration but remain in the background.

This is the process in which the specific function of the concentrative mind is fully activated. The nature of concentration is the holding of consciousness in a form which does not change, and to which perception, intellection, affection and volition do not reach. As the consciousness does not receive anything from the perceptive-intellective field but remains concentrated, in what is beyond perceptive-intellective, and unchanging, it is called the holding process. The first step of the process is dharana—the holding-concentration. The holding of consciousness in that form in which the 50 matrika-letters flow uninterruptedly is the dharana unit.

It is said: 'A well-controlled student should control the five forms of bioenergy by breath-suspension; (inspiration should precede suspension) and expiration through the nostril should follow suspension. When the throbbing of the bioenergy is controlled by breath-control, the mind, which is naturally restless to an extreme degree becomes fit, and should be made to undergo the process of dharana which should be done in the right way by the student who knows the secret of doing it' (—Shwetashwataropanishad, 2.9). Here it is stated that breath-suspension is an intrinsic part of holding-concentration.

Holding-concentration has been defined as: 'By controlling the desiring mind, a wise yogi should hold the Divine Spirit in his consciousness in concentration; this is dharana' (—Amritanadopanishad, 15).

It has also been said: 'A student of yoga, being prepared by abstention and other practices, should hold in his mind the five forms of super-matter (in their respective centres) within the body; this is the holding-concentration' (—Tri-shikhibrahmanopanishad, Mantra Section, 133–134). Narayana said: 'The withdrawing of consciousness from the perceptive field and holding it in the superconscious field is dharana' (—Mandalabrahmanopanishad, 1.1.8). In other words, the elevation of consciousness from the sensory level and its transformation by holding in it superconscious forms should be done. Atharwana said: 'Dharana is of three kinds: the holding-concentration on the divine aspect of self; holding-concentration on the void in the hrit-centre; and holding-concentration on the five divine forms in the five intra-spinal subtle centres' (—Shandilyopanishad, 1.9.1).

An advanced form of holding-concentration was expounded by Wishnu. He said: 'Whatever is seen with the eyes should be thought of as Divine Being; Whatever is heard with the ears, whatever is smelt with the nose, whatever is tasted with the tongue, and whatever is touched with the skin should be thought of as Divine Being. In this manner the objects of the senses should be transformed into Divine Being and are held in consciousness' (—Yogatattwopanishad, 69–72). Here, the sensory objects are given a divine form by thinking and are held in the consciousness in concentration.

About the Tantrika form of holding-concentration, Ishwara said: 'Concentration on the following points with breath-suspension is termed dharana; the points are: great toe, ankle, knee, scrotum, genitals, navel, heart, neck, throat, uvula, nose, eyebrow-space, breast, and head' (—Gandharwatantra, ch. 5, p. 25). So holding-concentration should be done while doing breath-suspension.

It is said: 'The knowers of yoga say—the holding in the consciousness of certain vital points along with breath-suspension is dharana' (—Prapañchasaratantra, 19. 21–22). The mind should be concentrated on a certain vital point with breath-suspension. It is further stated: 'The experts in breath-control say that those vital points through which one can leave one's own body and can enter another's body and can reenter one's own body are suitable for dharana;

they are: great toe, ankle, knee, anus, perineum, genitals, navel, heart, neck, uvula, nose, and eyebrow-space' (—Prapañchasaratantra, 19.51–53).

Shiwa said: 'The holding of the mind, with breath-suspension, on the great toe, ankle, knee, thigh, genitals, navel, heart, neck, uvula, nose, eyebrow-space, forehead, and top of the head is termed dharana' (—Wishwasaratantra, ch. 2, p. 11). Further, 'Concentration on the six subtle centres ... (and) the Coiled Power (Kundali) ... is termed dharana' (—Rudrayamala, Part 2, 27. 34–35).

The distinction between holding-concentration and deep concentration (dhyana) has been explained. It is said: 'Concentration on the whole divine form is dhyana, while only on one part at a time is dharana' (—Bhutashuddhitantra, ch. 9, p. 8). The matrika-letters are very suitable for holding-concentration. Only in deep concentration, can a divine form be the object. In fact, an appropriate divine form arises from mantra in deep concentration. Now we come to dhyana.

2 Dhyana (Deep Concentration)

Dhyana is the seventh stage of yama (control) and the second phase of mental control or concentration. The word 'dhyana' is derived from 'dhyai', to concentrate. Concentration is the holding of an image in consciousness continuously and without interruption by the penetration of any other images. When this concentration becomes very deep by an uninterrupted and continuous holding of an image in consciousness for a sufficiently long time, it is called dhyana. It is the specific function of that aspect of the mind, called dhi—the concentrative mind. The uninterrupted and continuous holding is the process of concentration. So the new term dhyana has been used in the seventh stage of control to mean deep concentration.

It is said: 'Eyes cannot receive the Supreme Spirit, nor can words express it, nor can it be reached by other senses and conative faculties or by ascesis or any other actions. The Supreme Spirit is revealed in dhyana; dhyana is only possible when consciousness is spiritualized by the purity of knowledge' (—Mundakopanishad, 3.1.8). Knowledge at the sensory level is manifold in character—a writti-form. The realization of Supreme Spirit is not possible through such knowledge. This is why it has been said that the senses cannot reach it. A mind which is only conscious because of perception, intellection and volition cannot reach the Supreme Spirit. When the manifoldness of knowledge is transformed into uniformness, consciousness becomes purified and spiritualized. In such a state of consciousness dhyana develops into its highest point in which Supreme Spirit is revealed. It is the development of dhyana into samadhi (superconcentration). However, to attain such a state of consciousness the practice of concentration is absolutely necessary.

It is said: 'As the two pieces of wood are used in kindling the sacred fire by attrition, so the body and the pranawa (first mantra) are as if two pieces of wood, and they should be used by dhyana for the realization of the luminous Supreme Spirit' (—Shwetashwataropanishad, 1. 14). This means that the body should be made motionless by posture and breath-control and then concentration should be practised in conjunction with mantra.

The hrit-centre is a very suitable point for the practice of deep concentration. So it has been said: 'Controlling the senses ... concentrate on the Divine Being who is quiescent, luminous, pure and blissful and in the hrit-centre' (—Kaiwalyopanishad, 5). Here is a particular mode of concentration for the students of yoga: 'Having assumed a (folded-leg) concentration posture, and with the hridayañjali mudra (a mode of alignment of hands and fingers to make them hollow) placed in the region of the heart, and with the eyes retracted from the world, applying pressure on the rima glottidis with the tip of the retroverted tongue, not allowing the upper teeth to touch the lower, keeping the body erect, and with the mind concentrated, control the senses. Then with the purified and spiritualized mind he should concentrate on Wasudewa (a divine form—Krishna) who is the Supreme Spirit. When concentration is so deep that the whole consciousness is moulded into the Wasudewa form, then that concentration will lead to libera-

tion. All sins of worldliness are destroyed by the concentration on Wasudewa with breath-suspension for three hours' (—Trishikhibrahmanopanishad, Mantra Section, 145–9).

Concentration on the universal form of God has been advised (—Darshanopanishad, 9. 1–2). But it is not possible until the Deity is realized by the mantra way of concentration. The final stage of dhyana is the concentration on Brahman (God) without form (—Darshanopanishad, 9. 3–5).

Narayana says: 'When concentration reaches the phase of "ekatanata", monoformity (of consciousness) of the Divine Being abiding in all, that is dhyana' (—Mandalabrahmanopanishad, 1.1.9). Ekatanata is that form of consciousness in which a chosen image is held continuously and without any interruption. The consciousness is in the form of a chosen image and this form continues without any change. So, ekatanata is very deep and continuous concentration. This deep concentration is dhyana.

There are two main types of dhyana: saguna (with form) and nirguna (without form). Wishnu says about concentration on form: 'Dhyana should be practised while concentrating on the Deity ... and at the same time breath-suspension should be done (in a natural manner). This is saguna-dhyana' (—Yogatattwopanishad, 104– 105). Here breath-suspension is the first stage of kewala kumbhaka, that is, normal suspension without inspiration and expiration. However, it is an advanced form of concentration. After the saguna-dhyana (concentration on form) is mastered, a yoga student should start with the nirguna-dhyana (concentration without form). Wishnu said: 'Nirguna-dhyana leads to samadhi (superconcentration)' (—Yogatattwopanishad, 105).

Now we shall consider the Tantrika form of dhyana (deep concentration). Sadashiwa said: 'Dhyana is of two forms: sarupa (with form) and arupa (formless). The object of the formless concentration is the Supreme Power-Consciousness which is beyond mind and speech, unmanifest, omnipresent, and unknowable; it cannot be identified as this or that; the yogis with great difficulties and through the processes of control attain it. I will now speak of concentration on form in order that the mind may be able to concentrate and the *yoga* practitioner may get the desired results quickly in concentration, and to develop the power of concentration of the subtle type. Actually, the Supreme Power-Consciousness, who is above time, is formless and splendid; this reality manifests itself by will in relation to mind-matter phenomena' (—M*ahanirwanatantra*, 5. 137–140).

The above statement clearly indicates that formless concentration is extremely difficult to obtain. A yog*i* can attain it only when he has been able to develop the power of concentration to a very high degree through the prolonged practice of concentration on form. So, concentration on form is the first step to formless concentration. Formless concentration is very near to superconcentration. When consciousness becomes highly rarefied and illuminated by spiritual light through the practice of concentration on form, the formless aspect of the Supreme Power-Consciousness reflects on, and shines forth in, that consciousness. The s*arupa* and *arupa* dhya*na* are the same as the W*aidika* s*aguna* and nirgu*na* dhya*na* respectively.

Concentration on form has been defined as: 'Experts on yog*a* say that dhya*na* is to make the form of Deity held (continuously) in consciousness' (—Pr*apañchasaratantra*, 19. 22–23). The holding process is concentration. So it is said: 'Dhya*na* is the concentration on the Deity of m*antra*' (—Kul*arnawa*, ch. 17, p. 83). It is clearly explained here: 'Deep concentration on the conscious form of the Deity of m*antra* in your consciousness is dhya*na*' (—Gandharwa-tantra, ch. 5, p. 26).

3 S*amadhi* (Superconcentration)

S*amadhi* is the eighth or the final stage of y*ama* (control). The word s*amadhi* is derived from 'dha' to mean dhar*ana*, that is holding. To maintain in the consciousness an image of an object without letting it slip or disappear from the consciousness is holding. It is the specific function of the concentrative mind (dh*i*) to hold an object in the consciousness without having it loosened and escaping from the

consciousness. This action of holding is in the nature of binding or restraining, because, without being bound or fastened together, the object may be lost. Therefore, the mental action of holding is an action of binding (b*andhana*), which means y*ama* (control).

Let us explain it in greater detail. Dhar*ana* or holding is a process by which only one object is retained in consciousness, or consciousness is shaped only in one form—the form of one object only, which is held in it; or holding the consciousness fixed on only one object; or, in other words, to bring or concentrate consciousness on one form or into one-pointedness. So the process of holding is the process of concentration. It is the process by which the multifarious consciousness is transformed into a monoform, and is in a state of concentratedness. That the holding is concentration, is indicated by the fact that the word 'dhyana' has been used for complete dhar*ana*, that is, uninterrupted and continuous holding, or deep concentration.

Holding consists of three phases according to the depth of concentration. In the first phase concentration is not very deep and so it is interrupted now and then. This form of concentration has been technically called dhar*ana* or holding-concentration. In the second phase, concentration becomes so deep that it does not break at all but continues uninterruptedly. This is called dhya*na* or deep concentration. In the final phase, holding reaches its maximum point of development. In other words, at a point when dhya*na* reaches its highest development, the process of holding is so firm that consciousness, which is in a most rarefied state, is only in the form of the object held, in its subtle aspect; and concentration is so deep that even I-ness is lost. This is what is technically called s*amadhi*. Now, dhar*ana* has reached its maximum point, and 'sam' to denote super has been prefixed to 'dha' with 'a' between, and thus the word s*amadhi* is formed. Therefore, s*amadhi* is superconcentration.

The action of holding is intrinsically associated with binding (b*andhana*). Binding restrains an object held in the consciousness from leaving it. It also restrains the penetration of other objects into consciousness. Therefore, holding is in the nature of yama (control). There are other terms which have been used to mean control. Bandha, bandhana, nigraha, nirodha, niyamana and ayama are synonymous with yama and all of them mean control. Control also develops stage by stage and at the eighth stage it reaches its highest development. To indicate this, 'sam' has been prefixed to yama to form sangyama, to denote supercontrol.

Holding has also another aspect. During holding, there is a union between the consciousness and the object. If consciousness remains united with the object, the object is restrained from escaping from consciousness. At the point of superconcentration this union is complete. To denote this, the term sangyoga, meaning superunion, has been used.

Now let us study the Waidika form of samadhi. About the accomplishment of superconcentration it has been said: 'By controlling the senses (through sensory control), by controlling the outwardly directed tendency of the mind (by concentration), by controlling the desires of the mind, and by ascesis, a yogi will be in samadhi. In samadhi all love is directed to the Supreme Spirit, and one is fully attached to him, fully absorbed in him and experiences all bliss in him. From samadhi arises divine knowledge by which God, whose power-in-word-form is pranawa, is revealed and the yogi is in him' (—Nrisinghatapinyupanishad, 2.6.4).

Samprajñata samadhi (superconscious concentration) has been defined as: 'The continuous flow of consciousness in the form of Brahman—God in which the I-ness has been dissolved is samprajñata samadhi. It is attained by prolonged practice of dhyana' (—Muktikopanishad, 2.53). Samadhi is of two forms: Samprajñata and asamprajñata. When the term samadhi is used, it usually refers to the samprajñata type. In samprajñata samadhi mental concentration has been developed to its highest point and, consequently, through such concentration consciousness is only in the God-form and nothing else, and this form of consciousness flows normally, uninterruptedly and continually, and even the I-ness is not a part of consciousness. The I-ness, illuminated, godly consciousness, in a state of concentration at its highest degree, is the superconscious concentration.

It has been said: 'The mind operating at the sensory level is the root-cause of all the wordly knowledge. If the mind is dissolved, there will be no wordly knowledge. Therefore, keep the consciousness fixed on the Supreme Being in deepest concentration' (—Adhyatmopanishad, 26). In superconcentration, God is held by concentration, and consciousness becomes godly. The form of consciousness attained in superconcentration has been described as: 'Samadhi is that state in which consciousness is only in the nature of the object concentrated on, and is still like the flame of a lamp in a windless place, and from which gradually the feeling of the action of concentration and I-ness has disappeared' (—Adhyatmopanishad, 35). That is, consciousness in superconcentration assumes the form of an object concentrated on, and is without I-ness, and does not change but continues to be in that form only.

The nature of superconscious concentration has been more clearly stated here: 'That state in which consciousness is in concentration and is illuminated by the divine light, and without any desire—that superconscious state is samadhi' (—Annapurnopanishad, 1.48). It is further stated: 'That state in which the mind is devoid of restlessness, I-ness is absent, mind is unconcerned with worldly pleasures and pains, and consciousness is absolutely motionless like a rock, in deepest concentration, is samadhi. That state in which all desires have been completely eliminated, there is no liking or disliking, and consciousness is free from waves, and absolutely tranquil, that is samadhi' (Annapurnopanishad, 1.49–50).

The form of consciousness developed in superconcentration, is not void or nothing, though it is object-less and I-nessless, but there is that bliss which is beyond any worldly pleasure, and is full of power. So it is asserted: 'That state of consciousness in which there are no objects, no passion or aversion, but there is supreme happiness and superior power, is samadhi' (—Mahopanishad, 4. 62).

The process of transforming the multiform consciousness into a uniform state is superconcentration. It is said: 'When consciousness reaches a state in which it becomes uniform, it is samadhi' (—Amritanadopanishad, 16). About the consciousness in superconcentration, Dattatreya said: 'Samadhi is that in which consciousness is in deepest concentration associated with the knowledge of the union between the embodied spirit and the Supreme Spirit' (—Darshanopanishad, 10.1). Dattatreya further said: 'That concentrative consciousness in which arises the knowledge of being only in Supreme Consciousness is samadhi' (—Darshanopanishad, 10.5). When consciousness is in the deepest concentration, there is the realization of only Supreme Being in which there is no feeling of the body, no perception, no intellection, and this is superconcentration.

Now with the Tantrika form of samadhi. Shiwa has defined samadhi as: 'According to all Tantras, samadhi is that concentration in which the sameness (samata) of the embodied spirit and the Supreme Spirit is revealed' (—Wishwasaratantra, ch. 2, p. 11). Here, the word 'bhawana' has been used to indicate deepest concentration. Shiwa has also explained the nature of the sameness. He says: 'Samadhi is that in which arises the consciousness of oneness (ekata) between the embodied spirit and the Supreme Spirit' (—Gandharwatantra, ch. 5, p. 26). This means that in superconcentration, consciousness is in the deepest concentration and is fully illuminated by the divine light in which the realization of the oneness between the embodied spirit and the Supreme Spirit occurs.

We have already stated that samadhi consists of two forms: samprajñata and asamprajñata (non-mens concentration). When superconscious concentration develops to its highest point, non-mens concentration is achieved. It is said: 'As salt thrown into water becomes the same as water, so the state in which the oneness between consciousness and the Supreme Spirit occurs is called samadhi' (—Soubhagyalakshmyupanishad, 2.14). This means, that, when all the writtis (objective images) disappear and, consequently, consciousness is in the form of the Supreme Being in concentration and nothing else, this is the state of samadhi. This samadhi is superconscious concentration. Because consciousness in the concentrative form still exists,

though highly purified and illuminated by divine light. Again it is said: 'When the vital activities are under full control and the mind is in deep concentration, consciousness becomes uniform; this is samadhi' (—Soubhagyalakshmyupanishad, 2.15). This is also superconscious concentration.

About the non-mens concentration it has been said: 'When all desires and thoughts disappear and the sameness between the embodied spirit and the Supreme Spirit occurs, it is samadhi. When the senses and the intellective mind and even the concentrative mind are absorbed, and, consequently, the entire mind undergoes a phase of negativity, (and, therefore, the whole existence is only the beingness of Brahman, and that Brahman is without mind and matter), this is samadhi' (—Soubhagyalakshmyupanishad, 2.16 – 17). In this samadhi, there are no desires, no sense action, no intellection and no thought, and even the highly spiritualized concentrative consciousness has been completely absorbed; in this grand 'nonentity' there remains only Brahman—Brahman in its supreme state which is without mind and matter, and consequently in this state the embodied spirit, as an individualized being, is nonexistent; the embodiment has been completely dissolved and the spirit has been united with the Supreme Spirit and has become one and the same. This is asamprajñata samadhi—non-mens concentration, in which, at the highest point of concentration, the concentrative consciousness, which is merely in the form of divine knowledge-light, is transmuted completely into Supreme Consciousness. By this highest concentration a state is reached in which everything else has been absorbed, and only Supreme Consciousness shines in its supreme aspect. This is supreme concentration—asamprajñata samadhi.

Wishnu has also said: 'Samadhi is the sameness between the embodied spirit and the Supreme Spirit' (—Yogatattwopanishad, 107). Atharwana has said: 'Samadhi is that state in which the oneness (aikya) between the embodied spirit and the Supreme Spirit occurs. It is without I-ness, without objects and without the knowledge of objects; it is a state full of bliss and in it there remains only Supreme Consciousness'

(—Shandilyopanishad, 1.11.1). So the words 'samata' (sameness) and 'aikya' (oneness) indicate the same thing. It is a state of oneness between the embodied spirit and the Supreme Spirit. Moreover, the non-mens concentration is not the insensate, gloomy metamorphosis of the human mind, it is not a state of being dead-alive, but a borderland of human development, the highest possibility of man in his spiritual endeavour; it is a state of becoming Supreme Spirit, with supreme bliss and supreme power; it is to be free from the bondage of the body and mind, to become liberated-alive. This has been pointed out by Atharwana.

Narayana said: 'When concentrative consciousness is lost, it is (mind-transcendent) samadhi' (—Mandalabrahmanopanishad, 1.1.10). When the penetration of the objective world into consciousness is prevented by sensory control, then the Supreme Spirit in its divine form is held in consciousness in concentration. At the beginning, concentration does not go very deep, so it breaks and the one-pointedness of the consciousness is interrupted. But concentration quickly regains its power. This is holding-concentration. When concentration grows deeper, and interruption does not occur, it continues; consciousness is now only in the divine form which is continually being held. This single-pointedness of consciousness is deep concentration. When the deep concentration becomes deepest, I-ness is lost, the whole world is lost, what remains is only the spiritually illuminated consciousness of divine form, it is the state of superconscious concentration. When the light-like concentrative consciousness is absorbed into Supreme Consciousness in supreme concentration, there remains solely the Supreme Spirit, and nothing else. This is non-mens concentration.

Ribhu said: 'When the uniform concentrative consciousness is dissolved by the most intensified concentration, there remains only the being of Supreme Consciousness' (—Annapurnopanishad, 1.23). In other words, through the deepest concentration the final form of consciousness disappears and only Supreme Consciousness as a whole remains. This is the state of non-mens concentration. Now we come to yoga.

Yoga Defined and Explained

From a linguistic point of view, the word 'yoga' has been derived form the root 'yuja', denoting: (1) sangyama, that is, control developed to its highest degree—supercontrol; (2) samadhi, that is, concentration developed to its deepest form—superconcentration; (3) sangyoga, that is, union in its complete form—superunion.

We have already considered the control factor. Yama (control) is the basic form of yoga. It (yama) develops through eight stages. At the eighth stage yama develops into its highest form and this is called sangyama, that is, supercontrol. The yama power, as we have noted, is intrinsically associated with the process of holding, that is, concentration. The control is in the nature of concentration. So, as yama develops stage by stage, concentration also develops along with the control. At the eighth stage, control reaches its highest point of development and becomes supercontrol, and concentration also reaches its highest degree of intensity and becomes superconcentration. Unless the mind is at the state of supercontrol, it is not possible to attain superconcentration. So it is said: 'It is impossible to attain samadhi when the mind is attached to worldly objects; but it is easy to attain samadhi for the mind undergoing sangyama' (—Gandharwatantra, ch. 5, p. 26). That samadhi is intimately related to sangyama has been disclosed here.

Yoga has been defined as: 'A non-oscillatory state of the senses, sense-mind and sense-consciousness, developed by dharana, that is, deep concentration, is termed yoga' (—Kathopanishad, 2.3.11). Dharana is the process of holding in deepest concentration the mono-form consciousness which, in other words, is superconscious concentration; and this is yoga. So it appears that yoga here is defined as superconscious concentration.

Yoga has also been defined as: "The state of real absorption of consciousness, which is beyond all knowledge, is termed yoga' (—Akshyupanishad, 2.3). Here the non-mens concentration has been defined as yoga. It has been said:

'When the deepest concentration on Supreme Brahman (attained at the final phase of superconscious concentration) also disappears by itself within, there arises nirwikalpa samadhi in which all latent impressions of feeling are eliminated' (—Annapurnopanishad, 4. 62). Nirwikalpa samadhi and asamprajñata samadhi are synonyms, i.e. for non-mens concentration. Here it is said that superconscious concentration ultimately leads to non-mens concentration.

That both forms of samadhi are the stages of yoga has been stated here: 'By yoga (that is non-mens concentration) yoga (that is superconscious concentration) should be controlled, and the multiformed consciousness by the one-pointed consciousness in which God is held; thus being in Supreme Consciousness, which is beyond all knowledge, the yogi becomes that' (—Soubhagyalakshmyupanishad, 2.12). That yoga is non-mens concentration has been stated by Sadashiwa. He says: 'That which is merely being, changeless, beyond mind and speech, and the only truth in the transitory worlds of mind-power-matter, is Brahman in its real nature; that Brahman is realized directly in yoga in the form of nirwikalpa samadhi (non-mens concentration) by those who have developed the equanimity of the mind, who are beyond all contraries of the world and without the feeling of my-ness about the body' (—Mahanirwanatantra, 3. 7–8).

That yoga is also superconscious concentration has been said by Shiwa in the Wishwasaratantra. So it is clear that superconcentration is yoga. We are, therefore, justified in concluding that both superconcentration and non-mens concentration are yoga.

So far we have considered the concentration aspect of yoga. But yoga has also the control aspect, as concentration is intrinsically related to control. Atharwana said: 'Yoga is the control of the writtis (mentimultiformity)' (—Shandilyopanishad, 1.7.24). Here the control aspect of yoga has been clearly stated. Consciousness may become free from the writtis by the control of the perceptive, intellective, volitive and affective aspects of the mind, and becomes monoform and single-pointed, in which only the Supreme Being is held in concentration.

This is the state of writtiless superconcentration. It has been said: 'When the constantly changing consciousness is free from writtis, it becomes non-oscillatory and concentrated, in which is revealed the infinite and whole Supreme Spirit' (Annapurnopanishad, 1.55). This is adhyatma-yoga—spiritual yoga. It is said: 'That Supreme Spirit which is unknowable, invisible and eternal, lying in all beings, and hidden, but shines forth in consciousness, is attainable by spiritual yoga' (—Kathopanishad, 1.2.12).

Yoga is the state of deep concentration, so superconcentration is yoga. It has been stated: 'Deep concentration arises in yoga' (—Sharadatilaka, 25.1). Without concentration yoga is not attainable, so it was said: 'A yogi attains yoga only in superconcentration' (—Rudrayamala, Part 2, 27.43).

The non-writti state has another aspect. When consciousness itself is absorbed, along with the disappearance of all the writtis, it is the non-mens concentration. It is said: 'The real absorption of consciousness which is beyond all knowledge is termed yoga' (—Akshyupanishad, 2.3). From this it is clear that the non-mens concentration is also yoga. So it is stated: 'The state in which consciousness, which normally undergoes writtis, is completely absorbed and there is supreme bliss, is termed non-mens concentration; it is the favourite of the yogis' (—Muktikopanishad, 2.54). Ishwara has also said: 'Samadhi is that in which consciousness is completely absorbed into Supreme Being' (—Kularnawa, ch. 9, p. 42).

Now we come to the third aspect of yoga—sangyoga, that is, union. The word sangyoga is derived from 'yuja' to which is prefixed 'sam', meaning super. Yuja has three meanings: (1) concentration, (2) control, and (3) union. Therefore, sangyoga means—(1) superconcentration, (2) supercontrol, and (3) superunion. We are now going to consider the superunion aspect of yoga.

Maheshwara says: 'The union (sangyoga) of the embodied spirit and the Supreme Spirit is called yoga' (—Yogashikhopanishad, 1.68–9). It is also said: 'The embodied spirit that possesses a mind, appears to be different from the Supreme Spirit; the union (yoga) between them is yoga'

(—Tantrarajatantra, 27.53). Here the word 'yoga' is used to indicate union. Shiwa says: 'The union (yojana) between the embodied spirit and the Supreme Spirit, or between Supreme Consciousness and Supreme Power is yoga' (—Niruttaratantra, ch. 11, p. 22). Here the word 'yojana' has been used for sangyoga (union).

The sangyoga is aikya (oneness). So it is said: 'According to yoga experts, oneness between the embodied spirit and the Supreme Spirit is yoga' (—Kularnawa, ch. 9, p. 43). This oneness in union occurs in samadhi. It has two stages of development. At the first stage when the union occurs the knowledge of the oneness shines forth in superconcentration. It has been stated by Dattatreya (—Darshanopanishad, 10.1.). At the final stage, even the knowledge of oneness disappears along with consciousness, and the oneness becomes real in non-mens concentration. Atharwana explained this (Shandilyopanishad, 1.11.1).

Samadhi is intimately related to union. It is said: 'On the accomplishment of sangyoga (union) one can be in a state of samadhi' (—Rudrayamala, Part 2, 27.42). Therefore the union is associated with the deepest concentration. In the deepest concentration the sameness between the embodied spirit and the Supreme Spirit occurs. So long as consciousness remains, it is in the deepest concentration which is saturated with the knowledge of the sameness. This is why it has been said: 'That deepest concentration in which arises the knowledge of the sameness between the embodied spirit and the Supreme Spirit is samadhi' (—Sharadatilaka, 25.27).

From the above study we come to the following conclusion.

Yoga is fundamentally based on yama—control. Yama develops stage by stage and finally reaches its highest limit and becomes sangyama—supercontrol. Yama is intrinsically related to concentration, and at the sangyama stage, concentration develops into samadhi—superconcentration. Concentration is also related to union and when concentration is deepest, the union becomes sangyoga—superunion. At the supercontrol level, concentration develops into superconcentration and union into superunion. And this state is yoga. So, yoga has three aspects—supercontrol, superconcentration and superunion. They are interrelated and inseparable from yoga. At the final stage in yoga, superconcentration is transformed into non-mens concentration because of the absorption of the consciousness, and, consequently, the superunion becomes the real oneness between the embodied spirit and the Supreme Spirit through the absorption of the embodied spirit into the Supreme Spirit; at this stage supercontrol also disappears. Now yoga becomes Mahayoga—the supreme yoga in which only Supreme Consciousness remains.

To reach this final yoga, it is absolutely necessary to develop the power of control and concentration, stage by stage. The stages are eight. They are: yama, niyama, asana, pranayama, pratyahara, dharana, dhyana and samadhi. These eight practices constitute Ashtangayoga—eightfold yoga. Layayoga is based on the eightfold yoga.

CHAPTER 2
Layayoga—
Its Significance and Method

Layayoga is that form of yoga in which yoga, that is samadhi, is attained through laya. Laya is deep concentration causing the absorption of the cosmic principles, stage by stage, into the spiritual aspect of the Supreme Power-Consciousness. It is the process of absorption of the cosmic principles in deep concentration, thus freeing consciousness from all that is not spiritual, and in which is held the divine luminous coiled power, termed Kundalini.

Wishnu says: 'Layayoga is that in which chitta (sense-consciousness) undergoes laya, that is, becomes absorbed in deep concentration; there are many methods for achieving this: but the most effective is dhyana (deep concentration) on God in form, which can be done also while walking, standing, eating, and resting. This is layayoga' (—Yogatattwopanishad, 23–4). Sense-consciousness which is the field where sensory images are constantly being formed, becomes transformed, through the process of concentration, into a form where the penetration of sensory images stops and, consequently, consciousness is free from image-undulations and, therefore, in a state of concentration. This state of consciousness is termed superconsciousness. So, sense-consciousness is transformed into super-consciousness by deep concentration. To achieve this end, concentration is practised by taking the divine form as the object of concentration. The divine form is made living in Ishtadewata, who appears from the living mantra. Under this condition, concentration becomes real and deep.

Maheshwara says: 'When one is established in layayoga, there is the union between the embodied spirit and the Supreme Spirit; and because of this, consciousness becomes complete-ly absorbed and along with it the cessation of respiration takes place' (—Yogashikhopani-shad, 1. 134–5). Here the final stage of layayoga has been explained. In the first stage of laya, all sensory images from the consciousness are eliminated and, therefore, the sense-consciousness becomes highly refined and is transformed into superconsciousness. This is the stage of samprajñata samadhi (superconscious concentra-tion). Thereafter the real union of the embodied spirit and the Supreme Spirit takes place when superconsciousness is absorbed. It is the stage of asamprajñata samadhi (non-mens concentra-tion). This is the final stage of layayoga. At this stage, the normal cessation of respiration occurs. This is kewala kumbhaka (normal cessation of respiration). It clearly indicates that when consciousness undergoes complete absorption in layayoga kumbhaka arises automatically.

In hathayoga, deep concentration is attained through the process of kewala kumbhaka, and, in layayoga, through deep concentration, kewala kumbhaka is normally attained.

Laya Process

In the Waidika laya process, the conative facul-ties, namely, speech, prehension, locomotion, excretion and reproduction, are to be controlled by the will-mind in concentration, stage by

68

stage. These actions become unmanifested owing to their tranquillization by control. The stages of control are as follows: (1) reproduction, (2) excretion, (3) locomotion, (4) prehension, and (5) speech. These control processes are carried out in the lower five subtle centres. In this way the body becomes motionless and the mind becomes free of all thoughts about the body.

Smell, taste, sight, touch, and sound are the senses. They are controlled in concentration in the lower five subtle centres, stage by stage, while the sense-mind, residing in the sixth subtle centre, is also controlled. Consequently, the sense-mind does not radiate the object-substance to . sense-consciousness. This results in sense-consciousness becoming free from objective images. This is the state of pratyahara (sensory control). When this is established, consciousness undergoes dharana and dhyana and finally samprajñata samadhi. Then samadhi consciousness is completely absorbed into the power aspect of Supreme Consciousness in time. This is the stage of asamprajñata samadhi (non-mens concentration).

By the process of control, the cosmic principles, namely, conative faculties, senses, sense-mind, sense-consciousness and superconsciousness, become unmanifested and are absorbed into the spiritual Power-Consciousness in deep concentration. The absorption of the cosmic principles in deep concentration, which is associated with control, is laya. So, laya is that control process which causes absorption in concentration. The laya has two stages. First, the absorption of sense-consciousness and, secondly, the complete absorption of the superconsciousness into Supreme Power-Consciousness.

It has been said: 'Mind has two forms—impure and pure: the impure mind is full of desires, and the pure mind is free from desires. Mind is the cause of both our bondage and our liberation; the mind which is attached to sense objects causes bondage, and when it becomes free from objects it leads to liberation; ... therefore, he who desires to be liberated should make his consciousness free from all objective images' (—Brahmabindupanishad, 1–3). By the laya process all objective images are eliminated

from consciousness, which becomes pure. The purified consciousness becomes transformed into superconsciousness in a state of samadhi, arising from laya. Laya develops into samadhi.

It is stated: 'The non-rising of the absorbed multiforms of the consciousness is the limit of the control' (—Adhyatmopanishad, 42). This requires explanation. The term 'laya' is derived from li meaning 'be absorbed in'. Laya, in the technical sense of yoga, means absorption in deep concentration. When the multiforms of consciousness undergo absorption in concentration and do not arise again to interrupt it, concentration develops into samadhi. This process of absorption consists of various stages. The first of these is concerned with the absorption of the sensory images and all conative impulses. The next stage is the absorption in concentration of intellection and thoughts. In this way, when the perceptive, volitive, and intellective functions of the mind are fully controlled by absorptive concentration, sense-consciousness begins to be transformed into superconsciousness. When concentration becomes deepest, samadhi is attained. Samadhi in the superconscious field is termed samprajñata samadhi, that is, superconscious concentration. The control power has now reached its highest degree of development. It is then termed 'nirodha' or sangnirodha, that is, supercontrol. This is the limit of mental control.

'Speech should be controlled in manas, manas in jñana-atman, jñana-atman in mahan, and mahan in Supreme Atman' (—Kathopanishad, 1.3.13). Here speech stands for all organs of voluntary action and the senses. The organs of action are controlled in manas, that is, will-mind; the senses are controlled in manas, that is, sense-mind. Jñana-atman is sense-consciousness and intellect, and mahan is the I-less super-mind, that is, superconsciousness. The senses are controlled in the sense-mind; that is, in concentration, the power of control is developed which causes absorption of the senses in the sense-mind. In a similar manner, the sense-mind, the will-mind, the sense-consciousness and the intellect are absorbed in concentration. So, by the power of control manifested in concentration, the senses and the sensory aspects of the mind are absorbed. After this, the super-mind is manifested. Now concentration is developed into samadhi. Finally, the supermind is absorbed in supreme concentration into Supreme Spirit. This is the state of non-mens concentration.

Yama said: 'Manas is higher than the senses, intellect is higher than manas, mahan is higher than the intellect, the unmanifested, that is prakriti, is higher than the mahan and the infinite and supreme Purusha, that is, Supreme Consciousness, is higher than prakriti; one who knows him (in samadhi), becomes free from bondage and immortal' (—Kathopanishad, 2.3. 7–8). The different aspects of the sensory mind, the supermind and what remains beyond mind, have been stated by Yama. He also indicated the stages of absorptive concentration. Here manas is the sense-mind. The senses, sense-mind and intellect are the main aspects of the sensory mind. When these are absorbed in concentration, mahan (supermind) is reached. For attainment of non-mens concentration the supermind should be reduced to prakriti (primus) by the absorptive concentration. Prakriti is that fundamental principle in which the super-mind undergoes negativity. Then prakriti itself is absorbed into purusha (disembodied conscious-ness principle).

The various principles, which are to be absorbed in concentration by stages, have been explained here: 'The "earth", "water", "fire", "air" and "void" principles; subtle earth, water, fire, air and void principles; the principles of smell and its objects, of taste and its objects, of sight and its objects, of touch and its objects, and of hearing and its objects; the conative principles, viz., reproduction, excretion, loco-motion, prehension and speech; sense-mind and its functions; intellect, I-ness and sense-conscious-ness and their functions; supermind and its function; and the creative aspect of infinite energy—all these are to be absorbed' (—Prashnopanishad, 4.8).

The five forms of metamatter (mahabhutas) and five 'tanons' (tanmatras), five senses and their objects, five organs of volitional actions and will-mind, intellection, I-feeling, sense-consciousness, supermind and the energy aspect of Supreme Power-Consciousness, which is the source of all creative phenomena, are to be absorbed in deep concentration in order to reach Brahman.

When all principles are absorbed in concentra-tion, what remains is Brahman—Supreme Spirit. It has been stated: 'That (Brahman) is infinite, being by itself, beyond mind, subtler than the subtlest (that is, without form), far away and still near (that is, beyond any position); that Brahman is hidden in what has been manifested as life-mind-matter' (—Mundakopanishad, 3.1.7). Unless all the creative principles are absorbed, the realization of Supreme Conscious-ness is not possible. That Supreme Being is to be realized by superknowledge arising in samadhi. It is said: 'That formless Spirit should be realized by superconscious knowledge in the body in which the vital processes are opera-tive, (that is, the living body); sarwa chitta (that is, consciousness exhibiting multiformity) is vitalized by the bio-forces; when this sense-consciousness is purified, the Supreme Spirit shines forth in it' (—Mundakopanishad, 3.1.9). Here, it is said that, when sense-consciousness, which is associated with the living body, is spiritually purified, it is transformed into super-consciousness, and samadhi is attained. In samadhi, superknowledge arises by which the Supreme Spirit is realized. The spiritual puri-fication of the sense-consciousness is achieved by the absorption of various principles in concentration.

Brahman—Supreme Consciousness, in the creative aspect, manifests consciousness in three forms. The first form is the sensory, and it functions in cooperation with the physical body. Consciousness is awakened by perceiving ex-ternal objects through the senses. At this stage the experiences of the 'I' are essentially based on perception. The 'I' has seven main supports from where all its experiences are effected. The means of the experiences are nineteen, viz., five senses, five organs of volitive actions, five bio-energies, sense-mind, intellect, I-ness and consciousness. In the second form, consciousness is awakened by thoughts and dreams based on impressions and desires. In the third form, consciousness is not awakened, so it is a state of nonconsciousness (—Mandukyopanishad, 1.3–5).

The 'I' feeling is awakened and maintained by intellection and willing, the site of which is the soma centre, and perceptivity, which has its sites in the five lower subtle centres. 'I' functions through the instrumentation of five forms of bio-energy, five organs of volitional action, five senses, will-mind, sense-mind, intellect and sense-consciousness. Consciousness is brought into being sensorially; the living body, sense-mind, and I-feeling take part in this. It is the sensory form of consciousness, that receives external impressions through the sensory channels. Now, 'I' enjoys the external world. When the senses become inoperative, as in sleep, the sense-mind may still function without the help of the senses. This function of the sense-mind is stimulated by the post-conscious impressions and desires. The usual example of this is dreaming. In deep thinking, the senses may be inoperative to a great extent. But when the senses are absorbed in deep concentration, the sense-mind becomes free and can acquire knowledge extra-sensorially. This knowledge falls under three categories: the same type of sensory knowledge acquired without the help of the senses; that form of sensory knowledge which cannot be acquired by the senses; and a supra-sensory form of knowledge.

When the senses and the sense-mind become inoperative, sense-consciousness becomes masked, giving rise to apparent nonconsciousness. It happens normally in deep sleep. But in layayoga concentration, sense-consciousness is absorbed, and sense-mind, will-mind and intellect are also absorbed, and the undifferentiated conscious 'Substance' of the sense-consciousness is spiritually transformed into highly rarefied superconsciousness. This is the stage of superconscious concentration. The Supreme Spirit is 'seen' through superconsciousness. When superconsciousness is also absorbed in supreme concentration, what remains is infinite Brahman. At this stage, there is neither sense-consciousness, nor nonconsciousness, nor superconsciousness; it is neither a conscious state, nor an unconscious state, nor any intermediate state. The reality remaining in this state 'cannot be seen, as it is beyond the senses; it cannot be "taken", as it is

beyond the reach of the volitive faculties; so it is hidden in everyday life; it is without any attributes, and beyond thoughts and, therefore, unidentifiable; it is only the being of Supreme Consciousness where all creativity and the manifested universe have come to nothingness; it is that Supreme Reality which is one and the whole; that is to be known' (—Mandukyopanishad, 1.7).

The absorption of sense-consciousness in concentration is the principal part of layayoga, as the attainment of samadhi entirely depends on it. Aditya said: 'The real chittakshaya (that is, the complete absorption of sense-consciousness), which is superconscious in nature, is yoga' (—Akshyupanishad, 2.3). The absorption of sense-consciousness is associated with the absorption of the senses, sense-mind, will-mind and intellect. This absorption is not the dark state of the mind. It brings into being that consciousness which is divinely illuminated. This is superconsciousness.

The process of absorption, technically termed here apañchikarana ('dis-quintuplication') has been described as follows: The 'earth'-form is absorbed in the 'water'-form (in concentration); 'water'-form in 'fire'-form, 'fire'-form in 'air'-form, 'air'-form in 'void'-form, 'void'-form in I-consciousness (which includes sense-consciousness, intellect, will-mind and sense-mind), I-consciousness in the mahan-principle (superconsciousness), mahan in awyakta, that is prakriti (primus) and awyakta in purusha (disembodied consciousness principle) (—Paingalopanishad, 3.6).

It has been said: 'That Brahman in the creative aspect is Indra, that is, endowed with the great yoga power, and is Prajapati—the first being with attributes; all the dewatas—super-beings, the five mahabhutas (metamatter) and all beings, including those which are produced from eggs, which are viviparous, insects, plants, other animals and men—and their sources—all are absorbed in the superconscious knowledge; superconsciousness is the centre of the absorption of all these and lokas (worlds). Superconsciousness is illuminated by Brahman' (—Aitareyopanishad, 3.1.3).

Here the secret of absorption has been disclosed. In relation to mind-matter phenomena, Brahman, with its Supreme Power, is in the creative aspect. The universe and all beings are the manifestation of the creative force of Brahman. The lokas are the chakras—the sites of sensory and mental functions. The mahabhutas and tanmatras and the sense-principles are in the lower five centres. Consciousness and mental functions are in the upper centres. Consciousness becomes limited when it is a field of perceptivity, intellection and volition. This consciousness is nurtured by the penetration into it of the objective substances lying outside it. When the sense-principles and sense-mind are absorbed in concentration, this consciousness becomes a non-being, not by becoming non-consciousness but by being transformed into prajñana, that is, superconsciousness. When the sense-consciousness becomes inoperative, the picture of the external world vanishes. Therefore, the absorption of sense-mind, sense-consciousness, intellect and will-mind creates a state of consciousness which is beyond all these. It is now prajñana—superconsciousness which is super-refined and illuminated by divine light.

There is a Waidika process of absorption, termed 'Ekadhanawarodhana', meaning, Prana (bio-energy) –Control (—Koushitakyupanishad, 2.2). The sensory functions of the mind are based on the functioning of the bio-energy in the body. The concentrated state of consciousness is difficult to attain without the control of bio-energy. It is the process of developing concentration causing absorption of cosmic principles in which bio-energy-control plays an important role.

First, the five sensory forms should be reduced to their right mantra-forms with which are linked appropriate dewatas (deities). With the help of the mantras, the senses should be absorbed in concentration in the deities. Thereafter, the deities are dissolved in the central dewata in the form of Kundalini, aroused by the absorption of pranic forces in pranayama, while in concentration. After this, the sense-consciousness and, finally, superconsciousness are absorbed into Kundalini.

It has been said: 'From mind void-form, from void-form air-form, from air-form fire-form, from that water-form and from that earth-form, and from that in turn the entire universe and all beings have been manifested. (Beyond all there is) Brahman—the undecaying, immortal, immutable and whole reality. By controlling the prana-apana bio-forces, spiritual light should be ignited in the mind in deep concentration; this will lead to the attainment of Brahman' (—Sannyasopanishad, 4.6).

At the sensory level, our consciousness is in union with the sensory objects through the functioning of the senses. This contact is completely broken when consciousness is in union with that luminous Kundalini, radiating spiritual knowledge. This union is effected in stages. By appropriate practice, in which pranayama forms an intrinsic element, the consciousness is irradiated by the Kundalini-light and the mind is spiritually strengthened. Such a mind is able to display desireless will, by which concentration is maintained and developed to a deep form. Now it is possible to get the senses and sensory objects absorbed in deep concentration. When all the the senses and sense-mind are absorbed, consciousness is transformed into superconsciousness. Finally, infinite supreme Brahman is reached by getting superconsciousness absorbed into Kundalini. It is an ancient Waidika process of absorption in concentration.

It is stated: 'There is in the void of the mind a reality which is birthless, one and eternal. That Narayana—the Supreme Spirit, takes the forms of earth, water, fire, air and void and lives within them as a living being, but they do not know him; he is in the forms of sense-mind, sense-consciousness, intellect and I-feeling, abiding in them as a living being, but they do not know him; he is in the forms of awyakta (prakriti) and akshara (Supreme Being with attributes), and is in them as a living being, but they do not know him; and he is in the form of dissolution, lying in it, but it does not know him. He is the Supreme Spirit, lying within all beings; he is without impurities; he is divine being and one and luminous by his own splendour; he is Narayana—Supreme Consciousness' (—Adhyatmopanishad, 1–1).

Here the process of absorption has been described. Unless all the cosmic principles are absorbed, Narayana is not reached, though he is in everything in his supreme aspect. The first part of the process consists in the absorption of the sensory principles by stages. The second part is the absorption of sense-consciousness with sense-mind, intellect and I-ness. The third part is the absorption of prakriti and God in divine form. And finally, there is the recoiling of that grand power—Kundalini, who has absorbed into her everything, into Narayana—Supreme Being.

About the process of absorption it has been stated that: 'The earth-form is the heart of all smell (that is, the smell principle); water-form is the heart of all tastes; fire is the heart of all forms; air is the heart of all touch; void is the heart of all sounds; awyakta (primus) is the heart of all mental powers; mrityu (that is, the central spiritual power causing absorption) is the heart of all beings; (after absorption of all principles) mrityu becomes one and the same with the Supreme Being. Thereafter, there is neither being of anything nor nonbeing of anything, nor anything which is beyond being or nonbeing of anything. This is nirwana—liberation' (—Subalopanishad, 7.13.2).

The smell principle is intimately related to and supported by the earth form. The centre of the earth-form is the right place for the absorption of the smell principle. Similarly, the appropriate centres for the absorption of the taste, sight, touch and sound principles are the centres of the water, fire, air, and void forms. The senses should be absorbed in these centres stage by stage. Then the mind with all its powers or faculties should undergo negativity. Thereafter, mrityu (death) which is the heart of all beingness becomes united, as Kundalini, with Supreme Consciousness.

This is the picture of the Waidika process of absorption. The essential part of this process has been adopted in Tantrika layayoga.

Tantrika Form of Layayoga

The outer objective world is the effect of the materialization of the cosmic metamatter energy, existing in subtle form, which has its centres of operation in the individual organizations, and there is a senso-mental process which connects the external world with the individual inner world. The original cosmic energy principle in its inertia aspect is the root of the manifested phenomenon we call matter. Through the senso-mental process the outer world is brought into consciousness and is known. The price of acquiring senso-mental knowledge is the masking of spiritual knowledge. The latter arises in consciousness when it is not impurified and diversified by the penetration of sensory objects. The spiritualization of consciousness means the development of one-pointed consciousness. Unless the sensory principles are made inoperative by appropriate means, this cannot happen. The spiritual power is anti-multifarious and, consequently, is in the nature of concentratedness. The whole source of spiritual power in the individual organization is Kundalini—the coiled power.

Kundalini is the Supreme Power in her spiritual aspect. But when the eternal energy of the Supreme Power is directed towards assuming a finite form, Kundalini remains coiled, and mundaneness arises in consciousness. The method of arousing Kundalini and uniting her with Parama Shiwa—Supreme Spirit—is the essential part of layayoga. First of all, the aroused Kundalini moves towards the Supreme Spirit. This creates a spiritual flow to God in the consciousness, and, stage by stage, the various cosmic principles are absorbed into Kundalini. Then the spiritual consciousness itself is absorbed into Kundalini, and ultimately Kundalini herself is absorbed into Supreme Spirit. The awakening of Kundalini and the spiritualization of consciousness through the absorption of various cosmic principles stage by stage is the process of concentration of layayoga. That form of concentration, in which consciousness is completely free from nonspiritual elements by absorption, and is fully illuminated by the luminous Kundalini, is the highest stage of samprajñata samadhi (superconscious concentration). Thereafter, Kundalini absorbs the spiritual consciousness and finally she herself is absorbed into Supreme Spirit;

it is the stage of *asamprajñata samadhi* (non-mens concentration). This is the Tantrika form of *layayoga*.

Angira said: 'Knowing the intimate relation between the cosmic objective phenomenon and the individual consciousness, the conduction of Kundalini towards the Supreme Being and her absorption in that in concentration is the third, that is *layayoga*' (—*Daiwimimangsadarshana*, 3.32). The unspiritual mutation of consciousness is due to the senso-mental radiations of the objective substance into consciousness, thus producing a state of mundaneness. The unspiritualization of consciousness comes to an end when the central coiled spiritual power is aroused and absorbs into itself, in deep concentration, all the senso-mental principles; and ultimately the aroused spiritual power is absorbed into the Supreme Spirit. The absorption process of concentration, first developed to a state of superconcentration, and finally to supreme concentration, is *layayoga*.

Shiwa has disclosed innumerable absorption processes for the attainment of *layayoga*. It has been stated: 'Krishna-dwaipayana and other yogis practised *layayoga* through absorptive concentration in the nine subtle centres' (—Yogarajopanishad, 4–5).

Deep concentration is in the nature of absorption in which all the creative principles are absorbed stage by stage as concentration becomes deeper. *Ishwara* said: 'A yogi should try to attain, in concentration, union between the embodied spirit and the Supreme Spirit. In concentration, all the cosmic principles should be absorbed, from the effect to the cause, in a reverse order, in Supreme Spirit. In this manner, the earth principle should be absorbed in the water principle, water in fire, fire in air, air in void, void in sense-mind, sense-mind in I-consciousness, I-ness to supermind, and supermind to prakriti (primus), and prakriti to Supreme Spirit in concentration' (—Gandharwa-tantra, ch. 11, p. 50).

As the fundamental part of *layayoga* is the arousing of Kundalini and the absorption of the various principles in Kundalini during her course through the different subtle centres, so this yoga is also called Kundaliyoga (—Rudraya-mala, Part 2, 41.42), and Kundaliniyoga (—Shaktananda-Tarangini, ch. 4, pp. 21, 28). This yoga has also been termed shatchakrayoga (—Rudrayamala, Part 2, 29.9), because the six subtle centres become involved in it.

Limbs of Layayoga

Tantrika *layayoga* consists of nine limbs or parts:

1 Yama, abstention.
2 Niyama, observance.
3 Sthulakriya, muscular control process.
4 Sukshmakriya, breath control process.
5 Pratyahara, sensory control.
6 Dharana, holding-concentration.
7 Dhyana, deep concentration.
8 Layakriya, absorption process (absorptive concentration).
9 Samadhi, superconcentration.

That *layayoga* is essentially based on the eightfold yoga, is clearly seen from its parts. The specific characteristic of *layayoga* is the absorption process. The other eight parts have been dealt with in chapter 1. But, from the *layayoga* viewpoint, some of these parts need special consideration.

Muscular Control Process

The muscular process consists in asana, i.e. posture, and mudra, i.e. control exercise. In *layayoga*, lotus posture (padmasana), auspicious posture (swastikasana), and accomplished posture (siddhasana) have been adopted for the practice of concentration and breath-control.

Eight control-processes (mudras) have been adopted in *layayoga*, namely, shambhawi, that is internal gazing; pañcha-dharana, that is five forms of holding-control; shaktichalana, that is internal power-conduction; and yoni-mudra, that is anogenital control. Shambhawi is practised, especially in relation to sensory control. The chief feature of shambhawi is concentration of the mind internally in the ajña centre, while the eyes can be kept open, but without seeing, or closed. By the practice of shambhawi, sensory control becomes easier.

The five forms of holding-control are practised for the mastery of dharana—holding-concentration. In this control, concentration is done with breath-suspension (kumbhaka) in the five lower centres on the earth-water-fire-air-void principles (one at a time) with the associated bija-mantras and deities. Shaktichalana and yonimudra are practised in connection with concentration in layayoga. Shaktichalana is the first part of the control exercise which culminates in yonimudra. Shaktichalana comprises the following factors: application of pressure on the perineal region by the heel of the left leg by assuming the accomplished posture (siddhasana), or by the heels of both legs by assuming the adamantine posture (wajrasana), anal lock (mula-bandha), abdomino-retraction (uddiyana-ban-dha), breath-suspension (kumbhaka) and thoracico-short-quick breathing (bhastrika). The execution of pressure and control in a definite order and at different points with breath-control helps much in the rousing of Kundalini and in her ascent. In hathayoga, shaktichalana has been combined with great control-posture (maha-mudra), great-lock (mahabandha), great piercing control (mahawedha), and chin-lock (jalan-dhara-bandha). In layayoga shaktichalana is the first stage of control and it assists yonimudra.

Yonimudra is performed as follows: assume the accomplished posture, with pressure on the perineum by the left heel and a pressure on the hypogastric region of the abdomen (the median region of the abdominal wall), by the right heel; now concentrate your mind on the muladhara centre, and inspire through both nostrils or through the mouth by making the lips resemble the beak of a crow, and at the same time contract the anus and genitalia forcefully and do abdomino-retraction; at the end of inspiration suspend the breath with chin-lock; during suspension of breath maintain the genito-anal contraction and abdomino-retraction, and hold in consciousness the luminous form of Kundalini in concentration; suspend as long as you can without too much strain, and then slowly expire and relax the neck muscles, abdominal muscles, and genito-anal region. Repeat. Yonimudra is practised to rouse Kundalini.

Breath Control Process

Breath control process is pranayama (breath-control). In layayoga sahita (breath-suspension with inspiratory-expiratory phases) has been specially adopted and developed into bhuta-shuddhi pranayama—internal purificatory breathing. This is the main breath-control in layayoga.

Ujjayi (both-nostrils breath-control) and shi-tali (lingual breath-control) are also practised. Another important breath-control practised in layayoga. is kewala (automatic breath-suspension) achieved by concentration. Purificatory breath-control will be discussed in chapter 6.

Concentration in Layayoga

In layayoga there are three main forms of concentration: thought-concentration, bindu-concentration and absorptive concentration.

Thought-concentration is generally practised in the bhutashuddhi process. There are also five special forms of thought-concentration which help in bhutashuddhi concentration. They are:

First Form—Concentration in the muladhara centre. This concentration has three forms—concentration on the earth principle with its colour and shape; concentration on the earth-bija; and concentration on Deity Brahma. This concentration is done with breath-suspension.

Second Form—Concentration with breath-suspension in the swadhishthana centre on (1) water principle, (2) water-bija, and (3) Deity Wishnu.

Third Form—Concentration with breath-suspension in the manipura centre on (1) fire principle, (2) fire-bija, and (3) Deity Rudra.

Fourth Form—Concentration with breath-suspension in the anahata centre on (1) air principle, (2) air bija, and (3) Deity Isha.

Fifth Form—Concentration with breath-suspension in the wishuddha centre on (1) void principle, (2) void-bija, and (3) Deity Sadashiwa.

Bindu-concentration is actually the concentration on the aroused super-luminous Kundalini. Concentration-on-bindu consists of two phases: first, the rousing of Kundalini by concentration combined with shaktichalana and yonimudra; and second, concentration on the roused Kundalini. When Kundalini is first aroused, it appears as if she were 'shaking' and consequently concentration is interrupted. By applying specific concentration on Kundalini in the ajña centre, she then appears steady and concentration becomes deeper and deeper. In deep concentration, Kundalini may assume the divine form of Ishtadewata—Supreme Being in form. When Ishtadewata is 'seen' in concentration, it becomes so deep that absorption follows.

Those who are not able to arouse Kundalini in bindu-concentration, should first practise thought-concentration in the following manner.

The object of concentration should be held in consciousness in concentration without any interruption and an attempt should be made to prolong concentration. Either assume the accomplished posture or the lotus posture for concentration. The objects of concentration are as follows:

1 Deity Brahma in the muladhara centre.
2 Deity Wishnu in the swadhishthana centre.
3 Deity Rudra in the manipura centre.
4 Deity Isha in the anahata centre.
5 Deity Sadashiwa in the wishuddha centre.
6 Deity Parashiwa in the indu centre.
7 Guru in the twelve-petalled centre under the thousand-petalled centre.
8 Extremely rarefied, lightning-like, luminous Kundalini in three and a half coils round Swayambhulinga in the muladhara.

The third is the absorptive concentration. This is the vital part of concentration in layayoga. When the aroused Kundalini is made steady by bindu-concentration, concentration develops into absorptive concentration, that is, concentration becomes so deep that it causes absorption of various creative principles. In this manner, consciousness is freed from all senso-mental activities, and consequently reaches a stage which is beyond all mentation. So, consciousness is transformed into superconsciousness by absorptive concentration and samadhi is attained.

In absorptive concentration the senses, sense-mind, sense-consciousness, and intellect, are absorbed step by step, into Kundalini, and consequently the cosmic strata of consciousness vanish. Now consciousness assumes a new character in which perceptivity, intellection, volitiveness and affectivity are not recorded. It is now in a divine form and in deepest concentration. It is the state of samadhi—superconcentration.

The following are the levels of absorptive-concentration.

First, absorption of sex and smell principles; absorption of earth principle with its bija; and absorption of Deity Brahma and Power Dakini—all into Kundalini in the muladhara centre.

Second, absorption into Kundalini of excretion and taste principles; water principle with its bija; Deity Wishnu and Power Rakini in the swadhishthana centre.

Third, absorption into Kundalini of locomotion and sight principles; fire principle with its bija; Deity Rudra and Power Lakini in the manipura centre.

Fourth, absorption into Kundalini of prehension and touch principles; air principle with its bija; Deity Isha and Power Kakini in the anahata centre.

Fifth, absorption into Kundalini of speech and sound principles; void principle with its bija; Deity Sadashiwa and Power Shakini in the wishuddha centre.

Sixth, absorption into Kundalini of Power Hakini; and sense-mind in the ajña centre.

Seventh, absorption into Kundalini of sense-consciousness in the manas centre.

Eighth, absorption into Kundalini of intellect in the indu centre.

The absorption of sense-mind, intellect, and sense-consciousness into Kundalini occurs in the ajña, manas and indu centres. This is the last phase of absorption at the senso-mental level. Thereafter Kundalini passes into the thousand-petalled centre and consciousness becomes Mahan—superconsciousness in which superconscious concentration arises and the whole consciousness is lighted by the luminous Kundalini. There is nothing but Kundalini. This is the stage of samprajñata samadhi. At this stage absorptive-concentration is transformed into superconscious concentration. It is the fourth stage of concentration.

At the highest stage of superconscious concentration, superconsciousness is absorbed into Kundalini. Then Kundalini unites with Parama Shiwa—Supreme Consciousness and becomes one and the same with that. This is the state of asamprajñata samadhi. In layayoga, it is called Mahalaya—supreme absorptive concentration.

CHAPTER 3
Kundalini — the Coiled Power

It is not possible to say that Truth in its supreme form, which is the ultimate reality, 'is this and not that'. But through memory, the revealed truth can be transferred to the highly rarefied intellectual level where it takes a meaningful sound form—the spiritual language; and through this language, the seers have said:

Parama Shiwa—Supreme God—is Nishkala, that is, in which Shakti (Power) remains unmanifested. At this stage, Shiwa is not separate from Shakti and Shakti is not separate from Shiwa. In other words, when Shakti has been completely united with Shiwa, she has no separate entity, Shakti is all Shiwa, it is the stage of Nishkala Shiwa. The beingness of Shiwa is maintained by Shakti and Shakti belongs to Shiwa. This indicates the beingness of Shakti is in the beingness of Shiwa. So Shiwa is alone, one and without a second. This means that in Supreme Shiwa there is nothing but Shiwa; there is no universe but only Shiwa; even the Supreme Power does not exist as a distinct entity, her beingness is in Shiwa.

Is Shiwa then void—nothing? No! It is not. Shiwa is all, there is nothing else but Shiwa. Shiwa is full, perfect; how can there be anything else in the being of Shiwa? Shiwa is the only being, because he is all; anything else is null in the beingness of Shiwa. Because of this, anything which is limited does not exist in Shiwa, and so he is infinite, and in infinite Shiwa there cannot be anything but he.

What is the nature of the beingness of Shiwa? It is beyond the senses and intelligence; it is even beyond superknowledge arising from super-concentration. When the functions of the senses, sense-mind and intelligence completely stop owing to the operation of supercontrol, superconscious knowledge arises from the calm and one-pointed consciousness. Even this knowledge appears to be too gross in relation to supreme knowledge of Shiwa; so it does not reach Shiwa. The supermind (mahan manas) which is super-purified and illuminated by super-light of samadhi, appears to be much coarser than Supreme Consciousness. When superconsciousness is dissolved by the control developed to its highest point, then a state of mental negativity arises. This non-mental state is neither darkness nor nothingness. It is the state of Supreme Consciousness—the disembodied Consciousness at its highest level.

Knowledge of the world cannot penetrate into concentrated superconsciousness, because this knowledge is associated with the oscillatory form of consciousness. Also the most rarefied concentration-knowledge (samadhi prajña) is below the non-mental supreme knowledge which exists only in the form of Shiwa. The highest stage of one-pointedness of consciousness is samadhi—superconcentration. In this state, prana (power principle), functioning in relation to mind, becomes concentrated and, as a result, mind is transformed into supermind. The supermind is illuminated by superconscious light (prajñaloka) arising from superconcentration in which pranic concentration by supercontrol has reached a very high degree. This is the state of superconscious concentration. But when this pranic concentration reaches its supreme limit, then prana assumes a form technically called Bindu. At this stage superconscious knowledge disappears and along with it, mind becomes a negative factor. This non-mental and supremely concentrated state of Power develops from supreme control. At this stage, power, as Supreme Power, is in supreme union with Shiwa.

In the real nature of the being of Shiwa is supreme control which, in turn, is non-mens supreme concentration, and this is in the nature of supreme union. This supreme control, supreme concentration and supreme union constitute Mahayoga—supreme yoga. Shiwa is in the nature of Mahayoga. The knowledge of Shiwa is beyond the superconscious concentration-knowledge, and, therefore, it is ultra-super-consciousness-knowledge, or non-mens supreme knowledge. It is the state of non-mens supreme concentration.

In the supreme union of Shiwa and Shakti, the being of Shakti is the being of Shiwa, as Shakti is an intrinsic part of Shiwa. This supreme union is in the nature of love and bliss. This love is supreme love and the bliss is supreme bliss. So, mahayoga (supreme yoga) is in the nature of supreme love-bliss. Shiwa in union with his Shakti is in supreme concentration through supreme control. Shiwa is in supreme yoga. This is Nishkala (power absorbed in) Shiwa and the Supreme Power is one and the same with him. This is the fifth (final) stage of supreme concentration (asamprajñata samadhi).

Nishkala Shiwa also appears as Sakala Shiwa when the power aspect is more pronounced, though Power remains as the being of Shiwa. At this stage, the beingness of Shiwa, which is the beingness of Supreme Power, is experienced as non-minded full consciousness and full bliss in supreme concentration. The yogi with the experience of full bliss-consciousness is established in non-mens concentration. This is the fourth stage of supreme concentration. This stage of full bliss-consciousness merges into supreme oneness of Shiwa and the Supreme Power as Nishkala Shiwa in supreme blissfulness and consciousness in Supreme concentration. This is the final stage of non-mens concentration.

The third is the Shiwa-Shakti level. At this stage Shakti—Supreme Power, is without her

specific powerfulness being manifested, but remains as yoga-power of Shiwa in his being. And still there is a suggestion that Supreme Power is also the source of specific power over and above the yoga-power. This is the third stage of supreme concentration. At this stage, the yogi experiences the full expression of the yoga-power of the Supreme Shakti in the being-ness of Shiwa with, as it were, a faint trace of specific power in the form of destruction of anything which is not non-mind-non-matter consciousness, in supreme concentration. Here is a suggestion that Shakti (Power) has two aspects: first, the yoga-power which is in full expression in the being of Shiwa when Shakti is Shiwa; second, the specific power which flows away from Shiwa and manifests in creativity. In the Shiwa-Shakti phenomenon, there is an expression of yoga-power and the unmanifesta-tion of creativity, but there is a faint trace of this.

The fourth phenomenon is Nada. At this stage, the specific power of Shakti, which was latent in the Shiwa-Shakti phenomenon, is aroused. The Nada-power is the germ of that great power which manifests as divine creative power to effect the universe of mind and matter. The specific power aspect of Shakti, which remains as non-being in Nishkala and Sakala Shiwa and hidden in the Shiwa-Shakti phenomenon, is aroused at the nada stage as prana, which is the origin of the great creative power. The pranic force is concentrated to its supreme degree in what is called Bindu, in which the supreme creative power is about to manifest. Bindu is the fifth phenomenon.

From the yoga viewpoint, the yogi being at the highest level of superconscious concentration, causes absorption of the highly purified super-mind and super-knowledge, and reaches the bindu level. It is the first stage of non-mens concentration. This non-minded concentration is not a state of deepest darkness. It is a stage in which prana is free from the 'cover' of the mind and supremely purified and concentrated to its highest degree. This concentration is so immense that, as it were, at any moment, prana might burst out and become scattered. The pressure of this motionless pranic power is so great that it seems as if the yoga-power is forced into Shiwa, where it remains and shines. But, in reality, the yoga-power is awakened at the bindu level and, step by step, its unfoldment occurs. The yogi at first experiences great difficulties in becoming established on the bindu level. The tremendously powerful pressure of the concentrated pranic force, causes him to descend. But, at the right moment, he is able to obtain the support of the yoga-power, which grows step by step and, at a certain point, exhibits supreme control, by which prana is controlled. When this occurs, the yogi reaches the nada level. This is the second stage of supreme concentration. Prana, being controlled by supreme control, is transformed into the nada form. Now the yoga-power develops to such an extent that the nada form is absorbed into Supreme Power. At this point the yogi reaches the Shiwa-Shakti level. This is the third stage of supreme concentration. Now the yoga-power develops to the supreme degree by which the yogi reaches the final stage of supreme concentration and his being is nothing but the being of Nishkala Shiwa.

Shiwa-knowledge is beyond the mind in any of its forms, and so it is non-mental, supreme consciousness. It comes into being at the bindu level. Its arousing is caused by the control of prana, which is supremely purified and without the contact of mind. This control is effected by the yoga-power in the form of supreme control. At the nada level, Shiwa-knowledge reaches its second stage of development. Supreme Power, due to the predominance of Shiwa-knowledge, absorbs prana in the nada form and begins to express yoga-power. Supreme Power in which prana has been absorbed exposes Shiwa by its yoga-power. This is the third stage of Shiwa-knowledge. The expression of full yoga-power is only possible when Supreme Power withdraws completely its specific aspect of power, and is established in the being of Shiwa as Shiwa. It is the fourth stage of Shiwa-knowledge revealing the sakala aspect of Shiwa. Finally, the sakala Shiwa-knowledge is transformed into Nishkala Shiwa-knowledge. This is the last stage. It is supreme control, supreme concentration and supreme union. This is supreme yoga.

Prana is a complex phenomenon. It is the principle of eternal energy embedded in Supreme Power. It is said: 'Dewatamayi Aditi came into being as prana and with the mind-matter' (—Kathopanishad, 2.1.7). Aditi is the unlimited Supreme Power who is dewatamayi, that is, whose being is the being of Shiwa—Supreme God. The specific power of Supreme Shakti (Power) is seen in the expression of that aspect of her power which is prana, and the mind-matter phenomena arise from pranic creativity. This is why it has been said: 'The entire universe, everything, arises from prana and is maintained by prana' (—Kathopanishad, 2.3.2). So 'All are established in prana' (—Prashnopanishad, 2.6).

The Supreme Power has two modes of existence. First, Supreme Power as Supreme Consciousness, when its power is expressed as supreme yoga-power and prana is coiled in Supreme Power-Consciousness and remains as Shiwa. So it is said: 'Prana is Brahman—Supreme God' (—Chandogyopanishad, 4.10.4). Second, Supreme Power in its specific power aspect, expresses its power as prana, which in highest concentration is bindu. It is in such concentration that, as it were, power will flow out of it. Here Supreme Power expresses its specific powerfulness. At this stage prana in the form of bindu is endowed with creativity. The manifestation of the creative phenomenon is the specificality of Supreme Shakti.

When the creative energy of prana is manifested, three primary attributes (gunas) are exhibited. The first is the primary energy-principle. This is rajas. The second is that principle which exhibits sentience in the form of concentration, knowledge, intelligence and thought. This is called sattwa (primary sentience-principle). The primary energy-principle as force-motion undergoes an inertial transformation. This is tamas (primary inertia-principle).

The supremely concentrated prana-force which occurs at the bindu level may, as it were, manifest itself at any moment. Before this manifestation, the three primary attributes—energy-principle, sentience-principle and inertia-principle—are zero factors. This is called prakriti (primary creative principle)—a state of negativity. But along with the first manifestation of creative energy the three fundamental principles undergo a state of relativity 'desired' by Supreme Power-Consciousness. Supermind arises from the primary sentience-principle; I-ness, intellective mind, sense-consciousness, will-mind, sense-mind and five senses from sentience-energy principles; conative faculties from inertia-energy-sentience; and tanons, supermatter and matter from the inertia-principle.

Now the point is this: how can the universe of mind-matter arise from infinite and supreme Shiwa in which there is nothing but Consciousness, and even the Supreme Power of Shiwa is in the being of Shiwa as Shiwa-Consciousness? How can a finite phenomenon be present in what is infinite? On the one hand, Supreme Power in the form of yoga-power, is in the being of Shiwa as Shiwa; on the other hand, Supreme Power possesses that energy which is specific in nature—the prana-energy endowed with creativity. The Supreme Shakti has the capacity of manifesting the creative energy as the universe; and when she is doing so, she is also expressing her specific power Maya (negato-positivity), by which the appearance of the universe has been possible. Maya exhibits an unusual power by which a phenomenon which is unreal is made to manifest in infinite Shiwa; but, in reality, this does not exist in Shiwa. In other words, the universe does not exist in the being of Shiwa; the universe is not a fact in the Shiwa-Knowledge. The universe exists only in the knowledge of an embodied being (Jiwa). The embodied being is an accomplishment of Maya who is capable of making the impossible possible. It is that power of maya by which a limitedness has been attributed to what is limitless. In this way the universe has been made possible.

Prana, which is endowed with the power of creativity, is first aroused at the nada level. It becomes supremely concentrated in the bindu-form. This concentrated bindu-power is in the nature of Kamakala—the power of actualizing the 'desire' to create; and consists of fifty sound-emitting energy-units in substance. At a certain moment, prana unfolds and its energy is manifested as pranawa-nada (the sound of Ong), in which there is a summation of fifty

manifested mantra-sound units (matrika), and from which the universe of mind and matter emerges.

Now from the yoga viewpoint—the yogi who has been established in the superconscious field through superconscious concentration is endowed with that consciousness which is without sensory objects and without I-ness. When this concentration develops to its highest level, the yogi's superconsciousness is absorbed in prakriti, and as a result a stage of mental negativity is reached. Then the yogi passes from this stage to the bindu-level. Here the yogi first experiences non-mens supreme concentration.

The phenomena of mind and matter are the expression of the great creative power of Ishwara —God. Shiwa—the supreme God who is with both yoga-power and prana-energy at the bindu-level, appears as supremely powerful Ishwara in creation. In him yoga-power and prana-energy are in harmony. He is in samadhi because of his yoga-power, and also the creator of the universe because he is endowed with prana-energy. Prana-energy is fully under his control by his yoga-power. The embodied being does not play any role in the creation of the universe of mind-matter, because he has no Godly power of creativity. The prana-energy is uncontrolled and yoga-power is almost dormant in him. He is the possessor of only small power.

What is the nature of the embodied being? It is that organized life-sentience which is supported by I-ness with the help of senso-mental and intellectual consciousness in which perceptivity and intellection are the main forms of knowledge, and that knowledge is limited; and in that organized life-sentience, prana-energy is limited and yoga-power is feeble, and, consequently, it is without super- or non-mens knowledge; and all knowledge appears as non-Shiwa; this is the embodied being.

Ishwara manifests his great creative power as Brahma (God as creator), sustains the universe as Wishnu (God as sustainer), and absorbs the universe as Rudra (God who absorbs the universe). And that Ishwara, remaining beyond the manifested universe, is in samadhi as Narayana (God in his supreme aspect). As the embodied being is endowed with small power, he can create only very limited things. He cannot create mind-matter but can play a little in the mental and material fields. Because of his limited knowledge, the embodied being is unaware of his Shiwa-being, and even Ishwara remains unknown to him. The prana-energy is functioning in him in a very limited manner, and it is uncontrolled and wastes away before its appropriate time.

From bindu to matter, the flow of power has two forms—the prana-flow and the yoga-power-flow. In creation, the prana-flow is very strong and away from Shiwa, and the yoga-power-flow, which is directed toward Shiwa, is very feeble.

The embodied being is controlled by the Kañchukas (the powers of limitation). The kañchukas are the specific powers of maya. They are five in number: Kala (time principle), Niyati (regulatory principle), Raga (pleasure principle), Widya (knowledge principle) and Kala (life principle). The prana-energy which is functioning in the embodied being is limited by time, and controlled by the regulatory principle. His mind is full of desires due to the influence of the pleasure principle, and his knowledge and power are limited. His knowledge is essentially based on worldliness, and in it God remains unknown. The love-feeling which is flowing in him is a restricted and perverse expression of supreme blissfulness which is in Supreme Power, and is experienced by him as pleasure, which is often associated with pain and is the source of desires. The prana-energy in the form of life-force makes him a living and conscious being. By the influence of time his life is only of short duration.

Life in the embodied being is a limited expression of prana-energy, and is maintained by the five-fold function of prana. These are: pranana, which supports the other four functions; apanana, causing energy to operate centrifugally; udanana, causing energy to operate centripetally; samanana, which causes equilibrium among other force-motions; and wyanana, which causes energy to move in all directions. Life in the body and sentience of the mind depend upon these functions. Prana as wayu has three fields of operation—the force-field where the different forms of bio-energy are in operation; the matter-field where bio-energies operate in relation to the body; and the mind-field where the operation of bio-energies results in different mental functions.

In the force-field, the fundamental action of bio-energy occurs through ida and pingala. These two force-motion lines are not like tubes or wires through which bio-energy passes. Force-motion lines are not material things. They are merely directions, forming, as it were, invisible lines. Bio-energy flows mainly through white and red lines. Activities and consumption of energy occur through red line; and control of activities and accumulation of energy take place through the white flow. In the body, the red flow causes catabolism, and the white flow anabolism. In the mind, the red flow causes mental diversity and restlessness, and the white flow makes the mind calm, attentive and reflective.

Pleasure which we experience in everyday life is the semblance of supreme bliss associated with the being of Shiwa. Man experiences pleasure in his creative activities, even though they are limited in nature. In the mental field, man creates material and spiritual sciences. He also experiences much pleasure in the building of his body. The life-force, having limited expression in the body due to the influence of the time and regulatory principles, causes growth and development of the body only for a certain limited time, and thereafter gradual decline and finally death. It is possible for man to develop great physical strength and prolong youth by appropriate methods, but senility cannot be altogether prevented, and death is inevitable. This is why eternal youth and life remain as dreams.

Begetting a new being is the highest form of creativity of the embodied being, by which the race is perpetuated. The procreative power is usually plentiful in all beings. Great intelligence plays no part in it, though there is room for constructive thoughts in this matter for man. For procreation it is not necessary to have a highly developed and strong body, though health and vitality are very helpful. And above all, the highest pleasure is experienced in the enjoyments of this kind. Procreation is a natural fact in life; but the enjoyment, which is inseparably associated with it, is also a natural fact. It appears that in the procreative act enjoyment is the primary factor and begetting children is secondary. Experience shows that hunger for this enjoyment persists after the loss of procreative power. We also find that conception usually occurs after many such enjoyments. The object of creativity is fulfilled by having one child through many enjoyments. The pleasure experience drives the two sexes again and again to perform this act, and under all circumstances. Is this natural enjoyment of pleasure ugly, shameful and unspiritual? We also find so many artificially continent persons.

The most intensified desire, and the love associated with it, in sexual enjoyment cause violent agitations of the mind and body. The infatuated mind finally becomes absorbed in deep lust-love in enjoyment; and the whole body takes part in it and helps the mind to experience the greatest pleasure by bringing about consummation. Thereafter, there is contentment and relaxation.

Adamantine Control

The yogi sees that the yoga-power is involved in sexual enjoyment. He sees that the highly excited mind becomes fully absorbed in deepest pleasure by abandoning other thoughts. This mental absorption has been possible by the aroused powers of control and concentration through intensified lust-love in enjoyment. In the body, the retentivity aroused by control plays an important role in enjoyment. According to yoga, yoga-power is expressed naturally in enjoyment to a certain extent, and it is possible to utilize it for developing concentration. The yogi is able to get sexual desire absorbed in the mantra 'Kling' by a special process, and to be in a state of concentration.

The yoga-process consists in two main forms— sight-process and touch-process.
Sight-process—Concentration with sound-pro-

cess (japa) while seeing the desire-provocative points.
Touch-process—Concentration with sound-process while in contact with desire-provocative points. It has several stages: (1) with close contact; (2) with slight contact; (3) with direct contact—passive; (4) with direct contact— dynamic.

Dynamic contact becomes effective when ujjayi kumbhaka (both-nostrils breath-control) in combination with uddiyana (abdomino-retraction) and mulabandha (anal lock) is incorporated. At the final stage of enjoyment, the sexual desire, concentrated to its highest degree, is absorbed in the mantra-sound 'Kling' in the triangular process of the muladhara by concentration combined with sound-process; and this results in the development of a state of deep concentration. In this state, Kundalini, who is in yoga-sleep (superconcentration) in the triangle, is aroused and extends herself from muladhara to ajña. Then Kundalini comes to the sahasrara, and superconscious concentration is attained. Finally, Kundalini proceeds still further and is absorbed in Parama Shiwa— Supreme Being in non-mens supreme concentration.

This adamantine control process is extremely difficult and many practitioners are unable to execute it successfully. Unless the force aroused in the strongest desire is converted into spiritual concentration by control, Kundalini will not be aroused. This is why it is very necessary to prepare oneself by bhutashuddhi (purificatory thought-concentration). Now we have to study the nature of Kundalini.

Kundalini

'Kundalini' and 'Kundali' are both Waidika and Tantrika terms. They have been used extensively and are widely known. They are synonyms. Kundalini has one thousand and eight names (—Rudrayamala, Part 2, 36.6–192), and each name signifies her specific character. The word Kundalini is from kundala, meaning circular or spiral or coil. Kundalini is that power which is circular, or spiral, or lies in coils. The meaning of Kundali is the same.

It is stated: 'Kundali is a power' (—Yoga-kundalyupanishad, 1.7). Also, 'Kundali power lies in eight coils above the Kanda point' (—Yoga-chudamanyupanishad, 36); 'Here, i.e., in the triangle in muladhara, lies Kundalini—the supreme power' (—Yogashikhopanishad, 1.169); 'the yogis attain liberation when Kundalini power rises above the Kanda' (—Yogashikhopanishad, 6.55); 'here is Kundalini—the supreme power' (—Warahopanishad, 5.51); 'Kundalini power is in eight forms and in eight coils' (—Shandilyopanishad, 1.4.8). So, according to the Waidika viewpoint, expressed in the Upanishads, Kundalini or Kundali is the power. The Tantrika viewpoint is also the same.

It is stated: 'Shiwa (Supreme Being) is like a corpse without Kundali power' (—Gayatri-tantra, 3.131); 'Here lies Kundali power in a latent state, and is without form' (—Brihan-nilatantra, ch. 8, p. 62); 'Kundalini power is the Mother Goddess and lies in one hundred coils' (—Bhutashuddhitantra, ch. 16, p. 14); 'Pinda (basic force of the body) is Kundalini Power' (—Mundamalatantra, ch. 6, p. 10).

Now, the nature of Kundalini power should be investigated. It is stated: 'Lightning-like luminous and subtle Kundalini lies within it (muladhara); she is 'seen' in concentration, and as a result all sins are destroyed and liberation is attained' (—Adwayatarakopanishad, 5). So, Kundalini is subtle, that is, she has no material form, and she is super-luminous. Consequently, she is beyond the senses. But she is 'seen' or realized in concentration. This means, when the sense-consciousness is transformed into concentrated superconsciousness, it becomes illuminated by the luminous Kundalini. At this stage all worldliness vanishes and the yogi ultimately attains liberation. This indicates the spiritual nature of Kundalini.

It is stated: 'Kundali is in the form of eight coils around the eight cosmic principles. She remains veiled by encircling completely the entrance to brahmarandhra (passage to the sahasrara centre). When Kundali is coiled in this manner, the functioning of the life-force is

maintained, and, consequently, alimentary and other functions of the body are carried out. When the dormant and supremely splendorous Kundali is aroused by the control of bio-energy in combination with supra-heat-energy, she appears in the Hrit centre' (—Trishikhi-brahmanopanishad, Mantra Section, 63–65). This means that Kundali power remains in eight coils around each of the eight subtle centres from the muladhara to the indu, causing the manifestation of knowledge arising from the activation of five senses, sense-mind, sense-consciousness and intellect. This coiled state of Kundali also causes bio-energy and all organs of the body to function. The coil indicates the dormant phase of Kundali in which the spiritual consciousness remains unmanifested and the sense-consciousness is aroused. In this way, eight great creative principles are in operation. They are the five sense principles located in the lower five centres and the sense-mind, sense-consciousness and intellect in the upper three centres. In each centre there is a coil, and this makes a creative principle situated in an appropriate centre manifest in consciousness. So, Kundali is the spiritual power-consciousness. When she is in coils, spirituality remains hidden and worldliness comes into being. When Kundali is aroused from her coiled state, spiritual power and spiritual consciousness are manifested.

It is further stated: 'Very bright like ten million lightnings and extremely subtle like a lotus-filament, Kundalini is in that (i. e. the muladhara). There is the cessation of unspiritual knowledge. The "seeing" of Kundalini causes the destruction of all sins' (—Mandalabrahma-nopanishad, 1.2.6). Here also Kundalini is described as supremely luminous and subtle (without form). She is the central spiritual power-consciousness. When she is aroused, unspiritual knowledge and worldliness disappear.

About the coils of Kundali-power it is said: Kundali-power is of the form of eight coils above the Kanda; she is the cause of bondage for those who are unspiritual, and of liberation for the yogis' (—Yogachudamanyupanishad, 44). The coils of Kundalini cause bondage. The coils are the unmanifested spiritual power and consciousness. Consequently, eight coils release the senso-intellectual knowledge of an unspiritual character. This is the cause of bondage. But a yogi, by concentration, arouses Kundalini by causing her to uncoil and, ultimately, attains liberation. So, when Kundalini is coiled, spirituality is blocked, and when she is uncoiled, spirituality is manifested.

The two phases of Kundalini have been more clearly stated here: 'When the power in the muladhara (that is, Kundalini-power) is asleep (that is, coiled), the knowledge of the objective world appears due to sleep (that is, spiritual unconsciousness). When the power inherent in Kundalini is aroused, the true knowledge of the three worlds (that is, the spiritual knowledge at the three levels of mind, power and matter) is attained. He who has gained the knowledge of the muladhara (and Kundalini) goes beyond darkness' (—Yogashikhopanishad, 6.23-4). When Kundalini is in coils, the senso-intellectual knowledge is manifested, and when she is roused, spiritual knowledge appears. These are the two phases of Kundalini—coiled and aroused. The power aspect is intrinsic to Kundalini.

Highest spiritual knowledge arises when Kundalini-power is roused. It is said: 'The knowledge coming from the arousing of Kundalini and (the associated) state of actionlessness bring about automatically the sahaja state (samadhi)' (—Warahopanishad, 2.77). The arousing of Kundalini is associated with that spiritual knowledge which leads to samadhi. Therefore, Kundalini knowledge is the super-conscious spiritual knowledge which culminates in superconscious concentration.

It is said: 'Lightning is Brahman; as lightning removes the darkness in the sky, so Lightning-Brahman destroys the darkness of sins; he who knows Lightning-Brahman is able to remove sins which prevent the acquirement of Brahman' (—Brihadaranyakopanishad, 5.7.1). The lightning-like luminous Kundalini is Brahman, that is, the power of Supreme Being by which worldliness is removed. The luminous power inherent in Kundalini is in the nature of absorption. When Kundalini is aroused, her absorptive power is released in concentration, and all the creative principles are absorbed.

It is stated: 'Where (in the triangle of the muladhara) lies the supreme power called Kundalini' (—Yogashikhopanishad, 5.6). So, Kundalini is the Supreme Power. In other words, Kundalini is the spiritual aspect of Supreme Power, which is different from the creative aspect of Supreme Power. When Kundalini is manifested, the creative aspect is withdrawn and Supreme Power as Kundalini becomes united with Parama Shiwa and remains one and the same.

Let us now consider the Tantrika exposition of Kundali. It has been stated: 'Within the body is the muladhara and within the latter is a triangle which is the abode of luminosity (i. e. Kundalini). ... Within the void of the triangle which is as bright as ten million moons, lies Kundali—the Supreme Power-Consciousness (paradewata) who is splendorous like ten million suns, and as subtle as the lotus-filaments, and lies in three and a half coils' (Gayatritantra, 3.44-6). And also, 'The Supreme (para) Kundali is the only means to the attainment of Supreme Brahman; without Kundali all the universes are like a corpse (without spiritual life), and even Shiwa (Supreme Being) is like a corpse. She is eternal, and the fifty mantra-sound units are in her and she is Supreme Consciousness (purnawidya)' (—Gayatritantra, 3.130-1).

So Kundalini is formless and splendorous and lies in three and a half coils in the triangle of the muladhara. She is eternal, because she is with eternal Shiwa; she is Supreme Consciousness as she is supremely united with Shiwa and is one and the same with him. This is why it is said that Shiwa is like a corpse without her, that is, Shiwa is never without his power Kundalini. And through Kundalini only Supreme Being is reachable. Unless the human consciousness becomes fully illuminated by the spiritual light of Kundalini, Supreme Being is not realized. This is why she is called Parakundali—Supreme Kundali.

The Kundali power when unmanifested is in coils. So it is said: 'That power (i. e., Kundali) which is in the muladhara is coiled like a serpent' (—Matrikabhedatantra, ch. 3, p. 3). When Kundalini power is coiled, she is in a latent phase. It is stated: 'Kundali power is in a dormant state and without form' (—Brihannilatantra, ch. 8, p. 62). Kundalini remains coiled, that is, in a latent form, so long as our consciousness remains in an oscillatory state. Kundalini light is not reflected on the sense-consciousness. When Kundalini is not registered in our consciousness, owing to its being impure and multiformed, she remains coiled. When our consciousness is purified and in concentration, Kundalini power makes it spiritually illuminated by being uncoiled.

About the nature of Kundalini, it has also been stated that: 'Kundalini shines like ten million lightnings and is without form; she is with fifty mantra-sound units and mantras; she is endowed with thirty-eight forms of superpower (kala); she pierces the three knots (Brahma, Wishnu and Rudra granthis) and is in Muladhara; and she is all spiritual knowledge' (—Gandharwatantra, ch. 29, p. 112). Kundalini is formless, because she is not gross; she is only known in concentration as something very luminous. This luminosity is the spiritual knowledge-light which shines forth fully in concentration as the nature of Kundalini is all spiritual knowledge-power. She is the source of mantra power and through mantra she assumes an appropriate form and exhibits thirty-eight kinds of superpower.

Further exposition of Kundalini has been made in the following statements: 'Kundalini is as bright as ten million suns and as cold as ten million moons; ... she is without form and her being is the being of Supreme Being; ... she is in the nature of supreme yoga' (—Tararahasya, ch. 1, Shaktisara, p. 2). And: 'Sadashiwa (Supreme Being) is united with Supreme Kundalini' (—Bhutashuddhitantra, ch. 14, p. 12); 'Kundali is the root of all beings; she is divine and subtle, and she is all bliss and in the nature of consciousness; consciousness is she in the universe and is in the form of yoga' (—Rudrayamala, Part 2, 26.37–8); 'In the fire-light in the muladhara lies that living power Kundali, who is supremely luminous and endowed with eternal force; she is in a latent form in three coils' (—Tantrarajatantra, 30.64–5); 'In subtle form of dhyana (deep concentration), the knowledge of shakti (power) arises; the shakti is Supreme

Kundali who is in the nature of Supreme Consciousness' (—Shadamnayatantra, 5.388).

These statements have clearly expounded the nature of Kundalini. Kundalini is very luminous, but this luminosity is without heat, as she is also very cool like ten million moons. The implication is, that in deep concentration when consciousness, being free from restlessness and infatuation, becomes calm, uniform and one-pointed, it is then illuminated by splendorous Kundalini. The luminosity is not indicative of having any form, as she is formless. The luminosity is the spiritual light from Kundalini, glowing in concentration, by which consciousness is spiritualized. Kundalini is in the nature of eternal, living, spiritual power and consciousness. At the highest concentration of spiritual power, Kundalini becomes one and the same with Supreme Consciousness. Kundalini is the living spiritual power; not intellective or imaginative, but a real and most powerful entity in spiritual life. Consciousness is purified and completely spiritualized by the spiritual radiations from Kundalini. At the highest level of superconscious concentration, consciousness becomes wholly of Kundalini.

Kundalini is in supreme yoga, that is, in non-mens supreme concentration. This means that Kundalini as Supreme Consciousness is also in supreme concentration; Supreme Consciousness in any other form is an impossible phenomenon. It is a sealed book to those who are not in a state of supreme concentration. The nature of Kundalini is yoga, because consciousness associated with her is concentrated superconsciousness in which her form, as concentrated spiritual light, penetrates, and by which it is super-illuminated. At the highest level of superconscious concentration, the spiritually illuminated superconsciousness is finally absorbed into Kundalini herself, who is then in non-mens supreme concentration. This is why it has been said: 'Kundali is eternally the master of yoga' (—Rudrayamala, Part 2, 26.41). Kundalini power is the yoga-power. She is the source of yoga; so it is stated: 'We concentrate on Kundalini ... who is in the muladhara and all bliss and all yoga and the yoga-mother' (Rudrayamala, Part 2, 26.21). It is also stated that:

'Kundali is the bestower of yoga' (—Rudraya-mala, Part 2, 29.22). Yoga is attained through Kundalini.

Kundalini is called Mahakundalini. It is stated: 'Tripura is the primordial power; she is the Supreme Power; she is Mahakundalini; she also is in the triangle of the muladhara' (—Tripura-tapinyupanishad, 1.9). When Supreme Power is in her supreme spiritual aspect, she is Mahakundalini. In this aspect, Supreme Power as Mahakundalini is united with Supreme Shiwa; so it is said: 'Sadashiwa (Supreme Shiwa) is united with Mahakundalini (in the thousand-petalled lotus)' (—Bhutashuddhitantra, ch. 14, p. 12). She has been called Mahakulakundalini (—Rudrayamala, Part 2, 6.23), because Mahakundalini is also in the muladhara as Kulakundalini (—Rudrayamala, Part 2, 36.181) and Kulakundali (—Kubjikatantra, 1.54). Kundalini lies in the triangle within the muladhara, so she is called Trikonashakti (triangular power) (—Tripuratapinyupanishad, 1.10). Mahakundalini is also called Mahakundali (—Rudrayamala, Part 2, 36.6).

Kundalini-rousing

Kundalini lies in three fundamental forms. It is stated: 'Kundali is in three forms, viz., eternally conscious, latent, and in concentration (—Shadamnayatantra, 4.189). Kundalini as supreme spiritual power is also Supreme Consciousness; this is why she is never without consciousness. But Kundalini appears as unconscious when her spiritual power is not manifested and her spiritual consciousness does not penetrate into sense-consciousness, because of its impurity and many-pointedness. This is the latent form of Kundalini and she is in that form in the muladhara when consciousness is oscillatory owing to constant senso-mental radiations into it. But she is perpetually conscious in the sahasrara.

The latent form of Kundalini is actually the state of yoga-nidra (—sleep) in which all her power has been withdrawn into herself and she is supremely conscious of herself as Supreme Consciousness. The great rishi Atharwana said: 'From the practice of khechari mudra (an advanced control exercise) arises unmani (consciousness without oscillation) and from that yoga-nidra; when a yogi attains yoga-nidra, he goes beyond time' (— Shandilyopanishad, 1.7.17–1). Unmani is that state in which consciousness is free from all oscillations. It is the highest state of superconscious concentration which ultimately leads to yoga-nidra, that is, non-mens supreme concentration. Nidra means sleep, that is, a state in which consciousness becomes nonconsciousness. When sense-consciousness is transformed into super-consciousness, samprajnata yoga (superconscious concentration) is attained. When superconsciousness is coiled into Supreme Consciousness, it is the state of asamprajñata yoga (non-mens supreme concentration). As in sleep sense-consciousness is coiled into non-consciousness, so in asamprajnata yoga superconsciousness is completely coiled into Supreme Consciousness; therefore it is called yoga-sleep.

The only possibility of approaching Kundalini is when she is in a latent form in the muladhara. Only in muladhara, is it possible to arouse Kundalini from her yoga-sleep (samadhi) and get our consciousness illuminated with spiritual light. Her supreme conscious aspect is beyond sense-consciousness. But when she is in a latent form, sense-consciousness is not at all influenced by her. Because sense-consciousness is so im-purified and diversified by pleasure-seeking desires and enjoyments and all forms of worldliness, it is unable to receive spiritual light from Kundalini. The sensory mind is so strongly tied by various worldly principles that it cannot free itself unless those principles are removed by some other power. It has been so powerless by its strong attachment to worldly things that one cannot even think of abandoning them; rather one feels pain in being passionless. So long as this decontrolled mental state continues, Kundalini is naught. This state of affairs can only be overcome by the purification of the mind by abstention and observance and by the arousing of Kundalini.

The arousing of Kundalini is the process of the

spiritualization of consciousness. The aroused Kundalini manifests absorptive power by which all worldly principles are absorbed, and causes spiritual radiations into consciousness. In this way, the formation of all sensory pictures and thought-forms in consciousness are controlled and consciousness is illuminated by the spiritual splendour of Kundalini. Ultimately, consciousness becomes wholly of Kundalini, and then the spiritualized consciousness is absorbed into Kundalini, and Kundalini into Supreme Shiwa when supreme yoga is attained. So it is said: 'Bringing Kundalini power in the consciousness, and (then) consciousness (lighted by Kundalini) getting absorbed into Kundalini—in this manner transforming the multiform consciousness into a state of concentration, Shandilya, be thou happy' (—Shandilyopanishad, 1.7.18). When consciousness becomes fully of Kundalini by the absorption of all senso-intellectual forms by Kundalini, it is a state of superconscious concentration. Then, this superconsciousness is absorbed into Kundalini. This is the first stage of non-mens concentration. Finally, when Kundalini is absorbed into Supreme Consciousness, supreme yoga is attained.

The process of rousing Kundalini has two main forms—Waidika and Tantrika. Let us first consider the Waidika process.

Waidika Process of Kundalini-rousing

The process of rousing Kundalini mainly consists in concentration, breath-control (pranayama) and certain control exercises (mudras). Concentration is also done on aroused Kundalini in different chakras (subtle centres), the most important of which is the hrit centre at the region of the heart. It is stated: 'Hridaya (hrit centre) is like a lotus, hanging with its face downwards, and there is some sound phenomenon associated with the flow of life-energy. Within this centre is shining super-light, which appears vast and unrestricted. Within this super-light is luminescence which is subtle and aroused.

Within this luminescence lies Supreme Being' (—Mahopanishad, 1.12–14).

The hrit centre normally lies with its head downward. When the awakened Kundalini reaches it, the centre opens upward and is illuminated by a vast light within which is the formless and aroused luminous Kundalini. Within Kundalini is Supreme Consciousness. The rousing of Kundalini and its conduction into the hrit centre is the process of concentration. At the first stage, only a vast light is realized. At the second stage, when concentration becomes deeper, Kundalini is realized within that light. And, finally, when concentration is deepest Supreme Being is realized within Kundalini.

The seat of Kundalini in latent form is termed Kundali-sthana (seat of Kundali). It has been stated that the middle of the body is what is called kanda-sthana (perineal region), which is oval-shaped and the central part of which is called nabhi (centre). Therein lies a chakra (centre) having twelve spokes. Above the twelve-spoked centre which is above the horizontal line of nabhi is Kundali-sthana (Trishikhi-brahmanopanishad, Mantra section, 58–62). That is, at the central part of the perineal region, there is a twelve-spoked subtle centre (inside the coccyx), above which lies the seat of Kundalini (that is, in the muladhara).

It has been further stated: 'In the perineal region is the seat of light (shikhi-sthana), triangular in shape and shining like molten gold. ... It is situated two digits above the anus and two digits below the genitals. Two digits below from the centre is the seat of Kundali. That Kundali is in eight coils in relation to eight creative principles' (—Darshanopanishad, 4.1–2, 11). That is, the seat of Kundali is within a very bright triangle. The triangle is situated at the middle point of the perineum. The triangle containing the seat of Kundali is within the muladhara. This is why Kundalini is called Adhara-Shakti (Power in muladhara) (—Yogashikhopanishad, 6.23). The shining triangle at the perineal region is within the muladhara. It is stated: 'Muladhara is situated in the region (perineum) between the anus and the genitals and in it lies a triangle; ... where (in the triangle) lies

Supreme Kundalini Power' (—Yogashikhopanishad, 1.168–9). Therefore, the seat of Kundalini is within the triangle situated in muladhara. In this seat, Kundalini is in a latent form.

It is stated: 'In the posterior aspect of adhara (muladhara), the three nadis (pranic power-lines) (ida, pingala and sushumna) are united. . . . In adhara is Pashchima-Linga (that is, Linga situated behind in the triangle of muladhara and is called Swayambhu; Swayambhu-linga is Supreme Consciousness in a spiritual form) where lies the door (to the brahma nadi); one becomes free from all worldliness when this door is opened. In the posterior aspect of adhara, if the moon and sun (the ida and pingala flows) become still, there stands the Lord of the universe; the yogi becomes absorbed into Brahma in concentration. In the posterior aspect of adhara, there are different aspects of God in form. When inspiration and expiration through the left and right nostrils are controlled, the sushumna (central force-motion line) flow starts, and Kundalini is aroused and passes through the six chakras situated within the sushumna, and ultimately goes beyond brahmarandhra (the end point of brahma nadi, and consequently sushumna, to reach Sahasrara). Those who enter the brahmarandhra attain the highest spiritual state' (—Yogashikhopanishad, 6.30–4).

Here the arousing of Kundalini and her passing through the subtle centres have been described. In the posterior aspect of muladhara lies sushumna (fire-like central force-motion line) and there ida (white force-motion line) and pingala (red force-motion line) have been united with sushumna. There is the specific form of Shiwa (Supreme Consciousness) termed Pashchima-or Swayambhu-Linga, around which Kundalini is in coils. The door to brahma nadi is there. The entrance to sushumna is, as it were, in a collapsed state when Kundalini is in latent form. At this stage, the pranic force currents are creating ida and pingala flows, and as a result inspiration and expiration continue through the nostrils. By controlling inspiration and expiration by kumbhaka (suspension), the ida-pingala flows are stopped; and with the development of kumbhaka the entrance to sushumna is opened. Kundalini is also aroused by kumbhaka and enters sushumna, and, step by step, passes through all the chakras lying within the sushumna, and ultimately, passing through brahmarandhra—the end point of sushumna, reaches sahasrara.

Breath-control plays an important role in rousing Kundalini. When breath-suspension is developed to its highest point, it normally becomes non-inspiratory-non-expiratory suspension (kewala kumbhaka). Kundalini is awakened by this form of suspension. So it is stated: 'By kewala kumbhaka Kundalini is aroused' (—Shandilyopanishad, 1.7.13–15). But non-inspiratory-non-expiratory suspension is only possible when a yogi has ascended to the highest level of breath-control. The easier method is bhastra kumbhaka (thoracico-short-quick breath-control with suspension). It is stated: 'Bhastra kumbhaka causes the arousing of Kundali . . . and removes impurities and other unfavourable conditions in relation to the entrance to brahma nadi' (—Yogakundalyupanishad, 1.38). Moreover, 'The arousing of Kundali is effected by bhastra kumbhaka. . . . It also helps (Kundalini) to pierce the three knots; this breath-control should be specially practised' (—Yogashikhopanishad, 1.99–100).

To make breath-control effective, it is necessary to create a purified state in the force-field (nadi-chakra) for the forceful operation of prana. It has been stated: 'A yogi who is perfectly motionless in posture and is well-controlled and habitually taking a moderate and healthful diet, should practise left-inspiration-suspension-right-expiration and right-inspiration-suspension-left-expiration breath-suspension in the lotus posture to get the impurities in the sushumna nadi (central fiery red force-line) absorbed' (—Shandilyopanishad, 1.7.1). Here, sahita breath-control has been advised for its internal purificatory effects. The force-motion system (nadichakra) is purified and the sushumna flow occurs. So it is stated: 'When the force-motion system is purified by the right application of the control of prana (breath-control), bio-energy passes freely through sushumna; when this central vital flow occurs, the mind becomes calm and this leads to the state of deep concentration' (—Shandilyopanishad, 1.7.9–10). The central vital flow is very important for arousing and conducting Kundali power through sushumna. This is why sahita breath-control is the basic practice.

The control of apana is intimately related to the rousing of Kundalini. The apanic control is effected by anal-lock. It is stated: 'When the downward motion of apana is reversed by the powerful anal contraction, which is called mula-bandha, the apana-force reaches the heat-energy centre, heat-energy is stirred up, and then apana and heat-energy stimulate prana and the body is full of heat-energy. The coiled Kundalini, being excited by this heat-energy, is aroused and, like a beaten serpent, becomes uncoiled and animated, —and through the entrance passes into the brahma nadi' (—Yoga-kundalyupanishad, 1.42–6).

The entrance to sushumna, called Kundalini-kapata (door of Kundalini), is opened by anal-lock. It is stated: 'The yogi should pass through brahmarandhra by opening the door of Kundalini by (anal) contraction. The entrance to the sushumna path, through which the yogi has to pass, is covered by the sleeping and coiled Kundalini (that is Kundalini in latent form). He who is able to arouse that power (Kundalini), will attain liberation. If Kundalini sleeps above the throat (that is, if aroused Kundalini goes into the state of samadhi in Sahasrara), the yogi will be liberated; but it will cause bondage for spiritually ignorant persons, should Kundalini sleep below the throat (i.e., it is not possible to attain spiritual knowledge, if Kundalini remains in a coiled state in muladhara)' (—Shandilyopanishad, 1.7.36–1–36–3).

The process of arousing Kundalini consists mainly in breath-control, anal-lock and concentration. It is stated: 'A yogi endowed with the power of concentration can get sense-consciousness absorbed in sushumna and respiration under control. When impurities in the force-field are eliminated (by sahita breath-control) the pranic force flows towards the right directions (and with full strength); (under this condition) if the centrifugal bio-energy (apana) is made to flow upwards by forceful (anal-) contraction, termed mula-bandha, it radiates into the centre of central bio-energy (prana wayu), and then both these forces (prana and apana), together with heat-energy, radiate into the seat of Kundalini who is in a coiled form; Kundali is excited by fire-energy and aroused by the two forms of bio-energy (prana and apana), and passes into the sushumna. Then Kundali passes through the Brahma-knot arising from force-motion principle, and suddenly flashes like a streak of lightning in the sushumna.

'Then Kundalini passes upward and reaches the Wishnu-knot situated at the heart region (that is, the anahata centre); then (after passing through this knot) Kundali goes still higher and reaches the Rudra-knot situated in the space between the eye-brows (that is, the ajña centre), and then piercing through it, she goes into the moon-sphere (shitangshu-mandala) where the anahata centre lies with sixteen petals. (According to the Tantras, this centre is called indu and has sixteen petals.)

'Then Kundali absorbs the eight creative principles arising from the negativity principle (prakriti) and goes to her own abode (that is sahasrara), and finally becomes united with Shiwa (Supreme Consciousness) and is absorbed into him. At this stage prana and apana, which are functioning together, are neutralized, and breathing is normally suspended' (—Yoga-kundalyupanishad, 1.62–69, 74–75).

Here, the process of arousing Kundalini and her conduction through sushumna and her absorption into Shiwa (Supreme Consciousness) has been explained. It is a highly complex process. The first part of the process consists in the control of apana by kumbhaka (breath-suspension) in conjunction with anal-lock and concentration. The controlled apana ceases its normal activities and exhibits its super-function by which the fire-principle represented by 'Rang' (mantra) is excited, thus causing radiations of subtle fire-energy. The fire-energy and reversed apana-force stimulate prana to exhibit its hidden power. Now, the apana and prana forces under the power of control are transformed into a concentrated energy, and are represented by the mantra 'Yang'. By the right application of 'Rang' and 'Yang' in kumbha-ka, these forces radiate on the coiled Kundalini, and are absorbed into her, who is then aroused.

The kumbhaka will not be forceful enough unless it operates in a purified force-field. This force-purification (nadi shuddhi) is effected by sahita breath-control combined with internal cleansing and purificatory diet.

The aroused Kundalini, who appears splendorous, passes through the sushumna, first by piercing the Brahma-knot situated in muladhara, and then breaking through the Wishnu-knot in anahata and, finally, passing through the Rudra-knot in ajña, reaches the moon-centre. When Kundalini passes through different centres in the sushumna, she exhibits her absorptive power by which the main creative principles, viz., five sensory principles, sense-mind, sense-consciousness and intellect are absorbed. After the absorption is complete, Kundalini reaches sahasrara and, finally, is united with and absorbed into Shiwa—Supreme Consciousness. This is the stage of asampranata samadhi—non-mens supreme concentration. At this stage there is a natural suspension of animation. This supreme state is supreme bliss. So it is stated: 'This is the supreme state, full of supreme bliss' (—Yogakundalyupanishad, 1.87).

It has further been stated: 'Kundali who is in eight coils should be aroused by breath-suspension carried to a high level according to the process of shakti-chalana (power-conduction). The arousing of Kundali is done while performing anal-contraction (during breath-suspension) ... Assuming the wajrasana (adamantine posture), the upward contraction (i.e., anal-contraction) should be practised regularly. The fire-energy ignited by bio-energy (that is, the upward apana stimulates the fire-energy in breath-suspension with anal-contraction) radiates into Kundali; thus being "heated", she becomes awakened. Then she enters into chandra-danda (brahma nadi) lying within the sushumna, and pierces through the Brahma-knot with (concentrated) bio-energy and "fire". Then Kundali passes through the Wishnu-knot and reaches where the Rudra-knot is, and there she stays. The Rudra-knot is pierced through by repeated sahita breath-suspension carried to a high level' (—Yogashikhopanishad, 1.82–7).

After the Rudra-knot is passed through, Kundalini assumes more the nature of Shiwa (Supreme Consciousness). Then inspiration-expiration is neutralized and non-inspiratory-non-expiratory suspension (kewala kumbhaka) follows. Normally, at this stage, the supreme union of Shiwa and Shakti (Kundali) takes place in supreme concentration (—Yogashikhopanishad, 1.115–17).

The process, by which Kundali power is conducted from her seat—muladhara—to the space between the eyebrows, that is ajña, is called shakti-chalana—power-conduction. This process essentially comprises breath-suspension and a special process termed saraswati-chalana (-motion). Kundalini is aroused by breath-suspension and saraswati-motion. The following is the saraswati-motion process: Assuming the lotus posture, breath-suspension is done after inspiration through the left nostril, and at the same time throat-contraction (i.e. jalandhara-bandha—chin-lock), abdominal retraction and anal-contraction are executed. During breath-suspension, the central abdominal muscle (rectus abdominis) should be rolled (in nauli form) from the right to the left and from the left to the right again and again. Expiration should be done through the right nostril (—Yogakundalyupanishad, 1.7–16). The saraswati-motion is an extremely complicated process and should be learnt directly from a guru.

There is an advanced Waidika process of awakening Kundalini. It consists, first, in the execution of throat-contraction (chin-lock), powerful anal-contraction and the pressing of the laryngeal region with the fully elongated and retroverted tongue (that is, tongue-lock), assuming the siddhasana; and then the awakened Kundali should be conducted by wajra-kumbhaka (the special form of breath-suspension used for the conduction of Kundali in different centres and to pierce through the knots) until she passes through the moon-sphere (indu centre) and reaches sahasrara (—Brahmawidyopanishad, 72–5).

The great yogi Dattatreya expounded to his disciple Sankriti an advanced Waidika process of awakening Kundalini. He said: 'Pressing the perineum with the right or the left heel and placing the opposite heel on the other ankle (that is, assuming the siddhasana with a heel set against the perineum to exert strong pressure on it), (being seated in this manner) the yogi should draw in air through the urethra (by special pranayama), using the pranawa mantra, and then he should concentrate the force (developed from the most powerful ano-perineal contraction, thus causing the strong upward motion of apana) on (the triangle of) muladhara. Fire, being kindled by wayu (apana), arouses Kundali' (—Darshanopanishad, 6.38–42).

Here, a special pranayama (breath-control) has been explained. This pranayama causes the urethral suction of air when applied in conjunction with very powerful anal and perineal contraction. The pranayama together with ano-perineal contraction causes the upward motion of apana and is concentrated in the triangle of muladhara. The concentrated apana stimulates fire-energy there, and fire-energy, together with apana, arouses Kundalini.

Tantrika Process of Kundalini-rousing

Real spiritual knowledge does not arise if Kundalini is not aroused; the mantra-flame is not ignited if Kundalini remains coiled. It has been stated: 'In muladhara lies that power (Kundali) which is in the form of a serpent (that is coiled). When that power is aroused, (its coil is changed into) circular motion and then with radiating mantra-sound she goes to her own abode (that is sahasrara) through brahmarandhra ... where the absorption of mind takes place' (—Nilatantra, ch. 10, p. 28). The coiled Kundalini is Kundalini in latent form. The coil is uncoiled in a circular motion when she is aroused. The roused Kundalini passes through brahma nadi to the sahasrara where the absorption of mind takes place in samadhi.

Kundalini is in samadhi in sahasrara. It has been said: 'In the innermost part of the great lotus (centre) sahasrara Kundalini in the form of a garland of fifty matrika-units lies round Shiwa' (—Todalatantra, ch. 9, p. 17). This is the samadhi state of Kundalini. This state of Kundalini is only realizable in samadhi. A yogi, conducting Kundalini to sahasrara, attains samadhi in which the super-knowledge of oneness with God arises. So, it has been stated: 'After conducting Kundalini (to sahasrara), one realizes in concentration one's being as the being of Shiwa' (—Todalatantra, ch. 4, p. 8).

The aroused Kundalini manifests the power of absorption by which all creative principles are withdrawn. It has been stated: 'The divine, coiled Kundalini, arising from muladhara, passes through the sushumna path to the void-centre (wishuddha) and absorbs all creative principles, and then comes to her own abode (sahasrara)' (—Phetkarinitantra, ch. 14, p. 39).

Parwati said: 'It is not possible to effect kundali-motion (—changkrama) (that is, arousing Kundali and conducting her through the sushumna to the sahasrara) without yoga. So long Kundalini is sleeping (that is, in a latent form) in the mula-lotus (muladhara), mantra, yantra (special diagrams) and worship are not fruitful' (—Gandharwatantra, ch. 5, p. 24). This means that deep concentration is the fundamental factor in arousing Kundalini, and concentration is done on coiled Kundalini in muladhara with pranayama and ano-perineal contraction. It has been stated: 'In the triangle which is in the nature of will-knowledge-action and is situated within the muladhara, Swayambhu-linga is shining like a million suns. Above, is Kundali, red in colour, as the flame of Swayambhu-linga, supremely subtle, and the sentience of all beings is derived from her; and she is Supreme Power and is called Goddess in the form of mantra (shabda-brahma); she, in a coiled form, is within all beings. ... First, concentrate your mind on muladhara with inspiratory control and arouse that power (Kundali) by the execution of ano-perineal control' (—Gandharwatantra, ch.5, p. 27–8). So, in the arousing of Kundalini, concentration, pranayama and ano-perineal contraction are used. It is practically the same type of process as that used in the Waidika process.

More about Kundalini: 'In the muladhara, lies Kundalini, who is spiritual consciousness, very bright-shining like a million lightnings, in the form of mantra with fifty matrika-units, endowed with thirty-eight forms of superpower, supremely subtle and capable of passing through the Brahma-, Wishnu- and Rudra-knots' (—Gandharwatantra, ch. 29, p. 112). It is extremely difficult to hold in consciousness such a subtle form of Kundalini. At first, her lustrous form should be taken for concentration. Gradually, as concentration goes deeper, her subtle form emerges from her splendorous form. In time, her other aspects also arise in concentration in consciousness. That concentration should be done on Kundalini in muladhara has been stated: 'Concentrate on divine Kundalini who is in the nature of spiritual knowledge and in the form of matrika-units, lying in the triangle of muladhara, where resides the shining linga which is named Swayambhu; here mental japa should be done' (—Gandharwatantra, ch. 29, pp. 108–9).

Shiwa has explained the process of concentration on Kundalini. He has also stated that pranayama (breath-control) is absolutely necessary for deep internal purification (—Gandharwatantra, ch. 10, p. 47). About concentration, he stated: 'Concentrate every day on Kundalini ... who is red and shining like a million suns and subtle; she is that Supreme Power who also creates, maintains and dissolves the universe; she is beyond the universe in her spiritual form ... ; by the mantra "Hung" this supreme power of Shiwa will be aroused and led through the six-chakras to Parama Shiwa (Supreme Consciousness); then Kundalini who is in the nature of supreme bliss is made to unite and be one and the same with Shiwa in deep concentration; ... and then Kundalini should be brought back to muladhara; concentrate on Kundalini who is very bright like a thousand rising suns and extremely subtle and in the form of mantra and extends from muladhara to brahmarandhra (end of sushumna). Kundali is in three forms ... —Supreme (turiya) Kundali in sahasrara as Supreme Power (Mahatripurasundari); in muladhara, she is like molten gold and is in the nature of mantra, and she extends from muladhara to anahata and is called Fire (Wahni) Kundalini; concentration should be done on her; in anahata, she as Sun (Surya) Kundalini is as lustrous as

a million suns and full of love, and extends from anahata to wishuddha; one should concentrate on her in calmness. In ajña, Kundalini is shining like a million moons and radiating "immortality"; she extends herself from ajña to the end of brahmarandhra and is called Moon (Chandra) Kundalini. ... Supreme Kundali is in the form of supreme consciousness. Concentration should be done on her. Her complete spiritual form should be contemplated. ... Concentration should be done again and again. ... This is the process called antaryaga (mental worship) which leads to liberation' (—Gandharwatantra, ch. 10, pp. 47–8).

This is a specific Tantrika process of arousing and conducting Kundalini to sahasrara. The process consists of the following factors:

1 Concentration should be done on Kundalini as shining red and extremely subtle in muladhara.
2 Kundalini should be aroused by the mantra 'Hung' (with pranayama and concentration).
3 Kundalini should then be conducted to sahasrara to unite herself with Parama Shiwa.
4 Special concentration should be done on Fire Kundalini who is shining like molten gold, and extending from muladhara to anahata.
5 Special concentration should be done on Sun Kundalini, very bright like many suns and extending from anahata to wishuddha.
6 Special concentration on Moon Kundalini, shining like the moon and extending from ajña to the end of sushumna.
7 Special concentration on Supreme Kundalini in the form of supreme spiritual consciousness with all divine power in sahasrara.

This is the concentration on different aspects of Kundalini.

Kundalini in latent form has two aspects: Kundalini in three and a half coils around Swayambhu-linga, lying in muladhara, called Kulakundalini; and Kundalini in eight coils, lying in sushumna from muladhara to indu, each of her coils being in each chakra (subtle centre)—muladhara, swadhishthana, manipura, anahata, wishuddha, ajña, manas and indu. These two aspects of Kundalini have been explained in both Waidika and Tantrika forms of layayoga. That aspect of Kundalini, lying in the entire sushumna, has again been subdivided into three forms, each having a Tantrika name. Kundalini, extending from muladhara to anahata, shining like molten gold, is called Fire Kundalini. Kundalini who extends from anahata to ajña is as bright as one million suns and is called Sun Kundalini. Kundalini, extending from ajña to the end of sushumna and lustrous like a million moons, is termed Moon Kundalini. That aspect of Kundalini, which is beyond sushumna, being in sahasrara, and is always in super- and supreme conscious states and all spirituality, has been termed in the Tantra, Turiya (Supreme) Kundalini.

There are six forms of concentration on Kundalini in the Tantrika process. They are as follows:

1 Concentration on Kulakundalini as extremely subtle and shining red, or shining like lightning.
2 Concentration on shining molten gold-coloured Fire Kundalini.
3 Concentration on sun-like very bright Sun Kundalini.
4 Concentration on moon-like lustrous Moon Kundalini.
5 Concentration on very subtle and bright like the rising sun Kundalini inside sushumna, extending from muladhara to the end of brahma nadi.
6 Concentration on Supreme Kundalini in sahasrara.

However, for the rousing of Kundalini, concentration should be done on Kulakundalini in muladhara. It should be done in conjunction with pranayama (breath-control). At a certain stage of kumbhaka (breath-suspension), the sushumna-flow starts by which the blockage is removed that is caused by Kundalini who is in eight coils. It has been stated: 'Worldly consciousness and activities are due to the diverse forms of bio-energy; for this reason the yogis practise bio-energy-control. Kundalini power, which is in eight coils in the sushumna, causes

the blocking of the entire path; by the control of bio-energy, an internalization and concentration of prana-energy occurs within the sushumna, which causes Kundalini to uncoil herself' (—Shiwasanghita, 5.168–71). Kumbhaka in conjunction with concentration effects the sushumna flow and the uncoiling of Kundalini and her absorption into Supreme Kundalini. At this stage, the aroused Kulakundalini passes through the sushumna to reach the sahasrara. When Kulakundalini is aroused by concentration and pranayama, the eightfold coiled Kundalini becomes uncoiled and is absorbed into Supreme Kundalini. Now, the entire brahma nadi is free and the aroused Kulakundalini passes through it to sahasrara.

Mantra plays a most important role in the Tantrika process of arousing Kundalini. But mere letter-form mantra is ineffective. Therefore, mantra should be made living by appropriate processes. The enlivened mantra, technically termed Prana-mantra, is applied in conjunction with pranayama and concentration. Purnananda says: 'That divine Kulakundalini who is in the nature of the highest spirituality, and flashes like a million lightnings, who is very subtle and in a latent form with three and a half coils, situated in the muladhara, should be aroused by prana-mantra' (—Shaktakrama, ch. 1, p. 1).

There is a special process of concentration in conjunction with japa (sound-process) which is done in arousing and conducting Kundalini through different chakras (subtle centres). About this Shiwa says: 'Directing his mind to muladhara, the yogi should concentrate on divine Kundali who is in the nature of Brahman (Shabdabrahman—Brahman in mantra form), and make japa of four-lettered matrika-mantra ten times. ... Then Kundali should be conducted to swadhishthana ... where japa of six-lettered matrika-mantra with concentration should be done' (—Bhutashuddhitantra, ch. 1, pp. 1–2). In this manner, japa and concentration should be done in manipura, anahata, wishuddha, ajña, indu and sahasrara (—Bhutashuddhitantra, ch. 2, p. 2).

The importance of anal-lock in conjunction with tongue-lock in rousing Kundalini has been emphasized. It is said: 'According to the Merutantra, Kundalini should be aroused by inspiration through the left nostril, along with anal contraction to a moderate degree, and the tongue pressing on the palate (tongue-lock) from muladhara and united with Parama Shiwa in the thousand-petalled lotus' (—Purashcharyarnawa, ch. 3, p. 191). It has been stated in the Tripurasaratantra that Kundalini and Swayambhu (-linga) are aroused by pranayama when they appear in their real forms (—Sarwollasatantra, 15.16).

Pouranika Exposition of Kundalini

Lastly, let us study what the rishis have said about Kundalini as recorded in the Puranas. Ishwara says: 'The Shakti (that is, Kundalini-shakti), should be aroused from muladhara by mula-mantra (the mantra imparted to the disciple by the guru) while suspending breath through the pingala path' (—Shiwapurana, 3.5.21). Here, mula-mantra in conjunction with breath-suspension has been used in rousing Kundalini. The pingala path indicates that surya kumbhaka (right-nostril inspiratory breath-control) should be adopted.

Wayu has said: 'The principle of Shakti (Power) from which arises all forms of energy, is the root of the manifested worlds. She is Kundalini (in her pure spiritual aspect); she is maya (in her creative aspect); she is pure and only in union with Shiwa (in her supreme aspect)' (—Shiwapurana, 5 a, 25.6–7). From this it is also clear that Supreme Shakti in her spiritual aspect is Kundalini and is in supreme union with Parama Shiwa (Supreme Being) at the highest level of spiritual yoga; and that Supreme Shakti in her creative aspect is maya, by which a finite phenomenon has arisen from an infinite reality.

Shankara has expounded the real nature of Kundalini. He said: 'It is stated that Kundali, coiled like a serpent, is unknown; and though she is in the apana region (that is in muladhara), she is not seen; that Kundali is also in the summit (that is sahasrara), and is glorified in the Wedas;

that she is the root of all spiritual knowledge, and is the secret spirituality in the form of Gayatri (the Goddess of mantra-sounds); that eternal Kundali is in all beings and endowed with the power of moving upward (when aroused); that she is seen and unseen, moving and unmoving, manifested and unmanifested, perpetual; that she is both beyond the matrika sound-units and also with the garland of letters; that the yogis "seeing" her constantly become contented for ever' (—Shiwapurana, 6.48.13–16). So, Kundalini is the eternal, unqualified, supreme, spiritual power lying dormant in all beings, and in that state she is unrealized. She is aroused by yoga and then 'seen'.

Ishwara says: 'That power which is like the lotus filament (that is, subtle), is to be aroused by pranayama in which inspiration and expiration are done through the right nostril, and then that aroused power should be conducted through the void-path (that is, sushumna) in concentration' (—Agnipurana, 96.106–7). Here, Surya Kumbhaka (right-nostril inspiratory-expiratory breath-control) and concentration are applied for arousing Kundalini and for her passage through sushumna.

Agni has said: 'The Ajapa Gayatri is conjoined with moon, fire and sun, and is called primary Kundalini. She is in the region of the heart as a sprout' (—Agnipurana, 214.27). Ajapa is the automatic repetition of the Hangsah mantra—the natural sound phenomenon connected with respiration—along with inspiration and expiration. When inspiration and expiration are changed to suspension (kumbhaka), the sound-emitting divine power known as Gayatri is awakened. This aroused power in muladhara is called primary Kundalini. She passes through sushumna to the hrit centre where she is realized in concentration.

That the Supreme Shakti (power) is Kundalini is clear from the statement made by King Himawan when glorifying Supreme Shakti (—Kurmapurana, Part 1, 12.125). Kundalini is the spiritual aspect of Supreme Power. In explaining the nature of yoga-knowledge (knowledge arising from and in relation to yoga) Krishna said: 'Organic control, such as of hunger and thirst, internal purification, nadi-shodhana (pranic purification), piercing through the chakras (power-centre), sensory control and mental control—being prepared by all these things the yogi should concentrate on Kundalini power united with Ishwara—Supreme Being' (—Brahmawaiwartapurana, Part 4, 110. 8–9). First a disciple should prepare himself by internal purification and control of the body, pranayamic super-purification, and sense-control, and then arouse Kundalini and cause her to pass through all the chakras and, finally, concentration should be done on Kundalini united with Shiwa.

According to Shiwa, as quoted by rishi Ourwa, Kundali shakti (power) is in the form of 'ou' (—Kalikapurana, 57.95). This means that Kundalini in muladhara is in the form of 'ou'—three and a half coils around Swayambhu-linga. It is the modified form of 'Ong'. In glori-fying Shakti (Power), Brahma said: 'she is straight as well as Supreme Kundalini' (—Soura-purana, 25.16). Kundalini is coiled in muladhara, but when awakened, she becomes straight and passes through the sushumna and reaches the sahasrara where she is Supreme Kundalini. Rishi Wyasa also glorified Shakti in the form of Gouri by saying: 'You are straight and you are Kundalini (coiled), you are subtle and the bestower of success in yoga' (—Sourapurana, 8.16). So, Kundalini exists in two forms: the coiled, when she is latent, and the straight, when she is aroused.

Parwati explained the process of rousing Kundalini and conducting her to sahasrara. She said: 'First with inspiration concentrate your mind on adhara (muladhara); then the region between the anus and external genitals (that is, the perineum) should be contracted to arouse the Power (Kundalini power). Then the (aroused) Power should be conducted to bindu-chakra (sahasrara) by piercing through the three lingas. Now concentration should be done on the Supreme Power who has become one with Shambhu (Shiwa) in union. From this union arises red-coloured life-substance, full of bliss, and the yogi satisfies the maya power (here: the power in the form of the mantra Hring, that is, Kundalini)—the bestower of success

in yoga, and all the deities in the six-chakras (—power-centres) with that life-substance (amrita), and then he brings back Kundalini through that path (sushumna) to the muladhara' (—Dewibhagawata, Part 7, 35.48–51). The process of the awakening of Kundalini is as follows: at first, inspiratory breath-suspension with concentration should be done, and along with it ano-perineal contraction (yoni-mudra) should be executed. The ano-perineal contrac-tion when executed during inspiratory suspen-sion causes the apana and prana forces to operate in the muladhara on the coiled Kundalini, by which she is ultimately aroused.

The concentration form of Kundalini, as stated by Narayana, is: 'Kundalini, who is in the red-coloured muladhara, is all red, like lotus filament (that is subtle), and is designated by the mantra Hring; her face is radiating sun-power, and her breasts are fire and moon powers (these are technical terms)' (—Dewibhagawata, Part 11, 1.44). And, 'When Kundalini passes first (that is, from the muladhara to sahasrara) she is splendorous like lightning and when she comes back (to muladhara), she is wet with life-substance (amrita). When Kundalini passes through the sushumna, she is all bliss' (—Dewi-bhagawata, Part 11, 1.47).

It has been stated that 'A spiritual disciple who is vital, sound in mind and body, and calm, attains God when he is able to bring Atman (here: I-consciousness merged in Kundalini) to the head (sahasrara) through the yogi-path (sushumna)' (—Mahabharata, 3.179.17).

The great rishi Washishtha stated: 'As strong streams in circular motions fill the river Ganga, so all the pranas fill the internal Kundalini (that is, Kundalini situated in muladhara) through the process of pranayama in combina-tion with pranawa mantra and concentration)' (—Yogawashishtha-ramayana, 5, 54.26). This process was adopted by Uddalaka. The ex-ternalization of prana forces are controlled by pranayama. Then they coil themselves into Kundalini when she is aroused.

About Kundalini Washishtha says: 'Within the tender plantain bud (muladhara), situated in the sushumna, lies that Supreme Shakti (power) having lightning-like splendour and speed. That power is called Kundali, because she is coiled. She is the Supreme Power lying in all beings and the source of all forms of energy. The pranic functions are due to that coiled power, but when she is aroused pranas cease to function. . . . She is the seed of all consciousness (sangwid), (—Yogawashishtha-ramayana, 6 a, 80.41–8). So, Kundalini is the basic power which supports livingness and consciousness in the embodied beings, when she is in a coiled state, and when she is aroused, she becomes the basis of spiritualized superconsciousness.

CHAPTER 4
Mantra —
Supra-sound Power

We are living in a world of sounds. As fish move through water, we move through sounds. Sounds are producing very many kinds of impressions on us. Some sounds are agreeable, others are annoying; some are sweet, others are harsh. Sounds are produced in nature—thunder in the sky, sounds from storm, from rainfall, breaking of the waves in the ocean, flowing of rivers; and innumerable other sounds occurring in nature. There are also the sounds made by birds and other creatures; the sounds of the human voice—language, even sounds within our bodies. Then, there are artificially created sounds—from planes, trains, cars, and machines. We hear all these, but we do not hear mantra-sounds amidst them.

Is it because these sounds destroy the mantra-sounds? If we go to a lonely place—a mountainous region, a deep forest, or some very solitary place where all these sounds are absent, and we feel calmness there, do we hear the mantra-sounds? No, we do not. Are we then to conclude that the mantra-sounds are merely a fiction? No, this is not the case. The human ear is only able to perceive sounds of certain frequencies, beyond that it cannot go. Therefore, because of these limitations the human ear cannot be taken as a criterion of the authenticity of the mantra-sounds.

Yogis say that the mantra-sounds are heard by a 'perfect ear'. They also say that the 'perfect ear' develops when sense-consciousness is transformed into non-undulatory, one-pointed consciousness by the process of concentration. When concentration becomes so deep that it continues without any interruption at any point and, finally, the sense-objects and the everyday I-ness vanish from the conscious field; and a 'super-I' is awakened, the mantra-sounds arise and are 'heard'.

If we accept the experiences of the yogis as facts, then we have to accept that sounds exist in three forms—audible, inaudible and audible in concentration. But this simple statement does not explain the sound phenomenon; it requires further clarification.

Sound

Sound is regarded as a disturbance or wave, produced by a vibrating object in a material medium, usually air, in which one molecule, when it collides with another, transmits sound. In this manner, the sound waves travel in the air, at an approximate speed of 1100 feet per second, and are perceived by the auditory mechanism as sound. The transmission of sound waves through the external aspect of the auditory system occurs in this way: The sound waves are collected by the external ear and are transmitted through the external auditory meatus to the tympanic membrane, and thence through the ossicles to the cochlea of the inner ear where the auditory receptors are located. Sound vibrations are converted into nerve impulses in the cochlea, and pass as waves of electrical negativity along the acoustic nerve to the temporal cortex.

The capacity of the human ear to receive sound vibrations is limited. Out of practically an infinite range of vibrations occurring in nature, the human ear perceives sounds only from 16 to 20,000 complete vibrations per second. Below 16, only discontinuous pulsations are perceived and above 20,000 nothing is heard. But there are some animals, especially bats and dogs, who are able to perceive sounds of frequencies higher than 20,000.

The brain is not the seat of consciousness, nor do brain functions effect consciousness. The brain is a quantity of matter consisting of molecules, atoms and elementary particles, where no trace of consciousness is found. But when it is vitalized by the functioning of bio-energies, it becomes a highly sensitized instrument for the operation of consciousness.

Neural-neuronal impulses, which are electrical by nature, are converted into a non-material force—the wayu-energy—at a certain area of the brain and are conveyed to the sense-centres and then through the ida-path to the sense-mind. The sense-mind finally radiates it to the sense-consciousness where it develops into a conscious form and the 'I' feels it as a sensory object. In this way sound is experienced. This is the internal aspect of the auditory system. That this aspect is not merely a fanciful appendage, but a more intrinsic part of sensory phenomena is indicated by the following facts. The sense-mind, elevated to the Dhi level, is able to perceive a sensory object directly without using the external sensory mechanism. There are many instances of this. Moreover, in pratyahara (sensory control), all sensory impulses are normally stopped and none of them penetrate into sense-consciousness. The external mechanism remains intact, only the connection is severed. Sense factors from the outer world may penetrate through the nervous paths and reach the brain, but no sensory perception is experienced in this state.

Let us now return to the consideration of sound.

The Sound Phenomenon

A vibrating object emits vibrations which in turn set up vibrations—waves of sound—in the surrounding air. The range of air-vibrations is wide. But only a limited number of air-vibrations (10 or 11 octaves) can produce vibrations in the mechanism of the human ear; the other vibrations do not affect it. These vibrations are transformed into nerve impulses in the cochlea and pass through the acoustic nerve to the cerebral cortex and thence to a certain area of the brain. Thereafter we experience a conscious sound form—the perception of sound—in the sense-consciousness through a complex power-line system in which sense-mind plays a dominant role.

An object, when vibrating, produces sound waves in the air. But when the object is not vibrating it cannot emit any sound. This indicates that an object in a quiescent state ceases to emit sound. This can be interpreted to mean that the sound power is inherent in an object and remains in it in a latent form; when an object is made to vibrate by striking, the latent sound power becomes sound vibrations. Or, sound vibrations are simply a gross manifestation of subtle vibrations of sound which are not registered in a material medium.

Our recognition of an external world is essentially due to sense-impressions radiating to our consciousness. We know the objective world mainly through our senses. Objects which were outside consciousness penetrate through the sensory channels into it, where they develop into conscious images. The senses of smell, taste, and touch operate when they are in direct contact with objects. The sense of hearing is activated by the sound waves in the air; and sight is due to light falling on the retina from the objects in the environment. Knowledge of an external world, acquired sensorially, is incomplete and only meaningful in a desire-bound existence.

The senses are limited in their power. First of all, they cannot receive any impressions from the outer world if these fall below the threshold of sensation. This refers to both size and distance.

The perception of smell is not effected by a single molecule of a fragrant object or the perception of taste by a single molecule of sugar; we can neither hear nor see, if the objects are situated at a far distance. We also fail to establish sensory contact with an obscured object. These are the limitations of our senses. These limitations can be overcome to a certain degree by extending the range of our senses with the help of super-sensitive instruments. We have been able to see objects very far from us with the aid of a telescope, to see minute objects through a microscope, and to see what is obscured by X-rays. But scientific instruments have also their limits. The objective world appears to be larger and more complex than what we experience through our senses even when their range is greatly extended by the use of instruments.

So, our knowledge of the outer world is restricted because of the sensory limitations. When 'seeing' through the senses, objects appear to be linked with space-time. Perhaps this incomplete seeing gives rise to space-time phenomena. A material object can be seen in three dimensions in space. There is no possibility of the senses receiving any impressions of more than three dimensions. In our seeing of objects, time also becomes a factor.

The space factor appears to arise in our 'seeing' the outer world through the senses. The material objects are seen in space, at rest or in motion. Space is that which affords the possibility of the existence of material objects to be perceived by us. But consciousness, in which the images of the objects are formed and apprehended, does not know space. It has no length, breadth or thickness; it cannot be measured quantitatively; it is not located in space. But images in consciousness are seen in space. The time factor operates both in consciousness and with regard to objects outside consciousness. Time indicates changes which the object of the outer world are undergoing constantly. Some changes are very rapid, some are slow. The influence of time on consciousness is not exactly like that exerted on material objects. The changes which are going on in consciousness can only be assessed by the rising and disappearing of the writtis (images in consciousness) in succession. So, the influence of time on consciousness is not exactly on consciousness, but on the writti-flows; on the other hand, time puts permanent marks on the material objects.

Space exists in relation to objects. Space by itself amounts to nothing. Space forms a part of the knowledge of an object. But without this objective knowledge space is zero. Time is also a factor in objective knowledge. Time by itself if interpreted as that moment when there are no forms in consciousness, is also zero. So, the space-time phenomenon is a relative truth, only applicable when the objective forms flow in consciousness.

How does the writti-consciousness arise? It is a mode of our being and is maintained by sense-functioning. Sense-impressions originate not in the senses but in events in matter. These impressions are received by the senses and are transformed into sensory impulses which are conducted to the cerebral cortex and thence to a certain area of the brain, where they are converted into matter-free energy and passes the body-mind bridge and reaches consciousness where objective knowledge develops. This consciousness is chitta—sense-consciousness. The sensory knowledge, as writtis, is continually flowing in sense-consciousness. The writtis flow in succession, and may be termed—writti 1, writti 2, 3, 4, etc. The duration of one writti at a time in consciousness is generally short and the continuous flow causes an undulatory form of consciousness.

When writti 1 flows in consciousness, the knowledge of writti 1 arises, and this knowledge is only of that particular writti. When writti 2 comes, writti 1 has been obliterated from consciousness, and the knowledge of only writti 2 shines forth in consciousness. This indicates that only one writti and its knowledge is possible at one time. But as the writtis flow in succession, our knowledge pattern is also in the nature of flowing, consisting of many forms. Usually our thoughts are composed of many forms fused together to constitute a more complete knowledge of certain things.

However, connected with the writtis or 'knowledges' is an entity which knows what is flowing in consciousness as *writtis*. In fact a *writti* is a form of knowledge due to the knowingness of that entity. If the knower disappears, *writtis* or 'knowledges' disappear. This entity, which establishes a conscious relation with objective images in consciousness, becomes the knower of the objects. This knowingness presents three facts: an objective form in consciousness, a conscious exposition of that object, and the presence of something which exhibits its quality as selfhood. This gives rise to the phenomenon of I-ness expressing 'I am this, I am that' feelings. This is *abhimana* (I-feeling). These feelings are intrinsically associated with I-ness. All these feelings originate from and are supported by the I-ness in relation to objective images. There are three main forms of these feelings: I as knower, I as doer, and I as supporter (as of the body). Sensory perception is the basic knowledge pattern appearing as 'I know this object, that object', etc. This may be associated with thoughts, feelings or volition.

There is another aspect of 'I' which is expressed on rare occasions. 'I' has the possibilities of knowing, thinking and doing unusual things which are not possible at the sensory level. This phenomenon is due to a conscious contact between 'I' and some post-conscious impressions (*sangskaras*) stored in the nonconscious aspect of mind, called *hridaya*. In fact, all knowledge, thoughts, actions and feelings which have been experienced by the 'I' are transformed into post-conscious impressions and stored in *hridaya*, and can be brought back to consciousness by memory. However, the 'I' which knows what is arising in consciousness remains always in the same form and maintains its I-ness in all experiences. So, the objective forms are multifarious and transitory, whereas the I-ness is unchanging and stable.

Does the complete picture of the outer world penetrate into consciousness through the sensory channels? It is only a part—a superficial layer—that known through the senses. We know the solidity, liquidity, luminosity and airiness of matter. We experience the material world in smell, taste, colour, touch, and sound forms. But all these are in the superficial stratum.

Material substance is reducible to molecules, molecules to atoms, and atoms to elementary particles, such as electrons, protons, etc. It is now considered that the particles are the ultimate constituents of matter. However, in addition to the particles, there is also energy in matter. Energy may exist either in association with matter, or may make itself free from matter to become radiation. These particles are considered to be exceedingly small, indivisible and ultimate units of matter. But these particles are not minute pieces of hard matter of permanent size. They have two aspects—particles and waves. Electrons, which are negatively charged particles, and protons, the positively charged particles—both may appear as particles at one moment and as waves at another. Both particles and waves appear to be the same thing, or two aspects of the same thing.

Have we any direct experience of all these phenomena in relation to matter? No, they are beyond our senses, and also beyond the reach of the sensitive instruments. How then are they known? They are known indirectly from the experimental evidence obtained in laboratories and by the mathematical interpretation of the results of these experiments. In other words, it is an intellectual interpretation in which inference plays an important role, and which is based on knowledge acquired through the senses, instrumental observations, and other experimental evidence.

However, what escapes our observation is that the energy which is active in the superficial material field is continuous with that subtle energy system which is operative in the substratum where our senses do not reach, into which material instruments do not penetrate, and which our intellect does not grasp. This substratum is the subtle power-field over which is superimposed the gross material field. The subtle power operation is the basic part which sustains matter. Mainly two kinds of forces are active in the power-field: *mahabhuta* (metamatter) as forces and pranic forces. There are five *mahabhuta* forces and five pranic forces. *Mahabhuta* forces are reducible to highly concentrated sense forces, termed *tanmatras*, or *tanons*. The *tanons* are intrinsically associated with the phenomenon of the emission of lifeful ultramini-sound—Swanana, or Swanon. Swanana is derived from swana, meaning sound, to which is suffixed ana, meaning life. Swanon is the abbreviated form of swanana. Swanon is the germ-mantra.

Metamatter forces in combination with pranic forces constitute a subtle energy organization, arranged in five levels. They are:

1 Smell-energy organization, in which the fundamental aspect is the 'earth' metamatter which assumes a particular form and around which is a circular wave-motion. When the earth metamatter is reduced to its smell tanon, it emits a specific swanon.
2 Taste-energy organization, containing 'water' metamatter, a circular wave-motion and the taste tanon, emitting a specific swanon.
3 Sight-energy organization, containing 'fire' metamatter, a circular wave-motion and the sight tanon, emitting a specific swanon.
4 Touch-energy organization, containing 'air' metamatter, a circular wave-motion around it, and the touch tanon, emitting a specific swanon.
5 Sound-energy organization, containing 'void' metamatter, a circular wave-motion around it, and the sound tanon, emitting a specific swanon.

The sound tanon (shabda tanmatra) is the subtlest and perfect form of sound which can be 'heard' only by a perfect ear. It is here where swanons are formed. The sound swanon becomes transformed into the radiant (pashyanti) sound beyond the sound tanon level, and finally into sound-principle (para shabda).

Four Forms of Sound

Sound exists in four forms. It has been stated: 'Sound is in four forms; the Brahmanas (the seers of Shabdabrahman) who have controlled their minds fully, know these four forms. Of these, the first three are hidden and unknown; the fourth form of sound is used by human beings' (—Rigweda-sanghita, 1.22.164.45).

The four forms of sound are Para (supreme), Pashyanti (radiant), Madhyama (subliminal) and Waikhari (acoustic). The human beings hear only a part of acoustic sounds. The yogis 'hear' the other three forms in samadhi.

About the four forms of sound it has been stated: 'Sound is about to sprout in para (supreme) form; it becomes two-leafed (that is first manifested) in pashyanti (radiant) form; it buds in the madhyama (subliminal) form; and it blooms in the waikhari (acoustic) form. Sound which has been developed in the above-mentioned manner, will become unmanifested, when the order is reversed' (—Yogakundalyupa-nishad, 3.18–19). Here, the stages of development of sound, from the supreme form to the acoustic form, and in reverse order, have been described.

Maheshwara said: 'What is called Shabda-brahman, the nature of which is nada (causal or unmanifest sound), is an aspect of Supreme Infinite Being. Shabdabrahman as shakti (power) is in the form of bindu (supremely concentrated conscious power), and being in muladhara that shakti becomes Kundalini. From that arises nada (sound), like a sprout from a minute seed, called pashyanti by means of which the yogis see the universe. In the region of the heart (that is, in anahata), it becomes more pronounced, resembling thunder in the atmosphere. It is called madhyama. Again it (madhyama) becomes swara (voice) by the expiratory help and this is called waikhari' (—Yogashikhopa-nishad, 3.2–5).

It has been disclosed above that Shabda-brahman is the source of sound. Shabdabrahman is in the form of sound which is unmanifest. So it is called para. The power in Shabda-brahman is bindu, from which issued the universe that is in the nature of pranawa (the first manifested sound). The cosmic bindu in an individual being resides in muladhara as Kulakundalini who is the source of all sounds. From Kundalini arises pashyanti nada. Pashyanti becomes more pronounced and particularized in anahata and is called madhyama. The madhyama sound is expressed as voice, and this is waikhari.

This Waidika exposition of sound has been

adopted in the Tantras with explanations in greater detail. Shiwa says: 'The source of nada (sound) which is called para (causal) arises in muladhara; that sound being in swadhishthana, becomes manifested and is called pashyanti; that sound going up to anahata, becomes reflected in the conscious principle and is called madhyama; then going upwards in wishuddha in the region of the neck, by the instrumentation of the larynx, palate, the root and tip of the tongue, teeth, lips and nasal cavities … it becomes waikhari' (—Tantrarajatantra, 26.5–9).

Further, 'That eternal Kundalini in her Shabdabrahman aspect is the source of power in which is dhwani (power as supremely rarefied sound) that develops as nada (sound), then nirodhika (fire-energy expressed in control), ardhendu (the crescent moon), bindu (point) and para (supreme); and from para arise pashyanti, madhyama and waikhari sounds' (—Sharadatilakatantra, 1.108–9).

Kundalini as Shabdabrahman is endowed with power which is in the nature of sound-substance, having the possibility of developing as sound-power (nada), which is associated with fire-energy in the form of control-power, that is, higher spiritual energy. The sound-power assumes a semilunar shape with which is connected concentrated divine power-consciousness. This is the latent sound which is unmanifest. This is para sound. From para arises pashyanti, and then madhyama and finally waikhari.

Para-sound

Kundalini has two aspects—supreme and sound. In her highest aspect Kundalini, as Supreme Kundalini (Mahakundalini), is united with Supreme Consciousness and is one with that. At this level there is a complete absence of sound in any form—ashabda (non-sound). Kundalini in this aspect is Infinite Supreme Consciousness, having no attributes. But in her specific power-fulness, Supreme Power is able to produce a power phenomenon from which emerges the universe of mind and matter. At this stage

Kundalini is Shabdabrahman and her power is in the nature of sound-substance (dhwani). Sound-substance is not manifested sound, it is the life-energy principle (prana) which creates and operates in what has been created. This living sound-power is the causal sound and is called para-sound.

Supreme Brahman appears as Shabdabrahman when Supreme Power, which is one and the same with Brahman as Mahakundalini, 'wills' to express the kinetic counterpart of the static quiescent eternal reality. This aspect of Brahman is called Shabdabrahman, because the power which is going to be expressed is in the nature of nada—a phenomenon in which willing is imbued with effectivity in the form of pre-sound which becomes Supreme Bindu—the supremely concentrated power. The concentration is such as is fully ready to actualize the 'willing' of Supreme Power in her purely power aspect. This concentrated power is Bindu, because it is non-magnitudinous and non-positional power, which, when magnified, appears as splendorous and permeated with sonority without manifested sound. This power is Kundalini as Shabdabrahman. Here lies the principle of sound— sound unmanifested and undifferentiated but power in maximum concentration and in the nature of sound-substance. This power-sound is para-sound.

In Shabdabrahman there is an arrangement in a latent phase, termed kamakala—the principle of the actualization of the power as sound. Supreme Bindu (supreme power-concentration) before the manifestation of creative power assumes a threefold character—the three specific power-points (bindus), termed bindu (second) (consciousness-point), nada (sound-radiating energy-point), and bija (sound-specificality-point), which constitute a triangular process. Each power-point emits a number of sound-potentials—the would-be sound units—arranged in a line, and the three lines form the triangle. All these are in a latent phase and unmanifest. This triangular process is kamakala (triangular process of power-points).

Pashyanti-sound

At a certain point of concentration of energy, Supreme Bindu bursts, as it were, and a great concentrated power in the form of sound emanates. This power-sound is Pranawa Nada and is 'heard' by the yogis in concentration. The power aspect is concentrated prana-energy from which the name pranawa is derived. The prana-energy in motion creates a series of force-motion-lines, consisting of four phases. On its first emergence from Supreme Bindu it creates 'A' line—the A-phase—which is transformed into 'U' line, called U-phase. It is then changed into 'M' line—the M-phase. Finally, it assumes 'O' (Tantrika letter O)-shaped line in which 'M' is changed into nada-bindu and 'O' becomes the bija to form ong, as it is 'seen' by the yogis in concentration. In this power-form the sound factor is inseparable. The power is sound and the sound is power. This is the first manifested power-sound phenomenon—pranawa. This is called pashyanti-sound—the first manifested radiant sound.

Pranawa is the first manifestation of para-sound. Para-sound is the source of pranawa. So, pranawa is the first manifested sound. From this arise all forms of sounds—mantras, Weda, language and all other sounds. All sounds are finally absorbed in pranawa and pranawa into para-sound. Para-sound is Shabda-brahman.

Pranawa is a complex organization of powers in which a basic power supports various powers. The prana-force, which is in motion in Pranawa, makes the three bindus (power-points), which are in a latent form in kamakala, operate, and the sound-potentials begin to be actualized as matrika-warna (sound-units). In Supreme Bindu, which is consciousness-power reality, there are concidynamism potentials in a massive concentrated state, that now begin to develop. The consciousness factor arises from Kundalini and power from Prana. Of the three bindus (power-points), nada is the centre of pranic force, which is the fundamental sound-factor and from which occurs an emission of a super-refined ray (rashmi) of red colour. This is termed Rajas-guna (primary energy-principle). The red-power at the bindu becomes yellow radiant conscidynamism, termed Sattwa-guna (primary sentience-principle). The sound factor of the red-ray becomes a specific sound at the bija. The red-power is changed here into black-power which is termed Tamas-guna (primary inertia-principle).

The red-ray emission creates a red-line—rajas-line, which releases sixteen sound-units. In a similar manner, yellow- and black-lines are created, and are called sattwa- and tamas-lines respectively. From each of them sixteen sound-units are released. These three lines form and equilateral triangle standing on its apex. The left side of the triangle is the red-line, the base is the yellow-line, and the right side is the black-line. These three lines are the three forms of power, termed Wama, Jyeshtha and Roudri. Wama is the red-line and consists of sixteen sound-units from A to Ah; Jyeshtha is the yellow-line, consisting of sixteen sound-units from Ka to Ta; and Roudri is the black-line, consisting of sixteen sound-units, from Tha to Sa. In the three angles of the triangle are three sound-units, named Ha, between the red-line and the yellow line, Ksha, between yellow-line and black-line, and La (Rhha) at the apex within the triangle between the black-line and red-line. Ha is the moon-point, Ksha is the sun-point, and La is the fire-point. Wama-power is associated with the Brahma-Consciousness; Jyeshtha with Wishnu, and Roudri with Rudra. The red-energy in the yellow field creates mind and senses, and in the black field it creates tanmatras and mahabhutas. Sound-units operate in madhyama-sound.

The emerged prana-force begins to throb in pranawa in its characteristic manner, causing to be emitted what is called pranawa sound. The sound-motion is in the nature of what has been termed samanya spanda—basic infinitesimal motion almost uniform in character, which shows insignificant change in form. It is more quiescent than motional. It is the motional totality without having any specificality. The prana-throbbing and sound-motion are the same thing, or two aspects of the same thing. Sound is the exact nature of throbbing prana. The manifestation of prana-force is in the nature of sound. Sound is the mode of apprehension of power which is in motion. The sound pattern of the motion is Ong—the pashyanti-sound. Ong is the whole sound. Sound is also the mode—the only mode—of the uncoiling of the coiled power.

Madhyama-sound

The pranawa power-sound-motion changes from its vast and vague character to a clearly defined specific pattern in which limitedness and changeableness are more and more marked. The one pranawa-sound now becomes many particularized sounds. Hence, they have been termed wishesha spanda—particularized motion. The singularity of sounds arises from the bija which is 'O', as there is only one sound which is Ong. Now the plurality of the bija develops. But the nada-bindu factor of pranawa is retained, which becomes an intrinsic part of the newly developed bijas. This manifold specialized sound phenomenon is madhyama-sound developed from pranawa. Pashyanti-sound becomes madhyama-sound.

Pranawa is the original sound which is one and without parts and represents the manifested power as a whole. In detailed manifestation of power which occurs at the madhyama level, there is an expression of specialization and plurality. The original sound homogeneity existing in pranawa begins to change into sound heterogeneity existing in madhyama. Here matrika-warnas or matrika-arnas (primary sound-units) come into being. The word 'matrika' usually means mother, but here it is used in a technical sense. It stands for the warnas (particularized sound-forms) as a whole. Warna is usually translated as a letter of the alphabet. But the technical meaning of it is a particular sound-form. There are fifty warnas or sound-forms. Collectively, all fifty sound-forms are called matrika. So it is called a garland of fifty (mala panchashika).

The fifty sound-forms are from A to Ksha. The sound-forms from A to Ksha are collectively named Matrika. As there are fifty matrika letters from A to Ksha, matrika is also called fifty-matrikas (panchashanmatrikah). These sound-forms (from A to Ksha) are the bijas, that is, specialized sounds. So it is stated: 'A to Ksha sounds which are matrika are in the nature of bija' (—Kamadhenutantra, ch. 1, p. 1). These sound-forms are not lifeless letters; they are in the nature of consciousness and power. It is stated: 'The warnas (letters) from A to Ksha are Shiwa (Consciousness) and Shakti (Power); these warnas are (Shabda-) Brahman and exist always' (—Kankalamalinitantra, ch. 1, p. 1).

Matrika is living power and forms mantra. It has been stated: 'Matrika is living power and in the form of mantra' (—Kamadhenutantra, ch. 10, p. 12). Matrika is that power which leads to yoga. So it is stated: 'These are matrika-warnas (letters) which are within the sushumna and are in the nature of yoga; without the help of akshara (letter) spiritual yoga is not attained' (—Kamadhenutantra, ch. 12, p. 14). The matrika sound-forms are the detailed manifestation of pranawa-sound. It has been stated: 'Fifty-matrikas arise from nada (here pranawa-sound) in a regular order' (—Wishwasaratantra, ch. 1, p. 4).

Matrika-power is Kundalini. It is stated: 'The sound Ka is Kundali herself; Kundali is in the form of fifty-sounds matrika' (—Gayatritantra, 3.148). Further, 'Kundali is in the form of 50 sounds; she is nada and bindu; she is in the nature of consciousness; she is prakriti (primus)' (—Gayatritantra, 3,132), and 'Kundali who is in the form of fifty-sounds is eternal and the embodiment of highest spiritual knowledge. The attainment of Supreme Brahman is only possible through her; she is Supreme Kundali' (—Gayatritantra, 3.130).

It has been stated: 'The thread of what has been called a garland of fifty is in the nature of Power and Consciousness; Kundali-power (that is, the power in sound-forms) has (in this manner) been strung' (—Shaktanandatarangini, 8.8). This matrika-garland is also called the garland of spiritual knowledge. So it is stated: 'Fifty-matrika-power has been termed jñana-mala (a garland of spiritual knowledge)' (—Gayatritantra, 3.149).

Kundalini has two aspects: one is subtle which is beyond sound, and the other is the sound-form. There are fifty sounds and they are collectively called matrika. Sound is power. This power is in the nature of life-energy principle and manifest as sound. The sound-power is an aspect of Kundalini. Kundalini in her sound aspect is the principal Dewata (embodied divine consciousness) arising from appropriate mantra. The matrika-warnas are primary sound units. Matrika-sounds arise from Kundalini and are embedded in her. So, Kundalini is the root of matrika and in whom again matrika dissolves. After the dissolution of matrika into Kundalini, she remains in her subtle form.

Matrika-sounds

Matrika-sounds are primary sound-units, and each unit exhibits a specific form of sound. A sound-unit is composed of three fundamental parts: bija, nada and bindu. The bija part represents a specific sound of one kind, without being mixed with other sounds. Through the instrumentation of nada the bija-sound is rarefied, concentrated and conducted to bindu where the sound is transformed into spiritual consciousness. So a bija is always with nada-bindu. The bijas of matrika are fifty and therefore there are fifty forms of specialized sound. So, we have fifty primary sound-units.

Matrika-sound can be classified into two groups: principal and subordinate. The principal sound-forms are endowed with powers to activate or inhibit the powers of the subordinate sound-forms and to make the subordinate forms operate and cooperate with them or other subordinate forms. The subordinate matrika-sounds uncoil their powers with the help of the principal forms. The subordinate forms are able to exhibit great power when combined with appropriate principal matrika-sounds. The controlling mechanism lies mostly in principal forms. The subordinate forms cannot be successfully combined with each other without the help of the principal forms.

Principle sound-units are of two kinds—short and long. Short-power units inhibit the specific power of a subordinate sound-unit at short intervals in order to activate the specific power of another subordinate unit. Long-power matrika-units are able to activate a subordinate unit to its limit. The combination of matrika-units may be of the short-power type, the long-power type, or both types. In the short-power type, different units operate with short intervals between, and in the long-power type, the units operate at longer intervals. The nature of the combination of matrika-units determines the nature of the specific sound-motion. Tables 4.1 and 4.2 are the two tables of matrika-units: In all, there are fifty matrika sounds.

Table 4.1 Principal matrika-units—sixteen in number

Short type	Long type
a	a
i	i
u	u
ri	ri
lri	lri
	e
	ai
	o
	ou
common	
ang	ah

Table 4.2 Subordinate matrika-units—thirty-four number

k	ch	t	t	p	y	sh
kh	ch	th	th	ph	r	sh
g	j	d	d	b	l	s
gh	jh	dh	dh	bh	w	h
ṅ	ñ	n	n	m		ksh

Matrika-units exhibit certain general and specific characteristics. The following are the general characteristics:

1 Matrika-units contain three gunas (primary attributes)—sattwa, rajas and tamas. The

centre of sattwa is in bindu, of rajas in nada, and of tamas in bija.

2 Matrika-units may go beyond gunas when they are reduced to the principle of sound and become Kundalini.

3 Matrika-units are endowed with three forms of power—sentience-power, willing-power and action-power.

4 Matrika-units consist of bindu, nada, and bija.

5 Matrika-sounds are transformed into five forms of dewata (embodied divine consciousness) at the five tanmatra levels. The five dewatas are: Brahma, Wishnu, Rudra, Isha, and Sadashiwa.

6 Matrika-sounds are endowed with five forms of pranas. They are: prana, apana, samana, udana, and wyana.

7 Matrika-units constitute four forms of knowledge at four levels. They are:
(a) Highest spiritual knowledge at the sub-bindu level.
(b) Knowledge of tanmatras and mahabhutas.
(c) Super-sensory knowledge.
(d) Sensory knowledge.

Another important point is the colour phenomenon of matrika. Colour is an indication of the nature of energy predominating in a sound-unit. The bija-power when in motion creates a power-line which is seen in colour. The three fundamental colours are yellow, red and black. Sattwa predominates in yellow, rajas in red and tamas in black. Yellow indicates that bindu has greater influence on bija; red indicates the greater influence of nada on bija; and black shows the power of bija itself. The original colours are also changed to show the mixed character of the power-motion. The Table 4.3 shows the normal colours of the matrika-units.

When the matrika-units exhibit creative power, all of them become red at the sahasrara (thousand-petalled centre) level. But when they show the power of absorption or when they are going to be absorbed into Kundalini, they become white, that is transparent. From an evolutionary point of view, whiteness indicates a trace of the finest form of sattwa, and from the point of view of absorption, a white matrika

Table 4.3   Table of matrika colours

a	moon-white	ñ	shining red
a	white	t	shining white
i	white	th	shining yellow
i	shining yellow	d	shining yellow
u	yellow	dh	shining red
u	shining yellow	n	shining yellow
ri	shining red	t	shining yellow
ri	shining yellow	th	orange
lri	shining yellow	d	shining red
lri	moon-white	dh	shining yellow
e	deep red	n	shining red
ai	moon-white	p	moon-white
o	shining red	ph	shining red
ou	shining red	b	moon-white
ang	shining yellow	bh	orange
ah	shining red	m	orange
k	vermilion	y	smoke
kh	deep red	r	shining red
g	orange	l	shining yellow
gh	orange	w	shining yellow
n	smoke	sh	red
ch	white	sh	white
ch	shining yellow	s	white
j	moon-white	h	shining red
jh	shining red	ksh	white

N.B. All the matrika units are connected with nada-bindu and give the sound 'ng', except 'ang' and 'ah'.

is in a state where it is reducible to Kundalini. At the ajña level, the normally red 'h' becomes white and 'ksh' retains its normal white colour.

At the wishuddha level, the matrika 'h' becomes the sound-form of the sound tanon. The sound-form is called the bija of sound tanon. As a bija of sound tanon, 'h' with nada-bindu becomes 'hang' and its colour is white. In this centre there are sixteen matrika-units, from 'a' to 'ah', and all of them are red.

At the anahata level, the matrika 'yang' becomes the bija-sound of touch tanon and is in smoke colour. So it retains its original colour. It is in this colour that 'yang' is reducible to 'hang'. In this centre there are twelve matrika-units, from 'k' to 'th'. They are red. At the manipura level, the matrika 'rang' becomes the bija-sound of sight tanon and retains its original red colour. There are ten matrika-units in this centre, ranging from 'd' to 'ph', and they are blue in colour.

At the swadhishthana level, the matrika 'wang' becomes the bija-sound of taste tanon. It changes its yellow colour to white. In this centre there are six matrika-units which are golden in colour.

At the muladhara level, the matrika 'lang' is the bija-sound of smell tanon. This matrika-sound retains its original yellow colour. There are four matrika-units in this centre. They are of a golden colour.

Waikhari-sound

Madhyama-sound becomes waikhari-sound (gross aspect of sound) which operates as sound-energy in the material field and is transformed into sound (gross), a part of which is audible to the human ear. The audible part of sounds may be classified according to the following groups:

1 Language form—
   (a) spiritual and philosophical forms;
   (b) scientific forms;
   (c) common forms,
2 Music (vocal and instrumental).
3 Sounds from animals.
4 Sounds in nature.
5 Artificially created sounds.

Mantra

Mantra is in the nature of Kundalini and Consciousness. It has been stated: 'Mantra is in the nature of Shiwa (Supreme Consciousness) and Shakti (Kundalini power); mantra arises from the muladhara. Those who are able to hear mantra or to expound it are rare' (—Yoga-shikhopanishad, 2.5). Mantra comes into being from Kundalini who is in muladhara. Kundalini manifests herself as mantra. As Kundalini is never without Shiwa-consciousness, so mantra is of Kundalini and Consciousness.

Mantra is endowed with the power of transforming thinking into deep concentration and causing the life-power motion to be absorbed into sushumna, thus effecting effortless breath-suspension. It has been stated: 'Because of the power of concentration, of the conduction of central bio-energy into sushumna, of arousing divine consciousness, and of its being based on Supreme Consciousness, it is called mantra' (—Yogashikhopanishad, 2.7–8). Mantra which originates from Kundalini in muladhara is also called mula (basic) —mantra. Mula means root or basis. The mantra which originates directly from Kundalini in muladhara and is the root of all other mantras is called mulamantra. So it is stated: 'That which is the root of all mantras, which arises from muladhara, and because of the real form of the root (that is Kundalini) in its subtle nature is embedded in that (mula-dhara), it is called mulamantra' (—Yogashikho-panishad, 2.8–9).

It has been further stated: 'Through the process of concentration spiritual protection is effected; this is why it has been termed mantra. In all mantras power-in-sound-form (wachaka-shakti) is inseparably linked with power as Consciousness (wachya-shakti)' (Ramatapinyup-anishad, 1.1.12). Therefore, mantra is endowed with the power of protecting the practitioner spiritually through the process of concentration. Thinking develops into concentration by mantra, and this mantra-concentration offers spiritual protection.

Ishwara stated: 'It is called mantra, because deep concentration on the true form of the immensely lustrous dewata (embodied divine consciousness) and protection from all fear are effected by it' (—Kularnawa, ch. 17, p. 84). Mantra, technically, is derived from 'man' and 'tra'. 'Man' means manana, that is, concentration, and 'tra' means trana, that is, protection. This means that our consciousness becomes free from worldly thoughts and goes into a state of concentration by mantra. Or, 'man' = mana to mean consciousness, and 'tra' to mean protection, that is, as consciousness at the sensory level is multifarious in character, so its higher aspect is hidden. Mantra is that process by which superconsciousness is preserved by controlling oscillations of consciousness and developing concentration. Mantra is that sound-power by which the uncontrolled mind becomes controlled and concentration is established.

There is still another factor. In pranawa, the final sound-power of 'm' is transformed into nada-bindu, that is, the sound '*ng*' on which the effectivity of 'O*ng*' as a mantra depends. Then the matrika-sounds and all mantras formed by matrika are endowed with '*ng*' sound-power as an intrinsic part. As '*ng*' sound is the inmost constitution of mantra, and as '*ng*' sound has developed from the 'm' factor, so the sound-phenomenon has been termed mantra, the 'm' factor being used at the beginning of the word. Moreover, the bija-sounds of mantra are finally reduced to nada-bindu, therefore, the nada-bindu is the vital part of mantra, and, as this vital part develops from 'm', so 'm' has been used as the first letter in mantra. This is why 'm' is called mantresha—the lord of mantra; that is, the supercontrol-power of mantra lies in 'm'.

So we find that mantra is that form of power-sound which arises from Kundalini, first as concentrated, uniform single sound, termed pranawa, which develops as multiform specialized sounds—matrika—and their complex combinations that can be transformed into waikhari (gross)-sounds. To put it in another way, mantra is the uncoiling of Kundalini as sound-power from her subtle state. So Kundalini has two forms—the subtle luminous form, and the mantra-form. When the luminous form is aroused in muladhara, Kundalini absorbs mantra. On the other hand, when mantra is aroused, Kundalini manifests herself as a Divine Being in an appropriate form, and that finally leads to luminous form.

When pranawa-sound first issued from Supreme Bindu, there was an agitation in prakriti by which the minus gunas imbedded there became plus factors. At the sattwa point, mantra-sound-power has created mahan manas (superconscious mind), and at the tamas point shabda tanmatra (sound tanon) has been created. Pranawa develops into fifty matrika-sounds, and matrika creates bija(germ)-mantra, other forms of mantra and Weda-mantra. Bija-mantra is that form of mantra in which sound-power is

in great concentration and from which dewata arises. It is that concentrated sound-power which makes Kundalini manifest as dewata. Bija-mantra may be a simple matrika-sound, viz. 'Gang'—the bija-mantra of Dewata Ganesha. On the other hand, a bija mantra may consist of a combination of two matrika-units, viz. 'Houng'—the bija-mantra of Dewata Shiwa. A bija-mantra may be a combination of more than two matrika-units. A bija-mantra may have more than one bija and one or more sound-forms constituted by a number of appropriate matrika-units without nada-bindu to increase the power of the bija. In Weda-mantra, different matrika-units, generally without nada-bindu, constitute word-forms. Certain word-forms are used as mantra, while others present thought-knowledge-forms which are received and understood by one who has purified his mind and raised the level of intellection to the spiritual level. Many such minus nada-bindu word-forms are masked forms of matrika-units with nada-bindu. As, for example, the word 'yama' is the masked form of matrika-unit 'yang'.

Pranawa is the first mantra. It has been stated: 'What all the Weda declares to be attained, what all ascesis is directed towards, and for what thought-emotion control is practised, is, in brief, that sound which is called 'Ong'. This Ong is Shabdabrahman and also Supreme Brahman. ... This spiritual practice is the best and highest. ...' (—Kathopanishad, 1.2.15–17). At first, by the practice of the pranawa mantra, Shabdabrahman is attained. Then the pranawa-sound recoils into Kundalini. Thereafter, by deep concentration on luminous Kundalini, non-sound Supreme Consciousness is reached.

Pranawa is a combination of three sounds which arise from '*a*', '*u*' and '*m*'. As long as '*a*', '*u*' and '*m*' form three separate sounds, the yogi will not be able to reach the Shabdabrahman level. Each separate sound does, of course, produce results, but this does not lead to Kundalini. When the three sounds become one sound, it is the pranawa-sound as it is manifested in Ong. It is an extraordinarily grand sound, which contains the germ of the summation of all fifty matrika-sounds. It is called pashyanti-sound. When concentration is not deep, the penetration of outer objects into consciousness cannot be completely eliminated. When concentration is interrupted the one sound appears as three sounds. But in deep concentration the three sounds become one and inseparable. This is possible when the external, the internal and their connecting links are under control. This has been termed bahyabhyantara-madhyama-kriya (externo-interno-median process) (—Prashnopanishad, 5.6). By the external is meant the outer objects, and by the internal, consciousness, and the middle is their connecting links—the senses. This is the process of senso-mental control.

At the sensory level, the three sounds are actually two sounds—that of 'a' and 'u'; the 'm' sound disappears after the 'u' sound. The 'a' and 'u' sound-powers are transformed into pingala and ida power-lines which maintain inspiration and expiration. The silent 'a' sound expresses itself as inspiration, and the silent 'u' sound as expiration. The third sound 'm' disappears at the interval between expiration and inspiration. The 'a' ceases because the ida-flow causes expiration. The 'u' ceases because inspiration is induced by the pingala-flow. So 'a' and 'u' can never be united unless the pingala-ida flows are transformed into sushumna-flow. In sushumna-flow inspiration and expiration are changed into kumbhaka (breath-suspension). In sushumna-flow 'a' and 'u' are united to effect 'o' which is a long sound starting from the muladhara and passing through the swadhishthana, manipura, anahata, and wishuddha, where the genuine 'o'-sound is heard. Then 'o' passes the ajña and thereafter the subdued 'm'-sound appears as nada-bindu and becomes linked to 'o' and effects one sound. The one sound now passes the sushumna and enters the sahasrara and is absorbed into Shabda-brahman, and samadhi is attained.

From the pranawa-sound matrika-sounds arise at the madhyama level. There are 50 matrika-sounds, from 'ang' to 'kshang'. The matrika-sounds can again be transformed into pranawa-sound, and pranawa-sound into Kundalini by the mantra-process. In this process the matrika-sounds are combined with ong, viz., ong ang, ong ang, ong ing, etc. By this process, the matrika-

sounds are gradually absorbed into pranawa-sound.

However, matrika-sounds possess specialized powers which are aroused by the mantra-process. The matrika-sound 'ang' has the death-conquering power; at the spiritual level it gives immortality by bringing the disciple beyond matter-mind, and, at the material level, it promotes health and longevity. It is present also in all sounds; it is all-pervading. The 'ang'-sound is all-pervading, and in the nature of attraction. It creates affection in the mind and the disciple becomes the centre of attraction. The 'ing'-sound promotes growth of the body and general welfare, but it also causes great disturbance and pain to those who slip from the spiritual path. The 'ing'-sound develops the power of higher speech and is in the nature of purity. The 'ung'-sound imparts vital vigour and is the essence of strength. The 'ung'-sound causes spiritual strength through unbearable pain and sorrow. The 'ring'-sound is the power causing agitation and is tremulous in character. The 'ring'-sound presents charming splendour. The 'lring'-sound causes enmity and bewilderment. The 'lring'-sound is also bewildering. The 'eng'- and 'aing'-sounds are pure sentience and charming. The 'ong'-sound is in the nature of all speech and purity. The 'oung'-sound is all speech and is endowed with the power of subjugation. The 'ang' (that is 'ng') -sound has the power of control over animals and is bewildering. The 'ah'-sound prevents death and is violent in nature.

The 'kang'-sound gives happiness and prosperity. The 'khang'-sound causes agitation. The 'gang'-sound removes all obstacles and is great. The 'ghang'-sound gives good fortune and stops what is not good. The 'nang'-sound is mighty. The 'chang'-sound is destructive in nature. The 'chang'-sound is formidable. The 'jang'-sound destroys all evil and causes fear. The 'jhang'-sound destroys unspirituality. The 'ñang'-sound is the conqueror of death. The 'tang'-sound is endowed with superpower and is the destroyer of all diseases. The 'thang'-sound is moon-like and is helpful in concentration, and bestows pleasure. The 'dang'-sound is very powerful and splendid. The 'dhang'-sound gives wealth and good fortune. The 'nang'-sound is the bestower of all success and causes infatuation. The 'tang'-sound is kindly disposed and a wealth-giver. The 'thang'-sound leads to religious attainment and to purity. The 'dang'-sound is pleasing and promotes growth. The 'dhang'-sound is great and the conqueror of disease. The 'nang'-sound develops tranquillity and gives enjoyment and liberation. The 'pang'-sound is auspicious and the remover of all obstacles. The 'phang'-sound is lustrous and leads to superpowers. The 'bang'-sound is the destroyer of all evils and splendid. The 'bhang'-sound is frightful and the destroyer of worldliness. The 'mang'-sound causes temptation and enmity. The 'yang'-sound is all-pervading. The 'rang'-sound causes pain and sickness. The 'lang'-sound is splendid and all-sustaining. The 'wang'-sound promotes welfare and gives purity. The 'shang'-sound is pure and bestows success. The 'shang'-sound is pure and leads to virtue and causes wealth and the fulfilment of desires. The 'sang'-sound is the root of knowledge. The 'hang'-sound is pure and bestows knowledge. The 'kshang'-sound gives spiritual and worldy knowledge and is splendorous. It is, as it were, a crest-jewel.

We find that a matrika-unit is a specific power operating in its individual characteristic manner. The power-line created by the operation of the power is called a specific warna, which is at the same time emitting specific sound. So, a matrika-unit is a specific power in specific sound-form. Each matrika-unit is a mantra. Some of these matrika-units, when combined in a definite manner, create specific sound-power in a highly concentrated form. These are the bija-mantras— concentrated powers in sound forms. Other mantras are also created. And finally, the Weda has been created. All spiritual potentials and creative elements contained in the matrika-units grow through the Gayatri mantra and culminate in the Weda. Here the arrangements of the matrika-units have taken a characteristic course to form words and, at the same time, they become mostly minus nada-bindu. These words appear to be more like a language at the sensory level. The mantra-power of matrika has been transformed in the Weda into a rarefied form of sentience containing the knowledge patterns of both cosmic and spiritual phenomena by specialized letter-arrangements. Here, mantra-power has lost its specificity, and is changed into cosmic and spiritual knowledge patterns. The real meanings of these knowledge-buds cannot be deciphered with the help of mere linguistic knowledge. The highly technical letter- and word-combinations are only known to the yogis who have realized mantra and its power transformation.

Mantra has two forms of power: wachaka-power and wachya-power. Wachaka-power is Kundalini in sound-form. Kundalini herself is mantra. It is in this power that mantra exists as a vital force. By the mantra-process the mantra-sounds are reduced to Kundalini-power; and then Kundalini assumes the appropriate divine form—dewata—and is revealed to yoga disciples in that form. So mantra-sounds can be transformed into Kundalini when she appears as dewata. When a disciple is able, at this stage, to transform concentration on the dewata form into superconcentration, and is fully established in it, dewata will, step by step, be recoiled into Kundalini; and Kundalini will be Mahakundalini and will shine forth as attributeless Supreme Consciousness. This is the wachya-power of mantra—Mahakundalini as Supreme Brahman.

If the mantra is bija-mantra and is imparted by a guru directly to his disciple, it will produce quicker and better results. A bija-mantra is the depository of immense power in a most concentrated form which remains latent in it. This latent power is aroused by the mantra-process disclosed to the disciple by his guru. The sound aspect of the power gradually becomes more and more rarefied and, ultimately, is absorbed into Kundalini. At this stage Kundalini herself assumes the form of Ishtadewata. Ishtadewata is that divine form which arises from the bija-mantra when it is absorbed into Kundalini. When the latent mantra-power in the bija is aroused by the mantra-process, the sound is absorbed at a certain stage of concentration into Kundalini; and Kundalini manifests herself as the dewata linked to the bija. So Ishtadewata is the divine form of mantra. Ishtadewata is the manifested Kundali-power in form. This divine form is intrinsically related to the bija. Bija is dewata.

Dewata—the divine form—is not an imaginary form, but a form which Kundalini herself has assumed. It is the form which arises from bija-mantra. In deep concentration, mantra-sounds are recoiled into Kundalini and Kundalini appears as Ishtadewata. In the sound-process, concentration gradually becomes uninterrupted and deep. In this manner, holding-concentration is transformed into deep concentration. At a higher stage of deep concentration Ishtadewata arises from mantra. Ishtadewata is not a passive phenomenon. Ishtadewata becomes living when concentration reaches the stage of samadhi. When this superconscious concentration is fully established Ishtadewata is seen also in a deconcentrated state. The devotee, who is in the dewata-consciousness, sees, hears and feels Ishtadewata in a post-concentration state, and is absorbed into that divine form in concentration. Ishtadewata finally leads the devotee to his or her formless infinite Supreme Being experienced in non-mens supreme concentration. This is wachya-power. The wachya-power is Mahakundalini (Supreme Kundalini) as Supreme Consciousness.

Bija-mantra is a very specialized mantra. If bija-mantra does not harmonize with the birth-bija, it will not be fruitful. The birth-bija is the germ of the substance that causes the repeated births, growth, activities, decline and death of embodied beings. It creates a natural tendency toward spirituality or worldliness, morality or immorality, constructiveness or destructiveness. The birth-bija is a miniature mirror upon which the whole being is reflected. A guru should know all this by close contact with his disciple for a long period, so as to be able to choose the right bija-mantra for him. When the right mantra is chosen it will produce remarkable results within a short time. All bad and unspiritual tendencies will begin to change toward spiritual development, strength will replace weakness, disease will be displaced by health. There will be more and more happiness and less and less pain. If these things do not happen, either the wrong mantra has been chosen or the disciple is stone-hearted.

There is another unusual factor in relation to bija-mantra. When a yoga disciple first ascends to non-mens supreme concentration, he is unable to stay there and descends. When the ups and downs go on again and again, Mahakundalini, who is one with Parama Shiwa (Supreme Consciousness), exhibits her spiritual creativity, unlike the creativity of prana by which the universe has been evolved. Mahakundalini, masking everything that is not Consciousness, and only being in Consciousness, manifests herself through Supreme Nada and Supreme Bindu as bija-mantra and Ishtadewata at the sahasrara level. Bija-mantra arises from the Supreme Nada aspect of Mahakundalini and from the Supreme Bindu aspect. At one point bija-mantra becomes Ishtadewata, and at another point Ishtadewata becomes bija-mantra. It is Mahakundalini who shows her two aspects— bija-mantra and Ishtadewata. There is no difference between bija-mantra and Ishtadewata. The disciple at the sahasrara level, through bija-mantra, develops deepest concentration in which the entire consciousness is of Ishtadewata. When concentration is less deep, mantra-sound is heard and the mantra-sound makes concentration deeper and, at a certain point, it is transformed into Ishtadewata when concentration becomes deepest. In this manner, superconscious concentration becomes established in the disciple. He gradually becomes master. Then it becomes easier for him to pass through Supreme Bindu and Supreme Nada to Mahakundalini in her supreme spiritual aspect, and to attain stable non-mens supreme concentration.

There are two power-flows in mantra: one is the prana-flow and the other is the Kundalini flow. Kundalini exercises control over prana, both partially and completely. In partial control, the general creative activities of prana are restrained and the pranic energy is utilized in exhibiting superpowers. When prana is fully controlled, spiritual power arises in mantra by which Kundalini is aroused and her spiritual yoga power is released. This causes the absorption of all creative principles. So in mantra lie both spiritual yoga and wibhuti (superpower). In one aspect, mantra is a means to acquire superpowers; and in another aspect, mantra leads to spiritual yoga. This is why it has been stated: 'When the principle of mantra is known, a person becomes freed-alive and attains animan power (the power of transforming the material body into subtle body) and other superpowers' (—Yogashikhopanishad, 2.6–7).

Mantra in Waikhari-form

Mantra does not normally occur in the material field. Mantras are formed at the madhyama level where they exhibit their creative omnipotence under the full control of Ishwara—Supreme Being in his aspect of supreme powerfulness. On the other hand, mantras retain their basic spiritual power of arousing Kundalini. The mantra-sounds are heard at the shabda tanmatra level. Shabda tanmatra is all sound. Shabda tanmatra itself has its sound form. It is the bija 'Hang'. When Shabda tanmatra evolves akasha (void) mahabhuta and sparsha (touch) tanmatra by its sound-power, it becomes more specialized. In this sound energy-organization there are 16 matrika-units with the central bija 'Hang'. In a similar manner, there are 12 matrika-units and the central bija 'Yang' in the touch energy-organization, 10 matrika-units and bija 'Rang' in the sight energy-organization, 6 matrika-units and bija 'Wang' in the taste energy-organization, and 4 matrika-units and bija 'Lang' in the smell energy-organization. Neither matrika-units nor bijas occur beyond this point. This is the borderland of the madhyama. So beyond madhyama there are no mantras. Matrika has progressively decreased in size and, at the 'Lang' level, there are only 4 matrikas. And thereafter there is nothing.

When this point is reached, there is no creation of new principles; the mahabhutas are combined with each other in a complex manner to form material energy and matter. Shabda tanmatra together with akasha mahabhuta produce sound-energy in the material field, which effects gross sounds. In a similar manner, sparsha tanmatra, rupa tanmatra, rasa tanmatra and gandha tanmatra together with wayu mahabhuta, tejas

mahabhuta, ap mahabhuta and prithiwi mahabhuta produce respectively the sensory phenomena of touch, sight, taste, and smell in the material field. However, Shabda tanmatra is the only source of sound-energy which produces all kinds of sound in the material field, and only a part of it is audible. These are waikhari sounds. They are without nada-bindu. So they are non-mantra sounds.

The non-mantra waikhari sounds cannot go beyond the senso-intellectual consciousness, so they are unable to reach the tanmatra level. These waikhari sounds, when arranged in certain forms, become the avenues of the expression of mental ideas. It may also be said that non-mantra waikhari sounds are elements which contribute in the formation of that aspect of mind which functions through the senses and exhibits intellectual, volitional and affective phenomena. These sounds only operate in the material field. Mantra-sounds operate at the superconscious level. The non-mantra waikhari sounds are the elements causing distraction of the mind. This means that consciousness at the sensory level exhibits multiformity and is limited in its power. The sense-consciousness is only able to picture the outer world as smell, taste, sight, touch and sound. On the other hand, mantra-sounds develop concentration.

At the sensory level, one does not hear the mantra-sound nor see Ishtadewata. Then how is it possible to develop concentration through mantra? It indicates the necessity of having a guru who has heard the mantra-sound and seen Ishtadewata. The mantra-sound is that sound which is unmodified, natural, pure sound arising from a power having both aspects—pranic creativity and spirituality; and this perfect sound is 'heard' at the shabda tanmatra level.

Through a process of concentration the guru reaches the shabda tanmatra level. The process consists of five stages. He first reduces smell tanon in deep concentration to taste tanon, and then taste tanon to sight tanon, sight tanon to touch tanon and, finally, touch tanon to sound tanon—shabda tanmatra. At this level mantra-sounds are reflected, registered, and 'heard' by his highly purified and concentrated consciousness. He first hears the Weda-sounds, then Gayatri, then bija-mantras, then matrika and, finally, pranawa-sound. When he is established in concentration at the shabda tanmatra level, he follows the course of the sounds in a reverse way so as to reach their origin. At a certain level of concentration the Weda-sounds arise. When concentration becomes still deeper, the Weda-sounds vanish and the Gayatri-sounds arise. In this manner when Gayatri vanishes, bija-mantras arise and then bija-mantras merge into matrika. At this stage, the fifty specialized sounds are heard separately. Then there is a summation of these fifty sounds from which arises the sound 'ong'. Then through 'ong' the source of the mantra-sound is reached. The sound 'ong' is finally absorbed into Kundalini in muladhara, and the guru experiences only Kundalini in her lightning-like splendorous form. Again he comes back to the sound-form of Kundalini and follows the course of the mantra-sound—pashyanti and then madhyama through sushumna, and reaches the shabda tanmatra level. In this manner, by going up and down through sushumna again and again he becomes established in mantrayoga.

Now the guru desires to give mantra a waikhari form. Mantra is the seat of both prana and Kundalini. When prana is operative, the yoga-superpower is manifested, and Kundalini becomes coiled; but when prana is controlled, Kundalini is aroused and spiritual concentration becomes a normal mode of being. To give mantra a Waikhari form it is necessary to add elements to the mantra-sound which will impart audibility. These elements come from prana. When the genuine mantra-sound is altered in this way both prana and Kundalini become coiled. The genuine mantra-sound is first transferred to the rarefied thought-intelligence level where mantra gets its sensory form and is reflected in the purified sense-consciousness. From sense-consciousness it passes to the will-mind and then it becomes conative impulse, then cerebral energy and, finally, motor impulses which activate the apparatus for voice production to produce a replica of the mantra-sound in a new sensory form—the waikhari mantra. The guru is able to reduce the waikhari mantra to its original sound-

form. The guru utters the waikhari mantra to his chosen disciple who hears it; the guru also imparts the prana and spiritual powers to his disciple to make the waikhari mantra work. The guru does not wish to utter the mantra to those who are not prepared for it, because to them mantra appears as meaningless sounds. Even if a person hears a mantra and tries to work on it, he will achieve very little unless guided by a guru.

The mere sound-form of the waikhari mantra is without spiritual power and superpower. Consequently it is possible to think that such a mantra is useless. But it is different when a well-prepared disciple hears a mantra from his guru. The guru knows how to arouse both prana-force and Kundalini-power, which reside in the mantra in coiled forms, by applying appropriate processes. This is the arousing of the mantra—imparting life to the audible mantra. According to the direction of the guru, the disciple is able to make the mantra live. A guru of a very high order is able to impart to his thoroughly trained disciple an enlivened mantra, called siddha mantra, which does not require any process of awakening.

The auditory sound factor of the mantra is not useless at the sensory level. First of all, it is the only form in which the mantra can be used by a disciple who is unable to reach the tanmatra level by deep concentration. But it must come from a guru. The powerlessness of the waikhari mantra is mainly due to the transformation of its genuine normal sound to audible sound. But there are processes by which the audible mantra is made powerful and its spirituality is awakened. If this is not done, the mantra will remain as dead. But when it is made living, it exhibits various powers. On the spiritual side, Kundalini-power is awakened and in a right moment Kundalini manifests in an appropriate divine form linked to the mantra as Ishtadewata. Ishtadewata is also made to appear in a living material form by the mantra.

By ritualistic worship, pranayama (breath-control) and japa (sound-process), the spiritual power of the mantra begins to be aroused and as a result concentration becomes uninterrupted and deep. In this way, first dharana (holding-concentration) is mastered, and then dharana begins to be transformed into dhyana (deep concentration). When mantra is made fully enlivened by japa, dhyana and worship, Kundalini residing in the mantra in latent form is aroused and finally she appears in a divine form as Ishtadewata.

Except in case of an enlivened mantra, all waikhari mantras should be aroused by certain specific processes. They are complicated and cannot be successful without the help of guru. These processes consist in japa of certain specific waikhari mantras in a certain order with a number of nyasa (a special method of purification by placing hands on certain parts of the body with mantras), pranayama, and certain modes of concentration. The most important is the arousing of real sound-power in a waikhari mantra in which it has been latent due to an alteration of sound-form. The natural mantra-sound has been changed to the vibrational gross sound effected by the action of a vibrating mechanism. This is waikhari-sound. The mantra-sound is the pure normal sound intrinsically associated with power which is capable of exhibiting superpower and spiritual power. In creating the waikhari-sound, the normal mantra-sound which is apprehended without any modification in superconsciousness, has to be transmitted to intellect and sense-consciousness, where a process of modification takes place. This modification is necessary to give the sound a shape which can be reproduced as a vibrational waikhari-sound. In this process, the power emitting mantra-sound becomes latent, and its sound factor is reproduced, in a modified form, as waikhari mantra-sound. The original natural mantra-sound is called anahata-mantra (—Nirwanopanishad, 3.13). The mantra-sound is not produced through instrumentalization, but arises normally from Kundalini-power, this is why the sound is anahata, that is, not produced by a vibrating body, but unmodified and normal. Our object is to retransform the waikhari mantra-sound to anahata mantra-sound by arousing the sleeping power. When the power is roused, the anahata-mantra-sound will arise normally.

There is a highly complicated Waidika method of transforming the waikhari-mantra by a special pranayama in conjunction with a sixfold-process by which the real mantra-sound is released from the gross sound and penetrates through sense-consciousness to the sound realm which is shabda tanmatra, where the natural mantra-sound arises; and all these things should be done according to the advice of guru (—Yogashikhopanishad, 2.13–14). The non-mantra waikhari-sounds give an intellectual interpretation in the conscious field or are reduced to mere impressions in the nonconscious field. They have no possibility of reaching the superconscious field. But the waikhari mantra-sound can be made to release the power, coiled in it, by special processes of breath-control and concentration, which then pierces through sense-consciousness and reaches the shabda tanmatra level, where this power becomes mantra in perfect sound-form.

Ishwara says: 'When the power of the mantra (waikhari-mantra) remains hidden, that mantra does not produce any effects. When the mantra is made living, it gives all results. The mantra without life is mere letters. Such a lifeless mantra does not produce any result even if one makes millions of japa' (—Kularnawa, ch. 15, p. 75). Therefore, first of all the coiled power of a waikhari-mantra should be aroused. This is what is Mantra-chaitanya—the life-impartation to mantra.

The waikhari-mantra is made efficacious by the purification of the nadis (power-lines) and concentration. This super-purification is attained by breath-control and internal purification of the body. It has been stated: 'An excellent means to make mantra efficacious is concentration on divine Kundalini, residing in muladhara at the end of sushumna, along with the purification of the nadis' (—Mundamalatantra, ch. 6, p. 12). In a general way, the purification of the nadis is necessary, and is attained by pranayama and internal purification of the body. But more specifically the purification of sushumna is the most important. It is effected by kumbhaka (breath-suspension). It is also possible to make mantra work by deep concentration alone. So it is stated: 'The mantra becomes effective by concentration alone, without any physical process. Concentration should be done in the hrit-centre on Kundalini in form. The power developing from concentration will make mantra efficacious' (—Mundamalatantra, ch. 6, p. 12).

The waikhari-mantra should also be purified. Otherwise japa will not be effective. An advanced process of mantra-purification is as follows.

First, assume siddhasana (accomplished posture) with the left heel set tightly against the perineum, and the right heel against the root of the genitals; the body is kept perfectly straight and motionless. Then the apana-wayu should be raised by anal contraction with breath-suspension. By deep thinking, make all the letters of the mantra one by one enter through the sushumna-path into muladhara and transfer them to Kundalini who is in the nature of divine consciousness; then make the mantra-letters, one by one, enter into swadishthana, then into manipura, anahata, wishuddha, ajña and sahasrara. Think deeply that in the moon-sphere of this centre, the mantra-letters are fully saturated with life-substance (amrita). Again, by deep thinking, bring the mantra to ajña through sushumna, and then to wishuddha, anahata, manipura, swadhishthana and muladhara. Thereafter perform rishi-nyasa and other nyasas and, then make japa of the mantra one thousand and eight times. By this method the mantra should be purified (—Purashcharyarnawa, ch. 2, p, 90–1).

A mantra which has been purified and aroused by life-impartation, and strengthened by secret processes of japa produces astounding results. Mantra becomes effective by japa. Japa of a living mantra should be done to get the desired effects. Japa is of three forms; wachika (verbal), upangshu (muttering) and manasa (mental). When a mantra is clearly uttered and is heard by others, it is wachika; when a mantra is uttered in voice so low that only the person himself and nobody else hears it, it is called upangshu; and thinking of or concentrating on the letters of mantra is called manasa. Japa is that process by which a chain of the waikhari mantra-sounds is formed in consciousness. Sounds should first be correctly produced and a clear picture of the correct sound should be established in the mind. The guru utters the correct sounds of the mantra and the disciple hears them. By hearing again

and again from his guru, he learns how to produce correct sounds. He himself then utters the mantra in an audible manner. When he has mastered the correct sound production, he practises the production of correct sounds in a low voice. He concentrates on the sounds of the mantra when he utters the mantra. Mantra-sounds uttered in this manner develop concentration. He then practises to produce very low and rhythmic mantra-sounds, concentrating on the sounds. This develops the power of concentration to such an extent that he is able to make mental japa.

In mental japa, a faultless sound-form of the mantra is created in consciousness by thinking of the mantra-sounds. These sounds are of thought-forms based on correctly uttered sounds. One thought-form of sound follows another. There should be concentration on one thought-form of sound, and consciousness must hold it without letting it disappear. This is the mantra unit of concentration. At the end of one sound-thought-form there is a brief interval, and then the second form is created. In this way, when one-hundred sound-thought-forms are created, and the intervals are almost zero, and concentration is such that this whole chain of one-hundred sound-thought-forms without any break anywhere is held in consciousness, the concentration is called holding-concentration (dharana). The concentration of one-hundred units is the lowest type. Concentration of 10,000 units is of the medium type; and above it is the higher type. In any type of holding-concentration, the image of the sound-form should be firmly held in consciousness; the second image will replace the first, but it will occupy the whole consciousness, similarly with the third, fourth, fifth, etc., until 100 are completed. Concentration should not be broken off between the intervals of image formation, but pass from one to another, until the whole chain is complete. First, 100 chain-formation should be practised. Then 1,000, 10,000 and upwards, should be done in a graduated manner.

To explain it more clearly: one mantra unit concentration is this: concentration on the sound unit when uttered once or, concentration on the thought-form of the same when not repeated. When concentration is done on fifty mantra units, one after the other, that is, on the first unit, the second unit, the third unit to the fiftieth unit in succession, they constitute the unit of holding-concentration. Concentration consisting of twenty holding-concentration-units raises holding-concentration to the first level; 200 holding-concentration units make the second level, and above it is the third level. In one mantra unit concentration, the sound-form of the entire mantra should be held without any other objects impinging on it or replacing it partially or completely. In other words, the sound-form should occupy consciousness fully and without moving. This is the mantra unit of concentration. When fifty mantra units are linked to each other, they form a holding-concentration unit. The fifty mantra units are linked in this manner: the first unit is held in consciousness; when the final phase of the mantra-sound is thought, a new sound-form of the same mantra is to be created and held in consciousness in place of the first. When the third is created, the second will disappear. But the intervals between the units are so brief that there is no complete break in the sound-forms in the consciousness, and each sound-form is exactly the same. Still it goes on in succession, one form is replaced by another of exactly the same form. In this manner holding-concentration continues.

At a certain point, concentration becomes so deep that the successive formation of mantra-sound is changed into one continuous mantra-sound without any intervals, without any break at any point; there is no changing of form, no replacement, no penetration of any other objects —this long continued sound-form held in consciousness firmly and fully and without the manifested I-ness and without any other objects —is termed deep concentration (dhyana). Here is only one sound-form and nothing else. At a certain point of deep concentration, the sound factor of the mantra is transformed into a divine form. That is, the mantra-form of Kundalini is transformed into a divine form of Kundalini, which is called Ishtadewata. Now, Kundalini as mantra becomes Kundalini as Ishtadewata. With the arising of Ishtadewata, concentration becomes deeper and deeper, and finally it is transformed into superconcentration (samadhi).

In superconscious concentration (samprajñata samadhi), Ishtadewata becomes living. Deep love of God (bhakti) arises and flows toward Ishtadewata. Love becomes most intensified and flows only toward Ishtadewata by the strength of concentration, and concentration becomes deepest and prolonged by intense love. In this state, the whole consciousness is of Ishtadewata; any separate I-ness is absorbed into Ishtadewata. Finally, Ishtadewata changes into formless luminous Kundalini, into which superconsciousness is gradually absorbed, and Kundalini as Mahakundalini enters Parama Shiwa (Supreme Consciousness) and becomes supremely united with him to be one with Shiwa in non-mens supreme concentration (asamprajñata samadhi).

CHAPTER 5
Bhutashuddhi—
Purificatory
Thought-concentration

Bhutashuddhi is a process of deep thinking, of the rousing of Kundalini and of the absorption of all creative principles, stage by stage, into Kundalini and, finally, Kundalini into Parama Shiwa— supreme consciousness. Deep thinking gradually develops into concentration through this process. The thought-forms, that is what are thought of in this process, are exactly what actually happens in kundaliniyoga. So that it is not by any means fanciful thinking, but thinking of what is a fact; it is a series of phenomena which occurs when Kundalini is actually aroused in kundaliniyoga, and the same phenomena are imitated in thought by a disciple in the process of bhutashuddhi.

When concentration is not deep enough and often interrupted by the penetration of sensory objects into consciousness, this thinking process will be very helpful. The thinking will gradually become deeper by practice; and deep thinking will be changed into concentration in time. At this stage, control-power is developed to the extent that only one object is held in consciousness up to a certain time without any interruption. This is holding-concentration (dharana). Holding-concentration will gradually be transformed into very deep continuous concentration (dhyana) and, at a certain point, the thinking of rousing Kundalini will become a fact— Kundalini will be actually aroused. From now, the whole absorption process is accomplished automatically, that is, no thinking of absorption is necessary, Kundalini herself will absorb all principles, and this fact will be reflected in consciousness which is in a state of concentration.

When concentration develops into superconscious concentration (samprajñata samadhi) the whole consciousness is of Kundalini, and there is a complete absence of anything but Kundalini. Finally, divinely illuminated consciousness is absorbed into Kundalini and Kundalini into Parama Shiwa in non-mens supreme concentration. Therefore, bhutashuddhi leads to kundaliniyoga.

This thought-concentration process is purificatory. Consciousness is purified of all objective thoughts. When consciousness becomes free from thoughts, the I-ness also becomes unexpressed. The I-nessless and object-less consciousness is super-purified superconsciousness which is illuminated by splendorous Kundalini. Unless there is a complete elimination of all objective thoughts from consciousness, it will not be able to receive any light from Kundalini. The objective phenomena are due to the creative principles. When they are absorbed into Kundalini, consciousness becomes purified. As the process of thought-concentration develops real concentration, so bhutashuddhi is a purifying process.

Purusha and Prakriti

Supreme Reality—the eternal static whole Consciousness—is inconceivable at any stage of evolution. Supreme Power which is inseparable from Supreme Consciousness, in its power aspect, evolves creative principles. The seed of duality is born with the emergence of two great principles—Purusha (consciousness principle) and Prakriti (primus), and duality becomes an established fact in sense-consciousness. In purusha, consciousness is not tinged with what is not consciousness. This means that though prakriti has emerged, it is nonexistent in the purusha consciousness, and, consequently, there is no prakriti while one is in purusha. Prakriti is unmanifested here. Unmanifested to whom? To purusha, or when one is in purusha, that is in one's own conscious form. The three primary attributes of prakriti are in a negative phase.

But prakriti is not nothing; it is the source of all created phenomena. But how are its creative possibilities actualized? Can we say when prakriti is 'seen' by purusha? What is it that is 'seen'? Purusha consciousness is that in which there is nothing but consciousness. Prakriti is not consciousness, so it does not exist in purusha consciousness. Though prakriti is negated in purusha consciousness, it none the less exists. It exists as an aspect of Power (Shakti), and that Power itself is inseparable from, and one and the same with, Supreme Consciousness. So, it is Supreme Power. The Supreme Power as the power of beingness of Supreme Consciousness is infinite; but its power-manifestation is only possible when the power becomes finite. It is only possible when an unreal phenomenon—unreal in relation to Supreme Reality—is made to appear as real. This is effected by Maya—the specific power of Supreme Power. By the influence of this power, Supreme Consciousness appears as purusha and Supreme Power in its bindu (supremely concentrated power) aspect, appears as prakriti.

Prakriti is that aspect of bindu-power in which creative energy is in three forms as minus factors. These three forms are called gunas (primary attributes). In prakriti, the gunas are negative factors, but there is the possibility of the gunas being patent when prakriti becomes the source of creation. But the gunas remain negative in prakriti, unless they are aroused by something from outside prakriti. From where does this 'something' come?

Purusha and prakriti may be interpreted differently when there is no experience above the purusha-prakriti level. Purusha is consciousness in which there is no trace of anything else. As this consciousness is not analysable or reducible, so purusha is the ultimate principle. And prakriti exists as an independent principle, which is not consciousness. If we accept this, we have to explain the nature of the relation between consciousness and what is not consciousness. It is said that purusha is lame but can see, and prakriti can move but does not see. It is as if purusha sits on the shoulders of prakriti and shows the way, and prakriti moves blindly. This means prakriti in contact with conscious purusha undergoes evolutionary changes. But what does it actually mean? Does it not indicate that purusha is also endowed with power that makes prakriti evolve? If it is assumed that consciousness itself is the stimulus to make prakriti evolve, then we have also to assume that purusha consciousness exerts some influence on prakriti, either consciously or unconsciously. This purusha influence on prakriti cannot altogether be denied. This means consciousness as power, which is not without motive, is the root cause of the evolutionary changes of prakriti. If prakriti remains infinitely as an independent principle tending to develop as different cosmic principles in relation to purusha, then we have to admit that the ultimate picture of consciousness is that form of consciousness which is associated through its power with prakriti which is evolving. This form of consciousness cannot be the irreducible ultimate Supreme Consciousness, but it is a form which appears at a transitory phase of realization that ultimately culminates in the experience of the eternal static whole consciousness.

If the mere presence of purusha causes prakriti to evolve, then prakriti can never be in a state when the gunas are negative, and under this condition the absorption of prakriti is not possible and, consequently, non-mens concentration is an impossible phenomenon. Supreme Bindu is both Consciousness and Power. In its creative aspect, the power is prana-energy in a supremely concentrated state. On the other hand, Kundalini-power is associated with Supreme Bindu in its spiritual aspect. When creative prana-energy is manifested, the spiritual Kundalini-power remains in a coiled state. To make a finite phenomenon possible in infinite Supreme Consciousness-Power, Maya—negato-positivity principle—arises from Supreme Bindu. By the influence of maya prakriti appears as a separate principle in which is imbedded the creative germ consisting of three primary principles as minus factors, and from the mantra viewpoint prakriti is kamakala in which lie the pre-matrika units in a latent form. With the evolution of prakriti, also arises purusha as consciousness separate from, but related to, prakriti.

Purusha consciousness is Shiwa Consciousness, as if, isolated from Supreme Consciousness-Power by maya. The emergence of purusha is a most important phenomenon. The passivity of purusha does not stir prakriti directly, but as purusha consciousness is the consciousness of Supreme Bindu which, as Ishwara (Supreme Being in his creative aspect) 'wills' to express his (or her) creative omnipotence, it is this 'will' which acts on prakriti silently to make the gunas operate. The gunas operate on the principle of bindu-nada-bija. The nada or sound-emitting power becomes rajas (primary energy-principle) which is the source of all energy in the mental and physical fields. The same power becomes transformed into sattwa, (primary sentience-principle), which exhibits mental consciousness. The same nada-power becomes tamas (primary inertia-principle) which creates metamatter and matter.

Through the omnipotent 'willing' of Ishwara, purusha consciousness is reflected on sattwa, causing an 'artificial' consciousness which is expressed as mental consciousness; and the nature and degree of the expression depend on the concentration of sattwa. This reflection of puru-sha on sattwa does not change its passive nature. Sattwa itself is not consciousness; it is unconscious. But sattwa is in such a rarefied form that purusha consciousness becomes reflected on it. This reflection is mental consciousness. When mental consciousness is embodied, it begins to function, and the whole organization is called jiwa—an embodied being. Mental consciousness is also unconsciousness, if it is not enlivened by

life-force. Life-force is manifested in an embodied being. Mental consciousness is the source of all knowledge of embodied beings. This knowledge is attained only through the instrumentation of the body, senses and mind, and is limited. It does not reach beyond the sensory realm. Mental consciousness plays a predominant role in the functioning of the senses. As mind can also function without the help of the senses, so Ishwara's 'will' functions without mind or body.

As prakriti is not conscious, so the three gunas are not conscious factors. But sattwa cannot function without a background of life-force. It is clearly seen in embodied beings. If life-force ceases to function in an embodied being, mental consciousness is also brought to an end. The 'will' of Ishwara which stirs the minus gunas, also provides the life-background. The 'will' of Ishwara is the concentrated power of Supreme Bindu which is also Shiwa-consciousness. The power aspect is prana, which is living energy. In Ishwara's 'will', prana is fully controlled. The controlled prana is expressed as omnipotence in creation. Prana as energy gives rise to the three primary principles rajas, sattwa and tamas to constitute prakriti. These three gunas are unconscious. Through Ishwara's 'will' not only comes the directing impulse to rouse the gunas, but also the life-force which serves as a background for the functioning of sattwa, which, as mental consciousness, is manifested in a living organism.

The evolution of the universe is an expression of the highest yoga-wibhuti—omnipotency—by Ishwara. In Ishwara, prana-force is supremely concentrated and is fully under conscious control. In evolution, three fields are created: a mental conscious field, created by sattwa, a material field created by tamas, and a power field created by prana as life-force. Rajas creates energy which operates in the mental and material fields. Rajas-energy is transformed into elements of sentience in sattwa, and material energy and matter in tamas. Life-force transforms inorganic matter into living matter. In life-force lies also conscious power by which appropriate matter is selected that is made living, and is transformed into a pattern most suitable for the manifestation of mental consciousness. This transformation is a highly complicated process by which an apparently simple substance becomes highly complex. Every part of the process is purposeful, properly timed and wholly controlled. Cell activities and functional activities of the organs are parts of the activities of the organism as a whole. All these suggest that there is a conscious factor in the life-force. The life-force is the specific expression of prana. Prana, in creation, becomes wayu-force in five forms, namely prana-wayu, apana-wayu, samana-wayu, udana-wayu and wyana-wayu.

To summarize: purusha is the disembodied consciousness principle, arising from Supreme Bindu when it is about to evolve. When purusha consciousness becomes embodied and in-dividualized by the influence of maya and kanchukas, it is jiwa—embodied conciousness or being. So jiwa is purusha with modifications. Here purushas are many. On the other hand, when purusha becomes embodied cosmically and at the same time he is the master of maya and kanchukas (five forms of the power of limitation derived from maya), he is called Ishwara. Ishwara is an aspect of Supreme Bindu. So Ishwara is also purusha.

Prakriti, which is the unconscious power prin-ciple, also arises from Supreme Bindu. When Bindu is about to evolve, the power of Bindu as-sumes trifurcate creative power principles, which are in a state of negativity when the value of each principle is zero. This is called prakriti. Prakriti is the latent phase of creativity in the form of power principles as primary attributes in a negative state. This negativity is transformed into a state of relativity when the primary attributes become plus factors by the direction of Ishwara. At the pre-creative state, Ishwara is beyond prakriti—nirguna (without attributes). After creation, Ishwara becomes saguna (with attri-butes) and the entire cosmic mind-body is the embodiment of Ishwara.

Evolution of Creative Principles

Power in Supreme Bindu exists in two forms—prana and Kundali. Prana is the energy principle of Supreme Power in its omnipotent aspect, which is expressed as creative omnipotency. Supreme Power in its spiritual aspect is Kundalini. In Supreme Bindu energy is in a supremely concentrated form ready to manifest its creative omnipotence. Therefore, the prana-energy flow is away from Supreme Consciousness.

Prana is the living energy. At the prakriti level, a part of prana-energy is released which trifurcates as non-living gunas. Kundali-power is conscious spiritual power which flows most powerfully only towards Supreme Consciousness when prana-flow is controlled. But prana at the bindu point is also controlled by Kundali-power. This Kundali-control makes prana-energy ex-hibit highest yoga-wibhuti—creative omni-potence. Supreme Power in her power aspect is Supreme Bindu; and Supreme Bindu in its creative aspect is Ishwara.

Before prana manifests its creative omni-potence, a power called maya arises from Supreme Bindu by the influence of which the infinite power of Supreme Bindu appears as finite, and then evolution becomes possible. At a certain point, maya makes consciousness, which is united with the power in Supreme Bindu, appear as purusha—consciousness prin-ciple. Maya also causes prakriti to appear as unconscious power principle. But purusha and prakriti exist in relation to each other. When prakriti emerges from Supreme Bindu, Kundalini, as it were, radiates its power in the form of sound as kamakala (coiled creative omnipotency in sound-form) in which lie the germinal matrika-units.

In fact, kamakala and prakriti are not fundamentally different. The nature of the powers inherent in prakriti is in the sound-forms that are represented in kamakala. The three gunas in prakriti are the three lines of an equilateral triangle, consisting in latent sound-units which form kamakala. When the gunas begin to operate, the kamakala triangle, as it were, bursts and emits sound known as pranawa-sound. The power which is involved in trans-forming the minus gunas into plus ones, thus effecting their operations, is in the nature of pranawa-sound. The pure energy is from prana and the control of that energy is from Kundali-

121

power expressed as pranawa-sound.

Prakriti does not exist above the purusha level. The existence of prakriti is due to maya, and with the absorption of maya, prakriti is also absorbed, and what remains is bindu-power-consciousness in Supreme Bindu. The absorption of maya is a great step towards arousing the Kundali-power to the extent when it absorbs all sound-forms as well as prana. Now all creative impulses cease. Now, Kundalini as Supreme Kundalini is the spiritual aspect of Supreme Power. But Supreme Power in its creative aspect is Supreme Bindu in which prana-energy is supremely concentrated and on which Kundali as Shabdabrahman exerts control through sound-power to raise it to the level of creative omnipotence. The Kundalini-control over prana remains at the pashyanti and madhyama levels.

Kundalini, as Supreme Kundalini, ascends from Supreme Bindu to Supreme Nada. Nada is the power of Supreme Power in its power aspect, which is infinite, but with a trace of something which may develop as finite power. At this point, prana as infinite energy-principle is a part of Kundali. The possibility of being 'motional' is most pronounced in Supreme Bindu, in which prana becomes concentrated to the highest degree; but it is also controlled by Kundalini.

Nada is predominantly Kundali-power where there is a faint indication of sound element, which is neither evident, nor traced, nor manifested. This sound element becomes sound principle at the bindu level when Kundalini is Shabdabrahman. At the nada level, when Kundalini is towards Supreme Shiwa (Consciousness), sound is completely coiled into her. But when the power-flow is away from Shiwa, a faint indication appears. This untraceable sound element may develop into specific bija-mantra by which Supreme Kundalini, united with Supreme Shiwa, appears as Ishtadewata in the thousand-petalled lotus. The sound element develops into matrika in latent form at the bindu level, when Supreme Power is in its creative aspect.

When Supreme Kundalini is at the Shiwa-Shakti level, Shiwa shines forth in Kundalini.

At this stage, there is nothing but Shiwa in Kundalini. Thereafter Kundalini is in union in supreme love with Parama Shiwa—infinite Consciousness. This occurs at the Sakala Shiwa stage. Finally, Kundalini in supreme union becomes one and the same with Parama Shiwa. Now there is only Shakti (Power) as Shiwa, and Shiwa as one with his Shakti. Mahakundalini is now Parama Shiwa.

When bindu-power as prana first manifests its creativity, Kundali-power bursts through the kamakala triangle and appears as pranawa-sound which exercises control over the manifested pranic force. In fact, the pranawa-sound is the intrinsic part of the first manifested pranic force. The manifestation of pranic force is associated with the changes of minus gunas to plus gunas in prakriti. Now Kundali-controlled pranic force begins to operate at the rajas point. This occurs just at the end of pranawa-sound, that is, at the junction between pashyanti and madhyama. Pranic force exhibits circular motions, making twenty circles, and at each circle fifty matrika-units appear. In this way sahasrara (the thousand-petalled centre) comes into being. Here, each matrika-unit is twenty units strong.

Thereafter, the rajas-line, the sattwa-line and the tamas-line are manifested. In the rajas-line, where rajas is the predominant factor, prana bifurcates into rajas-energy and life-energy. Rajas-energy at the sattwa point is transformed into sentience, and at the tamas point it becomes matter and material energy. Life-energy at the sattwa point forms the vital basis for the functioning of sattwa, and at the tamas point forms living matter. At the rajas point, life-energy as wayu-energy creates force-field.

From sattwa arise, stage by stage, the following principles:

1 Mahan (supermind).
2 Ahang (I-ness).
3 Buddhi (intellective mind).
4 Chitta (sense-consciousness).
5 Jñanendriyas (senses).
6 Karmendriyas (conative faculties).

In mahan, there is a maximum concentration of sattwa. When the traces of rajas and tamas in the sattwa-line are neutralized, the absorption of mahan into prakriti takes place. The maximum concentration of sattwa gradually diminishes with the penetration of more rajas. Mahan is that form of consciousness in which there is absolute calmness without any undulations. This consciousness is where there is no objective phenomenon, and it is in a state of deepest concentration, that is, the final phase of super-conscious concentration. This consciousness is illuminated by the splendour of divine Kundalini.

When more of the rajas begins to penetrate into the sattwa point, consciousness begins to show oscillations. At the same time more of tamas also concentrates in it, causing a limitation of consciousness. All these occur step by step. In this way, ahang (I-ness) is created. Now, the conscious field is divided into two parts: I-consciousness and objective consciousness. The objective consciousness is that in which things remaining outside the I-consciousness become reflected. The objective consciousness has two aspects: dhi (concentrative mind) and chitta (sense consciousness). Along with chitta are created buddhi (intellective mind), manasyana manas (will-mind) and indriya manas (sense-mind). Then with more rajas and tamas, five jñanendriyas (senses) and five karmendriyas (conative faculties) come into being.

To summarize.

1 Mahan: consciousness which is without I-ness and objects. In this most rarefied consciousness there is the full reflection of purusha. Consciousness is in a state of the fourth stage of superconscious concentration. Mahan consciousness is the culmination of dhi consciousness.

2 Ahang. First level: consciousness which bifurcates into I-consciousness and objective consciousness. The objective consciousness is dhi consciousness which is in a state of the third stage of superconscious concentration in which Ishwara in form is reflected. Second level: Dhi is in a state of the second stage of superconscious concentration. Objects are five mahabhutas and five tanmatras. Third level: Dhi is in a state of the first stage of superconscious concentration. Objects are sensory. Fourth level: Chitta is in an oscillatory state (writti state). Intellective mind, sense-mind, senses, will-mind and conative faculties

are involved in this state. Objects: material objects. Functions: (1) sensory perception; (2) thought and intellection; (3) affectivity; (4) volition and conation.

From concentration viewpoint: 1 Mahan: superconscious concentration, final stage.

2 Ahang. First level: superconscious concentration, third stage. Object: Ishwara in form. Second level: superconscious concentration, second stage. Object: five mahabhutas and five tanmatras. Third level: superconscious concentration, first stage. Object: sensory. Fourth level: writti state. Writtis are derived from: (1) perception; (2) thought and intellection; (3) affectivity; (4) volition and conation.

Tamasa Evolution

Tamasa (relating to tamas—primary inertia principle) evolution arises from the primary inertia-principle from which develop five tanmatras (tanon), five mahabhutas (metamatter) and matter. The first development from tamas is sound tanon (shabda tanmatra). Sound tanon is the germ of all madhyama sound. It is itself in the form of the germ-mantra 'Hang'. Sound tanon develops into void metamatter (akasha mahabhuta), with which are related sixteen matrika-units from 'Ang' to 'Ah'.

From sound tanon arises touch tanon (sparsha tanmatra), the sound-form of which is 'Yang'. It develops into air metamatter (wayu mahabhuta), which is related to twelve matrika-units from 'Kang' to 'Thang'. From touch tanon arises form tanon (rupa tanmatra), the sound-form of which is 'Rang'. It develops into fire metamatter (tejas mahabhuta) represented by ten matrika-units from 'Dang' to 'Phang'. From form tanon is evolved taste tanon (rasa tanmatra). Its sound-form is 'Wang'. It develops into water metamatter (ap mahabhuta) represented by six matrika-units from 'Bang' to 'Lang'. Smell tanon (gandha tanmatra) arises from taste tanon. Its sound-form is 'Lang'. It develops into earth metamatter (prithiwi mahabhuta) represented by four matrika-units from 'Wang' to 'Sang'.

123

At this point the five forms of metamatter are combined to form matter.

Bhutashuddhi

It has been stated: 'Brahman is without manifested power (wiraja), (that is, static), and in it Supreme Power is absorbed (nishkala); that is, pure (shubhra), (that is, Brahman is in itself, there is nothing in it except Brahman); it is the splendour of all splendours, (that is, the splendour of Kundalini is from Brahman); Brahman is in supreme splendorous abode (that is, Brahman is in supreme void in splendorous Kundalini in the triangular process of moon-sphere in sahasrara); Brahman is reached by those who have realized (in samadhi) the supremeness of his being' (—Mundakopanishad, 2.2.10). Nishkala (with absorbed Power) Brahman is nishkala Shiwa—Parama Shiwa (Supreme Consciousness). The aim of layayoga is to reach nishkala Brahman. This is achieved by getting Supreme Kundalini absorbed into Parama Shiwa in non-mens supreme concentration.

About Brahman, it has been further stated: 'Brahman is beyond sound, touch, form, taste and smell; beyond the reach of the organs of speech, prehension and locomotion, Brahman is untouched by organic activities and carnal pleasures; Brahman is beyond mind, intellect, I-ness and sense-consciousness. Brahman is without prana, apana, samana, wyana and udana, without sense organs and sense objects, and mind; Brahman cannot be defined; Brahman is free from bondage, without attributes, unchangeable' (—Nrisinghatapinyupanishad, 2.9.20). Brahman is beyond the senses, all actions, sense-mind, sense-consciousness, intellective mind, and I-ness consciousness. Therefore, layayoga aims at the absorption of all these principles through Kundali-power to reach Brahman.

It is stated: 'They say that there was only Narayana (Supreme Consciousness) without a second; there was no Brahma, no Ishana (that is, God in forms); no water, fire and air; no heaven and earth; no stars, no sun and no moon.

It was he who was alone and motionless. Then he, being in himself, was in concentration, and then yajñastoma (creative energy in germ form) came into being. From this creative energy there issued fourteen purushas (forms of consciousness), one girl (primus), ten indriyas (senses and conative faculties), manas (sense-mind) as the eleventh, tejas (here: intellective mind) as the twelfth, ahangkara (I-ness) as the thirteenth, prana (bio-energy) as the fourteenth, atman (jiwatman) as the fifteenth, who is endowed with intelligence. The other principles are: five tanmatras (tanons), five mahabhutas (five forms of metamatter): twenty-five in all, and that purusha (consciousness principle) is one' (—Mahopanishad, 1.2–5).

Narayana is Parama Shiwa—Supreme Consciousness. He is infinite and all, and so, he is beyond the universe of mind-matter. But when he is in concentration, being established in his own secondless static form, he is also conscious of the beingness of his own power which, as Supreme Power, is one and the same with him. This beingness of power in him gives rise to the phenomenon of Shiwa-shakti in which there is a faint awakening of power which is of Shiwa. But in that power there is the possibility of expressing it in a finite form. The first step towards that manifestation is the supremely concentrated power in which is embedded the spiritual control factor. This has been termed 'Yajñastoma'—the germ of power-manifestation which in Tantrika terms consists of Supreme Nada and Bindu.

Form yajñastoma the following creative principles arise:

1 Purushas, which are fourteen; that is, divine forms of consciousness.
2 Purusha (consciousness principle).
3 Prakriti (primary creative principle; primus).
4 Ahang (I-ness).
5 Buddhi (intellective mind).
6 Manas (sense-mind).
7 Indriyas, which are ten. These are: five senses and five conative organs of action.
8 Prana (bio-energy).
9 Jiwatman (embodied being).

10 Tanmatras (tanons), which are five in
   number.
11 Mahabhutas (metamatter), which are five.

Here we find the fundamentals of kundaliniyoga and bhutashuddhi. The fourteen purushas
are deities, of which six are Shiwas. The first
Shiwa is Deity Brahma situated in the muladhara
centre; the second is Wishnu in the swadhishthana centre, the third is Rudra in the manipura centre, the fourth is Isha in the anahata
centre, the fifth is Sadashiwa in the wishuddha
centre, and the sixth is Parashiwa in the indu
centre. These Shiwas are also called Brahmas.

The Waidika process of kundaliyoga has been
briefly described here : 'Hridaya (hrit or anahata
centre in the heart region) is like a lotus with the
pericarp which hangs down in a deconcentrated
state. This centre should be turned upward by
sitkara (i.e. sitkara breath-control) and other
means. Within this centre is super-light (mahan
archi) with all-pervading flame, which radiates
in all directions. In the middle of this is subtle
Fire-flame (Kundalini), which has been brought
upward (that is, splendorous subtle Kundalini,
who resides in the muladhara centre, should be
roused and conducted to the hrit or the anahata
centre). Inside the flame (splendorous Kundalini), lies purusha as Supreme Being; he is
Brahma, Ishana (Shiwa), Indra, Akshara (imperishable) and supreme Swarat (Ishwara—
God)' (—Mahopanishad, 1.12–14).

In the Tantrika process, Kundalini is aroused
in the muladhara centre, conducted to the
sahasrara centre and is then absorbed into
Parama Shiwa; thereafter, the infinite Shiwa-
Kundalini is given a form having two aspects—
mantra-sound derived from Supreme Nada and
power-form from Supreme Bindu; this is Ishtadewata; then Ishtadewata is brought down to the
hrit or the anahata centre for concentration. In
the Waidika process, Kundalini is aroused in the
muladhara centre and then brought to the hrit or
anahata centre where concentration is done, first,
on mahan archi, that is, super-light emanating
from Kundalini; when concentration becomes
deeper : on Kundalini who is within the light;
and finally, concentration on Supreme Being—
Narayana or Parama Shiwa—within Kundalini.

At the first stage of concentration, super-
light is the object. When concentration becomes
deeper, the super-light is not recorded in
consciousness, but Kundalini herself shines forth
there. At the last phase of concentration,
Narayana emerges from Kundalini. In the Tantrika process, both Parama Shiwa and Kundalini
are transformed into Ishtadewata and concentration is done either in the sahasrara or the anahata.

There is also a Waidika process in which
Kundalini is brought from the muladhara centre
to the sahasrara centre where union between
them takes place. It is stated: 'Soma (here
Shiwa) is with that power which operates in the
upper region, and Anala (fire, here Kundalini)
is endowed with that power which operates
from below. The worldly knowledge is enclosed
between the two (that is, sensory knowledge is
due to the different situations of Soma-power
and Anala-power). When Agni (= Anala = Kundalini) rises up (from muladhara) and is united
with immortal Supreme Soma (Shiwa), Soma
becomes in the nature of Agni, and amrita
flows downwards (from the union). When the
power (Kundali-power), situated in the lower
region (that is, muladhara), passes upward, it is
called Kalagni (because that power, then,
absorbs time; that is, that power exhibits
absorptive power); when Kalagni-power goes
upward, it expresses its purifying and burning
effects (that is, the upwardly going Kundalini
purifies and absorbs all creative principles).
That power situated in adhara (i.e. muladhara)
is Kalagni (i.e. Kundalini); when it goes upward, Soma (Shiwa) turns downwards, and in
this way the union between Shiwa and Shakti
(Kundalini) takes place. Shiwa is in the upper
region (i.e. sahasrara); when Shakti goes into
the upper region, Shiwa becomes united with
Shakti (that is, when Kundalini goes up from
muladhara to sahasrara, Shiwa and Kundalini
become one and the same); everything is pervaded by Shiwa-Shakti. The universe arises
from that energy of Agni (when Agni as Kundalini is latent in muladhara, and prana is aroused);
by Agni (as Kundalini being aroused) the knowledge of the world is burned to ashes; the creative
energy is reduced to ashes (i.e. completely
absorbed). The energy of creativity evaporates

(when it is absorbed into *A*gni)' (—B*r*ihajjabal-op*a*ni*s*had, 2.8–13).

Also: 'Shiwa-fire (that is, Ku*n*dalin*i* as fire who is situated in the m*u*ladhar*a* around Shiw*a* as Swayambhu-ling*a*), after burning the body (that is, the five m*a*habhut*a*s and five t*a*nmatr*a*s which produce the material body and, as creative principles, are in the fi*ve* centres from m*u*ladhar*a* to wishuddh*a*), becomes united with Som*a* (that is Shiw*a*), in s*a*hasrar*a*, and as a result *a*mr*i*ta (deathless life-stream) flows; when a yog*i* is able to flow that *a*mr*i*ta from Shakti (Ku*n*dal*i*-power) and Som*a* (Shiw*a*), through the yog*a*-path (i. e. su*s*humn*a*-path), he attains immortality (that is, when the su*s*humn*a*-path is made free from all creative principles, and is full of only *a*mr*i*ta, immortality is attained)' (—B*r*ihajjabalop*a*ni*s*had, 2. 19).

Here is the W*a*idik*a* process of ku*n*dalin*i*yog*a*. When Ku*n*dalin*i* is actually aroused and conducted upwards, it is ku*n*dalin*i*yog*a*; and when it is not possible, the whole process, either W*a*idik*a* or Tantrik*a*, is done through thought-concentration and it is called bh*u*tashuddhi. This term has been used in Ramatapinyup*a*ni*s*ha*d* (1.5.1). It has been stated there: 'Bh*u*ta-dikang shodhayet', that is, bh*u*tas (five subtle elements) and other principles should be purified. This is bh*u*tashuddhi. Bh*u*tashuddhi is a fundamental process in the Tantrik*a* form of l*a*yayog*a*, and, consequently, it has been elaborated there.

*R*ishi Narada said: 'The purification of the t*a*nmatr*a*s-m*a*habh*u*tas of which the body is composed is by the union with changeless Brahm*a*n; this is called bh*u*tashuddhi. Splendorous Atm*a*n lies within the mind, and this is called the mental body by the yog*i*s who have realized truth. When it is purified, all is purified' (—Goutam*i*yatantra, ch. 9). Here, bh*u*tashuddhi has been defined. It is a process of purification of the principles of the body and mind. About the process, it is stated: 'By deep thinking, Shakti (Ku*n*dal*i*-power) situated in her own abode (i. e. m*u*ladhar*a*) should be aroused by the mantra 'H*u*ng' and conducted from m*u*ladhar*a* through swadhi*sh*thana, m*a*nipura, anah*a*ta, wi-shuddh*a* and ajña which are situated in the anal, genital, navel, cardiac, cervical and eye-brow regions respectively. Think of m*u*ladhar*a*,

the golden lotus with four petals; think that there is a triangle which shines like moon, sun and fire in m*u*ladhar*a*; then think deeply of j*i*watm*a*n (embodied being) in concentration; think of Ku*n*dalin*i* who is deep red, as bright as ten million lightnings and ten million suns, and as cool as ten million moons, and like the (motionless) flame of a lamp. By thinking, Ku*n*dalin*i* should be conducted through the path of su*s*humn*a* to unite herself with Paramatm*a*n in the region of Shiw*a* in s*a*hasrar*a* by the mantra 'Sohang'. During the process of conduction, five m*a*habhut*a*s (and t*a*nmatr*a*s), the organs of speech, feet, hands, anus and genitals which cause speech, locomotion, prehension, excretion and reproduction, and the organs of hearing, touch, sight, taste and smell and their functions—these twenty-five principles and puru*s*ha; and I-consciousness, sense-mind, intellective mind, sense-consciousness—all these should be absorbed (into Ku*n*dalin*i*) by thinking.... Finally, going down through the su*s*humn*a*-path, all these principles should be replaced in their appropriate places by the mantra 'Sohang'; this is bh*u*tashuddhi which is followed by matrikanyasa (a hand-process with mantra)' (—Goutam*i*yatantra, ch. 9).

*I*shwara has said about bh*u*tashuddhi that: 'Supreme Ku*n*dalin*i*-power should be made to pass with j*i*watm*a*n by the mantra 'Hangsah' from m*u*ladhar*a* by piercing all centres, step by step, to s*a*hasrar*a* and to unite her with Supreme Brahman (by thinking); senses and conative organs of actions, bh*u*tas, etc. and their functions, intellective mind, I-consciousness, sense-consciousness, etc.—all should be united (by absorption)' (—N*i*latantra, ch. 4). Also: 'Oh Mother of gods, j*i*watm*a*n along with Ku*n*dalin*i* and twenty-four principles should be made to be absorbed into Paramatm*a*n by the mantra "Hu*ng* Hangsah" along with inspiratory breath-control by the practitioner' (—T*o*dalatantra, ch. 4).

It has been stated: 'The purification of five bh*u*tas (i.e. five m*a*habh*u*tas and five t*a*nmatr*a*s) and indriyas (five senses and five conative organs of actions) is very carefully done; this is why it has been termed bh*u*tashuddhi' (—Gayatritantra, 1.202). So, the process of purification of creative principles is termed bhutashuddhi. This purification is effected by absorption. The roused Kundalini is alone able to exhibit the full and effective absorption-power. So, it is very important that Kundalini first should be aroused. About the rousing of Kundalini, Ishwara has said: 'Supreme Kundalini-power should be aroused by making apana go upward by pranayama in conjunction with prana-mantra ("Yang"); then Kundalini with jiwatman from anahata should be conducted by piercing all the centres to sahasrara above and unite her with Supreme Brahman' (—Bhutashuddhitantra, ch. 3). The fire-energy should also be applied to rouse Kundalini as has been stated by Mahadewa (—Sammohanatantra, ch. 4).

Sadashiwa, in expounding the process of bhutashuddhi, says: 'The earnest practitioner should place his hands with the palms upwards in his lap (sitting in a concentration posture); focussing his attention on muladhara, he should rouse Kundali by the mantra "Hung"; he should then conduct Kundali with all the principles associated with the "earth" to swadhishthana by means of the mantra "Hangsah", where these principles should be made to be absorbed in the "water". Having the "earth" together with the smell principle and its objects and others thus absorbed into the "water", he should get the "water" together with the taste principle, its objects and others absorbed into the "fire"; then the "fire" together with the sight principle, its objects and others into the "air"; then the "air" and the associated touch principle, its objects and others into the "void"; then the "void" together with the sound principle and its objects into I-consciousness, I-consciousness into supraconsciousness, supraconsciousness into primus, and primus into Brahman' (—Mahanirwanatantra, 5. 93–7).

It has been stated: 'Thereafter bhutashuddhi should be done. Placing his hands with palms upwards in his lap, the calm practitioner should concentrate on Kulakundalini who is the source of spiritual knowledge and is in muladhara; she is coiled like a sleeping serpent (that is, in a latent form) with three and a half coils around Swayambhu-linga, subtle, splendorous like ten

million lightnings and all knowledge. After the concentration, Kundalini should be roused by the mantra "Hangsah", or Pranawa, or Kurcha-bija ("Hung")' (—from Yamala, quoted in Tarabhaktisudharnawa, ch. 5). Here, one of the three mantras has been advised for rousing and conducting Kundalini.

Apana-raising, pranayama and mantra are most important factors in the process of rousing Kundalini. It has been stated: 'By inspiring through the left nostril and at the same time contracting slightly the anus and pressing the palate with the retroverted tongue, Kundali-power should be united with Shiwa; expiration should also be done through the left nostril' (from Merutantra, quoted in Purashcharyarnawa, ch. 3). Here it is disclosed that Kundali-power which is in muladhara should be aroused by left inspiratory-expiratory breath-control along with anal-lock and tongue-lock. Then the roused Kundalini should be conducted to sahasrara to unite her with Parama Shiwa. Apana-energy is raised upwards by anal-lock.

About tongue-lock, Shiwa has said: 'A yogi should practise pressing the palate with the tongue by folding it. Gradually he will be able to reach the uvula. When the palatine region is pressed with the tongue, a kind of cool lifeful substance is secreted by the utilization of which the yogi is able to prolong his life. The tip of the tongue should press on the uvula. The life-substance secreted from the white lotus (i.e. Sahasrara) is in concentration. The yogi gains control over hunger and thirst and prolongs his life to a very great extent by bathing his body with this life-substance' (—Shiwapurana, 6. 47. 83–5).

To be able to execute tongue-lock correctly, the tongue should be made soft and elongated by milking-process and lingual exercise. Milking is the pulling of the tongue by wrapping it with a soft, fine, wet cloth. Lingual exercise consists in retroversion and stretching of the tongue, done alternately while assuming the adamantine posture (wajrasana).

Tongue-lock consists in pressing with the tip of the retroverted tongue the soft palate and uvula. This tongue-palate contact, when continued for a long time and with breath-suspension dries the part which is usually wet with mucus secreted by the palatine glands, and creates a state in which a radiation of life-force occurs through this part. An advanced yogi is able to reenergize his whole body with it, and, as a result, he attains a disease-free body and long life.

Pranayama plays an important role in rousing Kundalini. It has been stated: 'Subtle Supreme Kundalini should be roused from Muladhara by Kumbhakapranayama (breath-suspension)' (—Mantramaharnawa, 1. leaf 41). Pranayama is a fundamental part of bhutashuddhi. It is a special pranayama termed bhutashuddhi pranayama. But there is a modified form of bhutashuddhi which is done only by deep thinking and without pranayama. It has been stated: 'Divine Kundalini along with five bhutas should be united in thought-concentration; then "I am that" should be thought in concentration' (—Uddisha, quoted in Purashcharyarnawa, ch. 3). That deep thinking is the most important part of bhutashuddhi has been stated by Shiwa. He says: 'So, in bhutashuddhi thought-concentration (bhawana yoga) alone (is used)' (—Shaktisangamatantra, Tara Section, 12.13). Mind is purified by bhutashuddhi. It is stated: 'The purification of the mind and the embodied being is effected by bhutashuddhi' (—Shadamnayatantra, 4.151).

It has been stated: 'Sitting on a comfortable seat consisting of Kusha grass and on the top of which is spread the skin of the black antelope, the practitioner should assume the lotus posture and perform bhutashuddhi' (--Skandapurana, 2.5.4.20). So, lotus posture is considered a suitable posture for bhutashuddhi. But the posture to be assumed is mainly determined by the form of the process adopted. Accomplished posture is also very good, especially when apana-control is introduced in the practice.

Brahma has explained a form of bhutashuddhi in which pranayama in conjunction with the mantra pranawa has been used to purify all the principles—five forms of metamatter, five tanons, senses, conative organs, sense-mind, sense-consciousness, intellective mind, I-consciousness and others; pranayama is executed in a special manner with pranawa to control prana- and apana-energy (—Lingapurana, Section 1. 73. 11–16).

Absorptive Thought-concentration

Consciousness, when super-purified and in a state of superconcentration at its fourth stage, is of splendorous Kundalini. It is the final state of superconsciousness. This consciousness is finally absorbed into Kundalini. But before the attainment of the final form of superconsciousness, consciousness undergoes three stages of superconcentration: concentration-on-material-form (superconcentration, first stage), concentration-on-mahabhuta-tanmatras (superconcentration, second stage), and concentration-on-divine-form (superconcentration, third stage).

To transform concentration into superconcentration, it has first to be developed into dharana and dhyana. Dhyana is changed ultimately into the deepest form of concentration in which the I-ness feeling sinks, and only an object in its subtle form is held in consciousness, uninterruptedly and continuously. This is samadhi—superconcentration.

But dharana must be established in a form of consciousness which is multiform in character. This is due to the fact that this form of consciousness is maintained by the constant penetration into it of the sensory forms of smell, taste, sight, touch and sound through the sensory channels and in which sense-mind plays a fundamental role. The sensory images in the consciousness evoke intellection to a certain degree and also conscious thoughts associated with images. According to the types of sensory images, affectivity and conativeness or specific intellectuality are aroused. So sense-consciousness is the perceptual field (sangjnana) in which intellection, affectivity and conation play their roles, and, in this manner, sense-consciousness constantly changes its form.

In such an undulatory form of consciousness, concentration is not easy. Concentrative mind (dhi) does not radiate into such consciousness.

Conscious thoughts associated with perception often become the centre of exciting conative activities in which the organs of speech, prehension and locomotion, and organic and sexual functions are involved. When all these conative actions go on, consciousness is unable to exhibit holding-power to the extent of developing concentration. When the actions are controlled by appropriate postures (asanas), the body may be motionless, but the associated thoughts remain uncontrolled. Those thoughts directly concerned with the movements may cease to appear in that form; but, actually, they immediately change their character and begin to flow in consciousness in many new forms. But unless the flowing of thoughts is controlled, concentrative mind fails to operate in consciousness.

There are four main levels in perceptive consciousness: perceptual, conative, affective and intellective. Conative, affective and intellective phenomena are based on perception. At the conative level, all the five conative organs of action are in operation and conscious thoughts arising from perceptivity and conativeness are multiform and consciousness is in a state of restlessness. Such a form of consciousness is unfavourable to concentration. Holding-power is not maintained in such consciousness. But as such a form of consciousness is a fact in our common mode of existence, yogis have introduced two methods of developing concentration in a state when actions are a predominating factor. They are: karmayoga and mantrayoga.

Karma (action) may be divided into two categories: white and black. White actions are based on yama and niyama, and are done for the good of others, without having any self-interest. Black actions are those which are associated with hostility, falsehood, theft, discontent and excessive sexuality. In an ordinary life, man does both kinds of action. But only white actions are elements of karmayoga, while black actions impede it and impurify consciousness. These black actions which are habitually done should be controlled by doing the habitual white actions in a more intensified manner and often, and by the practices of yama, niyama and pranayama. Organic actions should be harmonized and sexual control should be achiev-

ed by the appropriate processes of hathayoga. Actions should be executed in the following manner: (1) dedication of all actions to God or Ishtadewata; (2) cultivation of unattachment to actions and their results. This is the path of karmayoga. Through it, consciousness becomes spiritually purified, and holding-power is developed.

Another means is mantrayoga. In mantrayoga, speech is transformed into the waikhari form of mantra. By japa (mantra-process of repeating mantra), the waikhari sound which is an approximate imitation of mantra-nada is correctly established in the mind. First of all wachika (verbal, which others can hear) japa should be practised for that purpose. Then upangshu (mantra is uttered in such a low voice that only the practitioner himself can hear, but not others) japa should be practised. Finally, manasa (mantra is uttered only mentally, without producing any sound) japa should be practised. In manasa-japa, the sounds of the matrika-units of the mantra should be thought. This sound-thought will be gradually established in the consciousness; that is, conscious thought is made of mantra-sounds by manasa japa. This can be achieved by repeated practice. From sound-thoughts will emerge holding-power.

Affectivity is an avenue through which concentration can be developed. This is possible through love (anuraga). What is love? It is an intense pleasurable feeling aroused in relation to a person for whom there is liking and who appears extremely attractive to that person, and for whom there is a strong attachment. Union with such a person gives highest pleasure and satisfaction. Separation causes sorrow, disturbances, anxiety and restlessness. When there is real and intense love, consciousness is saturated with love and in it the image of the object of love is held. In union, deep thought with deep feeling is evoked through pleasure and satisfaction, and, in separation, deep thoughts flow in sorrow. Qualities associated with real love are self-dedication and self-sacrifice, admiration and respect for each other, and a sort of deep intimacy, and a strong desire for union in which man or woman becomes fully absorbed in the object of love. Such an intense love is often

129

associated with sexual desire which is fully aroused in contact. Sexual desire may also go so far as to cause intense sexuality. At this point love becomes lust. However, love has other forms. Love in the form of affection is naturally expressed towards one's own children. It is very strong in mothers. There is also love for brothers and sisters, and for friends.

Is it possible to develop concentration in the centre of such emotionalized thoughts? First of all, concentration is based on a state of single-pointedness of consciousness. According to bhaktiyoga, love can be spiritualized to that degree when it assumes exclusively the form of only that object and nothing else. It is called ananyabhakti—single-pointed concentrated flow of love for God. This one object cannot be a material object. Because, material objects are seen in the diversified consciousness. Through the process of concentration, diversity is transformed into uniformity. The likeness of a material object in thought-form can be undertaken at the beginning as an object of concentration. As concentration develops, the thought-form changes and finally is reduced to what is an unknown phenomenon, never experienced in the material world. This is the experience of subtle elements—mahabhutas which can be farther reduced to tanmatras. These experiences occur when consciousness is in a state of concentratedness. Superconcentration is attained on mahabhutas and tanmatras. But when love is fully spiritualized, even mahabhutas and tanmatras are not registered in consciousness which is flooded by bhakti (divine love). In the most intensified love in concentration, only God in the form of Ishtadewata is held in consciousness. Love-concentration at its highest degree becomes ananda samadhi—superlove-concentration.

So, when bhakti flows, consciousness only receives and holds divine forms, and nothing else. Bhakti develops non-attachment to worldly objects, stage by stage. There are, of course, preliminary practices which help to arouse bhakti. First of all, thoughts should be purified and spiritualized by yama and niyama, especially, by ritualistic worship, japa (mantra-practice) and thinking of Ishtadewata. All these belong to waidhi-bhakti (ritualistic or devotional divine love) which ultimately leads to ragatmika-bhakti (all-love). This is the path of bhaktiyoga.

Those who are able to raise their intelligence and thoughts to a spiritual level, and whose thoughts are purified by yama and niyama, are fit for the practice of jñanayoga. By spiritual deliberation and reflection, they become unattached to mundane objects and are able to make consciousness free from worldly thoughts. By applying 'neti neti' (not this, not this) deliberation, they go beyond the world, and finally become established in Brahman (Supreme God) in asamprajñata samadhi. This is the state of rajayoga.

In layayoga, Kundalini is aroused by concentration in combination with mantra, pranayama and certain control processes of hathayoga. The aroused Kundalini exhibits absorptive power to the highest degree, by which she absorbs all the creative principles located in the chakras (subtle centres) when piercing through them. Absorption occurs in a certain order, and, finally, when all creative principles except superconsciousness are withdrawn, samprajñata samadhi is attained in sahasrara. This is the limit of Amakala. Thereafter, the stage of Nirwanakala is reached. Now Kundalini becomes Nirwana-shakti. After that Kundalini herself becomes united with and is absorbed into Parama Shiwa. This is the final stage of asamprajñata samadhi. This is kundaliniyoga.

In bhutashuddhi, the entire process of kundaliniyoga, in exact order, is rendered in thought-forms. What actually happens in kundaliniyoga is imitated in thoughts. In fact, kundaliniyoga in thought-form is bhutashuddhi. The Kundali-rousing which is the first part of the process of Kundaliniyoga is done in thought, that is, thinking deeply of the rousing of Kundalini. The absorption of various creative principles in the same order as actually takes place in kundaliniyoga is also done in thoughts in the same order.

In bhutashuddhi, thought is not mixed with intellectuality. Here, thought is merely a mental image of a certain form or action which requires no intellection, but is associated with attention and a certain degree of concentration. Concentrative-mind is brought into play for making thought forceful. When the thought is a conscious form of an image of an object, and the whole thought is of that image, and there is no interruption in the flow of that thought and there is no penetration of something else in it, it is called thought-form. A thought-form is to be maintained for a certain time without allowing it to slip, or mix with, or be replaced by, other thoughts. The minimum time a particular thought-form is to be maintained is the lowest kumbhaka-unit which is a four-matrika-unit (4-m-u). During kumbhaka (breath-suspension), an internal calmness develops. The calmness is frequently interrupted by organic and muscular disturbances. Organic harmony should be established by exercise, diet and internal cleanliness. Muscular relaxation and motionlessness should be developed by the practice of asana (static posture exercise).

Thought-form should be practised while assuming a concentration posture in which the body is fully relaxed and without any motion. Sit calm for some minutes. Then practise 4-m-u kumbhaka. It is done in this way: inspire in an effortless manner and suspend for four matrika-units, then expire slowly in an effortless manner without measure. When the 4-m-u kumbhaka becomes easy, and inner calmness remains undisturbed, and it can be repeated according to certain rules, then this kumbhaka should be considered as accomplished. Thereafter, higher-unit kumbhakas should be practised stage by stage.

The following are the stages of kumbhaka:

1 4-matrika-unit kumbhaka
2 6-m-u
3 10-m-u
4 12-m-u
5 16-m-u

Thought-form should be practised during kumbhaka. It is done in this manner: think of one object only, and nothing else. The depth of thinking will be such that the whole thought will be of that object only, and nothing else; and that thought will not be dim, but vivid and clear, nonundulatory, and unpenetrable and unreplaceable by other thoughts. That non-

moving steady single thought is mono-thought. The duration of mono-thought is the duration of kumbhaka. The practice is done stage by stage:

1 4-m-u kumbhaka together with mono-thought
2 6-m-u   — ditto —
3 10-m-u   — ditto —
4 12-m-u   — ditto —
5 16-m-u   — ditto —

This is the general limit of kumbhaka and mono-thought practice. When mono-thought with kumbhaka is practised in this way, thought becomes deeper and deeper, and, at a certain point, it is transformed into real concentration. At this stage, the power of control to hold an object in consciousness is so developed that that object becomes the whole of consciousness; consciousness, now, is of one form and single-pointed; the object held in consciousness becomes steady; and consciousness is now impenetrable by other objects, and does not change its form. Such holding-power of control is termed dharana —holding-concentration. As concentration goes deeper, it becomes uninterrupted normally, and continues for a longer period. This is dhyana —deep concentration. Finally, concentration becomes so deep that I-ness feeling disappears and only an object in its subtle form remains. This is samadhi—superconcentration. The first form of samadhi is samprajñata samadhi— superconscious concentration. It is also divided into four stages:

1 In which appropriate material forms are the objects.
2 In which mahabhutas-tanmatras are the objects.
3 In which God in form, or Ishtadewata is the object.
4 In which subtle Kundalini is the object.

Finally, samprajñata samadhi is transformed into asamprajñata samadhi after the absorption into Kundalini of samadhi-consciousness and primus. Now only Kundalini remains. Ultimately, Kundalini is absorbed into infinite Supreme Consciousness and remains as the being of Shiwa. This is the final stage of asamprajñata samadhi. This is the goal of kundalini-yoga, and bhuthashuddhi is the means to it.

In bhutashuddhi, the mono-thought formation is done in the chakras (subtle centres), starting from the muladhara and working up to the sahasrara. The chakras are the seats of creative principles. The lower five chakras, in addition, are the seats of sensory principles, principles of conative actions, bio-energies and deities. The yoga-processes practised in the chakras are summarized here.

1 In the muladhara:
  (a) Conative control—sexual control.
  (b) Sensory control—smell control.
  (c) Bio-energy control—apanayama to control apana-energy.
  (d) Anal control.
  (e) Concentration on Deity Brahma.
2 In the swadhishthana:
  (a) Conative control—organic control.
  (b) Sensory control—taste control.
  (c) Bio-energy control—apanayama.
  (d) Yonimudra and perineal control.
  (e) Concentration on Deity Wishnu.
3 In the manipura:
  (a) Conative control—locomotor muscular control.
  (b) Sensory control—sight control.
  (c) Bio-energy control—samanayama to control samana-energy.
  (d) Uddiyana process (abdominal retraction control).
  (e) Concentration on Deity Rudra.
4 In the anahata:
  (a) Conative control—prehensile control.
  (b) Sensory control—touch control.
  (c) Bio-energy control—pranayama to control prana-energy.
  (d) Concentration on Deity Isha.
5 In the wishuddha:
  (a) Conative control—speech control.
  (b) Sensory control—sound control.
  (c) Bio-energy control—udanayama to control udana-energy.

  (d) Jalandharabandha mudra.
  (e) Concentration on Deity Sadashiwa.
6 In the ajña:
  (a) Sense-mind control.
  (b) Will-mind control.
  (c) Concentration on the Goddess Hakini.
7 In the manas:
  Control of sense-consciousness.
8 In the indu:
  (a) Thought control.
  (b) Concentration on the God Parashiwa.
9 In the guru:
  Concentration on Guru—God in form.
10 In the sahasrara:
  Samprajñata samadhi.

In bhutashuddhi, all these different forms of control are not practised as specific exercises in different chakras. But the concentration on gods and goddesses situated in the chakras is a part of bhutashuddhi. A specific system, based entirely on what actually happens in kundalini-yoga, of mono-thought formation has been adopted in bhutashuddhi. At the beginning, the process is only of thought. Thought is of a non-intellective and non-deliberative character, of one image, non-undulatory, and impenetrable by other thoughts. The duration of each thought-form is willed and is immediately replaced by another specific thought-form. In this manner, a specific thought-chain is made. Thought gradually becomes deeper by practice, and finally is transformed into concentration in which holding-power is manifested. This is holding-concentration.

A thought, when composed of only one image without any intellective oscillations and remaining steady and deep, is able to express its hidden power by which it becomes a living phenomenon —a fact. So, deep thinking of arousing Kundalini and of absorption of different creative principles in different chakras becomes facts, when thought is transformed into holding-concentration, and that into deep concentration. In this way, bhuta-shuddhi becomes ultimately kundaliniyoga.

CHAPTER 6
Bhutashuddhi Pranayama—
Purificatory Breathing

Bhutashuddhi pranayama is a special form of sahita breathing which forms an important part of bhutashuddhi. This breathing effects deep internal purification by the mantra power. The purificatory effects of bhutashuddhi are enhanced by this breathing in which mantra and concentration are intrinsic parts. Mantra causes deep internal purification and its power is increased by breath-suspension and concentration. This is why Shiwa has said that bhutashuddhi should be done with pranayama (—Brihannilatantra, ch. 2, p. 5).

About the technique of bhutashuddhi pranayama, it is stated: 'Inhale air through the left nostril, 16 measures; then suspend breath, 64 measures; and finally expire through the right nostril, 32 measures; with smoke-coloured wayu-bija, that is, the mantra "Yang", situated in a hexagram. Then breathe in through the right nostril, 16 measures; suspend, 64 measures; with red-coloured wahni-bija, that is, the mantra "Rang", in a triangle with swastika sign. Now think of black-coloured "Personified Impurity" (papapurusha) lying in the left side of the practitioner ... and then think that it is burned by the fire arising from muladhara, and its ashes are then expelled from the body with expiration through the right nostril, 32 measures. Now, with the white-coloured chandra-bija, that is, the mantra "Thang" which is in the forehead (that is, indu centre), inspire through the left nostril, 16 measures, then suspend, 64 measures, and at the same time think that by the showers of deathless substance in the form of 50 matrika-letters a new body has been created. Then, make the body firm by the mantra "Lang" while expiring (through the right nostril) with 32 measures' (—Goutamiya-tantra, ch. 9, p. 27).

It has been stated: 'The whole body along with "personified impurity" should be burnt by the fire-flame arising from muladhara. Inspire through the left nostril with the japa of mantra (thinking mantra mentally) "Yang", 16 measures; suspend 64 measures with the japa "Yang" and then expire 32 measures with the japa "Yang" through the left nostril; again inspire with the japa of "Rang" 16 in order to burn the subtle body, suspend with the japa of "Rang" 64 and at the same time think that the body is burnt into ashes, then expire with the japa of "Rang" 32 and think the ashes are eliminated; then inspire with the japa of "Lang" 16 and (by thinking) irradiate the body ...; suspend with the japa of "Thang" 64 and make the body firm (by thinking); and expire with the japa of "Wang" 32 and vitalize the body with death-less substance' (—Tararahasya, p. 8). Here is a slightly different technique.

Ishwara said: 'Inspire through the left nostril with the japa of the air-germ-mantra, that is "Yang" 16; then hold in the manipura centre with breath-suspension and with the japa of "Yang" 64; expire with the japa of "Yang" 32 through the right nostril. In this manner do the breathing with the fire-germ-mantra ("Rang"), holding the breath in the anahata centre. Purification is effected by the mantra "Yang" and burning by the mantra "Rang". Thinking of the white-coloured water-germ-mantra (that is,

"Wang") in the forehead (that is, ajña), expiration should be done through the right nostril with japa 32. In this manner the process should be repeated twelve times. This is bhutashuddhi for the purification of the subtle body' (—Bhuta-shuddhitantra, ch. 6, pp. 5–6).

The technique described here is as follows: (1) left inspiration and suspension, right expiration, with mantra 'Yang'; measures 16–64–32; for the purification (drying purification) of the subtle body; (2) right inspiration and suspension, left expiration, with mantra 'Rang'; measures 16–64–32; for the burning (burning-purification) of the subtle body; (3) left inspiration and suspension, right expiration, with mantra 'Wang'; measures 16–64–32.

Another technique of bhutashuddhi breathing, which is done in modified bhutashuddhi, is this: 'Inspire through the left nostril and at the same time think of smoke-coloured air-germ-mantra ("Yang"), and do japa of the mantra 16 times; suspend and do japa of the mantra 64 times, and at the same time think that the black-coloured "personified impurity" in the left interior part of the body along with the (subtle) body, has been dried (by the mantra); then expire through the right nostril with the japa of the mantra 32 times; inspire through the right nostril with the japa of fire-germ-mantra "Rang" 16 times and at the same time think of the mantra as red-coloured; suspend with the japa of the mantra 64 times and at the same time think that the "personified impurity", together with the subtle body, has been burnt by the fire arising from muladhara; then expire through the left nostril with the ashes (produced by burning) and with the japa of the mantra; again, thinking of the white-coloured moon-germ-mantra "Thang", inspire with the left nostril and at the same time make japa of the mantra ("Thang") 16 times and think of the moon in the forehead (indu centre); then suspend with the japa of the water-germ-mantra "Wang" 64 times and at the same time think that the whole body which is of matrika-letters has been (newly) made by the deathless substance (amrita) flowing from the moon in the forehead (indu centre); then expire through the right nostril with the japa of earth-germ-mantra "Lang" 32 times and

at the same time think that the body has been made firm' (—Bhutashuddhitantra, ch. 16, p. 15).

The technique of bhutashuddhi breathing given here is complete. It is as follows: (1) left inspiration 16—suspension 64—right expiration 32, with the japa of the mantra 'Yang' along with concentration; (2) right inspiration 16—suspension 64—left expiration 32, with the japa of the mantra 'Rang' and concentration; (3) left inspiration 16, with the japa of the mantra 'Thang' and concentration; suspension 64, with the japa of the mantra 'Wang' and concentration; right expiration 32, with the japa of the mantra 'Lang' with concentration.

Here, concentration means deep thinking which is done along with the mental mantra-japa and with either inspiration, suspension or expiration. These respiratory acts are measured by the japa. Thinking becomes deeper when done with mantra and breathing. The purificatory process consists of internal drying and burning. Drying becomes effective by the mantra 'Yang' in combination with thinking and breathing. Similarly, burning becomes effective by the mantra 'Rang' in combination with thinking and breathing. The purificatory process is followed by the re-energizing process. It consists of two factors: body-remaking and body-firming. The remaking of the body is done by the mantras 'Thang' and 'Wang' with breathing and thinking, and the newly made body is made firm by the mantra 'Lang' with breathing and thinking. The power of 'Yang' is released when done with left, inspiratory and suspensive, right, expiratory breathing, and of 'Rang' in right inspiratory and suspensive, left expiratory breathing. The power of 'Thang' is awakened in left inspiratory breathing, that of 'Wang' in suspensive breathing, and that of 'Lang' in right expiratory breathing.

The process of drying (shoshana) is effected by the mantra 'Yang' in left inspiratory and suspensive, right expiratory breathing with 16–64–32 measures; and the process of burning (dahana) by the mantra 'Rang' in right-inspiratory-suspensive-left-expiratory breathing with 16–64–32 measures (—Wishwasaratantra, ch. 2, p. 23). It has been stated: 'Drying, burning and irradiation (plawana) should be done with the mantras "Yang", "Rang" and "Wang" respectively. In this manner, the practitioner should perform bhutashuddhi' (—Koulawalitantra, ch. 2, p. 6). Also, 'Oh Deweshi! the practitioner, for the purification of the body, should do drying, burning, ashes-removal, amrita (vital substance)-shower (warshana) and irradiation (aplawana) by the air-germ-mantra ("Yang"), fire-germ-mantra ("Rang"), water-germ-mantra ("Wang"), moon-germ-mantra ("Thang") and earth-germ-mantra ("Lang") respectively, in conjunction with inspiration-suspension-expiration (that is, pranayama)' (—From Tantragandharwa, quoted in Shaktanandatarangini, 7. 10).

Here the process of purification has been clearly defined. The purificatory process consists of five practices:

1 Drying with the mantra 'Yang' in conjunction with breathing.
2 Burning and ashes-removal with the mantra 'Rang' and breathing.
3 Amrita-shower with the mantra 'Wang' and breathing.
4 Irradiation with the mantra 'Thang' and breathing.
5 Body-firming with the mantra 'Lang' and breathing.

Thinking is an intrinsic part of the purificatory process. It is stated: 'In the left nostril, the thinking of smoke-coloured air-germ-mantra ("Yang") should be done (in inspiration through the left nostril). Then the body should be dried by "Yang" (in suspension) by thinking, and then think of "Yang" (while expiring) through the right nostril. Then think of red-coloured fire-germ-mantra ("Rang") (while inspiring) through the right nostril; burn the dried body into ashes by the fire from "Rang" (by thinking while suspending breath), and then expire through the left nostril (while thinking that) the ashes are removed. Then the white-coloured germ-mantra "Thang" should be placed in the forehead (indu centre), by which the lunar amrita (vital substance) will be made to flow downward (all by thinking). Then, thinking that the amrita-born body is pure and pleasing, bring the jiwat-man to its own place in a right manner' (—Sanat-kumaratantra, ch. 3, p. 2). Here, the whole process is done by thinking in conjunction with breathing. The sounds and colours of mantras are thought of and the purificatory processes are done by thinking.

Wayu is the subtle pranic energy which is in operation. The germ-mantra is in the form of wayu-energy, that is, wayu-energy forms an intrinsic part of the germ-mantra. The wayu-energy changes its character in left inspiration, right inspiration, left expiration, right expiration and suspension. The wayu-energy when operative during left inspiration and suspension, and right expiration, is the 'Yang'-energy by which the body is dried; the wayu-energy in right inspiration and suspension, and left expiration becomes 'Rang'-energy which burns the body along with impurities (—from Bhairawatantra, quoted in Tarabhaktisudharnawa, ch. 5, p. 153). It indicates that the wayu-energy becomes a germ-mantra-energy by appropriate breathing. The mantra-energy is subtle and radiates a particular colour-ray and is apprehended in concentration. So long as apprehension is not possible, the mantra should be thought of in the right colour.

It has been stated: 'In the navel region (manipura centre), think of the red-coloured maya-bija, and then burn the subtle impure body by the fire coming from it by thinking' (—Tarabhaktisudharnawa, ch. 5, p. 155). Here, it has been clearly stated that the purificatory processes should be done by thinking, and the body is not the physical body but subtle body. Again, 'Think of the smoke-coloured "Yang"-wayu (-energy) in the navel region (manipura centre) and make the subtle body dry by the mantra ("Yang") (by thinking) while doing the left-inspiratory-suspensive, right-expiratory breathing, 16–64–32. Think of the red-coloured fire-germ-mantra ("Rang") in the region of genitalia (swadhishthana) and burn the impure subtle body by the mantra ("Rang") (by thinking) and at the same time do the right-inspiratory-suspensive, left-expiratory breathing, 16–64–32. Thinking of the water-germ-mantra "Wang" in the region of the uvula, make the flow of amrita from the sahasrara centre by the mantra ("Wang") (by thinking) while doing left-inspiratory breathing, and irradiate the whole body by amrita by "Wang" (by thinking) while doing

135

suspensive breathing. Then think of the earth-germ- mantra "Lang" in the anal region (muladhara centre) and irradiate the body fully by "Lang" (by thinking) while doing right-inspiratory breathing. By this, a most excellent non-white-non-black divine body is attained' (—from Yamala, quoted in Tarabhaktisudharnawa, ch. 5, p. 156).

From the above exposition, it is clear that a germ-mantra is in the nature of wayu, that is, prana or vital energy which emits a particular-ray. In other words, a germ-mantra is a form of life-force which emits silent sound and colour radiation. The mantra-power is only approachable through deep mono-thought which, in time, develops into concentration. However, the power of the mantra is aroused by deep mono-thought, and is utilized in the purification of the subtle body to make it divine. The purificatory effects also extend to the physical body through thought and pranayama (breath-control). Thought becomes forceful and effective by breathing. So, mantra, thought and breathing— all three become intrinsic parts of the purificatory process.

It has been stated: 'The drying (process) done by air-germ-mantra ("Yang") is called body-drying. This (process) should be performed while doing left-inspiratory-suspensive, right-expiratory breathing. The. burning of the body by burning-germ-mantra ("Rang") is called body-burning. The process should be done in right-inspiratory-suspensive, left-expiratory breathing. The whole body should be irradiated by the currents of amrita flowing from the union of Kundalini and Shiwa (Supreme Consciousness). This process is called irradiation' (—Kularnawa, ch. 15, pp. 74–5). Here, it is indicated that the processes of body-drying and body-burning are the effects of specific germ (bija)-mantras and the mantras become effective when done in conjunction with appropriate breathing. The germ-mantra 'Rang' has been called burning-germ-mantra, (dahana-bija) that is, fire-germ-mantra which is 'Rang'. Certain germ (bija)-mantras are endowed with the power of purification, so it is stated: 'The purification of the body should be done by "Yang", "Rang", "Wang" and "Lang" (—Garudapurana, 1.12.2); and 'The

body of subtle elements is to be dried and burnt by the germ (bija)-mantras "Yang" and "Rang" respectively; and then think of amrita (vital substance) along with the germ-mantra "Wang"; finally, the whole body should be irradiated by amrita with the help of the germ-mantra "Lang" (—Garudapurana, 1.11.2–3). Here, it is clearly stated that the mantras have the power to effect purification of the subtle body.

That deep thinking plays a most important role in the mantra purification of the body has been expressed thus: 'Think of "Yang" in the heart region (that is, anahata) and of "Rang" which is like three bright flames endowed with the power of burning and purifying; then think in the moon centre (indu chakra) situated in the cerebral region of white-coloured amrita by the flow of which the earth centre (muladhara) is being irradiated; by this process, a divine body which is free from all impurities is attained' (—Brahmapurana, 61. 4–6). Here we find that the mantra and its specific purificatory action should be done by deep thinking. It has been further stated: 'The germs of the body are five elements. These subtle elements are earth, water, fire, air and void factor (akasha). For the purification of these elements, the processes of drying, burning, ashes-removal, amrita (vital substance)-shower and irradiation should be done (in succession); these purificatory processes are done by thinking' (—Kalikapurana, 57. 104–6). It has been clearly stated here that the purificatory processes should be done by thinking.

So, bhutashuddhi pranayama is a special purificatory process done as a part of bhutashuddhi. It is the mantra purification, as it is effected by mantra. The mantra purification consists of the specific processes of drying, burning, ashes-removal, amrita-shower, irradiation and body-firming. Each specific process is intimately related to a specific germ-mantra. The germ-mantra causes the specific purification. Drying is effected by the germ-mantra 'Yang', burning and ashes-removal by 'Rang', amrita-shower by 'Thang', irradiation by 'Wang' and body-firming by 'Lang'. The impure subtle body is dried by 'Yang' and burnt by 'Rang'. Amrita-flow is caused by 'Thang' and a new body is formed by the irradiation of amrita by 'Wang', and finally, the new body is made firm by 'Lang'. The power of the germ-mantra is aroused by japa, deep thinking and breathing. Japa is the repetition of the germ-mantra by thinking of the desired number during breathing. Verbal and semi-verbal japa should be practised first to master the correct sound of the mantra. In mantra-thought the correct sound-form is an important factor. Also the colour of the germ-mantra should be thought of. The specific action of the germ-mantra, namely, drying, burning, etc. should be done by thinking. Therefore, thinking is the thought of the mantra sound, mantra colour, mantra japa and mantra action. Thinking is done in conjunction with breathing. Mantra becomes effective and thinking deep by appropriate breathing. Each germ-mantra produces effects when practised in conjunction with a particular form of breathing. Now we shall consider the breathing aspect of the mantra purification.

Sahita Breathing

Sahita is a Waidika form of breath-control. It is stated: 'Kumbhaka is said to be of two kinds —sahita and kewala; so long as kewala is not attained sahita should be practised' (—Yoga-kundalyupanishad, 1.20). Moreover, 'Kumbhaka (breath-suspension) is of two forms—sahita and kewala. Sahita is with inspiration and expiration, and kewala is without inspiration and expiration. Sahita should be practised until kewala is attained' (—Shandilyopanishad, 1.7.13–15).

The two main forms of Waidika breath-control are sahita and kewala. In sahita, suspension is with inspiration and expiration. Therefore, it is inspiratory-expiratory suspension. It ultimately leads to the attainment of kewala. Kewala is non-inspiratory-non-expiratory suspension. This is the highest form of suspension. Sahita develops that power by which the suspensive phase is much prolonged and gradually the inspiratory and expiratory phases are fully controlled. At this stage the suspensive phase

develops into kewala-suspension—automatic suspension 'without inspiration and expiration' (—Yogatattwopanishad, 50).

The prolongation of suspension (kumbhaka) is extremely difficult. According to yoga, this is only possible when certain deep internal purification is effected. So it is stated: 'Thereafter (after the specific purification) the power of holding breath for a prolonged time is developed' (—Yogatattwopanishad, 49). This specific purification is termed nadishuddhi, that is, the purification of the subtle wayu-force (vital-force) operating as nadis—force-motion lines. These nadis are not physical channels but subtle radiation lines created by the motional wayu-forces. The motional directions of wayu-forces are the nadis. The nadis form a system technically called nadi-chakra—force-motion field, or force-field.

The term 'shuddhi', which means purification, in relation to the nadis has been used in a technical sense. Purification is that process which makes wayu-force free from what interrupts its full functioning. There are two main motions of wayu-force—ida and pingala. These two motions or flows are controlled by sushumna. Under sushumna control, the sun and moon lines are perfect and in harmony.

Pingala-force (that is, wayu-force radiating as pingala-line) causes the consumption of energy in the body by exhibiting actions, that is, the energy is transformed into activities. When there is excessive consumption of energy, the body becomes depleted of energy, weak and exhausted. On the other hand, if the body is unable to mobilize the necessary quantity of energy, there will be an impairment of functional efficiency of the body. Energy conservation is effected by ida-force. There is a certain limit of this process. When the ida-force is weak, the conservation of energy is below the normal level and, consequently, the body is in an adynamic state. When the ida-force functions excessively, the pingala-function is lowered. If both ida- and pingala-forces are under normal sushumna control, a balance will be established between the conservation and consumption of energy, and as a result, the body will be vital, healthy, vigorous and efficient.

In the mental field, pingala-force produces creative mental energy and ida-force mental relaxation and calmness. Excessive pingala influence causes uncontrolled and destructive thoughts, violent emotion and a general restlessness of the mind. Excessive ida-force causes dullness, mental torpor and decreased thinking power. When the forces are under sushumna-control the mental life is well-balanced and well-controlled. Under this condition, the mind is able to do intellective, constructive thinking and also to exhibit controlled thoughts; mental creativity and mental calmness and concentratedness go together. All these are only possible when sushumna-control is brought into play.

The harmonization of ida and pingala occurs when sushumna exercises its control over them in a normal manner. This is effected by the super-purificatory process called nadishuddhi. Under this state, sushumna radiates its control-power to ida and pingala by which their flows are normalized and harmonized. The ida-pingala power-flows are now forceful but well-controlled, neither in excess nor in deficiency, and the directions of force-motions are now normal, that is, they radiate in a right course enabling them to exhibit their full potency without any deviation or destruction. Nadishuddhi is the process of normalization of the wayu-forces when they are able to exercise their full power on the mind and body to effect rarefaction and concentratedness of the mind and purification and vitalization of the body.

According to yoga, sahita breathing plays the fundamental role in nadishuddhi. Because of this sahita breathing forms a very important part of pranayama, both of Waidika and Tantrika forms. It has been stated: 'The practitioner who has been practising regularly abstention, observance and (concentration) posture should perform pranayama; by pranayama the nadis (wayus or vital forces) become purified' (—Shandilyopanishad, 1.3.15). Here, the pranayama is sahita pranayama. When pranayama is done with inspiration, expiration and suspension it is called sahita. It is often called only pranayama, as it is stated, 'The process consisting of inspiration-suspension-expiration is called pranayama

(—Darshanopanishad, 6.1). It has been farther stated: 'Pranayama is that which consists of inspiration-suspension-expiration with the measures 16–64–32' (—Mandalabrahmanopanishad, 1.1.6). The measures of 16–64–32 are the regular ones used in sahita.

The technique of sahita has been given as, 'Inspire slowly through the left nostril, measure 16, suspend, measure 64, and then expire through the right nostril, measure 32; again do inspiration through the right nostril, suspend and expire as before with attentiveness' (—Yogatattwopanishad, 41–2). Here, the form of sahita and its regular measures have been given. So sahita is that breathing in which the breath-acts are executed in the following sequence: left inspiration 16—suspension 64—right expiration 32—right inspiration 16—suspension 64—left expiration 32. The sahita breathing causes nadishuddhi, so it is stated: 'By the practice of this breathing (sahita) for three months, nadishuddhi is attained' (—Yogatattwopanishad, 44). Nadishuddhi is also important for the practice of a higher stage of sahita in which power of suspension develops to a very high degree. It has been stated: 'The practitioner who is well-controlled by the practice of abstention, observance and posture, should first do nadishuddhi (by sahita) and then perform (the higher aspect of sahita) pranayama' (—Trishikhibrahmanopanishad, Mantra Section, 53). Nadishuddhi is only possible when inspiration-suspension-expiration is executed in right measures. It has been stated: 'When inspiration, suspension and expiration are done in right measures, then nadishuddhi is attained' (—Shandilyopanishad, 1.7.7.).

The general indications of nadishuddhi are 'lightness of the body, increased power of digestion and assimilation' (—Darshanopanishad, 5.11); 'reduction of body fat' (—Yogatattwopanishad, 46); 'comeliness' (—Shandilyopanishad, 1.5.4), and 'healthiness' (—Shandilyopanishad, 1.7.8). The fundamental effects of nadishuddhi are 'the increased power of breath-suspension' (—ibid., 1.7.8), and 'the easy entrance into sushumna of the wayu-force; when this is effected, tranquillity of the mind is attained' (ibid., 1.7.8–10).

In Tantrika pranayama, sahita and kewala are also the most important parts. It has been stated: 'Kumbhaka (suspension) is of two forms —sahita and kewala. Sahita suspension is that which is done in conjunction with inspiration and expiration. Sahita should be practised until kewala is accomplished. That natural suspension which is without inspiration and expiration is really pranayama, and that is kewala suspension' (—Grahayamala, Pranayama Section). The technique of sahita which has been given here is: 'Assuming the lotus posture, ... inspire slowly through the left nostril, then suspend as long as you can, and then expire slowly, not forcibly. Again, inspire slowly through the right nostril, suspend as long as you can, then expire slowly (through the left nostril). . . . This is harmless sahita suspension, (kumbhaka)' (—from Dattatreyasanghita, quoted in Pranatoshanitantra, Part 6, ch. 1, p. 407). This indicates that left-inspiration-suspension, right-expiration, right-inspiration-suspension, left-expiration type of breathing is sahita breathing. This breathing when practised for three months effects nadishuddhi (—ibid.). So, sahita breathing causes nadishuddhi.

The regular measures adopted in inspiration, suspension and expiration in sahita breathing is explained here: 'Inspire slowly through the left nostril with the measure 16, ... suspend 64, and expire slowly through the right nostril. Then the breathing should be done in a reverse manner, and again it will be reversed, and in this manner breathing should be controlled' (—Tripurasarasamuchchaya, ch. 3, p. 10).

All this indicates that sahita breathing causes nadishuddhi and when nadishuddhi is attained the body becomes vitalized and normally healthy and the mind purified and concentrative. And above all, nadishuddhi creates a state in which the power of suspension (kumbhaka) is enormously increased.

PART 2

THE CHAKRA SYSTEM

CHAPTER 7
Introduction to the System of Chakras

The word 'chakra' has many meanings, viz., the wheel of a carriage, a potter's wheel, an astronomical circle, a circular weapon, an army, a form of military array, etc. It has also been used in a more specific sense. There are some special chakras used for the selection of an appropriate mantra for initiation, namely, kulakula-chakra, akathaha-chakra, akadama-chakra, etc. Special chakras are also used in relation to worship, as, for example, kurma-chakra. In our study here, a chakra is an organization which is circular in form, having a specific centre. It is situated within the body, not as a part of the gross body, but as a supra-material power-form. It is imprinted undetectably in the body. Because of its subtle character a chakra is not seen by the eyes, even with the help of supersensitive instruments.

It has been stated: 'Body is of two kinds: gross (material) and subtle (extra-material). The material body is composed of flesh, bone, hair, blood, fat and marrow, excretes urine and discharges faeces, is endowed with vital activities (wata) and undergoes metabolism (pitta). The subtle body is composed of nadis (force-motion-lines), of which ida is that nadi which is moon-white and situated on the left side, pingala is like the sun and masculine, and between these two nadis is sushumna containing brahma-nadi. Sushumna is extremely fine and, turning from right to left, it extends from muladhara to brahmarandhra (—Bhutashuddhitantra, ch. 6, p. 5). From this it is clear that the nadi system belongs to the subtle body, it is not a part of the material body. The chakras are within the sushumna nadi. So it is said: 'Inside it (sushumna) is the extremely subtle chitrini nadi which is divine in character and is in the form of letters (matrika-units), and in which are strung the six chakras' (—Sammohanatantra, Part 2, ch. 2, p. 2). More clearly, 'Inside the sushumna is the shining nadi named wajra, and inside it is the subtle chitrini through which Kundali passes; the beautiful six lotuses (chakras) are in this nadi' (—Rudrayamala, Part 2, 25. 51–2). So the chakras are subtle centres within the innermost force-line of sushumna. They do not belong to the material body, and therefore they are not seen.

The material body is the effect of the metamorphosis of the basic energy which is made to operate on the surface stratum due to the influence of prana-force. That basic energy is entirely matter-free and active in the substratum, but is endowed with a specific quality which, under certain condition, gives it an inertial character. This basic energy exhibits a circular wave motion which is reducible to a subtle infinitesimal point. This energy pattern is the tanmatra-mahabhuta forces which exist in five forms. The fifth mahabhuta, prithiwi (earth metamatter) force on the surface stratum exhibits its inertial quality and, as a result, energy appears in a conjugated form—energy particles. But energy may appear also as free from particles. Here, the prithiwi factor becomes latent, and the tejas (fire metamatter) factor patent. Under this condition, energy appears as thermal, luminous or electrical. In the energy transformation, the ap (water metamatter) factor

143

plays an important role and is associated with the chemical form of energy and energy as waves.

The tanmatra-mahabhuta forces create inorganic matter, in which the influence of prana-force plays a most important role. Prana-force, appearing as wayu-forces, operates in relation to tanmatra-mahabhuta forces to create living matter. The creation of a living organized body is impossible without the wayu-forces being involved in combination with the basic tanmatra-mahabhuta forces. The chemical changes in the body are not able to create a living body, but they are an indication of and concomitant with life-force activities in the body. The inoperativeness of pranic forces makes the chemically intact body a corpse. Nothing can alter it. Different forms of energy—thermal, mechanical, electrical—which are active in a living body are entirely dependent on the operation of the pranic forces; they themselves cannot create living matter, or atomic energy. Energy in a more refined form appears as electrical. Energy associated with the elementary particles and radiation is electrical in nature. In muscular contraction, conduction of nerve impulses and cerebral activities, the electrical form of energy is manifested. But the pranic force is neither thermal, mechanical nor electrical; it is supramaterial. There must be a level at which energy becomes non-electrical in nature and is completely released from any material bondage. The living brain substance is associated with chemical energy, and electrical energy is patent in the cerebral activities. But there is no possibility of having either the vital force or consciousness manifested in the brain, unless there is a source of energy which is non-material.

The material body is living because the wayu-forces are operating in its substance in an intrinsic manner, but their centres of operation do not lie in it; they are beyond the matter-energy field; they are in the substratum. When the wayu-forces are withdrawn from the material substance, the body appears as lifeless and without consciousness. This inoperativeness of wayu-forces in the material body does not make them vanish. In the substratum, they function in a subtle organization—the immaterial subtle body—in which consciousness is held without

material substance. The truth of this statement is demonstrated by what is called 'Parashari-rawesha' (entering into another's body). A yogi can leave his own body by volition, and can enter into a body which is recently dead. When he leaves his own body, it becomes dead, and a dead body becomes alive when he enters into it. This superpower was exhibited by the well-known Shankaracharya.

The nadi-field has been created by the matter-free wayu-force-motion-lines. The wayu-forces are in motion in this field, and gliding as pingala-current to vitalize the material body on the one side, and, on the other, as ida-current it makes the mind operate. There is a central power-line called sushumna which exercises its control over ida and pingala flows, and in which the centralization of the wayu-forces has occurred. The wayu-forces are constantly oozing from the sushumna centres causing the ida-pingala currents. In these centres, the centrifugal wayu-forces can be controlled and harmonized, and can also be stopped.

The basic part of the sushumna centres are tanmatra-mahabhuta forces. Each centre consists of two parts—the centre itself and a peripheral aspect. The centre is an infinitesimal point which, from a material point of view, is zero. This point in the substratum is a power concentrated to its highest degree, which arises from the primary inertia-principle (tamas), and is called tanmatra-force. This force is in the nature of germ-mantra. The tanmatra-force, being transformed into mahabhuta-force, appears as circular radiant energy emitting certain matrika-units. This is the peripheral aspect. This is a sushumna centre and is termed chakra. There are five lower chakras in the sushumna which are formed of tanmatra-mahabhuta forces. The chakras are stabilized by the tanmatra-mahabhuta forces, because of their inertial nature. The inertial factor is more pronounced in prithiwi (earth metamatter)-force, wave character in ap(water metamatter)-force, brilliance and power in tejas(fire metamatter)-force, and highly purified energy is in wayu(air metamatter)-force. The akasha(void)-force is the base.

The tanmatra-forces are so subtle and con-

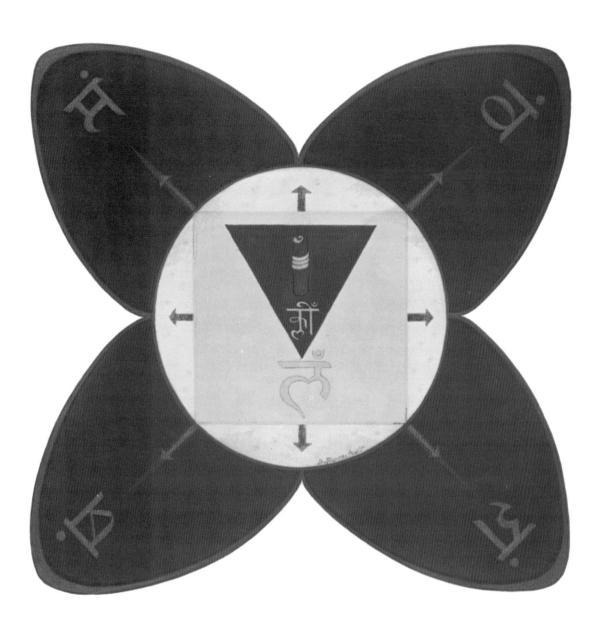

1   Muladhara Chakra

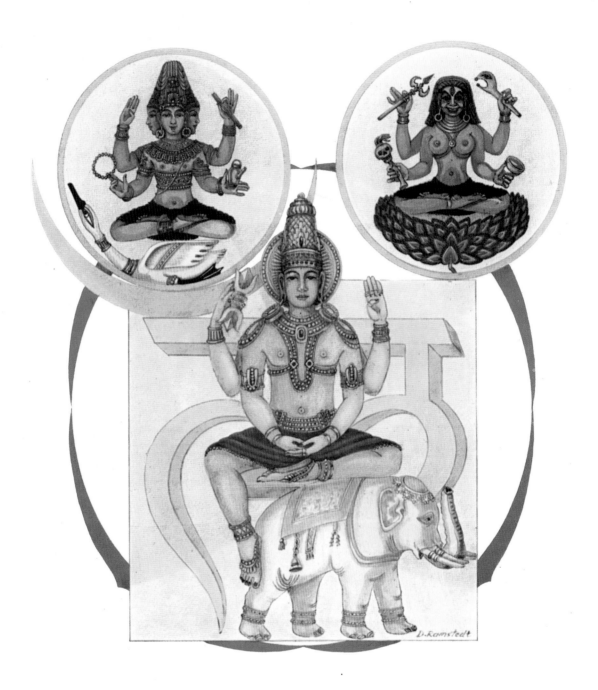

2   (above) Deities in Muladhara (A)

3   (opposite) Deities in Muladhara (B)

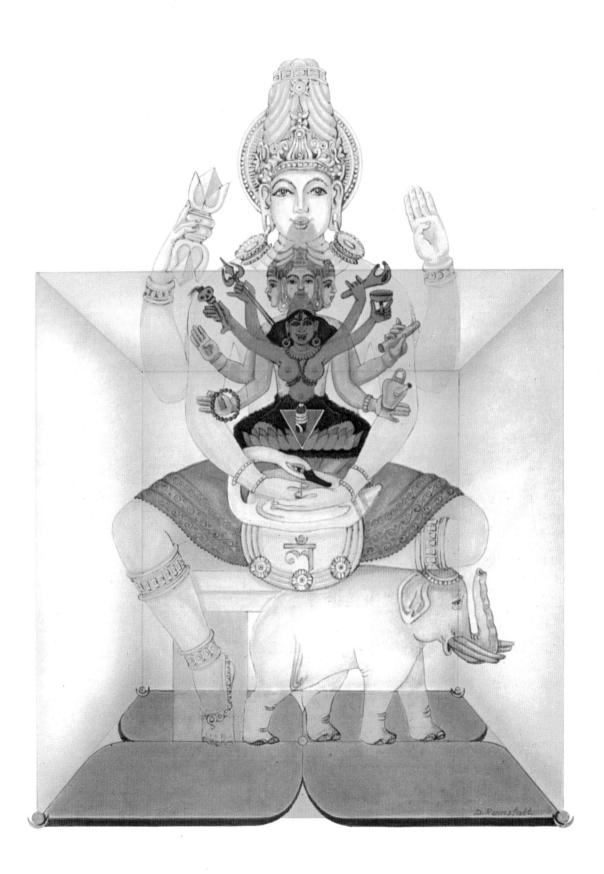

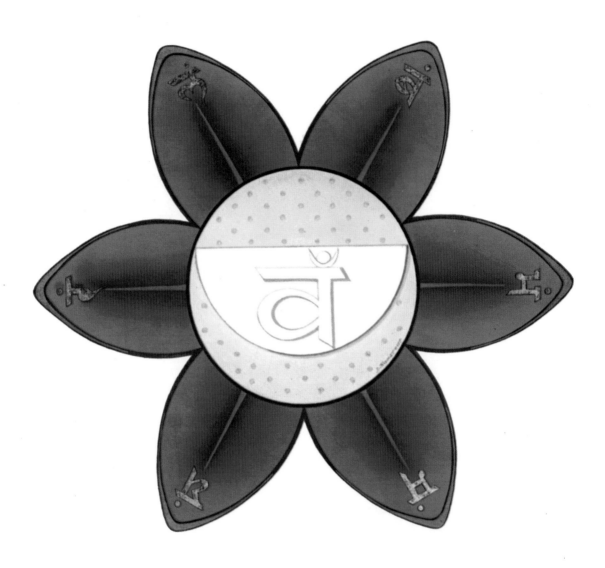

4   Swadhishthana Chakra

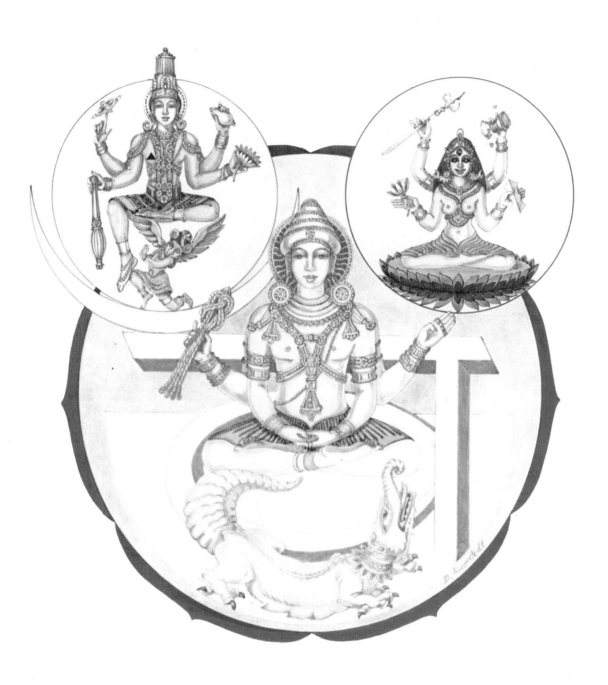

5   Deities in Swadhishthana (A)

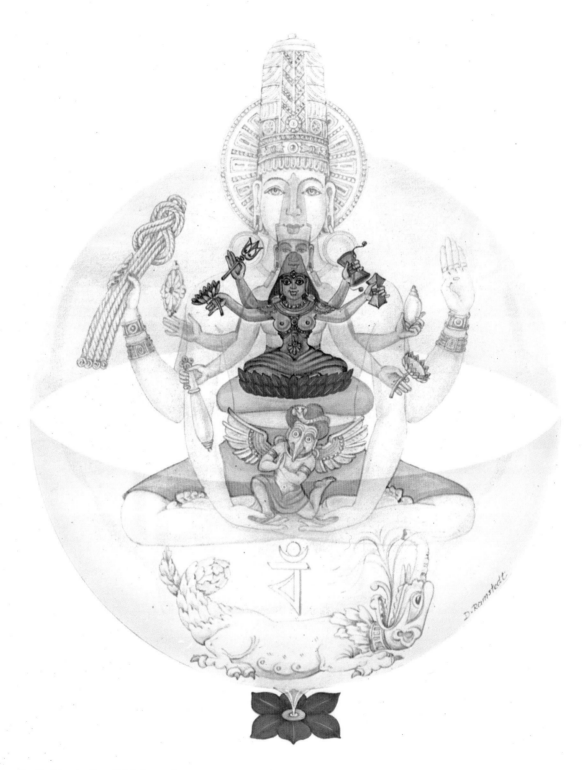

6 Deities in Swadhishthana (B)

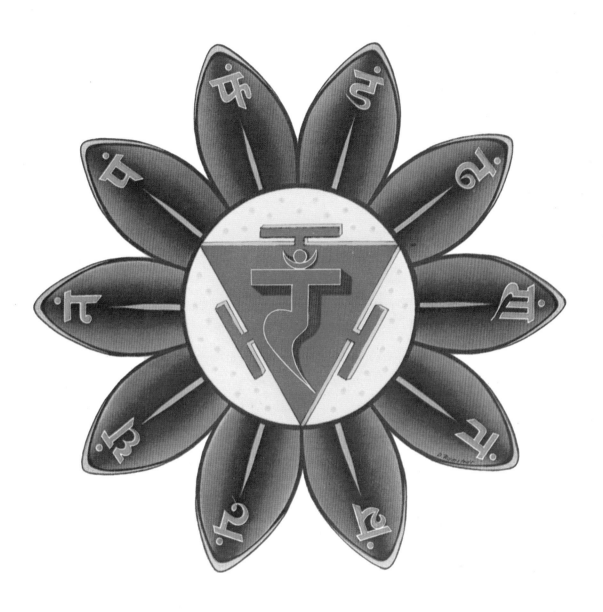

7   Manipura Chakra

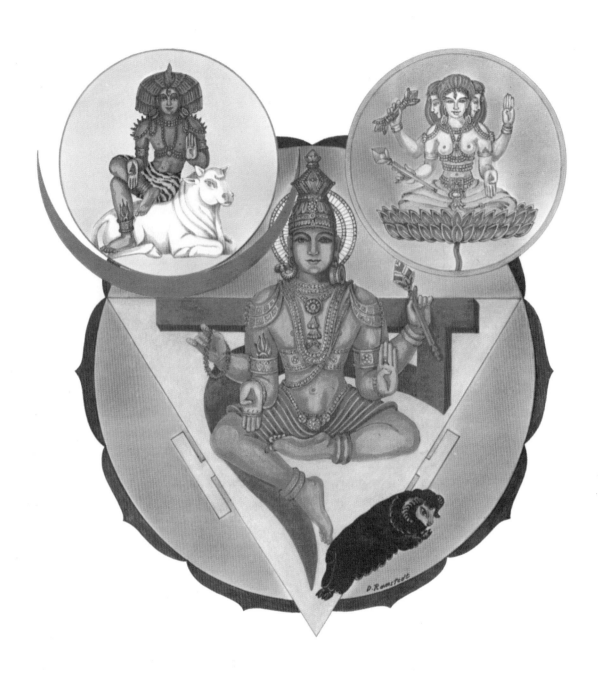

8   Deities in Manipura (A)

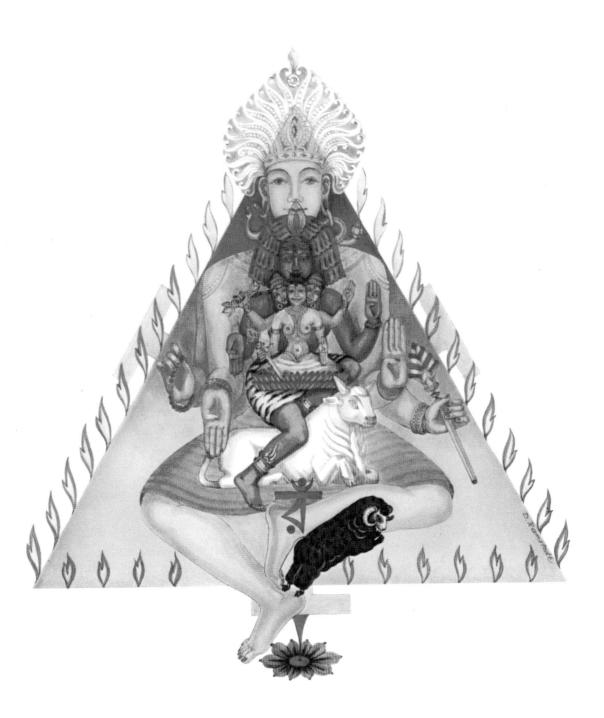

9   Deities in Manipura (B)

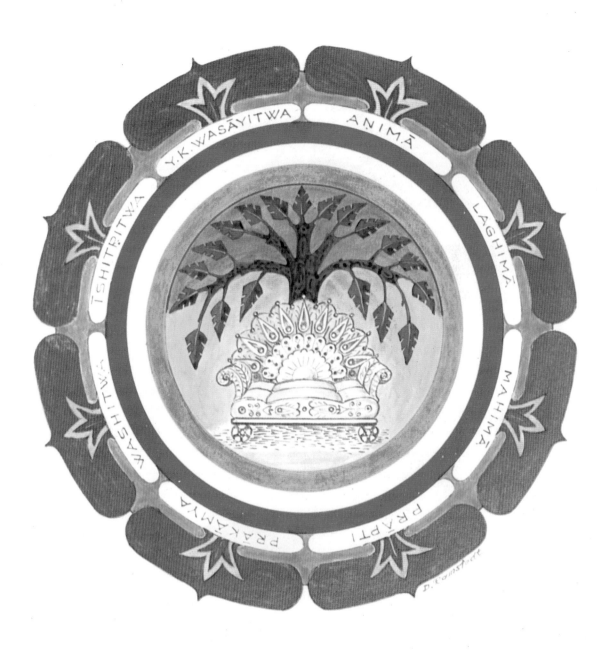

10   Hrit Chakra

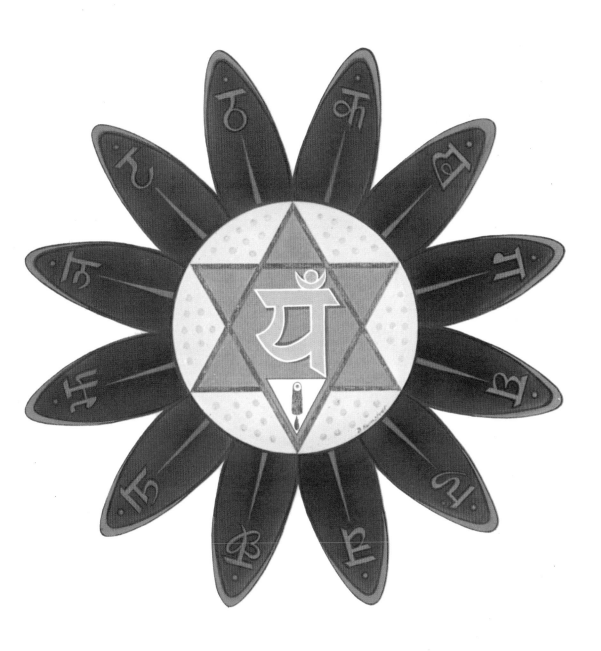

11   Anahata Chakra

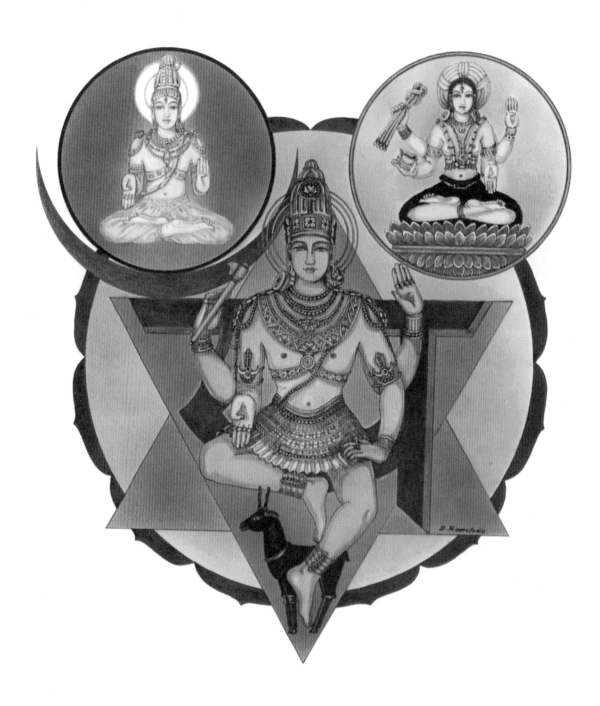

12   Deities in Anahata (A)

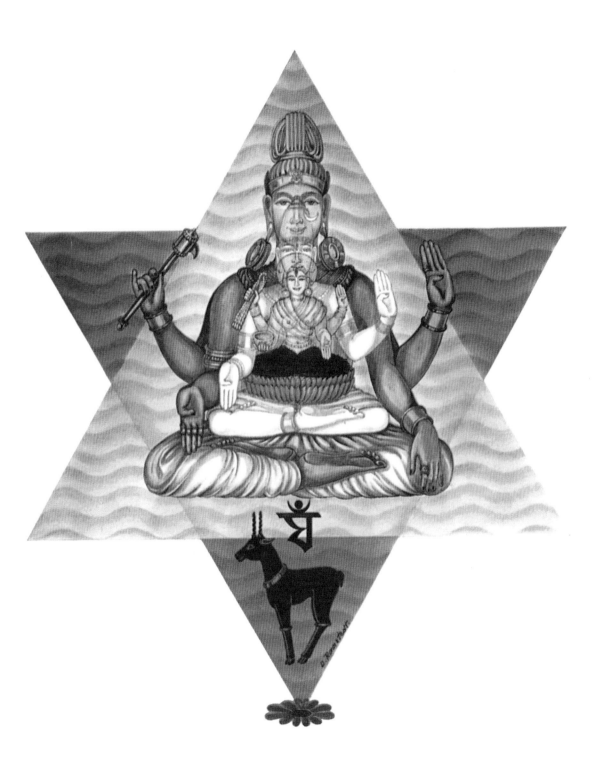

13   Deities in Anahata (B)

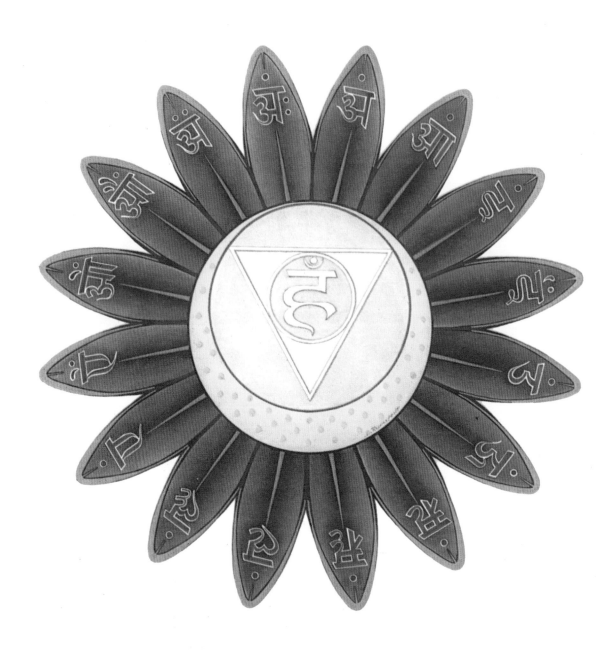

14   Wishuddha Chakra

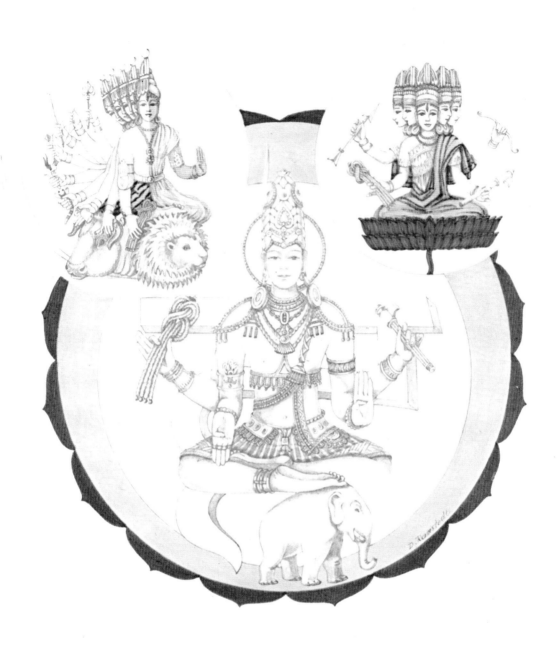

15   Deities in Wishuddha (A)

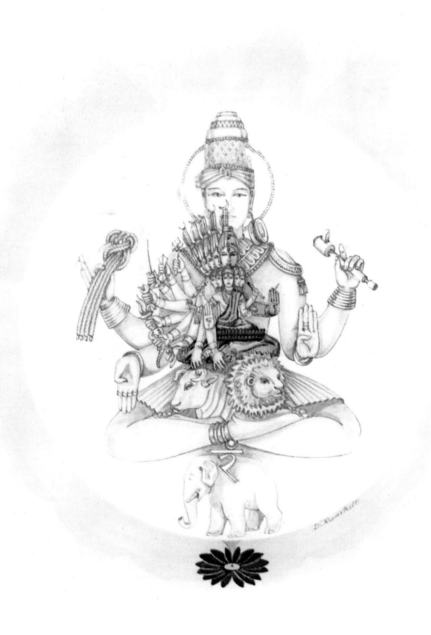

16   Deities in Wishuddha (B)

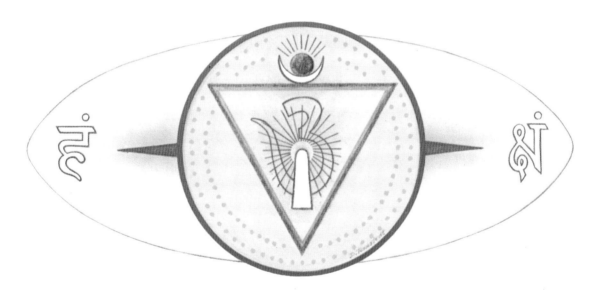

17   Ajña Chakra

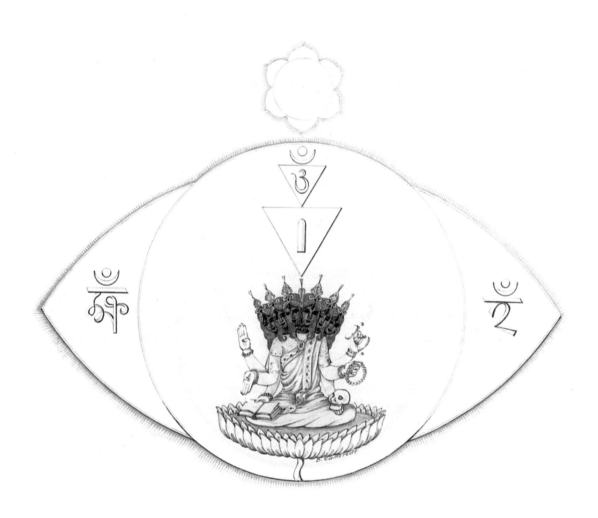

18   Hakini

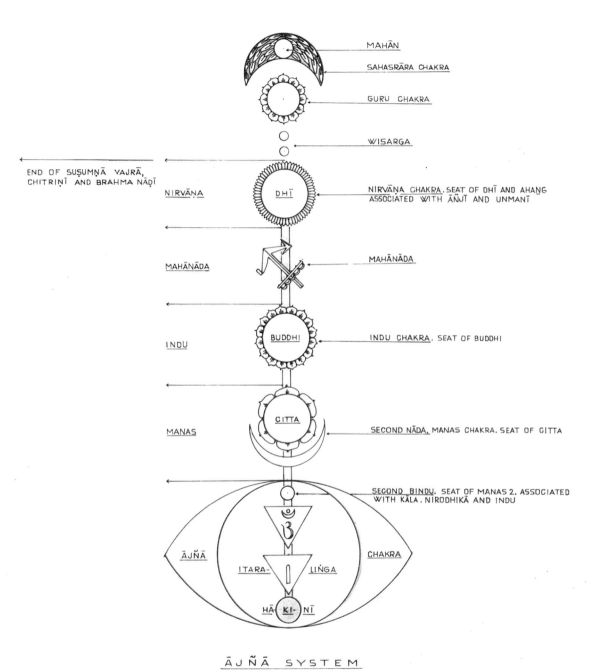

MAHĀN

SAHASRĀRA CHAKRA

GURU CHAKRA

WISARGA

END OF SUṢUMṆĀ VAJRĀ,
CHITRIṆĪ AND BRAHMA NĀḌĪ

NIRVĀṆA   DHĪ   NIRVĀṆA CHAKRA. SEAT OF DHĪ AND AHAṄG
ASSOCIATED WITH ĀÑJ̄I AND UNMANĪ

MAHĀNĀDA   MAHĀNĀDA

INDU   BUDDHI   INDU CHAKRA. SEAT OF BUDDHI

MANAS   CITTA   SECOND NĀDA, MANAS CHAKRA. SEAT OF CITTA

SECOND BINDU. SEAT OF MANAS 2. ASSOCIATED
WITH KĀLA. NIRODHIKĀ AND INDU

ĀJÑĀ   CHAKRA

ITARA-   LIṄGA

HĀ- KI- NĪ

ĀJÑĀ SYSTEM

19   Ajña system

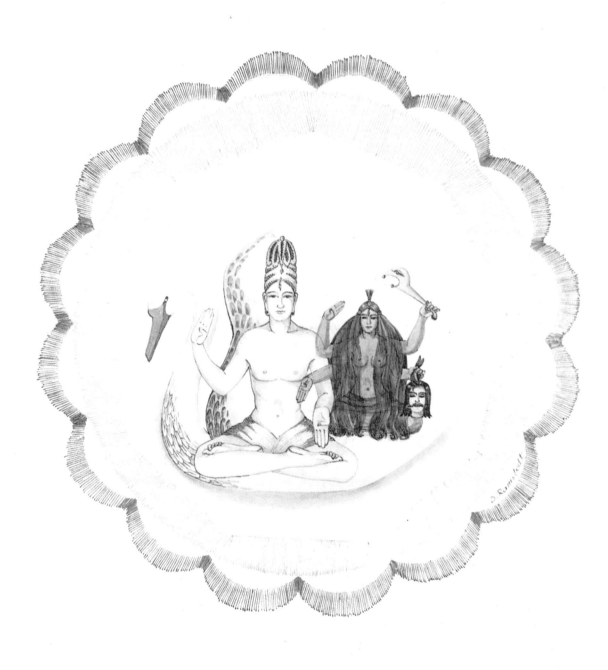

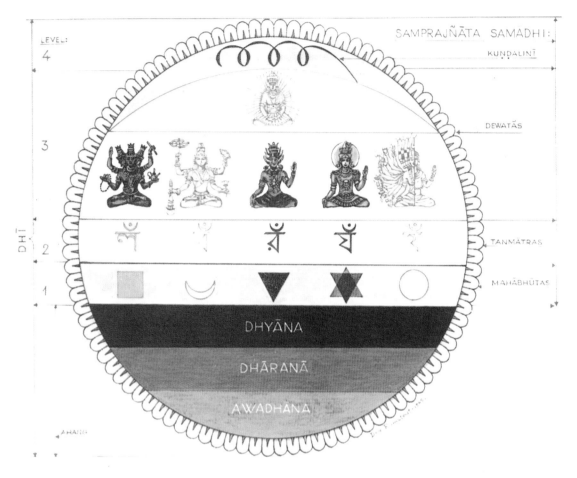

SAMPRAJÑĀTA SAMADHI:

KUŅDALINĪ

DEWATĀS

TANMĀTRAS

MAHĀBHŪTAS

LEVEL:
4

3

2

1

DHĪ

AHANG

DHYĀNA

DHĀRANĀ

AWADHĀNA

NIRWĀŅA CAKRA

21   Nirwana Chakra

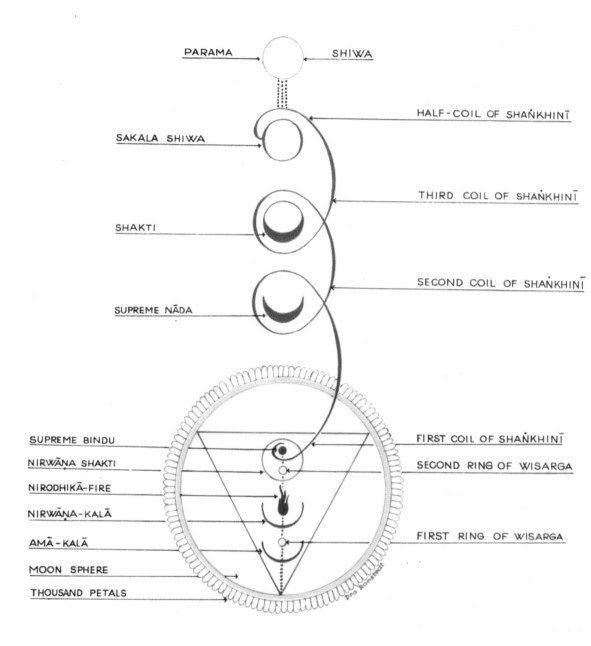

PARAMA →　　　SHIWA

HALF-COIL OF SHAŃKHINĪ

SAKALA SHIWA →

THIRD COIL OF SHAŃKHINĪ

SHAKTI

SECOND COIL OF SHAŃKHINĪ

SUPREME NĀDA

SUPREME BINDU ———　　FIRST COIL OF SHAŃKHINĪ

NIRWĀNA SHAKTI ———　　SECOND RING OF WISARGA

NIRODHIKĀ-FIRE

NIRWĀNA-KALĀ

AMĀ-KALĀ　　　　　FIRST RING OF WISARGA

MOON SPHERE

THOUSAND PETALS

SAHASRĀRA ORGANIZATION

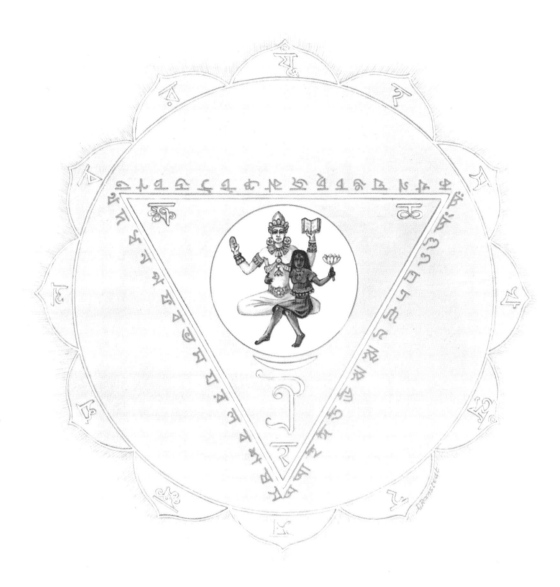

23   Guru Chakra

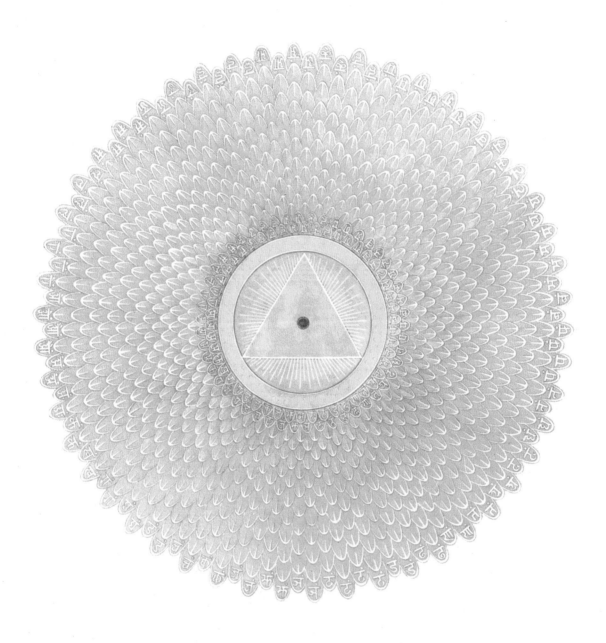

24   Sahasrara Chakra (A)

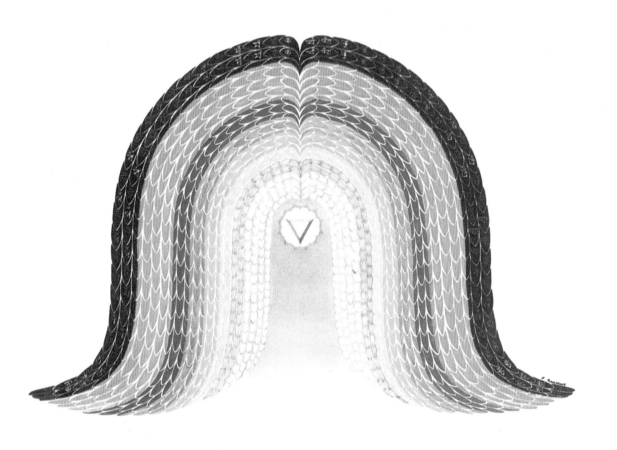

25   Sahasrara Chakra (B)

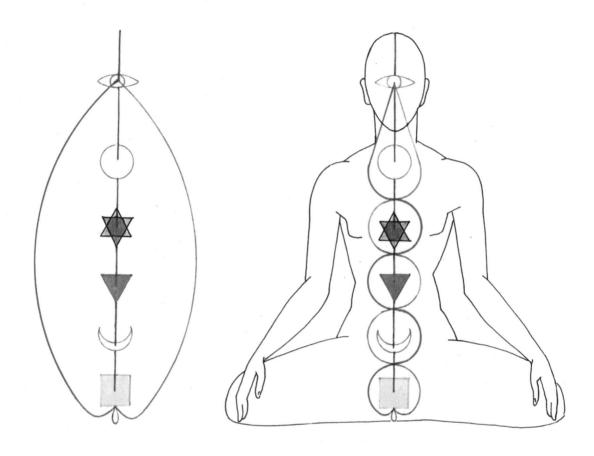

1 . BOW POSITION   2 . HALF-COIL POSITION

26   The Ida-Pingala Course. (i) Bow Position. (ii) Half-coil Position.

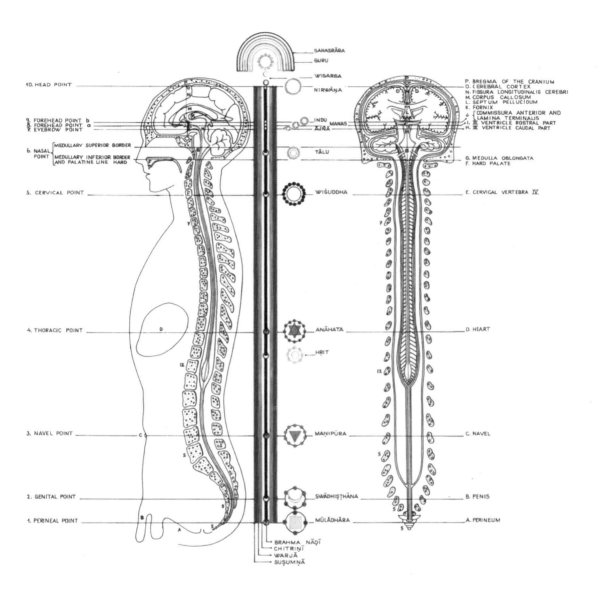

27 Location of Chakras in the Chitrin; the Surface—Vertebro Cranial Relations.

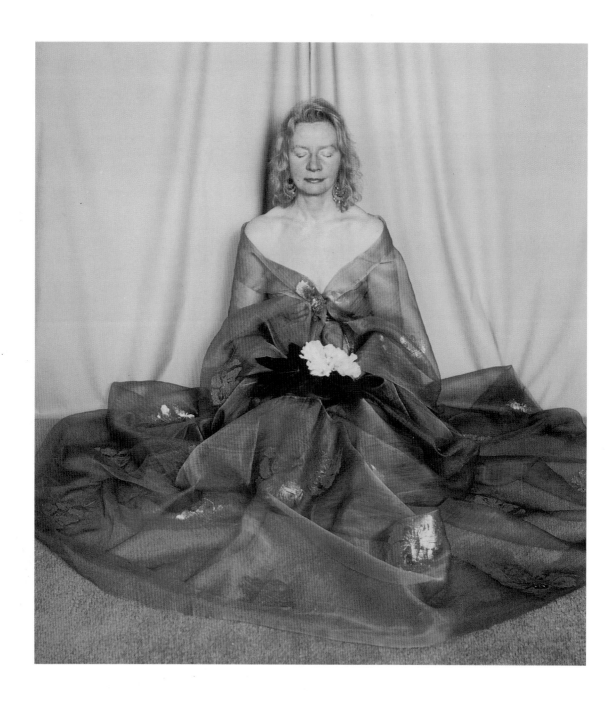

28   Concentration

centrated that they can only be realized in their mantra forms. Each tanmatra-force represents a specific germ-mantra. A germ-mantra consists of three fundamental parts—bija (sound-specificality), nada (sound-power) and bindu (conscious form). In a germ-mantra, sound-power assumes a specific character from the bija and is exposed as a divine form (dewata—deity) at bindu. So in each of the five lower chakras, is a germ-mantra from which arises a specific deity. Also in each chakra, there is a specific Power-Consciousness which controls all forces operating there. A sense principle is also connected with the tanmatra-forces. So each chakra is the seat of a specific sense principle. Prana, being manifested as wayu-forces, is linked to the tanmatra-mahabhuta forces. Each specific wayu force is located in a chakra. The conative principles are also in the chakras.

So we find that a chakra is the repository of powers of various forms—tanmatra-mahabhuta forces, wayu-force, mantra-power, a specific Deity and Power (Shakti), sensory principle, conative principle, and other forms of power. How is it known that all these powers are in the chakras? The chakras are subtle, so they are not seen even with the aid of a supersensitive instrument. This does not indicate that they do not exist. An atom is built up of particles which are so minute in size that they are not visible. The chakras are subtler than atoms and particles. If an atom can contain a tremendous amount of energy, why should not a chakra, which is infinitely subtle, contain energy which is practically unlimited in quantity and capacity? The chakra energy can be aroused and controlled by pranayama (breath-control) and dhyana (deep concentration).

When the specific energy residing in the muladhara centre is aroused by deep concentration, the power of levitation is developed (—Shiwasanghita, 5. 92). Deep concentration in the swadhishthana centre causes the body to be disease-free and long-lived (ibid., 5, 108–9). The power of entering into another's body (paradehapraweshana) is developed by deep concentration in the manipuraka centre (ibid., 5.114). The development of supersensory power and the power of the passing through air occur

by deep concentration in the anahata centre (—ibid., 5.120). All this indicates that chakras and powers located in them are not imaginary but facts. By the application of appropriate measures these powers can be aroused and made to manifest on the physical plane. The chakras with their mantras and deities can be seen in deep concentration. Deep concentration on the colour-form of a chakra at a particular location point produces a characteristic resonance—a response from an unknown region, and finally, a real living colour-form of the chakra appears there. The chakras are no more unreal than a nerve centre or a nerve plexus, though the former is extra-material, and the latter material.

The chakras form a system in the sushumna. The chakra system has been described both in the Upanishads and Tantras. There are also fragmentary descriptions of the chakras in the Puranas. This indicates that the subject is very ancient and was widely known in ancient India.

Pouranika Fragments on the Chakras

The thousand-petalled chakra, called sahasrara, is the first centralized power of pranawa emitted by Kundalini in her Shabdabrahman aspect, and in her supreme aspect she is one with Supreme Consciousness as Supreme Kundalini. It has been stated: 'From the navel of Narayana (Supreme Consciousness), lying in infinite water (in samadhi), arose a lotus with a large number (that is, one-thousand) of petals lustrous like ten-million suns' (—Shiwapurana, 1.2. 34–6). Here, the origin of sahasrara has been stated. It has been more clearly stated: 'The imperishable great lord Hari (Supreme Consciousness) who is the creator of the whole universe, while lying in infinite water, produced a finite phenomenon; he created a lotus from his navel, which contains 1000 petals, and is pure, golden and shines like the sun' (—Padmapurana, 1.39. 152–3). The great rishi Sanatkumara stated: 'That lotus which is at the highest part is yellow and shines like the sun and the moon' (—Shiwapurana, 4.40.26).

145

That lotus is sahasrara. It has been stated: 'The Supreme Power (in the form of Mahalakshmi) is in the pericarp of the thousand-petalled lotus' (—Dewibhagawata, 9.42.8). Concentration should be done on Mahalakshmi in sahasrara. Also, 'Eternal, splendorous, lotus-eyed Brahma, arising from primus, sat in the thousand-petalled lotus' (—Mahabharata, 12. 331. 21).

Sahasrara is the centre where concentration is developed into superconcentration (samadhi). Concentration is first made on Guru (God in form) in a white twelve-petalled lotus which is a part of sahasrara. It is stated: 'Getting up from bed in the early morning and changing dress, one should concentrate on Guru in the subtle, pure and life-giving thousand-petalled lotus which is in relation to brahma-line (-randhra)' (—Brahmawaiwartapurana, 1.26. 5–6). It has been said here that sahasrara is a subtle centre, that is, it is extra-material and endowed with prana-force. Concentration on Ishtadewata also is done on hritpadma or sahasrara. So it is stated: 'Concentrate on Ishtadewata in hrit-padma or the great pure white thousand-petalled lotus (chakra)' (—ibid., 1.26.8). Sahasrara is the centre where there is spiritual splendour. It has been said: 'In ancient time, Indra was able to "see" the spiritual splendour in the thousand-petalled padma by the japa of germ-mantra given by his guru' (—ibid., 4.21.174).

About ajña chakra, it has been stated: 'Ajña where concentration is done on Supreme Brahman (in form) is from Supreme Power' (—Shiwa-purana, 5 b. 8.7). Ajña chakra is in the form of energy, the source of which is Supreme Power. So ajña and other chakras are power-centres. Four chakras have been mentioned in a technical manner by Maitreya in describing the yoga process adopted by Sati when she desired to abandon her physical body. Maitreya stated: 'Assuming a (yoga) posture over which she had full control, Sati executed the pranayamic method of control of prana and apana wayus in the nabhi-chakra (that is, manipura chakra); then she raised slowly the udana wayu in pranayama with concentration to hrit (that is, hrit or anahata chakra), and then she conducted it through the kantha (that is, wishuddha chakra) to the bhrumadhya (the space between the eyebrows, that is, ajñachakra)' (—Bhaga-wata, 4.4.25).

Of 1000 names of Shiwa stated by God Wishnu, there are three names which are after three chakras. They are: Swadhishthanapada-shraya (the support of the position of the swadhi-shthana chakra), Manipura, Hritpundarikama-sinah (seated in the hrit chakra) (—Shiwa-purana, 1.71. 69–70). The muladhara chakra has been mentioned here: 'Starting from muladhara' (—ibid., 2.11.40). In explaining pranawa (Ong), Ishwara said: 'Oh Parwati! adhara (muladhara), manipura, hridaya (hrit or anahata chakra), wishuddhi (wishuddha), ajña, shakti, shanti and shan-tyatita are in due order the seats of pranawa, and of all seats shantyatita is the highest; only he who is intensely passionless is fit for it' (—ibid., 3.3. 27–9). Here, the swadhishthana chakra has not been mentioned. However, there are nine chakras if swadhishthana is included. Shakti, shanti and shantyatita are the new terms which are not common. Shakti chakra may stand for manas, shanti for indu and shantyatita for sahasrara.

Rishi Upamanyu gave a description of the chakras. He said: 'Making the body completely motionless with bio-energy fully controlled, worship Shiwa and Shakti with concentration seated in hrit padma (chakra) within the body. Concentration should also be done in mula (the perineal region, that is, muladhara), nasagra (the tip of the nose), nabhi (navel, that is, manipura), kantha (throat, i.e. wishuddha), talurandhra (lalana chakra), bhrumadhya (ajña), dewadashanta (brahmarandhra, that is nirwana chakra) and murdhan (highest part, that is, sahasrara) ... In dwidala (a chakra with two petals, that is ajña), shodashara (sixteen-petalled chakra, that is wishuddha), dwadashara (twelve-petalled chakra, that is anahata), dashara (ten-petalled chakra, that is manipura), shadasra (six-petalled swadhishthana chakra) or chatura-sra (four-petalled muladhara), concentration should be done on Shiwa. In the space between the eyebrows (that is, intra-cerebral region), there is a lotus (chakra) with two petals shining like lightning; the petals contain two matrika-letters ("Hang" and "Kshang"), arranged from the right to the left.

'The sixteen-petalled chakra contains 16 matrika-letters (from '*Ang*' to '*Ah*'), arranged from the right. The (twelve-petalled) lotus which is as bright as the sun is in the heart region; the matrika-letters from "*Kang*" to "*Thang*" are on its petals, arranged from the right; concentration should be done here. In the navel region within the spinal column, there is a milk-white lotus (ten-petalled) which contains in its petals the matrika-letters from "*Dang*" to "*Phang*" in due order. The lotus with 6 petals, with its face down, and red, contains the matrika-letters from "*Bang*" to "*Lang*" in its petals. The golden coloured muladhara contains the matrika-letters from "*Wang*" to "*Sang*" in due order in its (four) petals' (—Shiwapurana, 5 b. 29. 130–40). Here, the following chakras have been mentioned: muladhara, swadhishthana, manipura, hrit or anahata, wishuddha, lalana, ajña, nirwana and sahasrara. Practically the whole chakra system has been briefly described.

It has been stated: 'Upawarhana, at first, passed through the muladhara, swadhishthana, manipura, anahata, wishuddha and ajña—these six chakras' (—Brahmawaiwartapurana 1.13. 13). Here, the regular six chakras have been mentioned. Furthermore, 'Brahma controlled by yoga (that is, breath-control and concentration) with great care the six nadis (power-lines), viz., ida, sushumna, medhya, pingala, nalini and budha, and six chakras, viz., muladhara, swadhishthana, manipura, anahata, wishuddha and ajña' (—ibid., 4.20. 27–8). It indicates that there was a yoga process to control the nadis (power-motion-lines) and the six chakras. Krishna said: 'After achieving control over longings, senses, hunger and thirst, and effecting the internal purification and the purification of the nadis (superpurification of the power system), and piercing through the chakras, concentration should be done on Supreme Being united with Kundalini-power. The six chakras are: muladhara, swadhishthana, manipura, anahata wishuddha and ajña' (—ibid., 4.110.8–10). It has been disclosed here that concentration on Supreme Consciousness united with Kundalini is effective when the control of the body by exercise and ascesis, control of the senses and desires by sensory control, internal purification of the body

and the purification of the nadis, and the piercing of the chakras are done. The piercing of the chakras means the rousing of Kundalini and her conduction through the chakras to sahasrara where concentration should be done.

Here is a technical exposition of the chakras. It has been stated: 'Concentrating for a brief period on Supreme Power in the six chakras, the practitioner should concentrate on her in the chakra with 16 petals in which are located the matrika-letters from "*Ang*" to "*Ah*", and thereafter japa should be commenced with mulamantra (special mantra given in initiation). At the space between the eyebrows where lies the borders of the three nadis, and is known as the junction of the three power-lines, there is a centre which is red, hexagonal and magnified to four-fingers' breadth; it is called by the yogis ajña chakra. In the region of the throat, the three nadis—sushumna, ida and pingala form a coiling which is hexagonal and magnified to six-fingers' breadth, where lies the centre, belonging to six-chakras, which is white, sixteen-petalled, magnified to seven-fingers' breadth, and contain (the matrika-letters from) "*Ang*" (to "*Ah*"). The expert yogis make concentration and japa of mantra in this chakra. The three nadis are united in the heart region' (—Kalikapurana, 55. 28–33). Here only two chakras are mentioned: ajña and wishuddha. All six chakras are suitable for concentration. The wishuddha chakra is suitable for both concentration and japa. The chakras are magnified to a certain extent which is necessary for thought-concentration in the earlier stages.

In another technical exposition of the chakras, it has been stated: 'The practitioner should concentrate on an excellent lotus situated three-fingers' breadth below the navel point (at the perineal point, that is, the lotus is situated within the coccyx and is called muladhara), having (in its pericarp) a region with eight corners or five corners. There is a triangle (inside the region) which is in the nature of fire, moon and sun. Concentration, according to one's power, may be done in this order: triangle of sun, of moon, and of fire, or triangle of fire, of sun, and of moon according to the process instructed. He should think that there are spiritual action, spiritual knowledge, unaffectedness and yoga-power in the lower part of fire. He should think in due order of the three primary attributes (gunas) in the region of the lotus. Then he should concentrate on Rudra (a specific divine form) who is united with his Power lying in relation to the primary sentience-principle (sattwa). Concentration should be done properly in the navel region (that is, manipura chakra), the throat region (wishuddha chakra), the region between the eyebrows (ajña chakra), the region of the forehead (indu chakra), or at the highest point (that is, void, where lies sahasrara). Thought-concentration on Shiwa should be done in the lotus with 2 petals (ajña), with 16 petals (wishuddha), with 12 petals (anahata), with 10 petals (manipura), with 6 petals (swadhishthana), and with 4 petals (muladhara), in this order' (—Lingapurana, 1.8. 92–7). Most of the chakras —muladhara, swadhishthana, manipura, anahata, wishuddha, ajña, indu and sahasrara—have been mentioned here. A new technical description of the muladhara chakra has been given. That the chakras are the specific centres for the practice of concentration has been disclosed.

Again, 'Worship (with concentration) (to Shiwa) is done outside the body, and also in the square region (muladhara), the six-cornered (lotus, termed swadhishthana), the ten-cornered (or ten-petalled lotus, that is manipura), the twelve-petalled (lotus, that is anahata), the sixteen-petalled (lotus, that is wishuddha) and the triangle (ajña) (within the body)' (—ibid., 1.75.35). Furthermore, 'Those who are spiritually advanced, worship Shiwa, the great master of yoga, with godly love (bhakti) and spiritual concentration (shubha yoga) in the six-petalled lotus (swadhishthana). He who 'sees' Shiwa in the triangle (ajña) ... becomes absorbed into him' (—ibid., 1.75. 38–9). It has been stated: 'Immortal Shiwa who is joyous in his self is in the dwadashantabrahmarandhra (that is, nirwana chakra), the point between the eyebrows (ajña), the palate region (lalana), the throat region (wishuddha) and the heart region (anahata), in this order' (—ibid., 2.21.28). Here, nirwana and lalana have been mentioned along with other chakras.

The system of chakras as explained by Dewi is as follows: 'There is a lotus which has 4 petals of molten gold (that is red). On the petals are (the matrika-units) "Wang", "Shang", "Shang" and "Sang" which are yellow. It has a six-cornered region. It is the basic centre (mula) and the support (adhara) (of Kundalini), so it is called muladhara. This is a centre for concentration.

'Above it is an excellent (lotus called) swadhishthana with 6 petals which are like fire (that is red). On the petals are (the matrika-units) "Bang", "Bhang", "Mang", "Yang", "Rang" and "Lang" of the lustre of a diamond. The name swadhishthana is from "swa" to mean Supreme Shiwa in an apprehensible form (linga) (that is, this lotus is the seat of Shiwa in form, so it is called swadhishthana).

'Above it, in the navel region, is splendorous manipura which is dark like a cloud (that is, black) shining like lightning. It is of power. It has 10 petals on which are 10 letters from "Dang" to "Phang" (that is, the 10 matrika-units; and they are like lightning; the shining effects on the petals are due to this). This lotus is like a blooming gem, so it is called manipadma. Deity Wishnu is in this lotus. Here it is possible to "see" Wishnu (by concentration).

'Above it is the anahata lotus (chakra) with 12 petals which are red like the rising sun and on which are the 12 letters from 'Kang' to 'Thang'. Within it is in linga-form (a form effective for concentration) Bana (a form of Shiwa) who is splendorous like ten-thousand suns. This lotus is called by the yogis anahata because here arises that sound which is non-sensory and is in the nature of Shabdabrahman. In this lotus is Supreme Being (in appropriate form) and it is the abode of bliss.

'Above it is the lotus named wishuddha with 16 petals of smoke-colour on which are the 16 matrika-units form 'Ang' to 'Ah' of great lustre. The superpurification of the embodied being occurs in this lotus through the realization of divine being, this is why it is called wishuddha. This wonderful lotus is also called akasha (void) (because it is the centre of the void-principle).

'Above it is the beautiful ajña chakra with 2 petals on which are (the matrika-units) "Hang" and "Kshang". Here lies the Supreme Being. In this centre, spiritual force passes into the practitioner, so it is called ajña.

'Above it is what is called kailasa (chakra), and above that is rodhini (chakra).... Above it (rodhini) is sahasrara (1000-petalled chakra) in which is the seat of Supreme Bindu' (—Dewibhagawata, 7.35.34–47).

About the locations of the six chakras, it has been stated: 'In the perineal region (adhara = yonisthana), genital region, navel region, heart region, neck region (talumula = the root of the palate, but here it is kantha = neck—Nilakantha's commentary) and the eyebrow region (lalata = the forehead, but here bhrumadhya = the space between the eyebrows—Nilakantha), (are the six chakras) having 4 petals, 6 petals, 10 petals, 12 petals, 16 petals and 2 petals respectively' (—ibid., 11.1.43). About the regions and mantras of the subtle elements (mahabhutas), it has been said that the 'earth' region is square of golden (yellow) colour within which is 'Lang'-bija (germ-mantra of the same colour); that the region of 'water' is of the shape of a white half-moon, within which is 'Wang'-bija (of the same colour); that the region of 'fire' is triangular in shape and red and encloses 'Rang'-bija (of the same colour); that the region of 'air' is circular and smoke-coloured and encloses 'Yang'-bija (of the same colour); and that the region of 'void' (akasha) is circular and is white (or transparent) in colour, and encloses 'Hang'-bija (of the same colour) (—ibid., 11.8.3–7).

Concentration on deities in different chakras is an ancient spiritual process and was practised by the rishis. It has been stated that a group named Kurpadrisha, which followed the rishi-path, used to practise concentration on the divine being in the abdominal region (that is, the manipura chakra), while the Aruni group practised concentration on extremely subtle form of God in the heart region (either hrit or anahata chakra), connected with the nadi-system; but the abode of Supreme Consciousness is in the extra-cerebral region (parama shiras, that is sahasrara) (—Bhagawata, 10.87.18).

There was a process of dharana (holding-concentration) in which the vital force is held in different chakras with breath-suspension and concentration. The holding was done in the chakras with four petals (muladhara), with six petals (swadhishthana), in the navel region (manipura), in the heart region (hrit chakra), (the chakra) in the region of the lungs with twelve petals (anahata), (the chakra) with sixteen petals, in the region of the palate (lalana or talu chakra), the space between the eyebrows (ajña chakra), and in brahmarandhra in the head (nirwana chakra) (—Skandapurana, 1.2.55. 44–5).

The Pouranika System of Chakras

From the descriptions of the chakras given in the Puranas, the Pouranika system for chakras emerges. It is as follows:

1 Muladhara. The term 'muladhara' has been used in Shiwapurana, 2.11.40; 51.29.140; in Brahmawaiwartapurana, 1.13.13; 4.20.28; 4.110. 10; and in Dewibhagawata, 7.35.34. It is mentioned indirectly in Shiwapurana, 56.29.131 and 134; in Skandapurana, 1.2.55.44; and in Lingapurana, 1.8.92 and 97; 1.75.35. Muladhara is also called adhara, Shiwapurana, 3.3.28.

Description. The muladhara chakra is situated in the perineal region (adhara or mula = yonisthana), that is a certain intracoccygeal point. It has four petals of red colour. On the petals are four matrika-letters 'Wang' to 'Sang' of yellow colour. It has a square region inside. It has also been stated that the region is five-cornered, six-cornered or eight-cornered. However, the region is of 'earth', and is generally accepted as a square which is yellow in colour, and the 'earth' germ-mantra 'Lang' which is also yellow resides in the square region. Inside the region is a triangle which is in the form of fire, moon and sun. This chakra is called muladhara, because it is the basic centre (mula) which is the support (adhara) of Kundalini. It is a centre of thought-concentration and mental worship.

2 Swadhishthana. The term 'swadhishthana' has been used in Shiwapurana, 1.71.69; in Brahmawaiwartapurana, 1.13.13; 4.20.28; 4.110. 10; and in Dewibhagawata, 7.35.35. This chakra is mentioned indirectly in Lingapurana, 1.8.97;

1.75.35 and 38; in Shiwapurana, 5b. 29.134; and in Skandapurana, 1.2.55.44.

Description. The swadhishthana chakra is situated above muladhara, in the genital region (that is, a certain intrasacral point). It has six petals of red colour. On the petals are six matrika-letters from 'Bang' to 'Lang' of the lustre of a diamond. In the pericarp is a half-moon-shaped region of 'water' of white colour in which is 'Wang'-bija of white colour. It is also said that the region is six-cornered. It is the seat of Supreme Shiwa in a form effective for concentration, so it is called swadhishthana. It is a centre for thought-concentration and mental worship.

3 Manipura. The term 'manipura' has been used in Shiwapurana, 1.71.70; 3.3.28; in Brahmawaiwartapurana, 1.13.13; 4.20.28; 4.110.10; and in Dewibhagawata, 7.35.36. It is indirectly mentioned in Lingapurana, 1.8.96 and 97; 1.75.35; in Shiwapurana, 5b.29.131 and 134; and in Bhagawata, 10.87.18. This centre is also called nabhi (navel)-chakra (—Bhagawata, 4.4.25).

Description. Manipura is situated above swadhishthana, in the navel region (that is, a certain intralumbar point). It has 10 petals of dark colour or black colour. On the petals are 10 matrika-letters from 'Dang' to 'Phang' which are lightning (of lightning colour). In the pericarp, there is a triangular region of 'fire' of red colour. Within it is the red-coloured 'Rang'-bija. This chakra has also been said to be milk-white. In that case the petals are white in colour. It is a centre for thought-concentration and mental worship.

4 Hrit (-padma). The hrit chakra has been mentioned in Shiwapurana, 5b.29.131; and indirectly in Skandapurana, 1.2.55.44.

Description. The lotus (chakra) is situated in relation to the heart (that is, a certain intrathoracispinal point, below anahata and above manipura. It has eight petals which are white in colour. Pranic forces are located here. It is a sacred place for spiritual concentration (—Lingapurana, 1.86.62–64).

5 Anahata. The term 'anahata' has been used in Brahmawaiwartapurana, 1.13.13; 4.20.28; 4.110.10; and in Dewibhagawata, 7.35.39. It is mentioned indirectly in Lingapurana, 1.8.97;

2.21.28; in Bhagawata, 4.4.25; 10.87.18; in Skandapurana, 1.2.55.44; and in Shiwapurana, 5b.29.133.

Description. Anahata is situated, above manipura, (and above hrit) in the heart region (that is, a certain intrathoracispinal point). It has twelve petals of red colour. On the petals are twelve matrika-letters from 'Kang' to 'Thang'. In the pericarp is the region of 'air' which is circular and of smoke-colour. In the region is the smoke-coloured 'Yang'-bija. Within the chakra is splendorous Bana-linga (Shiwa in a special form which is suitable for concentration and worship). In it is 'heard' the non-sensory sound (anahata nada) of mantra, so it is called anahata. It is a centre for thought-concentration and mental worship.

6 Wishuddha. The term 'wishuddha' has been used in Brahmawaiwartapurana, 1.13.13; 4.20.28; 4.110.10; and in Dewibhagawata, 7.35.42. Another term 'wishuddhi' (for wishuddha) has been used in Shiwapurana, 3.3.28. It is mentioned indirectly in Lingapurana, 1.8.96 and 97; 1.75.35; 2.21.28; in Bhagawata, 4.4.25; in Shiwapurana, 5b.29.131 and 133; in Kalikapurana, 55.28 and 33; and in Skandapurana, 1.2.55.44.

Description. Above anahata is the wishuddha chakra, situated in the neck region (that is, a certain intracervicospinal point). It has sixteen petals of smoke-colour. On the petals are the sixteen matrika-letters from 'Ang' to 'Ah' which are lustrous. In the pericarp, there is the region of 'void' (akasha), which is circular in shape and white in colour (or transparent). The 'Hang'-bija, which is also white is in this region. This chakra is called wishuddha (which means purified), because here spiritual purification of the practitioner occurs through the realization of Supreme Being. It is the centre for thought-concentration, japa and mental worship.

7 Talu (chakra). This chakra has been mentioned in Skandapurana, 1.2.55.44; in Lingapurana, 2.21.28; and in Shiwapurana, 5b.29.131. The talu chakra has been termed lalana chakra in the Tantras. There is no description of the chakra in the Puranas.

8 Ajña. The term 'ajña' has been mentioned in Shiwapurana, 3.3.28; in Brahmawaiwarta-

purana, 1.13.13; 4.20.28; 4.110.10; in Kalika-purana, 55.30; and in Dewibhagawata, 7.35.44. It is indirectly mentioned in Lingapurana, 1.8.96; 2.21.28; in Bhagawata, 4.4.25; in Shiwapurana, 5b.29. 132; and in Skandapurana, 1.2.55.44. Ajña has been termed 'dwidala', because this chakra has two petals. Dwidala has been mentioned in Lingapurana, 1.8.97; and in Shiwa-purana, 5b.29.133 and 134. This lotus is also called 'trirasra' (triangle), as it has a triangular process inside the pericarp. Trirasra has been mentioned in Lingapurana, 1.75.39.

Description. Ajña is situated above talu chakra at the eyebrow region (that is, at a certain intra-cerebral point). It has two petals. The petals are like lightning. They are also mentioned as red in colour. On the petals are two matrika-letters 'Hang' and 'Kshang', arranged from right to left. It is a great centre for concentration and mental worship.

9 Shakti(-chakra). The term 'shakti' is a new one. It has only been mentioned in Shiwa-purana, 3.3.28. It may be the Tantrika 'manas' chakra. It is above ajña.

10 Kailasa(-chakra). 'Kailasa' is a new term. It has only been mentioned in Dewibhagawata, 7.35.46. Perhaps it is the same as the chakra 'shanta' used in Shiwapurana, 3.3.28. However, it appears that kailasa and shanta are identical

with the indu chakra. Kailasa is above shakti.

11 Rodhini(-chakra). The term 'rodhini' is a new one, and it has been mentioned in Dewi-bhagawata, 7.35.46. The terms 'dwadashanta', mentioned in Lingapurana, 2.21.28, and in Shiwapurana, 5b.29.132, and 'brahmarandhra', mentioned in Skandapurana, 1.2.55.45, appear to be synonymous with rodhini. The chakra which is in brahmarandhra has been termed nirwana in the Tantras. So rodhini is probably the Tantrika nirwana chakra.

12 Sahasrara. The term 'sahasrara' has been mentioned in Dewibhagawata, 7.35.47. This chakra also is called 'sahasrapadma' (lotus with 1000 petals), mentioned in Brahmawaiwarta-purana, 1.26.5, 'sahasrapatra' (1000-petalled), mentioned in the same Purana, 1.26.8, and 'sahasradala-padma' (lotus having 1000 petals), also mentioned in the same Purana, 4.21.174. The chakra named 'shantyatita', mentioned in Shiwapurana, 3.3.29, and sahasrara appear to be synonyms. Sahasrara has been indirectly called 'parama shiras', that is, supracerebral centre, mentioned in Bhagawata, 10.87.18.

Description. Sahasrara is situated above rodhini (at the supracerebral point). It has 1000 petals which are white in colour. It is the seat of Bindu (Supreme Bindu). Here concentration develops into superconcentration.

CHAPTER 8

The Waidika System of Chakras

The nadis are the subtle pranic force-motion-lines. They are created by the operation of the prana-wayus. The ordinary operation of the prana-wayus produces two effects: maintaining life in the body by their complex activities, and supporting mentation. But there is an extraordinary function of the prana-wayus in which the force-motions are centralized as the sushumna-line through which the central spiritual force passes and absorbs all principles which are the root causes of all nonspiritual phenomena. The centre of the nadi-system is in relation to hridaya, that is, the subtle hrit centre situated in the heart region. This subtle centre is not in the flesh of the heart, but at a point within the sushumna and that part of the sushumna is inside the thoracic spine in the heart region. The pranic energy passes externally to the mental and material fields as different nadi-lines to support mentalization and vitalization of the body. But when the hrit centre is aroused, a concentration of pranic energy occurs by which the dormant sushumna is energized.

Nadi-system

It has been stated: 'There are 101 nadis in relation to the hridaya (that is, the subtle hrit centre); among them that "one" nadi (that is, the sushumna) goes upward to the murdhan (the highest point, that is, brahmarandhra). Through this nadi the spiritual elevation (to

the sahasrara) is effected and, as a result, one becomes immortal. The passing through the other nadis causes deaths and births' (—Kathopanishad, 2.3.16). The 100 nadis indicate a large number of nadis. These pranic flows maintain worldliness. But that one nadi which is sushumna remains dormant when the other nadis flow strongly. The sushumna is aroused by the control of the flows through the other nadis. The sushumna passes upward from the muladhara to the brahmarandhra where lies the nirwana chakra. Kundalini passes through the sushumna to be in the sahasrara. The control factor appears to remain in the hrit centre.

This has been more clearly stated here: 'There are 101 nadis in relation to hridaya (hrit centre). Of these, one goes to the murdhan (brahmarandhra). Immortality is attained when one passes upward (to reach the sahasrara by piercing all the chakras). Death (and consequently birth) cannot be prevented when going through the other nadis. Of 101 nadis, the one is sushumna which is the highest. Within sushumna is concealed the nadi which is of the form of Brahman (that is, brahma nadi); this is pure in character. The ida is situated on the left side and the pingala on the right side. Between these two is the most excellent position (where the sushumna is located); one who knows that is the knower of the Weda' (—Yogashikhopanishad, 6.4–6). Here it is explained that of the 101 nadis, the 'one' nadi is the sushumna, and within it is the brahma nadi. On the left side of the sushumna stands the ida nadi and on its right side is the pingala nadi.

More about the sushumna: 'The winadanda (the vertebral column), made of bone and long, lying at the posterior part, extends from the anus and supports the body. The brahma nadi extends within. The sushumna which is sun-like is between the ida and pingala and is situated as a subtle line within the spinal column, and the brahma nadi is within the sushumna' (—ibid., 6. 8–9). Farther, 'The sushumna is the support of all nadis which are in all parts and spread in all directions. There are 72 thousand nadis along which wayu (pranic energy) operates. The wayu-paths are the empty lines of operation' (—ibid., 6.10, 14–15).

From all this emerges the following: the nadi-system consists of innumerable nadis which are all-directed and are in all places. The subtle hrit centre supports the function of the nadis. Of all the nadis, the one which is the sushumna is the greatest, because yoga is effected with the help of it. All other nadis are dependent on the sushumna for their controlled actions. The nadis are the directions of wayu (pranic force-motion). The sushumna is the central nadi and is situated within the vertebral column. On the left side of the sushumna is the ida and on the right side the pingala. Inside the sushumna lies the brahma nadi.

It has been stated: 'The oscillating prana-force which causes respiration becomes controlled when it is held in the sushumna' (—Yoga-shikhopanishad, 6.7). When the pranic force operates through the other nadis, the vitalization of the body is effected. But when it is held in the sushumna, it is fully controlled and there is natural breath-suspension, with no inspiration or expiration. So the sushumna is the central nadi where the control factor is situated.

When the sushumna flow occurs, the pranic force is withdrawn from other nadis and is concentrated within the sushumna and, as a result, breath-suspension (kumbhaka) occurs. This is very favourable for concentration. At this stage the sushumna centres are aroused. Both breath-control and concentration play a most important role in arousing the centres. Concentration on the sushumna centres is so important that it is denoted by a technical term 'sushumnadhyanayoga' (—Yogashikhopanishad,

6.43)—concentration-in-sushumna which leads to superconcentration.

It has been stated: 'The sun-coloured sushumna extends from the muladhara to the brahma-randhra. Within it (that is, within the muladhara to which is connected the sushumna), lies Kunda-lini who is lightning-like splendorous and extremely subtle' (—Mandalabrahmanopani-shad, 1.2.6). Within the vertebral column lies the sushumna as a subtle line of pranic operation, extending from the muladhara to the brahma-randhra, and is sun-coloured (that is, red). The junction between the muladhara and the sushumna is called the sushumnadwara, that is, the entrance to the sushumna (—Yoga-shikhopanishad, 1.75). The sushumna has been called the central nadi (madhyanadi) (—ibid., 6.41).

About the nadi-system (nadi-chakra) it has been stated: 'The sushumna being connected with the triangle of the muladhara is of twelve digit-length. When the sushumna is cut length-wise like a half-split bamboo, the innermost part is the brahma nadi. The ida and pingala stand on either side of the sushumna and are closely attached to the wilambini and have extended to the interior of the nadika. The golden (or yellow)-coloured wayu (pranic or vital force) moves through the ida on the left, and the sun (or red)-coloured wayu through the pingala on the right. The wilambini arises from the central part from where all nadis originate and ramify upwards, downwards and obliquely. This is called the nabhichakra, which is like a plexus the size of a hen's egg. Therefrom arise the gandhari and hastijihwa, which pass to the eyes; and the pusha and alambusa which go to the ears; and the great nadi shura to the space between the eyebrows; that nadi called wishwo-dari is concerned with the digestion of four kinds of food; the saraswati nadi extends to the tongue; the raka nadi causes thirst, sneezing and phlegm in the nostrils. The shankhini nadi originates from the region of the throat and turns downwards; it absorbs the essence of food and circulates in the brain. There are three nadis which, from the centre, go down-wards. Of these the kuhu nadi is involved in the evacuation of the bowels, waruni in making water; and the nadi in the frenum of the prepuce of the penis, called chitra, causes ejaculation of the semen. This is nadi-chakra' (— Yogashikhopanishad, 5. 17–27).

And 'the nadi-kanda (the central plexus of the nadis) is located nine digit-lengths above the genitals. It is (when magnified) four digit-lengths in thickness and four digit-lengths long, egg-shaped and concealed in fat, marrow, bone and blood (that is, physically invisible). There lies the twelve-spoked nadi-chakra (nadi-system) which supports the body. In nadi-chakra lies Kundalini who has kept concealed the brahmarandhra, which is to be reached through the sushumna.

'The alambusa and kuhu nadis are situated in relation to the sushumna. Adjoining them are the waruna and yashaswini where lie the two spokes. The pingala is situated in the right spoke. Between the spokes are situated the pusha and the payaswini. The nadi saraswati lies in the posterior spoke of the sushumna. Adjoining them are the shankhini and the gandhari. The nadi called ida stands on the left side of the sushumna. The hastijihwa and then the wishwodari lie adjacent to it. These nadis are in the spokes of the chakra (nadi-chakra), and are arranged from right to left. They are the twelve nadis which are the flows of twelve wayus (vital forces). These nadis are the vital force-motion directions (or lines) and are of different colours; they are like a piece of cloth, the central part of which is called nabhichakra (centre of the nadi-system). ... Ten wayus (vital forces) flow through these nadis (that is, the flows of the wayus are the nadis, or the subtle lines created by force-motions); thus the wise student having well understood the nadi-motion (-gati) which is (actually) wayu-motion' (— Warahopanishad, 5. 20–31).

Moreover, 'There (in the nadi-chakra) is the sushumna which is known as the bearer of cosmic principles (that is, there are various centres of cosmic principles within the sushumna) and the means to liberation (when these centres are absorbed in Kundalini). It (sushumna) dwells in the vertebral column (winadanda) (that is, sushumna is situated within the vertebral column), and extends from the back of the anal region (that is, the muladhara) to the head where is the brahmarandhra. This subtle divine nadi is manifested there. The ida is situated on the left side of the sushumna, and the pingala on the right side. ... The saraswati and kuhu are situated on the postero-lateral part of the sushumna. The waruni is between the yashaswini and the kuhu. The payaswini is situated between the pusha and the saraswati. Between the gandhari and saraswati is yashaswini. The alambusa is in the kanda (nadi-kanda). The kuhu extends to the genitals. The waruni, which extends in all directions, is in the superior and inferior aspects of Kundalini (that is, muladhara where lies Kundalini). The bright yashaswini extends to the great toe. Going upwards, the pingala extends to the right nostril. Behind the pingala, the pusha extends to the right eye. The yashaswini goes to the right ear. The saraswati goes to the tongue. Being upwardly directed, the shankhini goes to the left ear. The gandhari, lying behind the ida, extends to the left eye. The alambusa extends upwards and downwards from the anal region. There are other nadis in relation to the fourteen (chief) nadis, and besides them, there are many more nadis. As the leaf of the ashwattha (Ficus Religiosa—sacred fig tree) and other trees are full of vessels, so the body is pervaded by nadis' (— Shandilyopanishad, 1.4. 10–11).

To summarize—the nadi-chakra (nadi-system) is formed of innumerable nadis which are arranged in a plexus-like formation, having twelve spokes. The nadis arise from the spokes and they are also between the spokes. The nadis are essentially the subtle lines of pranic force-motions, and are of different colours. Of all nadis, fourteen are important, and of the fourteen, three are the most important. They are the ida, pingala and sushumna. Of these three nadis, the sushumna is the greatest. The sushumna is the central part of the nadi-system. It is within the vertebral column and extends from the muladhara to the brahmarandhra in the head. Inside the sushumna lies the brahma nadi. The ida and pingala are situated on the left and the right side of the sushumna respectively (outside the vertebral column).

Chakras

Surya—God, who in his infinite aspect is static, but in his power aspect appears as finite when he assumes the form of the universe. That Surya is the secondless divine knowledge-light who manifests his power as rays. The Supreme Power, which is the power of Surya, is splendorous, and so he is splendorous. The first manifested rays are centralized in a form of a lotus from which radiate 1000 rays, as if they were petals. The central Kundali-power emits power-rays which are in the nature of supra-sounds. These are the matrika-sounds containing fifty distinct sound-units, which, being summated, cause pranawa-sound. The fifty sound-powers in the thousand-petalled lotus are distinct, and each is twenty-fold strong. The matrika-sound-powers become more specialized in the six lower chakras, and the sound chain is formed from the regular and inverse manner, which makes the total sound strength 100, each sound being two-fold strong (—Prashnopanishad, 1.8).

It has been stated: 'Aditya (God) is father (in his creative aspect) and has five feet (that is, five creative principles—tanmatras-mahabhutas, represented by "Hang", "Yang", "Rang", "Wang" and "Lang") and twelve forms (that is, mahat, ahang, five senses and five conative faculties); he is beyond the sensory knowledge, but from him came the senses and other principles; he is in the seven chakras (as the presiding Deity in each chakra, that is, in the muladhara, swadhishthana, manipura, anahata, wishuddha, and indu as a Shiwa, and in the sahasrara as Parama Shiwa) and in six spokes (that is, the six principles—mind, and the five mahabhutas which are in the six chakras, from the ajña to the muladhara)' (—Prashnopanishad, 1.11).

From God in his creative aspect arise seven chakras where all creative principles are located. So it is said: 'From God seven worlds (lokas, that is, chakras) have come where the pranas move (—Mundakopanishad, 2.1.8).

The chakras are the subtle positions where Supreme Being is realized in his appropriate forms. The principal positions are within the sushumna, and their corresponding external locations are the navel, heart, throat and head. It has been stated: 'There are four (main) positions (for the realization) of Supreme Being. They are the navel, the heart, the throat and the head. Brahman in its four aspects (chatushpada) becomes manifested in these positions as Brahma in the waking state, as Wishnu in the dreaming state, as Rudra in the state of deep sleep, and as Supreme Brahman (akshara) in the samadhi (superconcentration) state (turiya), (—Brahmopanishad, 1). The waking is that in which the senses and mind are in action. At this stage the spiritual realization is not possible unless one is able to be in the position in the sushumna, which is the manipura chakra, which is at the same line of the navel. It is a suitable centre for concentration, and when concentration becomes deep (dhyana), Supreme Brahman as Deity Brahma is realized here. The dreaming state is the state of thoughts. So long as thoughts are not fully controlled, deep concentration (dhyana) is not possible. Under this state, one should be in the hrit chakra in the sushumna for concentration. This centre corresponds externally to the heart region. In the hrit centre, Supreme Brahman is realized as Deity Wishnu. In deep sleeping, the senses and mind are inoperative, and it is a state of unconsciousness. But when consciousness is turned into a state of deep concentration, the senses and sense-mind become actionless. Under this condition Supreme Brahman as Rudra is realized in the wishuddha chakra situated in the neck region. The fourth state (turiya) is the state of samadhi, when concentration develops into superconcentration. This occurs in the sahasrara—the extra-cerebral centre, when Supreme Brahman is realized in superconscious concentration (samprajñata samadhi).

About the hrit chakra, it has been stated: 'All deities, prana-wayus and the (main) prana, and the divine light ... are in the heart (hrit chakra); all these are in the heart which is in the nature of consciousness' (—Brahmopanishad, 4). The hrit centre is of consciousness, that is living. When a chakra is aroused by concentration, it becomes living. The hrit chakra is an excellent place for deep concentration (dhyana).

It has been stated: 'The immutable living divine light situated in the hrit lotus (chakra) becomes the Supreme Being in the kadamba (Stephegyne Parviflora Karth) which is like a spherical form (that is, the sahasrara chakra) (through super-conscious concentration); that Supreme Being is actually beyond samadhi; he is infinite, he is love, supreme consciousness, splendorous and all-pervading. The yogi who concentrates on this (divine) light as still resembling a lamp in a windless place and like a real gem, is sure to get liberation' (—Trishikhibrahmanopanishad, Mantra Section, 156–8). Here two stages of concentration have been mentioned. The first stage is deep concentration on the divine light in the hrit chakra. This divine light is Kundalini. When Kundali-concentration is mastered, it is transformed into superconscious concentration in the sahasrara, where Kundalini is ultimately absorbed into the Supreme Being in non-mens supreme concentration.

It has been stated: 'Cool light is experienced by internal focussing (antarlakshya) in the saha-srara' (—Mandalabrahmanopanishad, 1.4.1). Internal focussing is the concentrativeness of consciousness based on sense-withdrawal. Cool light is the Brahman-light which is revealed by internal focussing in the sahasrara. This light is from luminous Kundalini. Kundalini is the spiritual aspect of Supreme Power of Supreme Being. When Supreme Power manifests herself in a finite form from her supreme state of infinitude, the cosmic phenomenon arises. The embodied being, though a very minute part of the vast cosmos, exhibits all the creative principles which are operating cosmically. It has been stated: 'From Atman (Supreme Being) arise all pranas. All lokas, all dewas, all bhutas; the secret name of that Atman is the truth of all truths; the pranas are truth, but Atman is the truth of all truths' (—Brihadaranyakopa-nishad, 2.1.20). The pranas are the pranic forces which include also the sense-mind and senses located in the chakras; the lokas are the chakras in the body; the dewas are the deities within the chakras, bhutas are the tanmatras (tanons) and mahabhutas (five forms of metamatter).

The yoga-practitioner realizes in concentration Supreme Being as a Deity in a chakra.

The Deity appears as splendorous and living, and he, the practitioner, with the increased depth of concentration, becomes absorbed into the Deity and realizes the sameness of his form with that of the Deity. In the 'earth'-principle (which is in the muladhara chakra) is the splendorous living Deity. By deep concentration, the embodiment of the practitioner is transformed into the form of the Deity in the conscious field. Similarly, the splendorous living Deity is in the 'water'-principle (in the swadhishthana), in the 'fire'-principle (in the manipura), in the 'air'-principle (in the anahata), in the 'void'-(akasha)-principle (in the wishuddha), in the 'moon' (that is, the indu chakra), in the 'lightning' (that is, the nirwana chakra), and in the 'truth' (that is, the sahasrara), and the realization of the Deity and the absorption into it is possible by deep concentration and by the control of the specific principle lying in the chakra through concentration (—Brihadaran-yakopanishad, 2.5.1,2,3,4,7,8,10,12).

It has been stated: 'There is the hridaya which is like the bud of a lotus, and its face is turned downwards. ... In relation to it lies an infinitesimal void (sukshma sushira) where is situated the whole. Within that lies the great fire (mahan agni) with its all-pervading flame and its power on every side. ... Its rays are emitted upwards, downwards and obliquely. ... Within it is a very minute fire-flame (wahni-shikha) which shines like lightning in the blue sky, and is lightly yellow and subtle. Within this flame is the Supreme Spirit. He is Brahma, Shiwa, Hari, Indra; he is the imperishable Supreme God' (—Narayanopanishad, 50–52). Here the chakra system has been explained in an ancient technical manner. The hridaya is like a lotus, that is, it is the hrit lotus or chakra, which ordinarily lies with its head downwards. The chakra turns upwards during concentration. There is a void in relation to the hrit lotus. The void is subtle, that is, it does not exist in a material sense. Here the whole chakra system is situated. This void is the sushumna within which lie the chakras, including the hrit chakra. Within sushumna, at its lower end, is the great fire, that is the fiery triangle lying inside the muladhara. Within this fire sphere lies the extremely rarefied fire-flame, that is, Kundalini who is lightning-like splendorous and slightly yellowish and subtle. When Kundalini is aroused, the fiery sphere becomes illuminated and emits rays on all sides. Within Kundalini the Supreme Spirit is revealed. First, Kundalini is aroused in the muladhara and then conducted to the hrit chakra, where concentration on Kundalini is done. When concentration becomes very deep a divine form as Brahma, Shiwa or Hari is revealed. When Kundalini is brought to the sahasrara, deep concentration is transformed into superconscious concentration. The Supreme Spirit is realized in superconscious concentration in Kundalini. Finally, Kundalini is absorbed into Supreme Spirit and what remains is only He in a state of Supreme concentration.

In the first five chakras, are situated five mahabhuta-tanmatra-principles. Each has its own colour and sphere. They are described here: 'The "earth"-principle is yellow in colour, and its sphere is quadrangular in shape and with the emblem of wajra (thunderbolt) .... The "water"-principle is white, and its region is crescent-shaped and white .... The "fire"-principle is shining vermilion in colour .... The "air"-principle is smoke-coloured, and its region is shaped like a sacrificial altar where is strong Deity Maruta .... The "void" (akasha)-principle is shining black in colour' (—Trishikhi-brahmanopanishad, Mantra Section, 135–41).

The chakras are mentioned in connection with a Waidika process of pratyahara (sense-withdrawal) in which prana is held by breath-suspension in conjunction with concentration. It has been stated: 'The holding should be done in ... muladhara, nabhikanda (that is, manipura), hrit, neck region (wishuddha), talu (talu or lalana chakra), space between the eyebrows (that is, ajña), lalata (forehead; that is, manas and indu chakras), and murdhan (head; that is, nirwana chakra)' (—Darshanopanishad, 7. 11–12).

The acquirement of the knowledge of the chakras is absolutely necessary. It has been stated: 'Having acquired the knowledge of the six chakras, the yoga-practitioner should reach into the regions of the chakras by breath-control. Thereafter, the pranic force should be conducted upward (through the sushumna) by breath-suspension. This yoga should be practised in conjunction with wayu (that is, pranayama), bindu (that is, mantra), chakras, and chitta (consciousness). (This practice leads to) samadhi (superconcentration) by which the yogis attain immortality' (—Yogashikhopanishad, 6. 74–75). By concentration combined with breath-control and mantra, Kundalini should be aroused in the muladhara and conducted to the various chakras, and, finally, to the sahasrara where samadhi is attained.

Kundalini is the Supreme Power in her highest spiritual aspect when she is one and the same with Supreme Spirit. But when she is coiled in the muladhara, prana manifests as wayu (force-motion) and operates in the mental and material fields. So it has been stated: 'The muladhara triangle (that is, the triangular region inside the muladhara) which is situated between the anus and the genitals (that is, yonisthana = perineum) is the place where Shiwa (Supreme Being) manifests himself in the form of bindu (that is, Sway-ambhu-linga which becomes reflected in consciousness in concentration). In this place (triangular region) lies Supreme Power as Kundalini (that is, in a coiled form). From Kundalini arises wayu, fire is kindled, appears bindu (divine form), nada (suprasound) becomes gross, and hangsah (in the form of respiration) and mind originate. The six chakras from the muladhara (to the ajña) are said to be the seats of Shakti (Power). The place above the throat (that is, above the ajña) and which ends in the head (that is, the region from the ajña to the nirwana chakra) is said to be the seat of Shambhu (shambhawa sthana)' (—Warahopanishad, 5.50–3).

About the importance of the muladhara chakra, it has been stated: 'Some say that the adhara (muladhara) lies in relation to the sushumna and the saraswati (nadi). The (knowledge of the) world arises from the adhara and it is also absorbed there. Therefore, one should seek shelter with all efforts at the feet of a guru (who alone can disclose it). When the adhara-shakti (-power, that is, Kundalini) is asleep (latent) the knowledge of the world arises by the sleep (unspirituality). When Kundali-power is aroused, the true knowledge of the three

157

worlds (that is, the whole chakra system) is attained. He who knows the adhara goes beyond darkness. ... The brightness of the adhara chakra is like the radiance of a cluster of lightning; if the guru is pleased, liberation is attained undoubtedly (that is, the lustre of the adhara is due to the arousing of Kundalini; if a disciple learns from his guru the method of rousing Kundalini and her conduction through the sushumna, and practises it successfully, he will attain samadhi and then liberation). ... By doing kumbhaka (breath-suspension) in the adhara (by special pranayamic process), one is able to make absorptive concentration in the hrit or sahasrara. The kumbhaka in the adhara causes the shaking of the body, makes the yogi dance, (that is, to levitate), and the universe (in its subtle form) is seen there. The support of all creative principles is the adhara (because they are supported when Kundalini remains coiled in the adhara); in the adhara are all deities, all the Wedas. Hence one should choose the adhara (for one's spiritual practice).

'In the posterior aspect of the adhara (that is, the sushumna), there is a union of the three streams (triweni-sangama) (that is, the union of the ida, pingala and sushumna nadis). By bathing (performing deep internal purification) and drinking (assimilating life-substance by pranayama) there, man becomes free from all sins. In the adhara, there is Pashchima-linga (that is, Swayambhu-linga) where lies the entrance. As soon as it is opened (by rousing Kundalini), one becomes liberated from worldliness. In the posterior aspect of the adhara (that is, in the sushumna), if the ida (chandra) and pingala (surya) are controlled (that is, kumbhaka is done), there appears wishwesha (Shiwa, Supreme Being) (in a divine form); the yogi is absorbed into Brahman by concentration on him.

'In the posterior aspect of the adhara, is the living divine form (Deity Brahma). The prana-force enters into the sushumna when the ida-pingala flows are controlled (by kumbhaka). Then the six chakras are pierced (by Kundalini who then) enters the brahmarandhra (that is, nirwana chakra) and then comes out of it and attains the highest position (that is, reaches the sahasrara)' (—Yogashikhopanishad, 6. 22–34).

The muladhara is the most important chakra from the viewpoint of spiritual practice. In this centre lies Kundalini in her coiled form, and it is here she should be aroused. This is why Kundalini is called the adhara-power. When Kundalini is roused, her splendour makes the muladhara bright. Kundalini lies coiled around Pashchima-linga. When she is aroused, the entrance into the sushumna opens and she passes through the sushumna, piercing all the chakras situated there, and reaches the sahasrara. The process of rousing Kundalini consists of breath-suspension combined with mantra, concentration and certain internal control. The passing of Kundalini through the sushumna causes absorptive concentration which develops into samadhi (superconcentration) when Kundalini reaches the sahasrara.

About the passing through the sushumna of the roused Kundalini, it has been said: 'Then breaking through the Brahma-knot (Brahmagranthi) arising from primary energy-principle (rajas guna), Kundalini at once radiates into the sushumna-mouth (-wadana) (that is, the junction between the muladhara and sushumna) like a flash of lightning. Then Kundalini goes upward into the Wishnu-knot (Wishnugranthi) lying in the hrit (chakra; according to the Tantras, Wishnu-knot lies in the anahata chakra which is above but close to the hrit chakra). Then (piercing the Wishnu-knot) Kundalini goes still higher into the Rudra-knot (Rudragranthi) in the eyebrow-space (ajña chakra), and, breaking through it, reaches the moon-region (shitangshumandala); this is what is called anahata chakra having 16 petals (the moon-region has also been called the indu chakra—Yogakundalyupanishad, 1.71; the Tantrika term for the moon-region is the soma chakra which has also 16 petals; indu and soma are synonyms; they denote moon)' (—Yogakundalyupanishad, 1. 67–9). Finally, Kundalini reaches the sahasrara chakra. It has been stated: 'Absorbing into her the eight creative principles arising from primus (prakriti), Kundali reaches the (highest) region (that is, the sahasrara) where she is in contact with Shiwa; then she becomes united with and absorbed into Shiwa' (—ibid., 1. 74). The roused Kundalini absorbs various creative principles located in the chakras when passing through them. When she reaches the sahasrara, Kundalini alone shines forth in superconscious concentration. Thereafter, Kundalini becomes one and the same with Parama Shiwa in non-mens concentration.

About the six chakras, it has been stated: 'The muladhara, swadhishthana, the third manipura, anahata, wishuddhi and the sixth ajña are the six chakras. The adhara is in the anal region; the swadhishthana in the genital region; the manipura in the navel region; the anahata in the heart region; the wishuddhi in the throat region; the ajña chakra in the head' (—Yogakundalyupanishad, 3. 9–11).

Systems of the Chakras

There are several Waidika chakra systems. We shall now deal with these.

1 Chakra system as explained by Narayana

In the perineal region (adhara) is the brahma chakra (that is, the muladhara chakra). There is a triangle (trirawritta, or trirawarta, that is, turned round three times; the Tantrika term is traipura kona) which is a triangular region in the pericarp (of this chakra) where lies Shakti (Power, that is Kundali-power) which is in the form of lightning. Concentration should be done on this form. There (in the triangle) is the seat of kama (an aspect of apana-force) in the form (of the mantra 'Kling') which grants all desires.

The second is the swadhishthana chakra which has six petals. Inside the (pericarp of the) chakra is the linga (a divine form for concentration and worship) of the colour of a new leaf. Concentration should be done on this linga. Here is the place of udyana (that is, for the practice of lower uddiyanabandha control) which develops adamantine suction-power.

The third is the nabhi chakra (manipura chakra). Inside the pericarp is Kundalini who

is lustrous like ten-million newly-risen suns (that is, shining deep red) and splendorous like lightning and is in five coils like a coiled serpent. Concentration should be done on Kundalini (as deep red and very bright). The aroused Power (samarthya-shakti) (that is, Kundalini-power aroused by concentration) who is in the manipura chakra bestows all success.

The next is the hridaya chakra (that is, anahata chakra). It has eight petals and it lies with its face down. Inside (the pericarp) of this chakra is the shining linga-form (or lustrous jiwatman like the flame of a lamp). Concentration should be done on it. It is called hangsakala (that is, when jiwatman—embodied spirit, being purified, manifests its spiritual power), it is all love, and it exhibits the great power of control.

The next is the kantha chakra which is four fingers in size. On the left side of it stands the ida—the moon-nadi, and on the right side of it stands the pingala—the sun-nadi. Inside the (pericarp) of the chakra is the white sushumna on which one should concentrate. The anahata gives success to one who knows this. N.B.—Here the kantha chakra has been named the anahata chakra. But it is actually the wishuddha chakra.

The next is the talu chakra. It is situated (externally) in the uvular region (that is, pertaining to the uvula palatina), in the oral cavity, being supported by the front teeth. This chakra has twelve petals. The amrita (deathless substance) stream is flowing in this centre. Here, void-concentration should be done. This causes absorption of sense-consciousness (chitta). N.B.—The talu chakra has in the Tantras also been termed lalana chakra.

The seventh is the bhru chakra (ajña chakra). It is a subtle chakra. Here, concentration should be done on the knowledge-light as a still flame of the lamp (in a place without wind). This chakra is the root of the cranial centres (kapalakanda). Here, in the ajña chakra, the superpower of word-effectuality (waksiddhi) is attained.

The next chakra is the brahmarandhra which is also called the nirwana chakra. Here concentration should be done on Shiwa (Supreme Being) as a smoke-coloured flame (dhumrashikhakara). Here also is the seat of Power in form (jalandharapitha), granting liberation. Thus the parabrahma chakra.

The ninth is the akasha chakra (the sahasrara). Here is a sixteen-petalled lotus (chakra) with its face upwards. Inside the pericarp of this lotus is a triangular shaped region within which lies the raised Power (Urdhwashakti, that is, Kundali-power raised from the muladhara to this chakra) in relation to which is supreme void (parashunya). Concentration should be made here (as Kundalini united with Parama Shiwa). The Supreme void is the seat of Supreme Being (Purnagiripitha). All desires are spiritualized here (—Soubhagyalakshmyupanishad, 3. 1–9).

2 Chakra System as Exposed in the Yogachudamanyupanishad

The adhara (the muladhara chakra) has four petals; the swadhishthana has six petals; in the navel is the ten-petalled lotus (that is, the manipura); hridaya (that is, the lotus in the heart region named anahata) has twelve petals; what is known as the wishuddha has sixteen petals; in the space between the eyebrows is the dwidala (that is, the ajña which has two petals); in the great path of brahmarandhra (that is, where the line of conduction of brahmanadi, and consequently sushumna, ends) there is the lotus with 1000 petals (the sahasrara).

The first chakra is the adhara (muladhara), the second is the swadhishthana. Between the two (that is, the space between the anus and scrotum) is yonisthana (perineum), which is also called kamarupa and kama. The lotus situated in the anal region (that is, in the perineal region), having four petals (that is, the muladhara), contains within it (that is, inside the pericarp of the muladhara) what is said to be the yoni (triangle, a triangular-shaped region) which is also called kamakhya (because here lies the kama-germ-mantra 'Kling') which is worshipped by the yogis. In this triangle is the great linga (mahalinga), facing backwards (this linga has been termed in the Tantras Swayambhu-linga). (Around the great linga), lies (Kundalini) who shines like molten gold and is lightning-like splendorous; she is below the genitals (that is,

in the muladhara which is below the swadhishthana which is in the genital region). The supremely splendorous Light (Kundalini) is 'seen' in samadhi as infinite and all-pervading. When she is 'seen' in mahayoga (asamprajñata samadhi—non-mens concentration) (as Mahakundalini—Supreme Kundalini), the respiratory movements stop (that is, kewala kumbhaka is attained). In the navel region, there is the gem-like chakra (that is, the manipura chakra); he who knows it is a real yogi. Here is a triangle which is the region of 'fire'.

The word 'swa' denotes prana (prana-force); as it is the seat of prana, so it is called swadhishthana; and as it is the seat of sex-force, so it is also called the medhra (chakra—the genital centre). As a gem is stitched by a thread, so the chakra is strung by the sushumna; this is why the chakra situated in the navel region is known as manipuraka. Until the embodied being realizes the spiritual truth in the great chakra with twelve petals (the anahata chakra), which is beyond white and black actions he is not free from mundaneness. (—Yogachudamanyupanishad, 4–14).

Summary
The first chakra is the adhara (muladhara) which is situated in the perineal region. It has four petals. Inside the pericarp of the chakra is a triangle, also called kamakhya. Inside the triangle is the great linga, facing backwards, around which lies splendorous Kundalini who is 'seen' in superconcentration. In mahayoga (non-mens concentration), she is realized (as Supreme Kundalini).

The second chakra is the swadhishthana, (situated in the genital region), which has six petals. It is called swadhishthana, because it is the seat of 'swa' to mean prana (-force). It is also called the medhra (chakra—the genital centre), because it is also the seat of sex-force.

The third is the manipuraka. It is situated in the navel region and has ten petals. It is strung in the sushumna like a gem stitched by a thread, so this gem-like chakra is called the manipura. Inside the pericarp of the chakra is a triangle which is the seat of 'fire'.

The fourth is the twelve-petalled chakra

(anahata) where lies the embodied being. The fifth chakra is the wishuddha having sixteen petals. The sixth chakra, situated in the space between the eyebrows, is dwidala (that is, the lotus with two petals, called ajña). Then the thousand-petalled chakra (sahasrara) lying beyond brahmarandhra.

3 Chakra System as Exposed by Maheswara

The muladhara is situated in the space between the anus and genitals (that is, the perineum). There is a triangle (inside the pericarp of the chakra). Here lies the Supreme Power as Kundalini. Here is the seat of what is called kamarupa (that is, the power in the form of the mantra 'Kling'), which makes desires fruitful.

The swadhishthana chakra is situated in the genital region. It has six petals.

The manipura chakra is situated in the navel region. It has ten petals. The great chakra anahata is situated in the heart region and it has twelve petals. Here is the seat of what is known as Purnagiri (Supreme Being).

The chakra situated in the throat region is called wishuddha which has sixteen petals. Here is the seat of jalandhara (power to control breath by chin-lock). In the space between the eyebrows is an excellent chakra called ajña with two petals. Here is the great seat of what is known as udyana (udana-force control).

The 'earth' region is quadrangular, and the presiding Deity is Brahma. The 'water' region is half-moon-shaped and its presiding Deity is Wishnu. The 'fire' region is triangular, and its presiding Deity is Rudra. The region of 'air' is hexagonal, and its presiding Deity is Ishwara or Sangkarsha. The region of 'void' (akasha) is circular, and its presiding Deity is Sadashiwa, or Narayana. In the space between the eyebrows (in relation to and above the ajña) is the manas mandala (chakra) in the nada form. Here (that is, above the manas chakra) is the shambhawa sthana (chakra) (that is, the indu chakra). All these chakras in the body are in the form of power. (—Yogashikhopanishad, 1. 168–78; 5. 5–16).

Summary

Muladhara. The muladhara chakra is situated in the perineal region. It has four petals. Inside the pericarp is the quadrangular 'earth' region. Brahma is the presiding Deity of the chakra, residing in the square region. In the pericarp, there is also a triangle where Kundalini resides. Here is also the seat of kamarupa (kama-power in the mantra-form 'Kling').

Swadhishthana. The swadhishthana chakra is situated in the genital region. It has six petals. Inside the pericarp of this chakra is the semilunar 'water' region. The presiding Deity is Wishnu.

Manipuraka. The manipuraka chakra is situated in the navel region. It has ten petals. The triangular 'fire'-region is in the pericarp. The presiding Deity is Rudra.

Anahata. The anahata chakra is situated in the heart region. It has twelve petals. The hexagonal 'air' region is in the pericarp. The presiding Deity is Ishwara, or Sangkarsha. This chakra is the seat of Purnagiri (Supreme Being).

Wishuddha. The wishuddha chakra is situated in the throat region. It has sixteen petals. There is the circular 'void' (akasha) region in the pericarp. The presiding Deity is Sadashiwa, or Narayana. Here is the seat of jalandhara (the location for executing the chin-lock in breath-suspension).

Ajña. The ajña chakra is situated in the space between the eyebrows. It has two petals. Here, that is, in relation to and just above the ajña is the manas mandala (chakra) which is in the form of nada. The centre of udyana (udana-force control) is also here. Above this is the shambhawasthana (the indu chakra).

4 Chakra System as Explained in the Yogarajopanishad

The first is the brahma chakra where lies (in the pericarp) a triangle. In the apana (-force, which is situated in the triangle) is the germ-mantra (mulakanda) of kama form (that is 'Kling'). That (the triangle) is the place of fire (wahni-kunda) where lies Kundalini in three coils (trirawritta). One should concentrate on Kundalini who is Divine Light and living power.

The second is the swadhi*shth*ana chakra. Inside the (pericarp of the) chakra is the linga, facing backwards, and in shape and colour like a new leaf. There is also the seat of udr*iya*na (u*ddiya*nabandha) where concentration on it (linga) (along with u*ddiya*na) develops the great power of contraction-control.

The third is the nabhi chakra (that is, the ma*ni*pura chakra situated in the navel region). In this chakra, concentration should be done on Madhya-shakti (the roused and conducted Kun*dali*-power) who is in five-coils and as bright as lightning. It will give all success.

The fourth chakra (anahata) is in the heart region and lies with its face downwards. One should concentrate with great efforts on the hangsah (ji*w*atman—embodied being) in the form of (still) light.

The fifth is the ka*n*tha (throat) chakra (that is, the wishuddha chakra). There the i*d*a is on the left side and the pi*ng*ala on the right side (of the chakra), and the su*sh*um*n*a is in the middle. There, concentration on the bright Light gives success.

The sixth is the taluka chakra (talu chakra). It is in the region of the uvula. Here absorptive concentration in the void gives liberation.

The seventh is the bhru chakra (that is, ajña chakra). Here is the seat of bindu (bindu-sthan*a*). Liberation is attained by concentration on the circular Light in this centre.

The eighth is the brahma*ra*ndhra (chakra; that is, nirwa*n*a chakra). It is indicative of final liberation (nirwa*n*a). Liberation is attained by concentration on the subtle smoky light. Here. is the jala*n*dhara (breath-power in chin-lock); and the absorptive concentration in this chakra causes liberation.

The ninth is the wyoma chakra (sahasrar*a*), with which is connected (as its part) a chakra with sixteen petals. Inside it (wyoma chakra) is concealed what is known as Supreme Power-Consciousness. Here is the seat of P*u*rnagiri (Supreme Being). In this seat, concentration on Sh*a*kti (Ku*nd*ali-power) causes liberation.

Concentration should be done on these nine chakras stage by stage. Then one will attain success and liberation. (—Yog*a*rajopani*sha*d, 5–19).

Summary
1 Br*a*hma chakra (m*u*ladhara). In the pericarp of this chakra, is a triangle which is the fire-place. Inside the triangle lies the splendorous and living power Ku*nd*alini in three coils.

2 Swadhishthana chakra. Inside the pericarp of the chakra is the linga of the shape and colour of a new leaf, facing backwards. Here is the seat of udr*iya*na (that is, the practice of the lower aspect of u*ddiya*na control).

3 Nabhi chakra (ma*ni*pura). Inside the chakra lies lightning-like shining Ku*nd*alini as Madhya-shakti (power in the middle) in five coils.

4 Fourth chakra (anahata). Inside the chakra is the hangsah (ji*w*atman—embodied being) in the form of still light.

5 Ka*n*tha chakra (wishuddha). Inside the chakra is the bright Light.

6 Taluka chakra (talu). This chakra is situated in the uvular region. It is an important centre for absorptive concentration.

7 Bhru chakra (ajña). This chakra is the seat of bindu and of the circular Light.

8 Br*a*hmarandhra chakra (nirwa*n*a). In this chakra is the seat of jala*n*dhara and of the subtle smoky light bindu. It is a suitable centre for absorptive concentration.

9 Wyoma chakra (sahasrara). In this chakra is a sixteen-petalled chakra as a part of it. Inside the pericarp of the chakra is Supreme Power-Consciousness as Ku*nd*ali-power. Here is the seat of P*u*rnagiri (Supreme Being).

From the above fragmentary descriptions the W*a*idika chakra system has emerged.

W*a*idika Chakra System

1 M*u*ladhara chakra. The term 'm*u*ladhara' has been mentioned in the G*a*napatyupani*sha*d, 6; Darshanopanishad, 4.3; 7.7, 11; Mandala-brahma*n*opanishad, 1.2.6; Yogaku*nd*alyupani*sha*d, 3.9; Yogashikhopanishad, 1.168; 3.2; 5.5, 17; and W*a*rahopani*sha*d, 5.50, 53. The m*u*ladhara has been termed 'adhara' mentioned in the Yoga*ku*nd*alyupani*sha*d, 3.10; Yoga-chu*d*am*a*nyupanishad, 4, 6; and Yogashikhopa-

nishad, 6. 26–33; 'mulakanda', mentioned in the Yogakundalyupanishad, 1. 82; and 'brahma' (chakra) in the Soubhagyalakshmyupanishad, 3.1; and Yogarajopanishad, 5.

Description. The muladhara chakra is situated in the perineal region (intracoccygeal point). It has four petals. Inside the pericarp of the chakra is the quadrangular 'earth' region. The presiding Deity of the chakra is Brahma who is in the square region. In the pericarp, there is a triangle, called yoni. It is also called kama-khya. The triangle is the place of fire (and, consequently, it is red). Within the triangle is the seat of kama (desire), an aspect of apana-force, in the form of the germ-mantra 'Kling'. Inside the triangle, there is the great linga, facing backward, and around which lies lightning-like splendorous Kundalini in three coils, who is revealed in its true form in superconscious concentration, and as Supreme Kundalini in non-mens concentration (mahayoga).

2 Swadhishthana chakra. The term 'swadhi-shthana' has been mentioned in the Soubhagya-lakshmyupanishad, 3.2; Yogakundalyupanishad, 1. 84; 3.9, 10; Yogachudamanyupanishad, 4, 6, 11; Yogashikhopanishad, 1.172; 5.8; and Yogarajopanishad, 7. It is also termed 'medhra' (chakra), mentioned in the Yogachudamanyupa-nishad, 12.

Description. The swadhishthana chakra is situated in the genital region (intrasacral point). It has six petals. The semilunar 'water' region is inside the pericarp of the chakra. The presiding Deity of the chakra is Wishnu who is in the semilunar region. Here also lies the linga, facing backwards, of the form and colour of a new leaf. In this chakra is the seat of udyana (that is, a position for the practice of adamantine suction-power), which is also termed udriyana.

The term 'swadhishthana' is from the seat (adhishthana) of the prana (swa), that is, this chakra is the seat of wyana force.

3 Manipura chakra. The term 'manipura' has been mentioned in the Yogakundalyupanishad, 3.9, 11. The chakra is also termed 'manipuraka', mentioned in the Soubhagyalakshmyupanishad, 3.3; Yogachudamanyupanishad, 13; Yoga-shikhopanishad, 1.172; 5.9; and 'nabhi' chakra, mentioned in the Soubhagyalakshmyupanishad,

3.3; Brahmawidyopanishad, 68; and Yoga-rajopanishad, 9. It is indirectly mentioned in the Brahmopanishad, 1; Parabrahmopanishad, 5; Darshanopanishad, 7.12; and Yogachudam-anyupanishad, 5.

Description. The manipura chakra is situated in the navel region (intralumbo-vertebral point). It has ten petals. In its pericarp, there is the triangular 'fire' region. The presiding Deity of this chakra is Rudra who resides in the triangular region. Here also lies lightning-like splendorous Kundalini in five coils as Madhya-shakti (Kundali-power, roused from the mula-dhara and conducted into the manipura).

4 Hrit-pundarika (hrit chakra). The term 'hrit-pundarika' has been mentioned in the Trishikhibrahmanopanishad, Mantra Section, 156; and Maitreyyupanishad, 1.12. It has also been called 'padmakoshapratikashahridaya' (lot-us-bud-like hridaya, that is, the hridaya or hrit chakra) in the Mahopanishad, 1.12; and Narayan-opanishad, 50.

5 Anahata chakra. The term 'anahata' has been mentioned in the Yogakundalyupanishad, 3.10, 11; and Yogashikhopanishad, 1. 173; 5.9. It has also been termed 'hridaya' chakra (because it is situated in the heart region), mentioned in the Soubhagyalakshmyupanishad, 3.4; and Yogachudamanyupanishad, 5; and 'dwadashara' chakra (twelve-petalled lotus) in the Yogachudamanyupanishad, 13; and the 'fourth' chakra in the heart region in the Yogarajopanishad, 10. It has been indirectly mentioned in the Parabrahmopanishad, 5; Brahmopanishad, 1; and Darshanopanishad, 7.12.

Description. The anahata chakra is situated in the heart region (intrathoracispinal point). It has twelve petals. In the pericarp, there is the hexagonal 'air' region. Ishwara or Sangkarsha is the presiding Deity, residing in the 'air' region. Inside the chakra is the hangsah (em-bodied being) in the form of still light.

6 Wishuddha chakra. The term 'wishuddha' has been mentioned in the Yogachudamanyupa-nishad, 5; and Yogashikhopanishad, 5.10. It has also been termed 'wishuddhi', mentioned in the Yogakundalyupanishad, 3.10, 11; and Yogashikhopanishad, 1.174; and 'kantha' (throat) chakra, mentioned in the Soubhagyalakshmyupa-

nishad, 3.5; and Yogarajopanishad, 12. It has been indirectly mentioned in the Brahmopanishad, 1; Parabrahmopanishad, 5; and Darshanopanishad, 7.12.

Description. The wishuddha chakra is situated in the region of the throat (intracervicospinal point). It has sixteen petals. In the pericarp of the chakra is the circular 'void' (akasha) region in which is the presiding Deity Sadashiwa, or Narayana. Here is the seat of jalandhara (a postion for the execution of chin-lock).

7 Talu chakra. The term 'talu' has been mentioned in the Soubhagyalakshmyupanishad, 3.6. It has also been termed 'taluka' chakra in the Yogarajopanishad, 13. It has been indirectly mentioned in the Darshanopanishad, 7.12.

Description. The talu chakra is situated in the uvular region. It has twelve petals. It is a centre where amrita (deathless substance) flows. Here is the void for the practice of concentration.

8 Ajña chakra. The term 'ajna' has been mentioned in the Yogakundalyupanishad, 3.10, 11; Yogashikhopanishad, 1.175; 5.11; and Soubhagyalakshmyupanishad, 3.7. This chakra has also been termed 'bhru' chakra, mentioned in the Soubhagyalakshmyupanishad, 3.7; and Yogarajopanishad, 15; and 'bhruyugamadhyabila' in the Mandalabrahmanopanishad, 1.3.3; and 'baindawa-sthana' (-chakra) in the Yogakundalyupanishad, 3.8; and 'dwidala' in the Yogachudamanyupanishad, 5. It has been indirectly mentioned in the Darshanopanishad, 7.12.

Description. The ajña chakra is situated in the space between the eyebrows (intracerebral point). It has two petals. Here is the knowledge-light as a still flame of the lamp for concentration. It is the centre for the control of udana-force. And here also lies the seat of bindu (bindu-sthana). This chakra is the root of other cranial chakras.

In relation to, and just above, the ajña is the manas mandala (manas chakra). Connected with the ajña (and above the manas chakra) is the shambhawa-sthana (-chakra) (that is, the indu chakra).

9 Indu chakra. The word 'indu' means moon. The Tantrika term for this chakra is soma (moon) chakra. The term 'indu' is mentioned in the Yogakundalyupanishad, 1.71. It has also been termed 'shitangshu (moon)-mandala' (chakra) and anahata chakra mentioned in the Yogakundalyupanishad, 1.69; and 'shambhawa-sthana' (-chakra) in the Yogashikhopanishad, 5.16. It has indirectly been mentioned in the Darshanopanishad, 7.12; and Yogashikhopanishad, 6.48, 49.

Description. The shitangshu-mandala (-chakra), or indu chakra is situated in the forehead (lalata) region (above the manas chakra). It has sixteen petals. Here lies the deathless substance (amrita).

10 Nirwana chakra. The term 'nirwana' has been mentioned in the Soubhagyalakshmyupanishad, 3.8. It has also been termed 'brahma-randhra' (chakra), mentioned in the Yogakundalyupanishad, 1.83; and Soubhagyalakshmyupanishad, 3.8; and Yogarajopanishad, 16; and 'parabrahma' chakra, mentioned in the Soubhagyalakshmyupanishad, 3.8; and 'brahma-randhra mahasthana' (the great brahmarandhra chakra) in the Yogashikhopanishad, 6.47. It is indirectly mentioned in the Darshanopanishad, 7.12.

Description. The nirwana chakra is situated at the end point of the sushumna called the brahmarandhra. This is why it is also called brahmarandhra chakra. The petals are not mentioned. According to the Tantras, the nirwana chakra has 100 petals. Here lies the subtle smoky divine light suitable for concentration. Here is the seat of jalandhara (Power developed in breath-suspension with chin-lock). In this centre, Supreme Consciousness-Power resides.

11 Sahasrara chakra. The term 'sahasrara' has been mentioned in the Mandalabrahmanopanishad, 1.4.1. The other terms for the sahasrara are: 'sahasradala' (the chakra having 1000 petals), mentioned in the Yogachudamanyupanishad, 6; 'sahasrakamala' (the lotus or chakra with 1000 petals), mentioned in the Yogakundalyupanishad, 1.86; 'akasha chakra' (the chakra in the void), mentioned in the Soubhagyalakshmyupanishad, 3.9; 'wyoma chakra' (the chakra in the void), mentioned in the Yogarajopanishad, 17; 'wyomambuja' (a lotus or chakra in the void), mentioned in the Yogashikhopanishad, 6. 48; 'Kapalasangputa' (the

chakra which covers the cranium) mentioned in the Yogashikhopanishad, 1.76; and 'sthana' (to mean literally a place, an abode, a state, but technically it denotes a chakra; here sthana means Shiwa-sthana—the abode of Shiwa, that is, the sahasrara), mentioned in the Yoga-kundalyupanishad, 1.74. This chakra has been mentioned indirectly in this manner: 'Sun—the Supreme Being—exists with a thousand rays of light (sahasrarashmi) and in a hundred ways (shatadha)' (—Akshyupanishad, ch. 1, p. 1), that is, Parama Shiwa—Supreme Consciousness—being united with Kundalini is splendorous in the sahasrara, and he is also in a hundred-fold in the nirwana chakra.

Description. The sahasrara is situated in the region of void, that is, at the extracranial or extracerebral point. It has 1000 petals. There is a chakra with sixteen petals with its face upwards, under the sahasrara and forming a part of it. Inside the pericarp of the sahasrara is a triangle where lies the raised Supreme Power-Consciousness (Kundali-power). In relation to the Power lies supreme void (parashunya) where the seat of Supreme Being (Purnagiri) is.

The above description of the chakras indicates the incompleteness of the Waidika chakra system. It is mainly due to two factors: first, parts of the Waidika documents were lost during the course of time, and, consequently, the extant part is incomplete. Second, the Waidika chakra system is now less used by the laya-yogis in their spiritual practice. The Tantrika system has now been widely adopted.

CHAPTER 9
The Tantrika System of Chakras

The Tantrika chakra system is completer than the Waidika chakra system. The Tantrika system is based on the Tantras which are extant. It may not be quite complete, as a very large number of Tantras are lost. But from the viewpoint of spiritual practice, it is complete. Now, most of the layayogis have followed the Tantrika system. Many great layayoga masters have adopted it, and the Tantrika gurus teach it to their disciples directly and thoroughly.

Tantrika Nadi-system

Nadis constitute the nadi-system. It is said that the nadis are innumerous (—Wishwasaratantra, ch. 1, p. 6; Sharadatilaka, 1.43). Of these, the important nadis are numbered at 35,000,000 (—Kankalamalinitantra, ch. 2, p. 4; Gandharwatantra, ch. 5, p. 27; Todalatantra, ch. 8, p. 15; Shaktanandatarangini, 4.7; and Goutamiyatantra, 34.35). Of these, the more important nadis are 350,000 in number (—Shiwasanghita, 2.13), and still more important are 72,000 (—Sammohanatantra, Part 2, ch. 2, p. 1; Jñanasankalinitantra, verse 77; Niruttaratantra, ch. 4, p. 7; Shaktanandatarangini, 1.7), and of these are 70,000 (—Koulawalitantra, ch. 22, p. 79), and of these, the chief nadis are fourteen in number (—Sammohanatantra, Part 2, ch. 2, p. 1; Shiwasanghita, 2.13; and Tripurasarasamuchchaya, ch. 3, p.8). These fourteen nadis are: sushumna, ida, pingala, gandhari,

hastijihwa, kuhu, saraswati, pusha, shankhini, payaswini, waruni, alambusha, wishwodari and yashaswini (—Shiwasanghita, 2. 14–15).

Of these fourteen nadis, ten are more important; in fact, the ten nadis are considered the principals of all the nadis (—Kankalamalinitantra, ch. 2, p. 4; Niruttaratantra, ch. 4, p. 7; Goutamiyatantra, 34.35; Gandharwatantra, ch. 5, p. 27; Bhutashuddhitantra, ch. 6, p. 5; and Shaktanandatarangini, 4.7). The ten principal nadis are: ida, pingala, sushumna, gandhari, hastijihwa, pusha, yashaswini, alambusha, kuhu, and shangkhini (—Niruttaratantra, ch. 4, p. 7; and Shaktanandatarangini, 1.7). The gandhari flows in the region of the left eye, the hastijihwa in the right eye, the pusha in the right ear, the yashaswini in the left ear, the alambusha in the mouth, the kuhu in the genitals, and the shangkhini in the head (—Shaktanandatarangini, 1.7). The ida and pingala flow in the nostrils and the sushumna flows in the subtle path in the palatine region and up to the brahmarandhra (—Brahmasiddhantapaddhati MS).

Of the 10 principal nadis, three are the most important (—Kankalamalinitantra, ch. 2, p. 4; Gandharwatantra, ch. 5, p. 27; Bhutashuddhitantra, ch. 6, p. 5; Sammohanatantra, Part 2, ch. 2, p. 1; Tripurasarasamuchchaya, ch. 3, p. 8; Sharadatilakatantra, 25.29; Shaktanandatarangini, 4.7; Shiwasanghita, 2. 15; and Goutamiyatantra, 34.35). These three nadis are: ida, pingala and sushumna (—Tripurasarasamuchchaya, ch. 3, p. 8; and Shiwasanghita, 2.15). Of the three nadis again, one is the fundamental, and that is the sushumna

(—Kankalamalinitantra, ch. 2, p. 4; Gandharwa-tantra, ch. 5, p. 27; Tripurasarasamuchchaya, ch. 3, p. 8; Rudrayamala, Part 2, 25.51; Shiwa-sanghita, 2.16; and Goutamiyatantra, 34.36).

Nadis are of two kinds: gross or material, and subtle or non-material. The gross nadis are nerves, arteries, veins, capillaries, lymphatic vessels and other tubular organs of the body. The subtle or non-material nadis are called yoga-nadis (—Shiwapurana, 4.40.5). The word nadi is derived from 'nada' = bhrangsha, that is, falling down, running away; here, in a more technical sense, radiating. The word 'bhrangsha' is almost similar to the word 'bhresha' = motion. Kalicharana, the well-known commentator of Shatchakranirupana, a most authoritative work on the Tantrika chakra system, says, in explaining verse 2 of this work, that the word nadi is derived from nada = motion. Therefore, nadi is that which is motional or in motion; that is, whose nature is motion. The word 'wayu' has the same meaning. It is derived from wa = motion. That which is in constant motion is wayu. In a technical sense, wayu is the motional or active state of life-energy (prana), in which force-motions are exhibited. The principal force-motions are five, and they are termed prana-wayu, apana-wayu, samana-wayu, udana-wayu and wyana-wayu. The pranic wayus are in-separable from nadis.

It has been stated that the ten wayus—prana, apana, samana, udana, wyana, naga, kurma, krikara, dewadatta and dhananjaya, move in all the nadis (—Shandilyopanishad, 5.4.12; and also Warahopanishad, 5.31). As the nadis, termed yoga-nadis, are not material structures but subtle (—Shiwasanghita, 2.17), it should be interpreted in a technical manner. The nadis do not exist as tubules or wires, but are subtle lines of direction along which the wayus move. This means that the wayus which are constantly in motion are also nadis, as motion is associated with the lines of direction. It has been more clearly stated that the nadis are the prana-flows (pranawahini) (—Niruttaratantra, ch. 4, p. 7; Yogachudamanyupanishad, 16). In other words, the nadis are pranic force-radiation-lines, and their existence is inseparable from the existence of the pranic force-motions. The plexus-like arrangement of the nadis (nadimaya chakra) constitutes the power field (shakti-chakra) (—Niruttaratantra, ch. 4, p. 7). This is the nadi-system.

From the yoga viewpoint, the ida, pingala and sushumna are of great importance; and of the three, the sushumna is the highest. The sushumna is in the middle of the ida and pingala (—Todalatantra, ch. 2, p. 2; Niruttara-tantra, ch. 4, p. 7; Jñanasankalinitantra, verse 11; Tararahasya, ch. 1, p. 2). The ida is on the left side and pingala on the right side (—Niruttaratantra, ch. 4, p. 7; Gandharwa-tantra, ch. 5, p. 27; Tripurasarasamuchchaya, ch. 3, p. 8; Bhutashuddhitantra, ch. 6, p. 5; Sammohanatantra, part 2, ch. 2, p. 1–2); Wishwasaratantra, ch. 1, p. 6; Mundamalatantra, ch. 3, p. 5; Sharadatilakatantra, 25.30; Shaktan-andatarangini, 1.7). The positions of the ida and pingala have been more precisely stated here: outside the vertebral column are the ida and pingala, being on the left and the right, that is, the ida is on the left side of the spinal column, and the pingala on its right side (—Shatchakranirupana, verse 1). Also, on the left side of the vertebral column is the ida nadi, and on its right side is the pingala nadi (—Tararahasya, ch. 4, p. 22), and, outside the vertebral column, is the ida on its left, and the pingala on its right (—Koulawalitantra, ch. 22, p. 79).

The accurate position of the sushumna cannot be determined from the statement that it is in the middle of the ida and pingala. It has been stated: 'The principal nadi (sushumna) is in front of the vertebral column (merudandagre)' (—Kankalamalinitantra, ch. 2, p. 4). Here, the word 'agre' has been used, and it denotes 'in front of'. From this it can be assumed that the sushumna is outside and in front of the vertebral column. Apparently, this is supported by the following passage: 'O Shiwa, the ida nadi which is deathless substance of moon is on the left of the vertebral column, the sun-like pingala on its right side. Outside it (tadbahye) and between these two (tayormadhye) is the fire-like sushumna' (—Tantrachudamani quoted by Kalicharana in explaining verse 1 of Shat-chakranirupana). Kalicharana has rejected this statement on the ground that it contradicts verse 2. But 'tadbahye' can be interpreted as outside the ida and the pingala. In that case, it will mean that the sushumna is outside of and between the ida and pingala, not outside the vertebral column.

It has been stated: 'The sacred nadi sushumna which bestows all success is in front of the vertebral column (merupuratas)' (—Tararahasya, ch. 4, p. 22). The word puratas means in front of. It should be interpreted to mean that the sushumna is in the anterior part of the vertebral column. It has been stated: 'The sushumna, resting on the vertebral column (prishthawangshang samashritya), is between the ida and the pingala' (—Tripurasarasamuchchaya, ch. 3, p. 8); and 'The moon-sun-fire nadi (sushumna) rests on the vertebral column' (—Shiwasanghita, 2.17). Here, it should mean that the sushumna rests interiorly on the vertebral column. Raghawabhatta, the well-known commentator on the Sharadatilakatantra, has made this clear. The text says: 'The nadi sushumna, resting on the vertebral column (wangshamashrita), is between them (the ida and the pingala)' (—Sharadatilakatantra, 25.30). In explaining this verse, Raghawabhatta says: 'Wangsha means the spinal column, and ashrita denotes tadantargata = being in the interior of the spinal column', as it is said: 'She (sushumna) who is inside the void of the vertebral column (mundadharadanda), extending from the head to the adhara (muladhara).'

In commenting on the verse 'The nadi sushumna is in the middle . . . '(Shatchakranirupana, verse 1), Kalicharana says that 'in the middle' (madhye) means inside the void of the vertebral column. This is what Shatchakranirupana actually means, and that is proved by verse 2, in which it has been stated: 'Inside her (the nadi wajra) is chitrini . . . who pierces all the chakras lying inside the vertebral column and appears luminous because of these lotuses which are strung on her' (—Shatchakranirupana, verse 2). The chakras which are inside the spinal column are strung on the chitrini, and the chitrini is inside the wajra, and the wajra is inside the sushumna. The sushumna, consequently, is inside the vertebral column, not outside it.

The exact position of the sushumna has been more clearly indicated in the following passages: 'The principal nadi (sushumna) which is in the form of moon-sun-fire is in the vertebral column (merudande)' (—Gandharwatantra, ch. 5, p. 27). Here, 'in the vertebral column' means within the vertebral column, not outside it. 'That nadi (sushumna) which is absolutely calm (that is, realizable only through concentration) and which gives liberation, is inside the vertebral column (merumadhyasthita)' (—Todalatantra, ch. 2, p. 2). Here, it is clearly stated that the sushumna is inside the vertebral column, not outside it. Also, 'That (nadi) which is inside the vertebral column (merumadhye) extending from the muladhara to the brahmarandhra, and is all knowledge and in the form of fire, is sushumna' (—Sammohanatantra, Part 2, ch. 2, p. 2). Here also it is clearly said that the sushumna is inside the vertebral column. 'She who is inside the vertebral column (merumadhye) is the multiform sushumna' (—Rudrayamala, Part 2, 27.52). 'Sushumna is inside (madhyaga = being inside) the winadanda termed prishthawangsha (that is, the vertebral column)' (—Tantrarajatantra, 27.35). 'She (sushumna) is inside the vertebral column (prishthamadhyagata = being inside the spinal column), extending to the head' (—Koulawalitantra, ch. 22, p. 79). 'The principal (nadi sushumna) who is moon-sun-fire is inside the vertebral column (merudandantar = being inside the vertebral column), (—Shaktanandatarangini, 4.7). From all this we can come to the definite conclusion that the sushumna is inside the vertebral column.

It has been stated 'What is called wichitra (the nadi chitra or chitrini) . . . is inside her (sushumna)' (—Gandharwatantra, ch. 5, p. 27). 'That nadi which is inside the sushumna is the chitrini' (—Sammohanatantra, Part 2, ch. 2, p. 2). Further in Sharadatilakatantra, 25.34; Tripurasarasamuchchaya, ch. 3, p. 8; and Shaktanandatarangini, 4.8. These passages indicate that the chitrini is inside the sushumna, but that does not mean that the chitrini is next to the sushumna as the second nadi within it. Inside the sushumna is the nadi wajra, and inside the wajra is chitrini. So it has been stated: 'Inside the sushumna is the bright nadika (nadi) which is called wajra, and in it (within the wajra) is the subtle chitrini; and Kundali passes through it' (—Rudrayamala, Part 2, 25. 51–52). And, 'Inside the sushumna is the wajra nadi, and inside it (wajra) is the highest nadi called chitra (chitrini); and within it lies the supreme Kundali' (—Tantrarajatantra, 27.44). Also in Shatchakranirupana, verses 1, 2; Tararahasya, ch. 4, p. 22; Koulawalitantra, ch. 22, p. 79–80).

It has been stated: 'The brahma nadi is inside the chitrini' (—Todalatantra, ch. 8, p. 15). Moreover, 'Inside her (chitrini) is the brahma nadi, which extends from the oral orifice of Hara (here, Swayambhu-linga) to a point beyond which Adidewa (Paramashiwa in sahasrara) is situated' (—Shatchakranirupana, verse 2). And in Tararahasya, ch. 1, p. 2; ch. 4, p. 22; Koulawalitantra, ch. 22, p. 80; Shaktanandatarangini, 4.8. 'The brahma nadi has also been termed brahmarandhra' (—Shiwasanghita, 2.18). Further 'The supremely subtle brahmarandhra lies in her (chitrini)' (—Sammohanatantra, Part 2, ch. 2, p. 2, and in Sharadatilakatantra, 25.32. And 'Inside it (chitra nadi = chitrini nadi) is the exceedingly subtle brahmarandhra' (—Tripurasarasamuchchaya, ch. 3, p. 8).

According to some authorities, the brahmarandhra is within the brahma nadi. It has been stated: 'The brahmarandhra, which extends from the mouth of Hara (that is, the orifice of Swayambhu-linga in the muladhara) to Sadashiwa (that is, to the point beyond which lies the sahasrara in which lies Sadashiwa), is within it (brahma nadi)' (—Koulawalitantra, ch. 22, p. 80). Also in Shaktanandatarangini, 4.8.

There are other authorities who have not mentioned the brahma nadi or the brahmarandhra, but who speak about the movement of Kundalini through the chitrini. It has been stated: 'There lies the subtle chitrini through which Kundali moves' (—Rudrayamala Part 2, 25.52). Furthermore, 'The supreme Kundali is within it (chitra)' (—Tantrarajatantra, 27.44). This means that in the innermost part of the chitrini-power-radiation there is a void where there is no radiation. This inmost void has been termed brahma nadi, or brahmarandhra. The word randhra here denotes the vacuity deepest within. It is this void through which Kundalini,

who is Shabdabrahman, passes, or, it can be said that it is this void-path which leads to the sahasrara, the abode of Shiwa or Brahman. When it is said that the brahmarandhra is within the brahma nadi, it means that the immediate, outer aspect of the void is the brahma nadi, that is, the brahma nadi contains this innermost void termed brahmarandhra. The chitrini-power-radiation remains outside the brahma nadi. When the brahma or the brahmarandhra is not mentioned, it simply denotes that the inmost void is part of the chitrini.

Kalicharana (in his commentary on verse 2, Shatchakranirupana) says that the brahma nadi is the course along which Kundalini, who is in the nature of Shabdabrahman, moves to Paramashiwa; it is the void aspect within the chitrini nadi, and there is no other nadi inside the chitrini. The brahma nadi is the brahma-void, and so it is called brahmarandhra, and through it Kundali passes.

The sushumna extends from the mula to the brahmarandhra. So it has been stated: 'The sushumna, which is in the nature of fire and is endowed with all power, lying inside the vertebral column, extends from the mula (root) to the brahmarandhra' (—Gandharwatantra, ch. 5, p. 27). Also in Bhutashuddhitantra, ch. 6, p. 5; Shaktanandatarangini, 4.8; Tantrarajatantra, 27.36. It has also been stated that the sushumna 'extends from the middle of the kanda (the root or the origin of the nadis) to the shiras (the head, or cerebrum)' (—Shatchakranirupana, verse 1).

It has been stated: 'In the region below the genitals and above the anus (that is, the perineum), is the kanda-mula (central root) of oval shape, from which 72000 nadis have originated' (—Sammohanatantra, Part 2, ch. 2, p. 1). The kanda-mula is the source, resembling a bulb of oval shape, from which all nadis arise. The kanda-mula is externally in the perineal region, but, interiorly, it is inside the coccyx (the terminal part of the vertebral column), in a position just below the muladhara. When it is said that the sushumna extends from the mula, it does not mean from the muladhara, but from the kanda-mula which is the source of all nadis. The sushumna arises from the middle or the central part of the kanda-mula, which is just below the muladhara chakra. It then passes through the whole spinal column and the head to reach the brahmarandhra. It (sushumna) goes to the terminal point of the brahmarandhra ('brahmarandhranta'), that is, to the end of brahmarandhra (—Bhutashuddhitantra, ch. 6, p. 5; Tantrarajatantra, 27.36).

The kanda-mula has also been termed kanda. It has been stated that between the genitals and the anus (that is, in the perineal region) lies kanda, which is circular; and the nadis proceed from this kanda (—Sharadatilakatantra, 25. 28–9). The kanda is not actually situated directly in the perineum, as a physical organ, but inside the coccyx which is related to the perineal region. The word kanda has also been used in the Shatchakranirupana, verse 1.

The wajra nadi is inside the sushumna. It has been stated that the wajra extends from the genitals to the head (—Shatchakranirupana, verse 1; Koulawalitantra, ch. 22, p. 80). Here the genitals mean the perineal region connected with the genitals. It actually indicates the kanda within the coccyx. The wajra arises within the sushumna at its starting point below the muladhara. It passes along with the sushumna to the head, that is, the end point of the brahmarandhra where the sushumna ends. Inside the wajra is the chitrini. The chitrini extends from the point from which the wajra starts, and ends where the sushumna and the wajra end, that is, at the terminal point of the brahmarandhra.

It has been stated: 'Above it (the ajña chakra) is the splendid sahasrara where lies the end point of the sushumna with its void-part in the talumula (the end point of the palatine region). From here the sushumna, which supports all nadis, goes downwards to the triangular region of the muladhara.... In the talusthana (palatine region) is a lotus (that is, guru chakra) which is (the part of) sahasrara. In the pericarp of this lotus (guru chakra) is a triangle, facing behind, where lies the end point of the sushumna with its inmost void. This void is termed brahmarandhra, which extends from here to the muladhara lotus. Inside the sushumna (or more accurately, wajra), and around the brahmarandhra, always lies the power of the sushumna. This power is the chitra (chitrini). It is also termed sushumna-Kundali. The brahmarandhra and others (the chakras) are to be thought of in the chitra-power' (—Shiwasanghita, 5. 161–5).

It is indicated here that the end point of the sushumna and, consequently, the end of the brahmarandhra is in the palatine region in its upper border beyond which is the guru chakra, which is the lower part of the sahasrara. We have noted that the brahmarandhra or the brahma nadi starts from the orifice of the Swayambhu-linga, situated in the muladhara, and extends to reach the proximity of the guru chakra. But the sushumna starts from the kanda, which is just below the muladhara. The wajra and the chitrini also arise from the starting point of the sushumna. The brahmarandhra arises from the orifice of the Swayambhu-linga. So the sushumna, and along with it the wajra and chitrini, starting from the point just below the muladhara, extend upwards. At the point of the orifice of Swayambhu-linga brahmarandhra emerges within the chitra, and then the sushumna, wajra, chitrini and brahmarandhra, all extend upward and reach the terminal point of the head which is immediately adjoining to, but not continuous with, the guru chakra.

Chitra (chitrini) is in the form of power. The chitra-power has been termed sushumna-Kundali. The term indicates that the chitra-power creates the brahmarandhra through which Kundalini passes. The brahmarandhra is actually the Kundali-power-motion. When there is no Kundali-power-motion, the brahmarandhra remains in a potential form. The nature of the chitra-power is that it concentrates and centralizes to form chakras throughout its course at certain points. The chakras are in the chitrini. It has been stated that all the chakras are strung on the chitrini (—Rudrayamala, Part 2, 25.52; Shadamnayatantra, 5. 111; Koulawalitantra, ch. 22, p. 80). The chakras are not external objects attached to the chitrini. The chitra-power concentrates and develops into a chakra. The development of the brahmarandhra within the chitrini, and of the chakras in it, are the two specific power phenomena of the chitrini.

The chitrini is lustrous and radiates life-energy; in it are the deities (—Sammohanatantra, Part 2, ch. 2, p. 2; Gandharwatantra, ch. 5, p. 27); the five bhuta-principles and five deities are there (in the lower five chakras) and it is luminous with five colours (—Koulawalitantra, ch. 22, p. 80; Tripurasarasamuchchaya, ch. 3, p. 8); it is pure, deathless and blissful; it is the divine path (—Shiwasanghita, 2. 19–20); it is moon-bright and contains all deities, and is realizable by the yogis (—Shaktanandatarangini, 4.8); it is extremely subtle and pure intelligence, and is revealed through yoga to the yogis (—Shatchakranirupana, verse 2). It is in the nature of sentience (sattwaguna), but the brahma nadi which is inside it, is in the nature of inertia (tamoguna), and the wajra, within which lies the chitrini, is in the form of energy (rajoguna) (—Niruttaratantra, ch. 4, p. 7). This means, that the energy-principle predominates in the wajra, and owing to its influence its power radiates also centrifugally. In the chitrini, the power-radiations are essentially centripetal, concentrated and imbued with consciousness, because of the influence on it of the sentience-principle. Because of this, the chitrini is only realizable in deep concentration. Moreover, the chakras which are in the chitrini can only be known by concentration-knowledge-light (sukshmajñana) (—Shadamnayatantra, 5. 204). In the brahmarandhra, the inertia principle predominates and, consequently, all power-radiations cease, and a void is created where nothing but Kundalini can penetrate. This is why this tamas void is called the brahma-void (brahmarandhra).

It has been stated that the sushumna is in the form of moon, sun and fire (—Kankalamalinitantra, ch. 2, p. 4; Gandharwatantra, ch. 5, p. 27; Shaktanandatarangini, 4.7; Shiwasanghita, 2.17). This means that the sushumna exerts the influence of its moon aspect on the ida and that of its sun aspect on the pingala, and the control influence on both as fire. In the sushumna the control factor predominates because its basic nature is fire which exhibits the power of control. So it has been said that the sushumna is in the nature of fire (—Gandharwatantra, ch. 5, p. 27; Sammohanatantra, Part 2, ch. 2, p. 2; Shaktanandatarangini, 4.8). In the sushumna, both the moon and the sun radiations occur (—Sam-

mohanatantra, Part 2, ch. 2, p. 2; Sharadatilakatantra, 25.34), and they are conveyed to the ida and pingala. The sushumna assumes different forms (—Rudrayamala, Part 2, 27.52), because of its connection with the ida and pingala. The sushumna is all knowledge (—Sammohanatantra, Part 2, ch. 2, p. 2) and all power (—Gandharwatantra, ch. 5, p. 27; Shaktanandatarangini, 4.8; Goutamiyatantra, 34.39). In sushumna, three primary attributes (gunas) are operating (—Niruttaratantra, ch. 4, p. 7). The sushumna is exceedingly subtle (—Bhutashuddhitantra, ch. 6, p. 5; Rudrayamala, Part 2, 25.51), and this is why it cannot be known sensorially, but is 'seen' by the yogis through deep concentration (—Goutamiyatantra, 34.39). The sushumna is fit for yoga (—Shiwasanghita, 2.16), as it is non-undulatory (—Todalatantra, ch. 2, p. 2). Concentration on moon-and-sun-form is done in the sushumna (—Wishwasaratantra, ch. 2, p. 11). The sushumna is spiralled from right to left (—Bhutashuddhitantra, ch. 6, p. 5).

The ida is in the form of moon (—Gandharwatantra, ch. 5, p. 27; Bhutashuddhitantra, ch. 6, p. 5; Sammohanatantra, Part 2, ch. 2, p. 1; Wishwasaratantra, ch. 1, p. 6; Mundamalatantra, ch. 3, p. 5; Rudrayamala, Part 2, 27.51; Goutamiyatantra, 34.36), so it causes the conservation of energy in the body and calmness in the mind. It is in the nature of power (—Gandharwatantra, ch. 5, p. 27; Sammohanatantra, Part 2, ch. 2, p. 2; Shaktanandatarangini, 4.7; Rudrayamala, Part 2, 271. 51; Goutamiyatantra, 34.37), because the power is conserved there. In ida lies the deathless substance (amrita) (—Gandharwatantra, ch. 5, p. 27; Sammohanatantra, Part 2, ch. 2, p. 2; Shaktanandatarangini, 4.7; Rudrayamala, Part 2, 271.51; Goutamiyatantra, 34.37), so it is suitable for concentration and all spiritual activities. Ida is white (in colour) (—Gandharwatantra, ch. 5, p. 27; Bhutashuddhitantra, ch. 6, p. 5; Sammohanatantra, Part 2, ch. 2, p. 1; Rudrayamala, Part 2, 27.51; Goutamiyatantra, 34.36).

The pingala is in the form of sun and masculine in character (—Gandharwatantra, ch. 5, p. 27; Bhutashuddhitantra, ch. 6, p. 5; Sammohanatantra, Part 2, ch. 2, p. 2; Shaktanandatarangini, 4.7; Goutamiyatantra, 34.37). It indicates that energy is released and consumed in the activities, and muscular activities requiring great strength and speed are maintained by the influence of the pingala. The pingala also causes diversification of the mind. This is due to the sun-power. To overcome it, it is necessary to practise concentration-on-sun (—Wishwasaratantra, ch. 2, p. 11). The pingala is like the pomegranate flower in colour (that is, vermilion) (—Gandharwatantra, ch. 5, p. 27; Sammohanatantra, Part 2, ch. 2, p. 2; Rudrayamala, Part 2, ch. 27,52; Goutamiyatantra, 34.38).

The ida and pingala are the pranic flows (—Niruttaratantra, ch. 4, p. 7). The ida starts from the left side and the pingala from the right side of kanda-mula, and are on the left and the right side of the triangle situated in the muladhara (—Shiwasanghita, 5.172) when passing upwards. The ida is placed on the left and the pingala on the right side of the vertebral column. They are shaped like bows (—Sammohanatantra, Part 2, ch. 2, p. 2). They arise from the kanda, pass by the left and the right side of the muladhara-triangle, and during their course they are like bows and reach the ajña chakra. They also take another position. When they go upwards, they encircle the chakras (from the muladhara to the ajña) by alternating from left to right and right to left (—Yamala quoted by Kalicharana in his commentary on Shatchakranirupana, verse 1). In the bow position, the ida and pingala radiate independently, and in the circling position, they are energized and harmonized by the sushumna.

Summary

There are innumerable nadis which form the nadi-system. These nadis are subtle and are called yoga-nadis. From the yoga-viewpoint the three nadis—ida, pingala and sushumna are the most important. The nadis are pranic force-motions creating subtle lines of direction. All the nadis originate from the kanda-mula—the central root, lying below the position of the muladhara chakra (within the coccyx). The sushumna arises from the central part of the kanda, and goes upward through the vertebral column and the head and ends at a point which is externally cerebral and immediately adjoins the extra-cerebral guru chakra. There is no direct continuation of the sushumna with the guru chakra, which is the lower stratum of the sahasrara.

The wajra develops within the sushumna as its second internal nadi, and extends from the beginning of the sushumna to the point where the sushumna ends. The chitrini develops within the wajra as the third interior nadi, extending from the beginning of the wajra and terminates at the point where the sushumna ends. Within the chitrini, there is a void termed brahma nadi, or brahmarandhra, extending from the orifice of Swayambhu-linga situated within the muladhara, to the point where the sushumna ends. In fact, the sushumna itself is a system consisting of the outermost sushumna, interior to it the wajra, and inside the wajra is the chitrini. The chitrini has a void inside, which is called brahma nadi or brahmarandhra.

The sushumna has three aspects: moon, sun and fire. It radiates its power to the ida and pingala by its moon and sun factors respectively. It exercises its control influence on the ida and the pingala by its fire aspect. The fire power is fully awakened by the control of pranic radiations and is centralized in the wajra. The chitra-power is termed sushumna-Kundali, because it makes the brahmarandhra fully patent when the Kundali-power passes through it. The chakras are in the chitrini. The brahma nadi is in the nature of inertia (tamas), the chitrini in the nature of sentience (sattwa), and the wajra in the nature of energy (rajas). The three primary attributes (gunas) operate in the sushumna.

The ida is in the form of moon and power and its radiations contain deathless-substance. It is white in colour. The pingala is in the form of the sun, and its colour is vermilion. The ida originates from the left side of the kanda-mula, and the pingala from the right side, remaining to left and right respectively of the sushumna which is between them in the central position of the kanda. Then sushumna extends upwards through the vertebral column, but the ida and the pingala leave the vertebral column and extend upward to reach the ajña, remaining on the left and the right respectively of the vertebral column. When they go upwards, they assume two positions: bow and circling. The sushumna, when going upwards, assumes a spiral form.

Tantrika Systems of Chakras

According to the type of spiritual practice and, consequently, the mode of concentration, there are some differences in the systems. Here is the exposition of the main thirteen Tantrika systems of chakras, of which six systems are expounded by Shiwa.

1 The chakra systems as expounded by Shiwa

System A
The first chakra is the adhara, having four petals of molten gold (that is red). On the petals are the four letters from wa to sa, (i.e. wa, sha, sha, sa). Inside the pericarp of the chakra is a beautiful triangle which is in the nature of the deities Brahma, Wishnu and Shiwa, and of will, consciousness and action. Swayambhu-linga with Kundalini coiled around him is in the triangle. There is the desire-germ (Kamabija, that is the mantra 'Kling') in the triangle, which is to be concentrated on. Here are the centres of smell, locomotion and elimination principles. In this chakra lies Power (Shakti) Dakini, and concentration should be done on her. All these are in the 'earth'-region (lying in the pericarp of the muladhara). Concentration should be made on Kundalini in this manner: she is splendorous like ten-million moons and is in the nature of Supreme Brahman; she has three eyes and four arms and is mounted on a lion; she holds a book and a lute, and makes the gestures of granting boons and of dispelling fear.

The next is the swadhishthana which is situated in the genital region. It has six petals of vermilion colour. On the petals are the six letters from ba

to la (that is, ba, bha, ma, ya, ra, la) which are of shining coral-red. In the pericarp of the chakra is (the 'water'-region of) Waruna. Here lies the Power named Rakini. Concentration should be made on her. Here are also the centres of taste and sex principles.

The next chakra is the manipuraka. It has ten petals, dark blue in colour. The petals are ornamented with the letters from da to pha of lightning-like colour. In the pericarp of the chakra is the region of 'Fire'. Here lies Deity Rudra, endowed with the power of destruction, and with him is Power Lakini. Concentration should be done on Rudra and Lakini. Here is the centre of the sight-principle.

The next chakra is anahata. It has twelve petals of deep red. The shining letters from ka to tha are on the petals. In the pericarp of the chakra is 'air'. It is also the seat of jiwatman. Here is a triangle in which are situated Bana-linga. Power Kakini is also there. It is the centre of the touch principle.

The next is the wishuddha chakra situated in the neck region. It has sixteen petals which are smoke-coloured and contains the sixteen vowels (from a to ah) on its petals. In the pericarp of the chakra are the akasha (that is, the region of the void), and Deity Shiwa mounted on an elephant. It is the centre of the hearing and speech principles.

The next is the ajña chakra. It has two petals, white in colour, and ornamented with the letters ha and ksha. In the pericarp of this chakra is a triangle where lies Itara-linga. Power Hakini is situated here. Manas, buddhi, ahankara and prakriti are there (in separate chakras but closely connected with the ajña).

Then there is the great lotus sahasrara. This perpetual sahasrara is white and stands with its face turned downward. On its petals are the shining letters from a to ksha (that is, fifty letters). Connected with the pericarp of the chakra are the inmost spirit (antaratman) and Guru (in the twelve-petalled guru chakra which is the lower aspect of the sahasrara). (Below the guru chakra) there are the 'sun'-sphere (surya-mandala) (which appears to be the manas chakra, just above the ajña), and the 'moon'-sphere (chandra-mandala) (that is, the indu

173

chakra above the manas chakra). Then comes the mahanada-wayu (that is, the wayu in the form of mahanada—the great power of control) (that is, supremely controlled pranic power, effecting natural kumbhaka). And then (above the wayu) is the brahmarandhra (here is the terminal part of the brahmarandhra which bears also the same name; the chakra termed brahmarandhra or nirwana is here). Inside the (brahma) randhra (that is, the nirwana chakra) is the untinged and blissful Wisarga (that is, the Power which goes outside the brahmarandhra). Above it (that is above the sahasrara) is the divine Shankhini (Supreme Power who is in the spiral form and supremely tranquil in nature), and who (in her power aspect) creates, maintains and destroys. Below Shankhini is the 'moon'-sphere (within the sahasrara proper) where lies a triangle which is the abode of Shiwa (Kailasa). Here is the perpetual and unchanging amakala (that is, the power which maintains consciousness in a state of samadhi). Within it is the nirwanakala (the power named nirwana) in coil. Within it (nirwanakala) is the nirodhika (power of supreme control) in the form of fire. There is the supreme Nirwanashakti (Kundalini in her all-absorbing power aspect), who is the source of all. In this power (Nirwanashakti) is immutable supreme Shiwa. At this point, Kundali-power goes through the brahmarandhra back to the muladhara lotus (—Kankalamalini-tantra, ch. 2, abridged).

System B

The brahma lotus (muladhara chakra), which stands with its face turned downward, has four petals. Inside the pericarp of the lotus lies the beautiful 'earth'-region which is quadrangular and encircled by the seven 'seas'. There is a triangle on the square region, which is the seat of 'love-desire'. Inside the square region lies the bija (germ-mantra) 'Lang' which is in the form of Deity Indra, mounted on the king of elephants. Within the triangle is the great lord Shiwa in the linga form (a form suitable for concentration). The power, an aspect of which is maya (negato-positivity), in a coiled form like a serpent (that is, Kundali-power), encircles the linga by the three and a half coils,

and she has kept the orifice of the linga closed by her mouth. The bija of Indra (that is, 'Lang') is situated on the left side of the linga. Above the nada of the bija (the crescent aspect of the 'Lang' bija) is the seat of Deity Brahma who is the creator and the lord of all created beings. On his left side is Goddess Sawitri who is the source of the Weda.

Above this is a shining lotus called bhima (swadhishthana). It has six petals of vermilion colour. Inside the pericarp of the lotus is a circular region with four doors, wherein lies the bhuwar-world. Here lies Deity Wishnu with Shri (Goddess Lakshmi) on his left side, and Wani (Goddess Saraswati) on his right side. Wishnu is dressed in yellow raiment and is ornamented with a garland of flowers of all seasons (wanamala), and tranquil in appearance. He is the maintainer of the universe. His abode is called the waikuntha-world. On the right side of it is the goloka (a world) where Deity Krishna, holding a flute in his two hands, and Goddess Radhika are situated.

Above it is a great lotus (manipura) which has ten petals of black colour like rain clouds. On the petals are the letters from da to pha (ten letters) with nada-bindu (that is, matrika-letters). Inside the pericarp of the lotus is a triangle of red colour like the rising sun, and is ornamented with the swastika marks on its three sides. Inside the triangle is the wahni-bija (the 'fire'-germ mantra 'Rang'), seated on a ram. Here lies the abode of Rudra. Deity Rudra and Goddess Bhadrakali are here. This lotus is called the swar-world.

Above it, there is the beautiful wimala (pure) lotus (that is, the anahata chakra). It has twelve petals of deep red colour on which (are twelve letters from ka to tha) of the colour of pure vermilion. Inside the pericarp of the lotus is a shining hexagonal region where lies the beautiful wayu-bija ('Yang'). Here are Deity Ishwara and Goddess Bhuwaneshi (the mother of the universe), lying on his left side. This chakra is called the mahar-world.

Above it, there is the fascinating nirmala (free from impurities) lotus (that is, the wishuddha chakra). It has sixteen petals. In the pericarp of the lotus is the 'moon'-sphere (a circular region), where lies a hexagonal region. Inside it are (Power) Gouri and on her right side Deity Sadashiwa, seated on a bull-lion (one half bull and the other half lion). Sadashiwa has five faces and each face has three eyes. He is like a mountain of silver (that is, of white colour and motionless), and his body is smeared with ashes. He is clothed in a tiger skin and is ornamented with a garland of gems. He is in the form of the united Power-Consciousness (arddhanarishwara, that is, Power Gouri is the half of Sadashiwa's body). Sometimes he is only of lustre, and sometimes he is without any form. This chakra is called the jana-world.

Above it is the jnana (ajña) lotus. It has two petals. It includes the 'full-moon'-sphere (purnachandra-mandala, that is, the indu chakra) within which is a nine-cornered region, made of wishing-gem (chintamani). Here lies Shambhu-bija (that is, the germ-mantra of the God Shiwa—'Hang') which is in the form of a swan (hangsah). The 'swan' (the bija mantra) is Supreme Brahman (without any form) and also in the form of Shiwa (that is, wachaka-shakti—power-in-sound-form, of the mantra 'Hang' is Shiwa in divine form, and the wachya-shakti—power as Consciousness, of the mantra is Supreme Brahman). In the internal aspect of the 'swan' (that is, in the bindu of 'Hang') is Deity Para Shiwa and on his left is the all blissfull Goddess Siddhakali. This chakra (jnana) is called the tapas-world.

Above the jnana lotus is the sahasradala (thousand-petalled) lotus. It stands with its face downward and is situated in relation to the head (just beyond it). The petals of the lotus are endowed with all power. They are diversified and variegated, presenting white, red, yellow, black and green colours. Now they appear as white, the next moment they are red, and then yellow, and again white and then green. The lotus is called the satya-world. Inside the pericarp of the lotus, there is a vast ocean of nectar wherein lies the isle of gems (manidwipa). There is a wishing-tree (kalpadruma) where is situated a lustrous temple with four doors. Inside the temple is an altar made of fifty matrika-letters. On it lies a jewelled throne on which is seated Mahakali (Supreme Power) united with Maharudra

(Supreme Consciousness) as one. He who is Maharudra is Mahawishnu and Mahabrahma. The three are the one, only there is the difference in name (—Nirwanatantra, ch. 4–10, abridged).

System C
Muladhara. In the muladhara, there is a triangle called tripura which is in the nature of will, knowledge and action. Inside the triangle lies Swayambhu-linga shining like ten-million suns. Concentration should be done on his fourth aspect (turiya, that is, the concentration aspect) which is deep red. Above it is Kundali as his crest, and of red colour. Kundali is supremely subtle. She is the Supreme Power as Goddess Mahatripurasundari. She is the sentience principle in all beings. She is Shabdabrahman. She is splendorous and is in the nature of being-consciousness-bliss and eternal. She is within all beings in a coiled form. The lotus has four petals of red colour, and on the petals are the letters from wa to sa (four letters) of shining golden colour. It is the root and support of all chakras.

Above it is the lotus called swadhishthana which has six petals of fire-like red. On the petals are the letters from ba to la (six letters) of diamond-colour (that is, shining white). The name swadhishthana is derived from swa to mean supreme linga.

Above it is the great chakra—manipura, situated in the navel region. This centre is like mani (jewel), so it is called manipura. The lotus has ten petals of golden colour which shine like lightning. The petals have the letters from da to pha (ten letters) on them. (Deity) Wishnu is established in this lotus.

Above it is the anahata lotus which has twelve petals of red colour like the rising sun. The petals are ornamented with the letters from ka to tha (twelve letters) of red colour. Inside the lotus (in the pericarp) is Bana-linga (Shiwa in the linga-form named Bana), shining like 10,000 suns. The anahata-sound (non-sensory suprasound) arises in this lotus, so it is called by the yogis anahata. It is the abode of bliss where lies the divine spirit (parapurusha).

Above it is the lotus termed wishuddha which has sixteen smoke-coloured petals on which are placed the shining sixteen letters (from *a* to *ah*). In this lotus, the embodied being (*jiwa*) is purified because of his realization of Hang*sah* (Supreme Being), so it is called wishuddh*a*. It is also called akash*a* (because it is the seat of akash*a*—the 'void'-principle).

Above it is the ajña chakra where lies the Supreme Spirit. The lotus has two petals on which are the letters h*a* and k*sha*. They are moonlike white. The transference of divine knowledge (Guru's ajña) occurs here, so the lotus is called ajña.

Above it is the k*a*ilasa (chakra), and above the k*a*ilasa is the bodhin*i* (chakra). Above the bodhin*i* is the s*a*hasrara (having 1000 petals) lotus which is the centre of Bindu (bindu-sthan*a*) (—Gandharwat*a*ntra, ch. 5, abridged).

System D

The basic lotus is the m*u*ladhar*a* which has four petals of deep red colour. On the petals are the m*a*trika-letters from w*a* to s*a*. There is a beautiful bright triangle inside (the pericarp of) the lotus where lies the 'earth'-germ m*a*ntra (L*a*ng). Within the triangle is situated Shiw*a* (in linga-form) of a dark-green (shy*a*mal*a*) colour. Concentration should be done on him. Here (inside the triangle), lies K*u*ndalin*i* who is Supreme Power. The divine K*u*ndalin*i*, who is (Shabda-) Brahman, is splendorous like ten million lightnings and in a latent form, and in coils like a serpent around Shiw*a*.

The next is the swadhi*shth*an*a*, which is the seat of the 'water' (-germ-m*a*ntra). It has six petals of lightning-like colour, and on the petals are the letters from b*a* to l*a* which are white in colour. Here lies omniscient Shiw*a* who is to be concentrated upon.

The next is the m*a*nipura, which has ten petals of black colour. On the petals are the ten black-coloured letters from *da* to ph*a* with nada-bindu. Here lies Shiw*a*-linga (Shiw*a* in linga-form) of black colour like clouds.

Then, there is the anah*a*ta-puri (-chakra). It has twelve petals and on the petals are twelve letters from k*a* to th*a*. The colour of the petals and letters is white. This is (also called) h*ri*t-p*a*dma (heart-lotus) which is in the nature of pure sentience (s*a*ttw*a*). There, in front, lies

j*i*w*a* (the embodied being) in its divine aspect, like the flame of a lamp, in the form of consciousness and power, quiescent, pure and of golden colour.

The next is the smoke-coloured wishuddh*a* with sixteen vowels (letters from *a* to *ah* on its sixteen petals). Inside it lies akash*a* (void) which is in the form of power.

Thereafter is the ajña-puri (-chakra). It has two petals on which are two letters (h*a* and k*sha*). They (petals and letters) are white in colour. Here, divine knowledge (Guru's ajña) is imparted (to disciples), so it is called ajña.

Next is the s*a*hasrara. It lies in connection with (but beyond) brahm*a*randhr*a* where is situated Sadashiw*a*. The Supreme Power (as Mahak*u*ndalin*i*) is in union with Sadashiw*a*. This lotus has 1000 petals. Within the lotus is the region of power where lies Sadashiw*a*, who is pure consciousness and motionless like a corpse (—Bh*u*tashuddhit*a*ntra, ch. 1–3, abridged).

System E

The m*u*ladhara, swadhi*shth*ana, m*a*nipuraka, anah*a*ta, wishuddh*a* and ajña are the six chakras which are situated in the anal, genital, navel, heart, throat and eyebrow regions respectively. The basic chakra (adhar*a* pankaja) which is the m*u*ladhar*a* is above, but linked to the k*a*nda, with its face upwards. The m*u*ladhar*a* has four petals of red colour. On the petals are the letters w*a*, sh*a*, *sha* and s*a*, ornamented with filaments. There is the 'earth'-region which is quadrangular. Here is situated (the deity) Indr*a* mounted on an elephant named Airawat*a*. In the lap of the 'earth'-seed m*a*ntra (that is, within the bindu of the m*a*ntra 'L*a*ng') is the child creator (Brahma). Above it is a triangle composed of wama, jye*shth*a and roudr*i* lines. This triangle is the seat of Power (K*u*ndalini-power). Inside the triangle is the tremulous kama-wayu (desire-radiating power) in seed-form (that is, the kama-b*i*ja m*a*ntra 'Kl*i*ng'). Here is Swayambhu-linga (Shiw*a* in the linga-form named Sw*a*yambhu) with his face downwards. Divine K*u*ndali is of conch-shell colour (white), and like a creeper she is in three and a half coils around Sw*a*yambhu-linga and covers the face of the linga. Here also lies (Power) Dakin*i* with instruments in her hands as the door-keeper (that is, the presiding Divinity of the chakra).

Above is the swadhishthana with six petals of lustrous red. On the petals are the letters ba, bha, ma, ya ra, la, ornamented with filaments. There lies the watery waruna-bija (that is, the 'water'-germ mantra 'Wang') and above it is a triangle where is situated the great linga in the form of Wishnu. Power Rakini as a door-keeper is also there.

Above it is the manipura which has ten petals of a shining dark-blue (nila) colour. On the petals are the letters from da to pha. There lies the wahni-bija ('fire'-germ mantra 'Rang') in the triangle (which is inside the pericarp of the lotus) where is also Rudra-linga (linga in the form of Rudra) with six faces. In this chakra is situated Power Lakini as a door-keeper.

Above it is the anahata having twelve petals of yellow colour with the letters from ka to tha which are decorated with filaments. There is a triangle where is situated Bana-linga named Ishwara. There are also wayu-bija ('air'-germ mantra 'Yang') and jiwa (embodied being like the flame of a lamp and in the form of hangsah (that is, living). Here lies Power Kakini as the door-keeper.

Above it is the lotus wishuddha which has sixteen smoke-coloured, or sky-coloured (blue), petals. On the petals are the sixteen vowels (the letters from a to ah), decorated with filaments. There is a beautiful triangle (in the pericarp) where is situated Sadashiwa, and also Power Shakini as the door-keeper.

Above it is the ajña chakra which is without any principles of matter (shunya) and is the seat of mind. It has two petals of variegated (or white) colour on which are (the letters) ha and ksha. Here is situated the linga named Itara.

In the 'earth'-region (muladhara) lies the Power of Brahma; in the 'water'-region (swadhishthana) is Narayani (the Power of Wishnu); in the 'fire'-region (manipura) is the Power Waishnawi; in the 'air'-region (anahata) is Ishwari (the Power of Ishwara); in the 'void'-region (wishuddha) is Sadashiwa himself; and in the seat of mind (ajña) is the Itara-power.

Above it (ajña) is indu (that is, indu chakra, also known as soma chakra) which is situated in the region of the forehead (lalatadesha). Above it (indu chakra) is the nada in the form of half-moon. Above it (nada) is the shining mahanada which is in the form of a plough. Above it (mahanada) is the kala termed Añji, and above it is unmani. At the end of the kunda-lirandhra-kanda (that is, the nadi wajra, and, consequently, sushumna nadi; in other words where the sushumna ends), there is the twelve-lettered (twelve-petalled) lotus (dwadasharna) shining white in colour, where Guru is (this is called guru chakra). This chakra stands with its face upwards, being covered on the top by the lotus with 1000 petals of white colour mixed with red (rose or pink). There is a triangle (in the guru chakra) formed of three lines named a, ka and tha, and decorated with the letters ha, la, ksha (situated in the three corners) (—Sammohanatantra, Part 2, ch. 2, abridged).

System F

In the perineal region and in relation to the kanda is situated the adhara (muladhara) lotus. It has four petals and on the petals are 4 letters from wa to sa. This lotus is called kula (because of the seat of Kundalini). Inside the lotus are Swayambhu-linga and (Power) Dakini as the presiding Divinity. There is a triangle within the lotus where lies Kundalini. Above it is the quivering kama-bija (the desire-germ mantra 'Kling'), radiating light.

The second lotus which is called swadhishthana is situated in the genital region. It has six petals of red colour, and on the petals are the six letters from ba to la. The presiding Divinity is Rakini.

The third lotus which is called manipuraka is situated in the navel region. It has 10 petals of golden colour which are decorated with the letters from da to pha. The presiding Divinity is Lakini.

The fourth lotus is anahata, situated in the heart region. It has twelve petals of deep red which are decorated with the letters from ka to tha. Here is the wayu-bija (the 'air'-germ mantra 'Yang'). In this lotus is situated the lustrous Bana-linga. The presiding Divinity of the chakra is Kakini.

The fifth lotus is the wishuddha which is situated in the throat region. It has sixteen petals of smoke colour, and on the petals are the sixteen vowels (from *a* to *ah*). The presiding Divinity is Shakini.

In the eyebrow region is the ajña lotus with two petals of white colour which are decorated with (the letters) ha and ksha. The presiding Divinity is Hakini. Here is moon-like akshara-bija (Ong) which is Parama-hangsah (Supreme Being).

Above the ajña are three pithas (seats; here chakras, or auxiliary chakras), bindu, nada and shakti, situated (one upon the other) in the forehead region.

Above the three pithas, but outside the physical body (that is, cranium) is the brilliant lotus sahasrara (that is, the sahasrara is situated outside the cranium where the sushumna nadi ends). The sahasrara is also called kailasa where lies Mahesha (Supreme Shiwa) who is known as akula (Parama Shiwa—Supreme Consciousness—into which kula—Kundalini—has been absorbed)—the eternal, the immutable. Here, Kundalini-power named kula becomes absorbed (into Parama Shiwa) (—Shiwasanghita, 5. 80–205, abridged).

2 The chakra system as expounded by Bhairawi

The great lotus muladhara has four petals of red colour on which are the letters from wa to sa of golden colour. Here (in the pericarp) is the kshiti-mandala (the 'earth'-region). In the muladhara, there is a triangle (inside the 'earth'-region) which is in the nature of will-knowledge-action. Inside the triangle is Swayambhu-linga shining like ten-million suns. Above it is the kama-bija, and above that is the divine Kundalini in the form of a flame.

Above it is the shining swadhishthana which has six petals of red colour. On the petals are the six letters from ba to la which are like diamonds (shining white). (Power) Rakini and (Deity) Wishnu are situated in the pericarp. This lotus is situated in the genital region and is pervaded by the kandarpa wayu (an aspect of

the apana power which radiates love-desires).

Above it is the ten-petalled manipura, shining like ten-million gems. It is situated in the navel region. The lotus (that is, its petals) is like cloud (that is black in colour). On the petals are the lightning-like letters from da to pha. Here (in the pericarp of the lotus) lies (Deity) Rudra with (Power) Lakini.

Above it is the anahata lotus, situated in the heart region. It has twelve petals of red colour like the rising sun, or the colour of the bandhuka flower (Pentapoetes Phoenicea), that is, deep red. On the petals are the letters from ka to tha. Here (in the pericarp) are (Deity) Ishwara and (Power) Kakini. Inside it is Bana-linga shining like ten-thousand suns. The anahata is in the nature of Shabdabrahman which is realized here.

Above it is the sixteen-petalled lotus of smoke colour termed wishuddha, and on the petals are the sixteen vowels from a to ah of the colour of lightning. The lotus is situated in the throat region. It is the seat of akasha (that is, the 'void'-region). Here are situated (Deity) Sadashiwa and (Power) Shakini. This lotus is called wishuddha (which causes purification), because here the embodied being becomes purified through the realization of Hangsah (Supreme Being).

Above it is the ajña chakra situated in the eyebrow region. It has two petals of white colour. On the petals are the letters la and ksha with bindu. Here are the seats of hangsah and bindu. The transference of divine knowledge (Guru's ajña) occurs here, so it is called ajña.

Above ajña is what is called kailasa (chakra), and above kailasa is bodhana (chakra). Above the bodhana is the great white lotus sahasrara. It is the seat of Bindu. (—Rudrayamala, Part 2, 22. 2–13; 27. 53–70, abridged).

3 The chakra system as explained by Rishi Narada

The lotus termed muladhara has four petals of red colour on which are (the letters) wa, sha, sha, sa of golden colour. Inside the muladhara is a triangle which is in the nature of will-

knowledge-action. Inside the triangle is Sway-
ambu-linga, shining like ten million suns. Above
it is the kama-bija with kala-bindu-nada (Kling).
Above it is Kundali brilliant like a flame. Kundali
is shyama (that is black or deep green in colour),
and is in the nature of Krishna (Supreme Being).
She is established in Krishna.

Above it is the swadhishthana which has six
petals of red colour, and on the petals are the
six letters from ba to la, shining like
diamonds.

Above it is the lustrous manipura, situated in
the navel region. It has 10 petals of smoke colour.
This lotus is like gems, so it is called manipura.

Above it is the lotus termed wishuddha which
has sixteen petals. Above that is the ajña chakra.
Above ajña is kailasa (chakra), and above the
latter is bodhini (chakra). Above bodhini is
sahasrara where lies the seat of Bindu
(—Goutamiyatantra, 34. 40–54, abridged).

4 The chakra system as explained by Mahidhara

The muladhara has four petals which are decorated with the letters from wa to sa. Inside it is
situated (Deity) Brahma with (Power) Dakini.

The chakra named swadhishthana is situated
in the genital region. It has six petals decorated
with the letters from ba to la. Here is (Deity)
Wishnu with (Power) Rakini.

The manipuraka chakra has ten petals on
which are the letters from da to pha; it is situated
in the navel region. Here are (Deity) Rudra
and (Power) Lakini.

The anahata, which is in the heart region,
has twelve petals on which are the letters from
ka to tha. Here are situated (Deity) Ishwara
and (Power) Kakini.

The wishuddha is situated in the throat region.
It has sixteen petals on which are sixteen vowels
(from a to ah). In this lotus are (Deity) Sadashiwa
and (Power) Shakini.

The ajña chakra is situated in the eyebrow
region, and the letters la and ksha are (on its
two petals). Here lies (Deity) Parashiwa with
(Power) Hakini (—Mantramahodadhi, 4. 19–25,
abridged).

5 The chakra system as explained by Brahmananda

At the root of the vertebral column (that is,
at the lowest point of the sushumna nadi which
is within the vertebral column) lies the lotus
called muladhara. It has four petals of deep
red colour. Inside the pericarp of the lotus
is a triangle. Within the triangle is Swayambhu-
linga of golden colour and in the form of bindu
(supremely concentrated form which has no
magnitude but only position). He is with Power
Kakini. Supreme Kundali is in three and a half
coils around the great linga.

The six-petalled lotus (named swadhishthana)
is of whitish-red (raktapandara) colour. Inside
it is a linga of whitish-red colour and with
Power Hakini.

In the navel region is situated the eight-
petalled lotus (manipura) like a new cloud (that
is, black in colour). Here is a linga endowed with
the power of absorbing the universe, and it is
with Power Shakini.

There is a lotus (anahata) in the heart region
with sixteen petals of white colour. Here is the
great Maheshwara-linga with Power Lakini.

Thereafter is the great lotus (wishuddha)
with the ten petals of dark-blue colour. There is
a great linga named Kama lying with his
Power.

In the forehead region is the two-petalled
lotus (ajña) where is situated Brahma-linga
with the Power.

Above the topmost point of the sushumna
nadi, which is inside the vertebral column,
is the twelve-petalled lotus (guru chakra) where
lies a triangle which is in the nature of Brahma-
Wishnu-Shiwa, and above it is the sahasrara
lying with its face downward. Here (in the
sahasrara) is situated Parama Shiwa who is
Brahman (Supreme Consciousness). Guru (who
is in the twelve-petalled chakra) is in the divine
form and in the nature of mantra (—Tararahasya, ch. 4, abridged).

6 The chakra system as explained by Jñanananda

There is a lotus (muladhara) with four petals
of golden colour in the perineal region, which

are decorated with (the letters from) wa to sa, shining like gold. Here lies (Power) Dakini of red or white colour, three-eyed, and with fierce teeth, holding (in her two right hands) a shula (trident) and a khatwanga (a staff with a human skull at its top), and in her two left hands a khadga (sword) and a surakumbha (wine-pot). In the pericarp of the lotus is a triangle called kamakhya. Inside the triangle is kandarpa, an aspect of the apana (-power). Within the triangle is also Swayambhu-linga with his head downward, who is shining red and roving. There is the Kundali-power in eight coils around Swayambhu-linga.

The great lotus adhishthana (swadhishthana) is situated in the genital region. It is deep red and is decorated with the letters from ba to la of the colour of vermilion (on its six petals). Here lies (Power) Rakini who is of the colour of dark blue (shyama), holding in her hands a shula (trident), a wajra (thunderbolt), a padma (lotus) and a damaru (drum).

In the navel region is the manipura lotus of ten petals of the colour of deep blue (nila) on which are the letters from da to pha of the colour of lightning. Here is the 'fire'-region where is situated (Power) Lakini.

In the heart region is the anahata of twelve petals of the colour of mixed blue and yellow, or like the flame of a lamp (pingabha) with the letters from ka to tha of red colour.

In the eyebrow region is the lotus (ajña) shining like ten million lightnings which is the seat of mind. It has two petals with the bright letters (ha and ksha). Inside the triangle (which is situated in the pericarp of the chakra) abides Itara-linga the red colour (taruna aruna—the newly risen sun). Here is situated (Power) Hakini who is white in colour and three-eyed, and holds in her hands an akshamala (a rosary of rudraksha = Eleocarpus Ganitrus), a damaru (drum), a kapala (skull) and a pustaka (book), a chapa bow) and mudra (the gesture of granting boons). Within the lotus is situated the Inner-Atman (Supreme Being) bright with ongkara-light.

Then comes the sahasrara lotus standing with its head downwards. It is also called kailasa (—Koulawalitantra, ch. 2, abridged).

7 The chakra system as explained by Lakshmana Deshikendra

The muladhara has four petals. Inside it is a bright triangle where dwells Divine Shakti (Power, that is, Kundalini) who is splendorous like ten million lightnings, supremely subtle, in the nature of Shiwa-Shakti (Consciousness-Power) and in three-coils. She passes through the middle-path (that is, the brahma nadi which is within the sushumna) to Parama Shiwa (situated in the sahasrara). On the petals are the letters from wa to sa. Here is Kamalasana (Brahma, as the presiding Deity of the muladhara).

The six-petalled lotus swadhishthana has (on its petals) the letters from ba to la. Here is (Deity) Wishnu.

The navel-lotus (manipura) has ten petals with the letters from da to pha. Here abides (Deity) Rudra.

The heart-lotus (anahata) is decorated with the letters from ka to tha (on its twelve petals). Here is (Deity) Ishwara.

The throat-lotus (wishuddha) has sixteen petals on which are the (sixteen) vowels. Here lies (Deity) Sadashiwa.

The eyebrow-lotus (ajña) has two petals, decorated with the letters ha and ksha. Here is Bindu (which is Shiwa). Then, there is kala, then nada, nadanta, unmani, wishnu-waktra and guru-waktra (—Sharadatilakatantra, 5. 127-37, abridged).

8 The chakra system as explained by Brahmananda Giri

The basic chakra is what is known as muladhara which has four petals deep red in colour, and the petals are decorated with the letters from wa to sa of deep red colour. In the pericarp of the chakra is a triangle named kamakhya, which is in the nature of will-knowledge-action. In the triangle lies kandarpa (-power) named apara. Inside the triangle is also Swayambhu-linga of dark-blue colour, with a fissure, and his face downward. Divine Kundali, who is like a streak of lightning and supremely subtle, is in a latent form, and in three and a half coils from right to left around Shiwa (Swayambhu-linga).

The great lotus swadhishthana which is situated in the genital region has six petals on which are the letters from ba to la.

The manipuraka which is situated in the navel region has ten petals of red colour with the letters from da to pha.

The lotus anahata is situated in the heart region. It has twelve petals of red colour on which are the letters from ka to tha. Inside (the pericarp) is Bana-linga shining like ten-thousand suns. Anahata-mantra (mantra in the madhyama form, that is, the suprasound form) which is in the nature of Shabdabrahman (that is, Kundalini) is 'heard' here; and from this fact this lotus has been named by the yogis anahata.

In the throat region is what is called wishuddha, which has sixteen petals of smoke colour. The petals are decorated with the sixteen vowels from a (to ah). The purification of the embodied being is effected here, owing to the 'seeing' of Hangsah (Supreme Being); so it is called the wishuddha lotus. It is also called akasha (because it is the region of akasha—'void').

The chakra called ajña, which is situated in the eyebrow region, has two white petals on which are two letters ha and ksha. Inside the chakra is the great linga named Itara (that is, the great Itara-linga) of golden colour. Here, the transference of living divine knowledge (Guru's ajña) occurs, so its name is ajña.

Above the ajña is the kailasa (chakra) and above kailasa is the bodhini (chakra), and again above it, is the sahasrara, in which are situated Nada and Bindu. Here lies the Void (shunya-rupa) which is Shiwa (that is, the void is that where everything has been absorbed into Shiwa who, as Supreme Consciousness, only remains), and the circle (writta) around it (void, that is Shiwa) is splendorous Supreme Kundalini in three and a half coils. The thousand-petalled lotus stands with its face downward and is above the twelve-petalled lotus (the guru chakra, which is the lower part of the sahasrara), where lies Shiwa as Guru (infinite Supreme Being in divine form) (—Shaktanandatarangini, 4. 9–15, 31, abridged.)

CHAPTER 10
Exposition of the Chakras

This exposition of the chakras is essentially based on the Tantras and supplemented by the Waidika and the Pouranika accounts. The chakras are the centralizations of the chitra-power, occurring at certain points along the chitrini, and forming the chakra system. The chakra system consists of the muladhara, swadhishthana, manipura, hrit, anahata, wishuddha, talu, ajña, manas, indu, nirwana, guru, and sahasrara. The chakras will be considered under four subheadings: terminology, position, description, and explanation.

1 Muladhara

The muladhara is the first chakra occurring at the downmost point of the chitrini nadi. The principal term for the first chakra appears to be muladhara, which has been mentioned in the Upanishads, Tantras, and Puranas.

Terminology

The following are the Tantrika terms of the first chakra: (1) Muladhara which has been mentioned in the Todalatantra, ch. 2, p. 3; ch. 7, pp. 13–15; ch. 8, p. 15; ch. 9, p. 17; Matrikabhedatantra, ch. 15, p. 23; Kamadhenutantra, ch. 13, p. 16; Kankalamalinitantra, ch. 2, p. 6; Gandharwatantra, ch. 5, p. 27; ch. 10, p. 47; ch. 29, pp. 108, 112; Mantra-

mahodadhi, ch. 4, 20, 28; Shaktakrama, ch. 1, p. 1; Kubjikatantra, ch. 6, 280, 331; Tararahasya, ch. 2, p. 8; ch. 3, p. 18; ch. 4, p. 22; Tripurasarasamuchchaya, ch. 5.4; Bhutashuddhitantra, ch. 1, p. 2; ch. 3, p. 3; ch. 4, p. 4; ch. 5, pp. 4,5; ch. 8, p. 8; ch. 10, p. 9; ch. 14, p. 12; Sammohanatantra, Part 2, ch. 2, p. 2; ch. 4, p. 4; Mayatantra, ch. 6, p. 5; Purashcharanarasollasa, ch. 2, p. 2; ch. 9, p. 9; ch. 10, p. 11; Wishwasaratantra, ch. 1, pp. 6, 10; ch. 2, pp. 12,23; ch. 4, p. 44; Koulawalitantra, ch. 2, p. 6; ch. 3, p. 7; ch. 22, p. 80; Sharadatilakatantra, 5.127; Shaktanandatarangini, 4.10, 25,27,30,32,34; Rudrayamala, Part 2, 21.18; 22.2; 25.55; 27.53,58; 44.20; 45.6; Mahanirwanatantra, 5.104,115; Tantrarajatantra, 27. 35; 30,64; Puraschcharyarnawa, ch. 2, p. 90; ch. 5, p. 386; ch. 6, p. 490; Shaktisangamatantra, Tara Section, ch. 61.113; Mantramaharnawa, ch. 4. 1; Shadamnayatantra, 5.240; Shiwasanghita, 2.29; 5.92, 144; and Goutamiyatantra, 34.40.

(2) Adhara, mentioned in the Kankalamalinitantra, ch.2, p.6; Phetkarinitantra, ch. 14, p. 39; Kularnawa, ch. 4, p. 19; Jñanasankalinitantra, 67, p. 5; Kubjikatantra, ch. 6, p. 7; Bhutashuddhitantra, ch. 4, p. 4; Wishwasaratantra, ch. 2, pp. 11,12; Shaktanandatarangini, ch. 4. 9, 25, 29; ch. 9.16; Tantrarajatantra, 21.82; Shiwasanghita, 2.21; 5.89; Shatchakranirupana, 4; and Sammohanatantra, Part 2, ch. 3, p. 3.

(3) Mula chakra, padma, mentioned in the Nilatantra, ch. 5, p. 8; Gayatritantra, 3.44; Brihannilatantra, ch. 1, p. 2; ch. 6, p. 31; Gandh-

arwatantra, ch. 5, p. 24; Bhutashuddhitantra, ch. 1, p. 1; Koulawalitantra, ch. 22, p. 80; Shaktanandatarangini, 4.28; Rudrayamala, Part 2, 21.22, 23; 22.4; 29.11; Mahanirwanatantra, 5.93; Shiwasanghita, 5.98, 172; and Shatchakranirupana, 13.

(4) Brahma padma, chakra, mentioned in the Nirwanatantra, ch. 4, p. 6; Shadamnayatantra, 5.249.

(5) Bhumi ('Earth') chakra, mentioned in the Rudrayamala, Part 2, 21.27,28,40,49,50, 53,54,55.

(6) Chaturdala (four-petalled lotus), chaturdala padma (four-petalled lotus), mentioned in the Gandharwatantra, ch. 8, p. 39; Rudrayamala, Part 2, 60.27; Mundamalatantra, ch. 6, p. 9.

(7) Chatuh-patra (four-petalled lotus), mentioned in the Todalatantra, ch. 9, p. 16.

Position

The muladhara is situated in the region below the genitals and above the anus, and is attached to the mouth of the sushumna (—Shatchakranirupana, verse 4). The region between the genitals and the anus is the perineum. So externally, the muladhara is situated in the perineal region. Internally, the chakra is at the point of the opening of the sushumna, that is, at the beginning of the sushumna. The muladhara centralization occurs just at the point where the chitrini starts. The chitrini is inside the wajra, and the wajra inside the sushumna. It has been stated that kanda is situated above the anus and below the genitals (—Shiwasanghita, 5.80). This kanda is not the perineum, but the root from which all subtle nadis have originated. Externally, the kanda is in relation to the perineum, but internally it is situated inside the coccyx. The sushumna arises from the central point of the kanda. The mouth of sushumna is connected with the kanda. The mouth is the starting point of the sushumna and then it goes upward. The wajra, which lies inside the sushumna as the second nadi, arises from the starting point of the sushumna. The chitrini, which is inside the wajra as the third nadi, also arises from the same start-

ing point. At this starting point, which has been called the mouth of the sushumna, —and in fact, also the mouths of the wajra and the chitrini —the muladhara lies in the chitrini.

It has been stated: 'The four-petalled lotus (muladhara) is in the adhara' (—Gandharwatantra, ch. 8, p. 39). So, the region between the anus and genitals is called adhara, that is, the perineum. It has also been stated: 'The four-petalled lotus is in the adhara which is (connected with) the gudasthana (that is, anal region)' (—Koulawalitantra, ch. 22, p. 80). So, the adhara is the perineum. Yoni is another term for the perineum. It has been stated that the region between the anus and the genitals is yoni, where the kanda lies (—Shiwasanghita, 5.81). So the yoni is the perineum, and in the yoni-region lies internally (that is, in the coccyx) the kanda from which the sushumna arises. It has also been said that the muladhara is in the region of the anus (—Sammohanatantra, Part 2, ch. 2, p. 2), and so this lotus is also called gudapadma (anal lotus) (—Bhutashuddhitantra, ch. 10, p. 9). The exact position of the muladhara has been clearly stated in the Mridanitantra, which says that the muladhara is situated above the anus. This position of the muladhara has been approved in the Yogaswarodaya. The place above the anus means the place lying in that part of the perineum which is very close to the anus.

In the Waidika accounts, the same position of the muladhara has been described. It has been stated that the muladhara is in the region between the anus and the genitals (—Yogashikhopanishad, 1.168; 5.5). This region is the perineum. It has been stated that the yonisthana is between the muladhara and the swadhishthana and the muladhara is situated in the gudasthana (anal region) (—Yogachudamanyupanishad, Mantras 6–7). This means: the yonisthana is between the anus and the genitals, and, consequently, it is the perineum. The gudasthana is actually that part of the perineum which is close to the anus. Here, it is indicated that the position of the muladhara is in that part of the perineum which is closest to the anus. The term adhara for perineum has also been used. It has been stated that the brahma chakra (muladhara chakra) is in the adhara (—Soubhagyalakshmyupanishad, 3.1.). The adhara is the perineal region.

According to the Pouranika accounts, the muladhara is situated in the perineal region. It has been stated that the four-petalled lotus (muladhara) is placed in the adhara (—Dewibhagawata, 11.1.43). Adhara is the perineum. Also the term mula has been used for the perineum (—Shiwapurana, 5b. 29.131).

All the evidences—Waidika, Tantrika, and Pouranika—indicate that the position of the muladhara, when considered externally, is in that part of the perineum which is very close to the anus.

Description

The muladhara (Plate 1) has four petals (—Shatchakranirupana, verse 4). This has been supported by all Tantras as well as by the Waidika and Pouranika accounts. The arrangements of the petals are as follows: the first petal is situated in the north-east corner, the second petal in the east-south corner, the third petal in the south-west corner, and the fourth petal in the west-north corner of the lotus. The east and the west are considered to be on the right and the left side of the practitioner respectively.

The colour of the petals of the muladhara is shona (—Shatchakranirupana, verse 4). The commentators Kalicharana, Shankara and Bhuwanamohana say that the shona is the bloodcolour. According to Wachaspatyam (the great Sanskrit Dictionary, compiled by Taranatha Tarkawachaspati Bhattacharya), shona is the blood-colour. The blood-colour is the deep red colour like the jawa flower (the China rose or Bengal rose). That the petal-colour is deep red has been stated in the Bhutashuddhitantra, ch. 1, p. 1; Sammohanatantra, Part 2, ch. 2, p. 2; Tararahasya, ch. 4, p. 22; Mridanitantra, quoted in the Amarasanggraha MS and Shaktanandatarangini, 4.9. It has also been stated that the colour of the petals is like molten gold (—Gandharwatantra, ch. 5, p. 27; Kankalamalinitantra, ch. 2, p. 4; Rudrayamala, Part 2, 27.56; and Goutamiyatantra, 34.43). The molten

gold is the shining red colour. According to a certain Tantrika school the colour of the petals is pita (—Puraschcharyarnawa, ch. 6, p. 490). Pita is a yellow colour. It has also been stated that the adhara is of a golden colour (—Dakshinamurti, quoted by Wishwanatha in his commentary entitled Shatchakrawiwriti; Koulawalitantra, ch. 22, p. 80). The golden colour is the shining yellow. This school practises a different mode of concentration. However, in the generally adopted mode of concentration the petal colour has been accepted as deep red as taught by most of the gurus. In the Pouranika accounts, the muladhara has been described as of golden colour (that is, shining yellow) (—Shiwapurana, 5b.29.140) as well as of molten gold (that is shining red) (—Dewibhagawata, 7.35.34).

On the petals of the muladhara, are the four letters (wedawarna) from wa to sa which are of the colour of the shining udyat gold (—Shatchakranirupana, verse 4). The commentator Ramawallabha says that udyat gold means heated gold. The commentator Bhuwanamohana gives the same translation. The shining heated gold presents a mixture of shining red and gold colours. The commentator Wishwanatha explains 'udyat' as 'prasphutita', that is, blown or opened. The translation of the passage can also be: the letters are visibly shining as the colour of gold shines. Or, the lotus usually hangs with its head downwards; but when its head is upwards, it blooms and the four letters are seen shining like the colour of gold. However, let us see what other Tantras say about it. It has been stated that the letters (on the petals of the muladhara) are of the shining colour of gold (—Gandharwatantra, ch. 5, p. 27). This means that the letters shine like gold, i.e. the letters are gold or shining yellow in colour. This has been clearly mentioned by Bhairawi. She says: 'The letters from wa to sa are of the colour of gold (swarnawarna.= gold-colour)' (—Rudrayamala, Part 2, 22.2). Narada also says: 'The letters wa, sha, sha, sa (which are on the petals of the muladhara) are of golden colour' (—Goutamiyatantra, 34.42). It has been stated that the letters from wa to sa shine like gold (—Koulawalitantra, ch. 22, p. 80). There is another school which holds that the letters are of blood-colour (—Mayatantra, quoted by the commentator Wishwanatha; Shaktanandatarangini, 4.9). ' In the Pouranika accounts, it has been stated that the letters from wa to sa shine like gold (that is, gold-colour) (—Dewibhagawata, 7.35.34). So we find that the letters are of golden colour (or shining yellow colour) and also of blood-red or deep red colour. According to the mode of concentration, either golden or deep red colour should be adopted.

These four letters are wa, sha, sha and sa. This has been adopted in all Tantras. These letters are with nada-bindu (Ꙭ). It has been stated in relation to the manipura chakra that the letters should be with bindu (nada-bindu) (—Nirwanatantra, ch. 6, p. 8). This applies to all chakras. It has been stated that bindwardha (bindu + ardha : ardha-bindu = nada-bindu) should be added to the letters which are on the petals of the muladhara, swadhishthana, manipura, anahata, wishuddha, and ajña chakras (—Bhutashuddhitantra, ch. 1, pp. 1 and 2; ch. 2, p. 2). Wishwanatha, in his commentary entitled Shatchakrawiwriti, says that according to the Sarasamuchchaya, the letters which are in the six lotuses are with bindu (nada-bindu). So the letters wa, sha, sha and sa become wang, shang, shang and sang when nada-bindu is added. This indicates that the letters in the chakra are not the letters of the alphabet of the Sanskrit language. They are matrika-units which are the mantra-units.

The letters (matrika-letters) on the petals of the chakras are arranged from the right (to the left) (—Wishwasaratantra, ch. 1, p. 10). In connection with the wishuddha chakra, it has been stated that the letters are arranged from the right (—Shiwapurana, 5b.29.136). This applies to all chakras, as is stated in the Wishwasaratantra. So in the muladhara, the letters are arranged in this way: on the petal situated in the north-east corner, which is the first petal, is wang, on the petal in the east-south is shang, on the petal in the south-west is shang, and on the petal in the west-north is sang. Concentration on the letters is done both from right to left and in the reverse manner, depend-

ing on the purpose, evolution or absorption (—Wishwasaratantra, ch. 1, p. 10).

The petals of the chakras are the seat of specific qualities (writtis). Narayana, in his commentary on the Hangsopanishad, Mantra 7, has mentioned these qualities. He says that according to the Adhyatma Wiweka the specific writtis (qualities) are in the muladhara, swadhishthana, manipura, anahata and wishuddha, and these writtis are arranged on the petals from right (to left). Jaganmohana, (Jaganmohana Tarkalankara alias Purnananda Tirthanatha, a great authority on Tantra), in note eighty-seven in connection with his commentary on the Mahanirwanatantra, 5.104, also mentions the writtis which are on the petals of the chakras. Moreover, he has not only mentioned the writtis in the muladhara, swadhishthana, manipura, anahata and wishuddha as is done by Narayana, but also in the talu, manas and indu chakras. All these writtis will be mentioned in their appropriate place.

On the petals of the muladhara are the four writtis arranged from right to left. On the first petal (situated in the north-east) is greatest joy (paramananda), on the second petal is natural pleasure (sahajananda), on the third petal is delight in the control of passion (wirananda), and on the fourth petal is blissfulness in concentration (yogananda).

In this chakra is the quadrangular 'earth'-region, surrounded by eight shining spears (shulas), and within it ('earth'-region) is the dhara-bija (the 'earth'-germ mantra Lang) of the shining yellow colour and delicate like the lightning (that is, the bija is lightning-like and yellow in colour) (—Shatchakranirupana, verse 5). This translation (of verse 5) is according to Ramawallabha and Bhuwanamohana. But Kalicharana differs. He qualifies both the 'earth'-region and the 'earth'-germ mantra as yellow. He cites two passages in support of his explanation. In one passage, it is stated that the 'earth'-region is square and yellow in colour and surrounded by eight spears. The other passage says that inside it is the aindra-bija (that is, the 'earth'-germ mantra) which is yellow in colour. Let us investigate what other Tantras say. The Kankalamalinitantra (ch. 2, p. 4) mentions the 'earth'-region (prithwi) in the muladhara, but does not qualify it. The Rudrayamala merely mentions (Part 2, 22.3) the 'earth'-region (kshiti-mandala = 'earth'-region) in the muladhara without any description. Only the name of the 'earth'-germ mantra (prithwi-bija) has been mentioned in the Bhutashuddhi-tantra, ch. 1, p. 1. It has been stated that in the muladhara is the 'earth'-region (kshiti-chakra) where the 'earth'-germ mantra (dhara-bija) is situated, mounted on the elephant named Airawata (—Sammohanatantra, Part 2, ch. 2, p. 2). The colour of the 'earth'-region and its germ mantra has not been mentioned here. Also, the 'earth'-region (kshiti-chakra) is inside the pericarp of the lotus (muladhara), which is four-cornered (that is, square) and where the Lang bija lies in the form of Indra (the Deity) (that is, aindra-bija which is the same as the prithwi-bija) (—Nirwanatantra, ch. 4, p. 6). Here also colour has not been mentioned.

It has been stated that the 'earth'-region (prithwi-mandala) (lying in the muladhara) is yellow in colour and quadrangular and is surrounded by the eight spears; inside it ('earth'-region) is the 'earth'-germ mantra (dhara-bija) mounted on an elephant and four-armed (—Mridanitantra, quoted in Amarasang-graha MS). Here, the colour of the 'earth'-region has been mentioned, but not of the 'earth'-germ mantra. In the Waidika accounts, the 'earth'-region is only said to be a square (—Yoga-shikhopanishad, 1.176; 5.13). We find in the Pouranika accounts that the 'earth'-region (awani-mandala) is golden colour (that is, shining yellow), quadrangular and with a thunderbolt, and inside the region is the Lang-bija (prithwi-bija = the 'earth'-germ mantra) (—Dewibhaga-wata, 11.8.3). Here also the colour of the Lang-bija has not been mentioned.

The colours of the regions in the chakras are identical with their bijas. In the muladhara, the 'earth'-region is yellow in colour, so its bija Lang should be yellow also. In concentration, the colour of the 'earth'-region and that of the 'earth'-bija are thought of as yellow. This has been indicated in the Mantramaharnawa, 1,4, p. 41. Of the mantra Lang, 'la' is the bija part. It is the basic part which is intimately connected

with the particularized sound-form. The 'la' is the prithwi-bija (—Matrikanighantu, 53, p. 51). It has been stated that 'la' is yellow and like a streak of lightning (—Kamadhenutantra, 6.28). So, the colour of 'la' is shining yellow, and, consequently, 'la' with nada-bindu, that is, Lang, the 'earth'-bija, is of a shining yellow colour, as has been stated in the Shatchakra-nirupana, Verse 5. That the 'earth' (prithwi)-bija Lang which is in the muladhara is yellow has been clearly stated in the Mahanirwana-tantra, 5.104; also in the Shyamarahasya, ch. 1, p. 16. So both the 'earth'-region and the 'earth'-bija situated in the muladhara are yellow in colour.

The 'earth'-bija Lang has been explained in the Shatchakranirupana, Verse 6: 'the 'earth'-bija is ornamented with four arms and mounted on the King of elephants; on the lap of the bija is the child Creator, shining like the sun in the morning with four arms and four faces which are beautiful like lotuses. The King of elephants means the elephant named Airawata who is the bearer of Deity Indra. The 'earth'-bija and the aindra-bija are identical. From the viewpoint of the mahabhuta, Lang is the 'earth'-bija, and from that of the dewata (deity) it is aindra-bija. The Lang consists of the bija part and the nada-bindu part. The bija part is Deity Indra who has four arms and is mounted on the best elephant Airawata. On the lap of Indra is the Creator, that is, Deity Brahma who is the shining red colour like the rising sun, and who has four beautiful faces and four arms.

It has been stated that Lang-bija is in the form of (Deity) Indra (—Nirwanatantra, ch. 4, p. 6). So the bija aspect is Deity Indra, that is, Deity Indra arises from the bija aspect of Lang, when the mantra is made living by concentration and japa. Indra is seen mounted on the elephant named Airawata. So it is said that the king of the elephants (Airawata) is the carrier of the aindra-bija (—ibid., ch. 4, p. 6). Airawata is white and has four tusks (—Shabdakalpa-drumah). So it has been said that the seat of Indra, mounted on the elephant Airawata, is in the quadrangular 'earth'-region in the muladhara (—Sammohanatantra, Part 2, ch. 2, p. 2). In the concentration-form (the form arising from the mantra in concentration; and also the form which is thought of in concentration) of Indra, he is yellow in colour, thousand-eyed and holds in his hands the thunderbolt and a lotus, and is adorned with ornaments (—Tantrasara 3.52). The thousand eyes should not be taken in a literal sense. It means the fully aroused spiritual eyes. He has been described as having two eyes as well as three eyes. Indra should be considered as having four arms according to the text. He has also been described as having two arms. The thunderbolt and lotus are in his hands. If he is thought of as having four arms, then in the third hand he is holding a goad (ankusha), and the fourth hand may pass round his Power Indrani as in an embrace. But, in the concentration form, Indra is alone, and, consequently, he is holding the thunderbolt and a lotus in his two hands, and his other two hands are in the gestures of granting boons and dispelling fear. The lotus which is held in his hand is a blue lotus.

Brahma

On the lap of the dhara-bija Lang is Deity Brahma. So it has been said that on the lap of the dhara-bija is the child Creator (Brahma) (—Sammohanatantra, Part 2, ch. 2, p. 2). Also, Brahma, with Power Dakini, is in the four-petalled muladhara (—Mantramahodadhi, 4. 19–20); and, Kamalasana (Brahma) is in the muladhara (—Sharadatilakatantra, 5.130). The celebrated commentator Raghawabhatta says that Kamalasana is Brahma, who is the presiding Deity of the adhara.

In the Waidika accounts we also read that Brahma is the presiding Deity (adhidewata) of the quadrangular 'earth'-region (that is, the muladhara) (—Yogashikhopanishad, 1. 176; 5. 13). About the actual seat of Brahma, it has been stated that it is above the nada (the crescent aspect) of the aindra-bija (Lang) (—Nirwanatantra, ch. 4, p. 6). Above the nada of Lang is bindu (point), and, therefore, bindu is the seat of Brahma. This means that within the bindu lies Brahma in an unmanifested state. When the mantra is aroused, Brahma emerges from the bindu. So it is said that Brahma dwells there (that is, above the nada, which is bindu) (—ibid., ch. 4, p. 6). Kalicharana explains rightly that

'in the lap of dhara-bija' means within the bindu of the bija. He quotes a passage in which it has been stated: 'In the muladhara is the dhara-bija (which is) Amaradhipa (Indra) who is mounted on an elephant; in his (Indra's) lap, that is, in its bindu (i. e. the bindu of the dhara-bija Lang) dwells Brahma in the form of a child.' Here it has been shown that the dhara-bija and Deity Indra are the same. Kalicharana too says that the dhara-bija is identical with Indra. He quotes a passage which says: 'The mantra-letters are the dewata (divinity), and the dewata is in the form of the mantra.'

In the Waidika sandhya-yoga-process, concentration is done on Brahma during puraka pranayama (the inspiratory phase of breath-control). The Samaweda form of Brahma is as follows: Brahma is blood-coloured (deep red colour), with four faces and two arms, and holds a rudraksha rosary (aksha-sutra) in one hand, and a sacred water-pot (kamandalu) in the other hand, and is seated on a swan (hangsah). The Rigweda and the Yajurweda forms are the same as the Samaweda form. Concentration on Brahma is done in the navel region, that is, in the manipura chakra.

The concentration-form of the Divine Power Gayatri (Kundalini) as Brahmi (Power of Brahma) is this: as Brahma, she is (that is, she is of a deep-red colour, four-faced, and two-armed), with holy grass (kusha) in her hand, seated on a swan; she is in the stage of preadolescence—from her arises the Rigweda—and is in the sun-sphere (surya-mandala). This is the Samaweda-form. The Yajurweda-form is this: She is of a deep-red colour, clad in red raiment, three-eyed, holds (in her three hands) a goad, a rudraksha rosary and a sacred water-pot, and (the fourth hand) in the attitude of granting boons, is seated on a swan, in the stage of preadolescence, uttering the Rigweda, and in bhur-world, and she is the Divine Power of Brahma. In the Rigweda-form she is on a swan, and is assuming the lotus posture (padmasana); she is four-faced and deep-red in colour, her two arms are holding a rudraksha rosary and a sacred water-pot; she is in the stage of preadolescence; she is like Brahma; and she is Brahmani (the Power of Brahma). From all this, it appears that the form of Brahma and that of his Power are identical.

In *shatchakrayoga*, concentration on Brahma is done in the muladhara. In the Waidika process, the concentration form of Brahma is this: in the 'earth'-region with Lang is Hiranmaya (Brahma) who has four arms and four faces. In the sandhya process, there are greater details of his form.

The Pouranika form of Brahma for concentration is as follows: he is situated in the pericarp of the hrit lotus; his face is deep-red in colour (this means that he is of a deep-red colour); he has beautiful eyes, four faces and four arms, making the gestures of granting boons and dispelling fear, he has the sacred thread (brahmasutra) over his shoulder, and he is splendorous (—Padmapurana, 1.15.188–9). Brahma is also golden in colour, four-faced, and large-eyed (—Brahmandapurana, 24.15). Brahma has also been mentioned as having five faces (—Wamanapurana, 2.24). About the Powers (Shaktis) of Brahma, Wishnu and Rudra, it has been stated that Power Brahmi is of sattwa, and white in colour, Power Waishnawi is of rajas, and red in colour, and Power Roudri is of tamas, and black in colour (—Warahapurana, 96. 58–9). So the Powers of Brahma, Wishnu and Rudra appear to have the same qualities and colours.

The dhyana (concentration)-form of Brahmi (Power of Brahma) is as follows: Brahmi is deep-red in colour (as quoted by Kalicharana, or golden according to the text edited by Rasikamohana), clothed in the skin of the black antelope (krishnajina), and holds a staff (danda), a sacred water-pot (kamandalu) and a rosary of rudraksha, and makes the gesture of dispelling fear (—Wishwasaratantra, ch. 2, p. 22). According to Kalicharana, Brahma has the same weapons as his Power Brahmi; this conclusion he bases on the Saptashatistotra, which says that Shiwa and Shakti have the same weapons. The Pouranika accounts also support this view.

Moreover, it has been stated that Brahmani (Power of Brahma) is the real creator, and not Brahma, so he is (like) a corpse (—Kubjikatantra, 1.25–6). It indicates that the creativity of Brahma becomes manifested through his Power termed Brahmani or Brahmi. So, the

characters of both are identical.

The form of Brahma described in the Mridanitantra (quoted in the Amarasanggraha MS) is as follows: Shiwa named Brahma who is in the lap of dhara-bija is of deep-red colour and has four faces and four arms with different weapons. Also, Brahma is of deep-red colour, three-eyed, four-faced, holding (in his hands) the rosary of rudraksha and the sacred water-pot and seated on a swan (—Koulawalitantra, ch. 22, p. 80). Kalicharana quotes a passage from the Bhutashuddhitantra in his commentary on verse 6, which says that in 'its' lap is the child Brahma who is deep-red in colour, four-faced and four-armed and seated on the back of a swan. It has been stated that the Goddess Sawitri who is the 'mother' of the Weda is on the left side of Brahma (—Nirwanatantra, ch. 4, p. 6). It has also been stated that Brahma is with (Power) Dakini in the muladhara (—Todalatantra, ch. 7, p. 14; Mantramahodadhi, 4.19). (Concerning the form of Brahma for concentration, see Plate 2, left top figure).

Dakini

The Goddess (dewi) named Dakini is situated here (in the muladhara); she has four beautiful arms and bright red eyes; she is splendorous like the brilliance of many suns rising simultaneously; she always carries divine knowledge-light (to impart to the yogis) (—Shatchakranirupana, Verse 7).

Dakini is the Power of the muladhara. It has been stated that concentration should be done on Power Dakini who is fit to be worshipped (—Kankalamalinitantra, ch. 2, p. 4). Power Dakini is the presiding Divinity of the muladhara, so it has been stated that here (in the muladhara) is situated Dakini as the door-keeper (that is, the presiding Divinity) (—Sammohanatantra, Part 2, ch. 2, p. 2). That Dakini is the divinity of the muladhara has been stated in the Shiwasanghita, 5.90). Kalicharana quotes a verse in which it is stated that Dakini, Rakini, Lakini, Kakini, Shakini and Hakini are the queens of the six respective lotuses. So, Dakini is the presiding Divinity of the muladhara. Dakini is the Power which is linked to Brahma, the first Shiwa. It has been stated that Dakini, Rakini, Lakini, Kakini,

Shakini (and Hakini) are the Powers residing in the six lotuses, who are linked to six Shiwas (Brahma and others) (—Rudrayamala, Part 2, 25. 54–5). Because of this connection, concentration is done on Dakini along with Brahma in the muladhara (—ibid., 30.14).

Now we come to the form of Dakini for concentration. In the text (verse 7) Dakini has been described as having four arms and bright red eyes. About the colour of the body, it has been stated that she is shining like the lustre of many suns rising at the same time. Wishwanatha explains it as 'very red'. She is shining deep-red in colour. For concentration purposes we need greater details.

Forms of Dakini

'She appears like the autumnal moon (that is, she is shining white in colour), and has two arms; her eyes are smeared with collyrium and tremulous; she is bright with a mark on the space between the eyebrows (tilaka) of vermilion, clad in black antelopes skin and adorned with various ornaments; and her face is as beautiful as the moon' (—Kankalamalinitantra, ch. 5, pp. 22–3).

'Dakini is radiant and appears agile; she is the mother of wealth; she holds (in her hands) a sacred water-pot and a knife, and makes the gesture of granting boons' (—Kularnawa, ch. 10, p. 53).

'Dakini is shining white in colour and red-eyed; she holds a sword, a drinking vessel, a trident, and a skulled staff and has fierce teeth' (—Gandharwatantra, ch. 9, p. 42).

'Dakini who is the Power of Brahma is shining red in colour, four-armed, divinely dressed and holds varied weapons (in her hands)' (—Mridani-tantra, quoted in the Amarasanggraha MS).

'Dakini is red in colour, red-eyed, fearful to the unspiritual persons; she holds a skulled staff, club and a drinking vessel filled up with wine; she is fierce and has terrific teeth' (—Mahamukti-tantra, quoted in the Yogakalpalatika MS).

'Dakini shines like the morning sun (that is, red), (or) white like milk; she holds (in her right hands) a trident and a skulled staff, and in her left hands a sword and a drinking vessel; she has three eyes and fierce teeth' (—Koulawalitantra, ch. 22, p. 80). (For the form of Dakini for concentration, see Plate 2, right top figure.)

The Triangle

In the region where the moth of the wajra lies (and, consequently, the mouths of the sushumna and chitrini), in the pericarp (of the muladhara) is a triangle named traipura which is bright like lightning, beautiful, and is in the nature of love-desire (kama); wayu (vital force) named kandarpa (the energy associated with pleasurable desires) is present always and everywhere in the triangle; kandarpa is the controller of the embodied beings, very deep red and shines like ten million suns (—Shatchakranirupana, Verse 8).

It has been stated that inside the pericarp of the muladhara is a beautiful triangle (trikona) which is in the nature of will-knowledge-action and (the Deities) Brahma, Wishnu and Shiwa (—Kankalamalinitantra, ch. 2, p. 4). The triangle is the seat of love-desire (madana) where kandarpa is the presiding force (—Nirwana-tantra, ch. 4, p. 6). The triangle has been termed tripura (—Gandharwatantra, ch. 5, p. 27). The triangle is composed of three lines, called wama, jyeshtha and roudri and there lies the seat of Power (Kundalini-power); inside it is the tremulous desire-radiating force (kama-wayu) in the form of germ (bija) (that is, the kama-bija-mantra Kling) (—Sammohana-tantra, Part 2, ch. 2, p. 2). The triangle has also been termed yoni (a triangular process which is the abode of powers) where lies Kundalini, and in its upper aspect is situated the quivering and shining kama-bija (that is, the mantra Kling) (—Shiwasanghita, 5.91). In the mula-dhara is a triangle which is in the nature of will-knowledge-action where lies the kama-bija Kling (—Rudrayamala, Part 2, 27. 53–4). Also in the Goutamiyatantra, 34. 40–1). Yoni is a triangle. So it is said that the yoni (triangle) which is situated inside the pericarp of the muladhara is called kamakhya, inside of which lies kandarpa (force in the form of pleasurable desires) which is an aspect of apana (wayu) (—Koulawalitantra, ch. 22, p. 80). That the kandarpa-force is an aspect of apana-force has also been mentioned in the Shrikrama, quoted in his comment by Wishwanatha. The kandarpa has a special term —apara (—Shaktanandatarangini, 4.9). Kan-

189

darpa has also been called wahni-wayu (fire-force) (—Mayatantra, also cited by Wishwanatha).

It is mentioned in the Waidika accounts that there is a trirawritta region (that is a triangle) in the muladhara where lies the seat of kama in form (kama-rupa) (that is, kama in the form of the mantra Kling) (—Soubhagyalakshmyupanishad, 3.1). Inside (the pericarp of) the muladhara is yoni (the triangular region) which is kamakhya (the seat of kama) (—Yogachudamanyupanishad, 8). In the triangle is the seat of what is called kama-rupa (kama in form, that is, in the form of the mantra Kling) which makes desire fruitful (—Yogashikhopanishad, 1.171; 5.8). In the triangle is apana (-wayu) in which is what is called mula-kanda (germ form) and it is also called kama-rupa (kama-form); the triangle is the wahni-kunda (the place of fire) (—Yogarajopanishad, 6). Here it is indicated that an aspect of apana wayu is kama in germ-form which is Kling. The triangle is the seat of fire, that is, fire-wayu which is called kandarpa-wayu in the Tantras. So the kama or kandarpa-wayu is an aspect of apana wayu and is in the nature of fire, and it is called fire-force.

Swayambhu-linga

'Inside it (the triangle) is situated Swayambhu in the form of linga as pashchimasya (that is, "Ong"); he is beautiful like molten gold and is revealed by the knowledge arising in concentration (dhyana); he is of the shape and colour of new leaves; he shines like lightning and radiates cool rays like the full moon; as Kashi (the holy city of Benares) is the great seat of Shiwa, so the triangle (in the muladhara) is the seat of Swayambhu (a name of Shiwa); he is in union with Kundalini (wilasi); and he is like a whirlpool in the river (that is, in circular motion)' (—Shatchakranirupana, Verse 9).

The meaning of the word 'pashchimasya' is: with the face lying behind. But all the commentators—Kalicharana, Shankara, Wishwanatha, Ramawallabha and Bhuwanamohana—interpret it as: with the face downwards. Kalicharana quotes from the Kalikulamrita which says that Swayambhu is with his face downwards. The technical meaning of the

word is 'O' (—Warnabijakosha) which, with nada-bindu, becomes 'Ong'. On the basis of the technical meaning, it can be said that the linga is in the form of 'Ong'.

'Jñanadhyanaprakasha'—jñana is knowledge and dhyana means concentration. This compound word has been interpreted as follows. Kalicharana says: 'he who is realized by knowledge and concentration. The formless aspect of Swayambhu is revealed by knowledge, and Swayambhu in form is realized by concentration. Shankara says that the realization is caused by jñana yoga and dhyana yoga. According to Wishwanatha: he who is revealed by knowledge and concentration. Ramawallabha interprets jñana as tattwajñana and dhyana as chinta (reflection). Tattwajñana is the true knowledge; the knowledge of Brahman' (—Wachaspatyam); knowledge of the truth (—Apte). Bhuwanamohana also says that knowledge is the true knowledge and concentration is the reflection on the true nature; the jñanins by true knowledge and the dhyanins by concentration 'see' him. However, the senso-intellectual form of knowledge does not reach Swayambhu, so that knowledge which develops in concentration is the only means of his realization. So jñana-dhyana is the concentration-knowledge-light by which Swayambhu is 'seen'.

About the appearance (rupa) of Swayambhu, it has been said that it is like the appearance of a new leaf. According to Kalicharana, rupa includes both shape and colour. He says that as the pistil inside the champaka flower is broad at the bottom and tapers to a point at the top, so is the shape of Swayambhu, and he is shyama in colour. Shyama is black or green colour (—Wachaspatyam and Shabdakalpadrumah). Ramawallabha simply says that he has the colour of a new leaf. This has been explained by Ramakrishna Widyaratna as slightly red in colour (araktawarna).

Now, let us investigate what other Tantras say about Swayambhu. Swayambhu-linga is always with Kundali coiled around him (—Kankalamalinitantra, ch. 2, p. 4) and this explains why he has been called wilasi. It has been stated that inside the triangle is Swayambhu-linga, shining like ten million suns (—Rudrayamala, Part 2, 27.54;

Goutamiyatantra, 34.40). The colour of Swayam-bhu-linga has been more clearly stated here: he is as bright as the lustre of ten million suns and is of deep red colour (—Koulawalitantra, ch. 22, p. 80). And also, he shines like the lustre of ten million suns, and concentration should be done on his fourth aspect (that is, turiya—the concentration aspect) which is deep-red in colour (—Gandharwatantra, ch. 5, p. 27). These statements indicate that Swayambhu-linga is of shining deep-red colour. There is mention of his other colours too. It has been stated that concentration should be done on Divine Shiwa (here, in the linga-form, that is Swayambhu-linga) who is beautiful in the colour of shyamala (black or green colour), lying inside the triangle (—Bhutashuddhitantra, ch. 1, p.1). And in Shaktanandatarangini, 4.9. He is also of golden colour (shining yellow colour). It has been stated that inside the triangle is what is known as Swayambhu-linga who is of golden colour (—Tararahasya, ch. 4, p. 22).

About the linga-form of Shiwa. It has been stated that Maheswara (a name of Shiwa) in the form of linga is in the triangle (—Nirwanatantra, ch. 4, p. 6). The linga has also been called Mahalinga (the great linga; it is an epithet of Shiwa) (—Yogachudamanyupanishad, 8). In the linga-form, there is a fissure and it lies in pashchimanana (= pashchimasya, that is Ong-shaped) (—Shaktanandatarangini, 4.9). The linga-form is actually the bindu-form, so it has been stated that Swayambhu-linga is in the form of bindu (—Tararahasya, ch. 4, p. 22). The linga-form appears not to be in tranquillity. It has been said that Swayambhu-linga is roving (—Koulawalitantra, ch. 22, p. 80). This unquietness of the linga is due to the untranquil kamawayu-bija (kama-force in the germ-form, that is, the mantra Kling) (—Sammohanatantra, Part 2, ch. 2, p. 2). Kama-bija (Kling) itself is restless (—Shiwasanghita, 5.91). There is a close relation between Swayambhu-linga and kama-bija and the unquietness of the kama-bija is imparted to the linga. Their relation is still deeper. The linga-form appears from the kama-bija (—Mridanitantra, quoted in the Amarasanggraha MS). All this explains why it has been said that Swayambhu-linga is like a whirlpool.

Kundalini

Over it (on the body of Swayambhu-linga) is Kundalini who is subtle like the lotus-filament and splendorous like the lustre of young lightnings, and, like the spiral of the conch-shell, makes three and a half coils round Shiwa like a serpent, and keeps the sweet mouth (because of the amrita-flow in it) of brahma-dwara (brahma nadi) covered by her own mouth; she is asleep (in a latent form); she, like the indistinct hum of the excited bees, makes undifferentiated charming sounds (that is, the matrika-sounds which arise from Kundalini); she is the world-bewilderer (by her maya-power); she who preserves all the beings of the world by maintaining the functions of inspiration and expiration (in latency), being deep within the triangle of the muladhara, shines like a row of lights of excessive brilliance; within her (Kundalini, that is, in her inner aspect) is Parama Kala (Supreme Kundalini) (that is, Kulakundalini is really Supreme Kundalini) who is endowed with supreme yoga-power, supremely subtle (that is, her being is the being of Parama Shiwa), and (is the source of) para (shabda, that is, the principle of sound, or Brahmawidya—the Brahman-knowledge), and holds uninterrupted flow of the stream of amrita oozing from the constant joy (of being in supreme union with Parama Shiwa); she is Shriparameshwari (Supreme Power) who shines as eternal consciousness (that is, her consciousness is the eternal Shiwa Consciousness), and by her splendour the whole universe is illumined (that is, has come into being); and she remains supreme (—Shatchakranirupana, Verses 10–12).

Now, let us study what other Tantras say about Kundalini. It has been stated that Maya-shakti (Power, that is, Kundali-power who exhibits maya when coiled) is in coil like a serpent (that is, unroused) and the linga (Swayambhu-linga) is encircled by the three and a half coils by her, and she stays always by covering the orifice of the linga by her mouth (—Nirwanatantra, ch. 4, p. 6). Above the turiya aspect of Swayambhu-linga is the flame-like Kundali of red colour (that is, shining red) who is supremely subtle; she is Goddess Mahatripurasundari (Supreme Power), Shabdabrahman, splendorous, and in the nature of being-consciousness-bliss; and she is eternal and is in a coiled state within the embodied beings (—Gandharwatantra, ch. 5, p. 27). Divine Kundalini who is Supreme Power and (Shabda-) Brahman is coiled like a serpent and splendorous like ten million lightnings and lies by encircling Shiwa (Swayambhu-linga) in the muladhara-triangle (—Bhutashuddhitantra, ch. 1, p. 1). Divine Kundalini who is white as the conch-shell surrounds Swayambhu-linga by three and a half coils like a creeper and covers his mouth by her own (—Sammohanatantra, Part 2, ch. 2, p. 2).

'Supreme Kundali is splendorous like lightning and in three and a half coils, situated in the sushumna-path' (—Shiwasanghita, 2.23). 'Kundali who is Brahman is like a flame' (—Rudrayamala, Part 2, 27.55). 'Kundali is para (that is, the source of para sound) and shines like a flame, and black (or dark-green) in colour, and is in the nature of Krishna (God)' (—Goutamiyatantra, 34. 41–2). 'Kundalini who is Supreme Power and is in the nature of Brahman shines like ten million suns and is bright and cool like ten million moons and splendorous like lightning; she is not steady and, like a serpent, she is in three and a half coils around the great linga '(Swayambhu-linga)' (—Tararahasya, ch. 4, p. 22). 'Kundali-power in whom is embedded (the matrika-letters) a to ksha shines like lightning and is subtle like the lotus-filament, and is sleeping like a serpent, and is in eight coils (—Koulawalitantra, ch. 22, p. 80). 'Dewi (Divine Kundalini) is Shiwa-Shakti (that is, Kundalini is Supreme Power being one and the same with Parama Shiwa—Supreme Being) and in the nature of only consciousness; she is the power and is supremely subtle; she is splendorous like ten million lightnings and in three coils' (—Sharadatilakatantra, 5. 128–9). 'Divine Kundali who shines like a streak of lightning is, as a sleeping serpent, unroused, and in three and a half coils from right to left around Shiwa (Swayambhu-linga), and is supremely subtle like a lotus filament' (—Shaktanandatarangini, 4.10).

In the Waidika accounts, we find that Shakti (Kundali-power) is like fire (—Soubhagyalakshmyupanishad, 3.1). Kundali who is unroused and in coils (—Yogakundalyupanishad, 1.65). Kundali-shakti (-Power) is in eight coils (—Yogachudamanyupanishad, 36; Shandilyopanishad, 1.8; Trishikhibrahmanopanishad, Mantra Section, 63). Kundalini is the divine light and living power (—Yogarajopanishad, 7).

From the above statements emerges the following.

Divine Kundalini is in the nature of consciousness. She is the living power and is supremely subtle. She is like fire. She is splendorous like the lustre of strong lightnings, bright like many suns and cool like the moon. She is in three and a half coils around Swayambhu-linga, encircling him from right to left. She has also been described as being in three and eight coils. She is like a flame, not steady, and remains unroused in the muladhara. She is of shining red colour. She is also said to be white and black (or dark-green) in colour. She is Parama Kala (Supreme Kundalini) and also Supreme Power. She is Brahman. She is Shiwa-Shakti.

There are two forms of concentration on Kundalini—subtle and gross.

Concentration on subtleness
Kundalini is the living power and is consciousness, supremely subtle, lightning-like splendorous, moon-like cool, and in three and a half coils around Swayambhu-linga, from right to left.

Concentration on form
1 Kundalini who is Supreme Brahman shines like many million moons. She is seated on a lion, and has three eyes and four arms. She holds a book and a wina (Indian lute), and makes the gestures of granting boons (wara mudra) and dispelling fear (abhaya mudra) (—Kankalamalinitantra, ch. 2, p. 4).

Note: She should be thought of as red in colour.

2 Kundalini is red in colour, perpetually youthful with fully developed breasts and attractive eyes, and adorned with jewelled bracelets, small bells around the hip, anklets on the feet, and all kinds of ornaments and gems;

she is charming like the full moon and very beautiful (—Shaktanandatarangini, 4.34).

3 In the morning: in the muladhara. Kundalini is red like the rising sun in the morning; she has three eyes like the sun, fire and moon, and holds (in her four hands) a noose, a goad, a bow and a arrow.

At noon: in the hrit lotus. She is in early youth.

In the evening: in the ajña. She is splendorous, youthful and beautiful, and is Parama Kala (Supreme Kundalini) (—Shaktanandatarangini, 4.54).

4 Kundalini as Ishtadewata.

Note. The form of Ishtadewata is the form of Kundalini.

5 Special concentration on Kundalini, in the form of Goddess Dakshinakalika, in the muladhara. Goddess Dakshinakalika is four-armed, making the gestures of granting boons and dispelling fear with her right hands, and holding a sword and a human head with her left hands; she is possessed of three eyes which are like the moon, sun and fire; she is black in colour, perpetually death-less, youthful and naked, with a girdle made of hands of dead persons; she has dishevelled hair, a smiling face, long teeth and wears a necklace of skulls; her right foot is on the heart of Shiwa and stands on a great lotus; and she is in deep love-desire for union with the Supreme Being (—Kubjikatantra, ch. 6, p. 7).

Explanation

The chakras are the different levels of superconsciousness, so they are not reflected in sense-consciousness, because of its oscillatory character. It indicates that superconsciousness is not undulatory and is in a state of concentratedness. Therefore, the chakras are also the different levels of concentration. When concentration is very deep, the chakras appear in concentrated consciousness and are 'seen'. When concentration is practically a thought-form, it can be made deeper and transformed into real concentration comparatively easier when the thoughts are of the images of the chakras as seen in concentration. So the description of the chakras is vitally im-

portant for those students of concentration who are at the thought level.

The petals of the muladhara are the energy-radiations from the continuous circular energy-motions which maintains the prithiwi mahabhuta organization. The petals are deep red in colour. It indicates that there is the concentration of apana-energy which radiates red-rays. Each petal has its own specific concentration which is marked by a special matrika-letter. This mark is not artificial but occurs as an intrinsic aspect of the concentration. In the first petal is wang, in the second shang, in the third shang and in the fourth sang. The original colour-radiation of wang is yellow lightning-like, of shang golden, shang rose (red mixed with white) and sang lightning-like. In the muladhara petals, all the matrika-letters are of golden colour. So wang and shang retain their original colours, but the other two change their colours. The golden colour indicates that the mahabhuta-tanmatra-forces are concentrated in the petal-letters. When the petal-letters are blood-red (due to different mode of concentration), it indicates the apana-concentration.

From the viewpoint of concentration, the petal-letters form the mantra wang-shang-shang-sang which are utilized for japa for developing thought-concentration. At first, there is a petal-gap between the letters, and by the practice of japa the gaps become less and less and finally disappear and become conjoint with nada-bindu ('ng' factor). At this stage the four-lettered mantra becomes a four-matrika-concentration-unit. This is the unit for the muladhara. Now, the petal-concentration is reduced to circular concentration. At this stage, the four radiations (designated by the four-matrika-letters) cease and the circular energy-motion becomes more concentrated. The four-matrika-concentration-unit is that in which the four letters are seen simultaneously and as a whole in thought-form.

Thereafter, concentration is done on two main lines: mahabhuta-tanmatra concentration and concentration within the triangle. In mahabhuta-tanmatra concentration, the following forms are practised stage by stage: (a) meta-earth (prithiwi mahabhuta) concentration, (b) supra-smell (gandha tanmatra); (c) concentration-on-divine-form (-dewata).

In very deep concentration, meta-earth is 'seen' as a yellow square. When concentration deepens more and more, the square is reduced to an infinitesimal point which is the smell tanmatra, from which emerges the germ-mantra Lang of shining yellow colour. The original colour of the matrika-letter is yellow-lightning-like and the colour remains unchanged when it becomes the germ-mantra of supra-smell. When concentration becomes still deeper the bija aspect (that is, la) is transformed into Deity Indra. It is the beginning of concentration-on-divine-form. The Indra-form represents a higher order of powers to the point of most effectiveness and under the control of higher intelligence. The yellow colour of the form indicates that meta-earth and supra-smell (prithiwi mahabhuta and gandha tanmatra) is the predominating factor in the form. This is indicative of power.

Indra's great power is represented in the wajra (a thunderbolt) which he holds in his hand. The great control power has been concentrated in the wajra. Desire in its specific form is the creative desire which culminates in love-desire in which the senses function in relation to pleasurable objects and conative organs cause to heighten the pleasure-feeling and effect the union which is associated with the highest enjoyment. This longing for conjugal pleasure in which the strongest feeling is excited and the full organic cooperation becomes a fact, is an expression of strongest natural energy having a definite mental form and it becomes involved in organic activities at a certain point which is an elaboration of the original desire. From wajra comes the highest control power termed wajroli —the adamantine control, by which sexual energy in its mental and organic forms is fully controlled and transformed into a divine energy which increases the strength of concentration. The adamantine control consists of two main processes: development of reverse organic control and utilization of mental sexual energy in concentration. The apana-control plays an essential role in wajroli.

The fittest persons for the practice of this control are those who are endowed with great sexual vigour which is supported by general physical development. But usually these persons go in for sexual excesses, especially, when their spiritual qualities are in a rudimentary state. The wajra excites fear in them by causing disease and other sufferings. For all unspiritual persons, the wajra is the cause of fear. The sexually weak and physically undeveloped persons are unfit for the practice of adamantine control.

Indra is seated on an elephant. The elephant represents an excellence of physical development and strength. But Indra's elephant is not an ordinary one, it is a white elephant. It indicates that physical development need not impede spiritual growth but harmonizes with spiritual qualities. Indra's white elephant shows the spiritualized physical development. The Kuñjara (elephant)-process has been developed in relation to the white elephant of Indra. It is the process of purification and vitalization of the body. A person with such a development is the fittest person for the practice of adamantine control.

The wajra has other characteristic features. The sound associated with the wajra arises from the transformation of the madhyama sound (suprasound) into the waikhari (audible) sound. This means that the mantra is transformed into the waikhari form by the wajra-power, which is necessary for the practice of mantra. The wajra itself is the manifestation of the bija Lang or Mang. The Lang (or Mang) power is metamorphosed into the form of wajra in the muladhara. The wajra-power has also been manifested by Kundalini, by which she keeps concealed the great fire-energy lying within Swayambhu-linga. The light aspect of the wajra is the spiritual light by which consciousness is illumined. This consciousness becomes so purified and concentrated that the Deity Brahma appears in it and the whole consciousness is brightened by the lustre of Brahma. The Indra-form is derived from the bija Lang in the muladhara. The form can be reduced to Lang. The white elephant of Indra is from the bija Kang or Khang.

Concentration on Brahma

Brahma is one of the six Shiwas (Supreme Being in forms). It has been stated that Brahma,

Wishnu, Rudra, Ishwara, Sadashiwa and Parashiwa are the six Shiwas (—Rudrayamala, Part 2, 25. 53–4; also in the *Shad*amnayatantra, 5. 283–4 and the Gayatritantra, 3.146–7). Beyond the six Shiwas is Parama Shiwa (Supreme Brahman). It has been stated: 'Brahman has three aspects— gross, subtle and Supreme. The five forms (belonging to the five mahabhuta-tanmatras) of Brahman (that is, five Brahmas which are the five Shiwas of the Tantras) are gross and termed wairaja (belonging to Brahman forms). The subtle form is Hiranyagarbha characterized by the primary three bijas with nada (that is, the first mantra Ong). The Supreme Brahman is the ultimate truth, in the nature of consciousness, being and love, immeasurable, undefinable, beyond mind and senses, in itself, attributeless, without form, immutable, untinged, eternal, whole, incomparable and perfect' (—Yogashikhopanishad, 2. 14–17). The Waidika Supreme Brahman is the Tantrika Parama (Supreme) Shiwa. The five forms of Brahmans are the first five Shiwas. Hiranyagarbha is the sixth Shiwa named Parashiwa. The five Brahmans have been named Hiranmaya (Brahma) in the 'earth'-region (in the muladhara), Narayana (Wishnu) in the 'water'-region (in the swadhishthana), Rudra in the 'fire'-region (in the manipura), Ishwara in the 'air'-region (in the anahata), and Sadashiwa in the 'void'-region (in the wishuddha) (—Yogatattwopanishad, 84– 99). So the Waidika terms and the Tantrika terms are identical.

All the Shiwas or Brahmas are the six forms which arise, stage by stage, in concentration. They are the divine forms of Supreme Shiwa, also called Narayana. So it has been stated that Brahma and Shiwa are Narayana (—Tripadwibhutimahanarayanopanishad, 2.16). It has also been stated that Brahma is Narayana (—Kurmapurana, 1.6.3). Narayana is the Supreme Being, and Wishnu, Brahma and Maheswara are the same (—Warahapurana, 70.26). That the (Supreme) Brahman is Brahma, Shiwa and Wishnu has been stated in the Kaiwalyopanishad, Mantra 8. He who is Shiwa is also Hari (Wishnu) and Brahma—Brahman in three forms (—Garudapurana, 1.23.34). This means that Supreme Brahman assumes the forms of Brahma, Wishnu and Rudra.

According to the predominating primary attributes (gunas), the divine forms vary. Sattwa predominates in the Wishnu-form, rajas in the Brahma-form and tamas in the Rudra-form (—Shiwapurana, 1.6.20). Powers associated with Wishnu, Brahma and Rudra are of the same character. Lakshmi, the power of Wishnu, is in the nature of sattwa; Brahmi, the power of Brahma, in that of rajas; and Sati, the power of Rudra, in that of tamas (—ibid, 1.6.21). The rajas, sattwa and tamas attributes influence the mind and its concentration power. In the first stage of concentration rajas, which functions on the sattwa basis, develops the power which makes concentration deep, and consciousness is in the Brahma-form.

The basic aspect of the Brahma-form is the smell principle (gandha tanmatra) which is rarefied yellow in colour. When this aspect is predominant, Brahma appears as of golden (shining yellow) colour. But when the rajas attribute and apana-force predominate Brahma is deep red. In the usual mode of concentration deep red colour is applied. Brahma has four faces, each with three eyes, and four arms. Four faces indicate the four forms of sound: para (the principle of sound), pashyanti (radiant), madhyama (suprasound) and waikhari (audible). The first three forms are inaudible. The two ordinary eyes are the eyes which are endowed with full sensory power and coupled with a highly developed insight. The third eye in the forehead is the concentration-eye which 'sees' things which can only be seen in deep concentration.

Brahma holds in his hands a danda (staff), kamandalu (a sacred water-pot) and akshasutra (a rosary of rudraksha). Danda indicates the power of control exercised by Brahma over the nonconscious impressions (sangskaras) which maintain the body. Kamandalu indicates that the life-force symbolized in water, which is held in it, is under full control, that is, in a state of kumbhaka. Or the kamandalu is the expression of the indu chakra where amrita (life-energy) is reserved, and radiates to reenergize the whole organism in concentration on Brahma. Akshasutra is the sutra (thread) on which a-ksha, that is, the fifty matrika-letters from a to ksha, have been strung; the sutra is that on which all words have been strung; it is Brahman (—Brahmopanishad, 7–9). Also, it is called sutra because it (as Brahman) is within all beings and it awakens the Brahman-form (—Yogashikhopanishad, 2. 10–11). It has been stated that akshamala (the rosary of rudraksha) is in the form of fifty (matrika-) letters from a to ksha (—Guptasadhanatantra, ch. 11, p. 15). The akshasutra indicates the matrika-letters from a to ksha strung by Kundalini. Brahma makes the gesture of dispelling fear. Fearlessness is a spiritual quality. Real fearlessness arises when unspiritual knowledge is removed. Brahma dispels fear from the practitioner by bestowing spiritual strength.

Brahma is seated on the hangsah (swan). Shankara in his commentary on Kathopanishad, 2.2.2, says that he who moves everywhere is hangsah. This means that he who pervades everything is hangsah, that is Supreme Being (Paramatman). So it has been stated that hangsah is within all beings (—Nirwanopanishad, 1.24). Hangsah is without a second (Shwetashwataropanishad, 6.15), so he is Supreme Being. It has been stated clearly that hangsah is Paramatman (—Pashupatabrahmopanishad, Part 1, 13). On commenting on this, Upanishad Brahmayogi says that one who removes the delusion which is in the nature of nonself, by the realization of the true nature of Atman is hangsah. The commentator Narayana also says that he who removes ignorance (unspiritualness) is hangsah (his commentary on Chulikopanishad, Mantra 1).

The garland of letters, that is, fifty matrika-units, is in the form of hangsah who is Shabdabrahman, that is, Kundalini. Shabdabrahman is Ishwara when the matrika-sound-power has been manifested in which time becomes involved. Ishwara is Paramatman. The matrika-sound-power causes the attainment of the wealth of Brahman, that is, samadhi (based on Pashupatabrahmopanishad, Part 2,1). This is the hangsah process of the attainment of samadhi and this has been expounded in a technical Waidika language. So it has been stated that hangsah is the spiritual thread of manojajña (the spiritual process of concentration) (—ibid., Part 1, 17).

Hangsah is also jiwa (embodied being) when he moves in the worldly circle without the recognition of his infinite nature (—Shwetashwataropanishad, 1.6). This mode of existence ceases when the superunion of jiwatman and Paramatman occurs in manojajña (that is, samadhi) (—Pashupatabrahmopanishad, Part 1, 18). The real thread of connection is effected through the five forms of pranayama in which the five pranas are controlled. Jiwa as a conscious being is constantly undergoing changes because his consciousness is oscillating between the four main powers (chatushkala)—sensory, intellective, affective and volitive. These changes are expressed by the functioning of the five pranas as ha-sa movement which is automatic and in which consciousness itself remains unaffected, but it supplies all the power causing its undulatory form. When the normal cessation of respiration occurs, consciousness becomes free from oscillations and in a state of concentration (based on Brahmawidyopanishad, 16–19).

The hangsah-breathing is normal respiration with its rate and depth reduced to an almost imperceptible form by conscious relaxation, general effortlessness and mental calmness. Under this condition of breathing, concentration develops. Hangsah is here hangsah breathing as the basis for concentration on Brahma.

From the mantra viewpoint, Brahma is reducible to the matrika-letters kang, mang and kshang, and the bija-mantras Ong and Kang; danda to the mantra Namah; kamandalu to thang; and akshasutra to all matrika-letters from ang to kshang.

Concentration on Power Dakini

The power (shakti) of the Supreme Being is Supreme Power who is eternal and always with and in the being of Supreme Consciousness. Sometimes she is awakened and sometimes she is unroused. In one of her aspects, she is Shabdabrahman, and in another aspect she is beyond it. At times she manifests her specific 'powerhood', at other times she is tranquil. She is omnipotent. She manifests her conscious power (ichchashakti) in three forms: yogashakti (the samadhi-power), bhogashakti (the power involved in world-experience) and wirashakti (the heroic power). In samadhi-power one is able to reduce consciousness into the supreme form in *asamprajñata samadhi*. Bhogashakti is that power which operates when there is awareness of the outer world. In the spiritual practice of the eight-fold yoga, and in worship and other religious activities this power is fully operative. It is also operative in the activities of daily life and all humanitarian actions done with the purpose of pleasing God. Wirashakti is the power of formalization by which Shakti (Power) manifests herself in form. Shakti in form is endowed with eight superpowers (*aishwarya*) (—based on *Sitopanishad*, 34–7).

Shakti appears in many forms. In the chakras, there are six main forms. They are in the six chakras from the muladhara to the ajña. They are called Dakini, Rakini, Lakini, Kakini, Shakini, and Hakini (—*Shadamnayatantra*, 6. 261–2). They are the presiding Divinities of the chakras, that is, the chakras are fully controlled by them. They are also called the doorkeepers. They exercise their power for the selection of qualified practitioners who are able to practise in the chakras.

Power Dakini is situated in the muladhara. Her fierce appearance and weapons excite fear in man who is not spiritually prepared. The drinking vessel in her hand stimulates thirst for drinking and appetite for food. But the food and drink which man takes cannot prevent death. It is indicated in the skulled staff. While living, he often expresses a feeling of harmfulness because he is unable to love others, and the sword and trident are used as destructive weapons. But a practitioner with well-developed spiritual qualities sees in the drinking vessel deathless substance (*amrita*) which can be made to flow within him by deep concentration, and he proceeds towards immortality in spite of the death of the body as indicated in the skulled staff. The sword is the spiritual knowledge which destroys all mundaneness. The trident removes three forms of pain—pain arising in the body, pain caused by outside influences and pain from the invisible source. Concentration on Dakini develops spiritual qualities.

Dakini is reducible to her germ-mantra Dang, the mantra Khphreng, and the matrika-letters

ong, oung, *ah* and phang; the sword to the germmantra khang, and the trident to the matrika-letter oung.

Yoni in muladhara

Yoni is a triangular process, being formed by the triangular kandarpa-energy which is an aspect of the apana-force, and is shining deep red in colour. The mantra-form of this energy is kl*ing*. The nature of the energy is of fire which, when aroused, is expressed as love-feeling associated with the intense desire for enjoyment. The kandarpa-energy is always in motion, but its activities are intense when it is brought to the conscious level, and the whole apana system is accelerated by them. The triangular energy is associated with the three-fold controlprocess termed yonimudra—genito-control. It consists of three factors: (a) ano-genital contraction in which anal-lock develops into genitallock, (b) abdominoretraction, and (c) breathsuspension with chin-lock. Apana-force, including kandarpa-energy, is controlled by yonimudra. For deep concentration on Kundalini, it is very important for neutralizing the kandarpa-energy motions, which is effected by yonimudra. Yonimudra is also an important part of the process for rousing Kundalini. Moreover, it is the first step towards the practice of wajroli—adamantine control.

Swayambhu-linga and concentration

Shankara in commenting on Swayambhu (*Kathopanishad*, 2.1.1) says that Swayambhu is Parameshwara (Supreme Being) who always exists by himself—independently, never dependent on another. Swayambhu is the Supreme Being, and also the name of Brahma, Wishnu and Shiwa (—*Wachaspatyam*). So Swayambhu is he who exists always by himself, without depending on another or anything else—the eternal self-existing being, that is, the Supreme Being. In the triangle of the muladhara Swayambhu is in the linga-form.

The term linga has been used here in a technical sense. It has been stated: 'It is that which is called linga because it is subtle, it is the source (of everything), it is that into which all is absorbed, it is also motional, and it is a (specific)

form (for the realization) of the Supreme Being'
(—Yogashikhopanishad, 2.9–10). The linga
is a specific manifestation of Supreme Being,
subtle in character, endowed with omnipotency,
which in concentration becomes, step by step,
reduced from a subtle line-form to a subtle
bindu (point) when its motional aspect disappears, and into which all cosmic principles
are absorbed. The power aspect associated with
the linga is Kundalini which gives it a form
because of her coils around it, and this form is
most suitable for concentration. The nada
(suprasound) aspect of the linga is aroused and
'heard' as pranawa which are the coils of Kundalini, and the pranawa-concentration to its highest
point causes the uncoiling of Kundalini.

That the linga is the Supreme Being and in his
subtle aspect is realized by the yogis in concentration has been stated: 'The linga which bestows
all good and bliss is luminous, imperishable,
perfect and omnipresent, and is established
in the hearts of yogis' (—Shiwapurana, 1.26.14).
It has also been stated in the Skandapurana
that akasha (void) is called linga the base of
which is the earth and is the abode of the dewas
(deities) and into which everything is absorbed.
Here the akasha is the chidakasha. The chidakasha is what is undefiled as the akasha, and
the support of all—the Brahman (—Wachaspatyam). The base of the linga (Swayambhu-
linga) is the 'earth'-region in the muladhara
where lie Deities and Powers. Swayambhu-
linga is always with Kundalini in the muladhara,
and when Kundalini is roused all Deities and
Powers and cosmic principles are absorbed
into her.

It has been stated: 'The linga is of two kinds,
outer and inner. The outer linga is material,
the inner is subtle and bright. Those who are
devoted to religious rites worship the linga
of material forms. Those who are unprepared
take the gross form of the linga to be able to
concentrate on the subtle linga. One who is
unable to "see" the spiritual (adhyatmika) linga
should think of the subtle linga in the gross
forms. The subtle, shining and immutable
linga is "seen" by those who possess the knowledge (arising from concentration). The gross
linga made of earth, wood and other materials

is for those who have no such knowledge'
(—Shiwapurana, 1.26. 15–18). The real linga
is subtle and luminous and is 'seen' inside by
deep concentration. When a practitioner has
not the power of deep concentration, he will
have to take the gross linga for worship and the
thought-form of the gross linga for developing
concentration. So it has been said that the
worship of Swayambhu-linga develops (con-
centration-) knowledge by itself (—ibid, 2.16.34).

There is a void aspect (chidra) of Swayambhu-
linga where lies the great fire-energy which
becomes activated by prana-force by pranayamic
suspension. The entrance is guarded by Kundalini when in coils. This state maintains the ida-
pingala flows which effect respiration (based
on Todalatantra, ch. 8, p. 16). When the fire-
energy is released by pranayama, it plays an
important role in arousing Kundalini. It has
been stated: 'So long Kundalini and Swayambhu
are in an unroused state in the muladhara, no
spiritual work should be done. . . . That divine
Kundalini and that Divine Being (Swayambhu-
linga) who is the Supreme Being are roused
by pranayama and assume the wished for forms'
(—Tripurasaratantra, quoted in Sarwollasatantra, 15. 15–16). When the fire-force is ignited
by pranayama both Swayambhu-linga and
Kundalini are aroused.

The concentration-form of Swayambhu-linga is
diagrammatic. It has been stated that Shiwa-
linga is in the form of the diagram consisting
of a, u, ma, nada and bindu, and is surrounded
by pranawa from which arises the nada (pranawa-
sound) and thereafter it is absorbed (—Shiwapurana, 3.10. 14–16). The bright subtle line
which emerges from the Supreme Bindu assumes
the pranawa-form and emits pranawa-sound.
In the muladhara, the pranawa-form is the coils
of Kundalini around the bright line which is
Swayambhu-linga. By concentration, pranawa
is enlivened and the mantra-sound appears.
By deeper concentration the mantra-sound is
absorbed into Kundalini and she is then roused
along with Swayambhu-linga.

Concentration on Kundalini
After a practitioner is well prepared by con-
centration-on-Brahma, he can undertake con-

centration-on-Kundalini. The first stage is the concentration-on-form. The concentration-on-form of Kundalini is of red colour like the rising sun in the morning. When the form is clear and well established in consciousness by repeated and long practices, the red colour should be thought of as very bright. At first, the face should be thought of as very bright and gradually the whole body. Then the red form should get slowly absorbed in the shining red colour and finally there will be no form, but only the red light. Now Kundalini is in the form of red light.

The next step is to transform Kundalini, who is in the red light form, to the lightning-like splendorous form. Now Kundalini has no shape, but is only in her splendorous form. The practitioner is advised to see, in the lightning-like brightness the formless subtle Kundalini in concentration. There will be more and more perception of her subtleness through her brilliant lustre. These forms of concentration should be done in the muladhara.

In another of her aspects, Kundalini is situated in the brahma nadi and extends from the muladhara to the sahasrara, and is supremely subtle and in the nature of force (—Wishwasaratantra, ch. 2, p. 12). Concentration should be done on this supremely subtle Kundalini in the brahma nadi who extends from the muladhara to the sahasrara. To be able to accomplish this advanced concentration, the practitioner is advised to do the following forms of concentration:

1 (a) Concentration on Fire (Wahni)-Kundalini who is shining red like the molten gold in the muladhara.
(b) Concentration on Fire-Kundalini who is situated from the muladhara to the bottom of the anahata.
2 (a) Concentration on Sun (Surya)-Kundalini who is splendorous like many suns at a time, in the anahata.
(b) Concentration on Sun-Kundalini from the anahata to the Swadhishthana.
3 (a) Concentration on Moon (Chandra)-Kundalini who is lustrous like many moons at a time and in the form of amrita (deathless substance), in the ajña.

(b) Concentration on Moon-Kundalini, situated from the ajña to the end of brahmarandhra.
4 Concentration on Turya (the fourth aspect)-Kundalini who is only spiritual consciousness, in the sahasrara.

After the practice of all these forms of concentration, bhutashuddhi-concentration should be undertaken. After it is accomplished, the process of arousing Kundalini should be practised. At first, the mantra should be aroused according to the instructions of a guru. Then, the arousing of Kundalini should be practised. The roused Kundalini then goes to the sahasrara after absorbing all principles lying in the chakras, where samprajñata samadhi is attained. At this stage, consciousness is only in the form of Kundalini. When this stage is fully established, the Kundalini-consciousness is coiled into Kundalini when she alone shines in Supreme Consciousness and finally is absorbed into it in asamprajñata samadhi.

2 Swadhishthana

The swadhishthana is the second chakra, lying above the muladhara in the chitrini nadi.

Terminology

The following are the Tantrika terms of the second chakra.
1 Swadhishthana, mentioned in the Nilatantra, ch. 5, p. 9; Todalatantra, ch. 7, p. 14; ch. 9, p. 17; Kamadhenutantra, ch. 13, p. 16; Kankalamalinitantra, ch. 2, p. 4; Kularnawa, ch. 4, p. 19; Jñanasankalinitantra, verse 67; Gandharwatantra, ch. 5, p. 27; Mantramahodadhi, 4.21; Kubjikatantra, 6. 289; Tripurasarasamuchchaya, 5.11; Bhutashuddhitantra, ch. 1, p. 2; ch. 3, p. 3; ch. 4, p. 4; ch. 5, pp. 4,5; ch. 8, p. 8; ch. 10, p. 9; ch. 14, p. 12; Sammohanatantra, part 2, ch. 2, p. 2; ch. 4, p. 4; Mayatantra, ch. 6, p. 5; Purashcharanarasollasa, ch. 2, p. 2; Wishwasaratantra, ch. 1, p. 10;

Mundamalatantra, ch. 6, p. 9; Sharadatilaka-tantra, 5.131; Shaktanandatarangini, 4.11,29, 30, 34; 9.16; Rudrayamala, part 2, 15.35; 22.4; 25.55; 27.57,58; 37.14,35; 44.20,21; Maha-nirwanatantra, 5.94; Tantrarajatantra, 21.82; Purashcharyarnawa, ch. 2, p. 90; ch. 5, p. 387; ch. 6, p. 490; Shaktisangamatantra, 61.114; Shadamnayatantra, 5.262;423; Shiwasanghita, 5.106,107,213; Mridanitantra (quoted in Amarasanggraha MS); Goutamiyatantra, 34.44; and Shatchakranirupana, verse 18.

2 Adhishthana, mentioned in Sammohana-tantra, Part 2, ch. 2, p. 2; and Koulawalitantra, ch. 22, p. 80.

3 Bhima, mentioned in Nirwanatantra, ch. 5, p.6.

4 Shatpatra (lotus with six petals), mentioned in Todalatantra, ch. 9, p. 16; Sammohana-tantra, Part 2, ch. 4, p. 4; Gandharwatantra, ch. 8, p. 39; Shaktanandatarangini, 7.14.

5 Shaddala padma (lotus with six petals), mentioned in Tararahasya, ch. 4, p. 22; Rudraya-mala, Part 2, 45.6; 60.28.

6 Wari-chakra (chakra containing 'water'-principle), mentioned in Rudrayamala, Part 2, 21.97, 107,112,113.

Position

The swadhishthana is situated in the genital region, when considered externally. As the chakras are in the chitrini, and the chitrini is within the sushumna as the third nadi, and the sushumna is within the vertebral column, so the swadhishthana is within that part of the vertebral column which corresponds to the genital region. That the swadhishthana is situated in the genital region has been stated in the Shatchakranirupana, Verse 14; Jñanasankalini-tantra, Verse 67; Gandharwatantra, ch. 8, p. 39; Sammohanatantra, Part 2, ch. 2, p. 2; Wishwasaratantra, ch. 1, pp. 8,10; Koulawali-tantra, ch. 3, p. 8; Shaktanandatarangini, 7.14; Mahanirwanatantra, 5.114; Mridanitantra (quoted in Amarasanggraha MS), and in all other Tantras. That the position of the swadhishthana is in the genital region has also been mentioned in the Waidika as well as in the Pouranika accounts.

Description

The swadhishthana (Plate 4) has six petals (—Shatchakranirupana, Verse 14; and in all Tantras and in the Waidika and Pouranika accounts). The colour of the petals is vermilion-red (—Shatchakranirupana, Verse 14; Kankala-malinitantra, ch. 2, p. 5; Nirwanatantra, ch. 5, p. 7; Shiwasanghita, 5.106; Mridanitantra, quoted in Amarasanggraha MS). The colour has also been stated to be fire-like red (—Gandharwa-tantra, ch. 5, p. 27; Rudrayamala, Part 2, 27.56; Goutamiyatantra, 34.43), lightning-like (—Bhutashuddhitantra, ch. 1, p. 2), lustrous red (—Sammohanatantra, Part 2, ch. 2, p. 2); whitish red (—Tararahasya, ch. 4, p. 22); and deep-red (—Koulawalitantra, ch. 22, p. 80). In the Parwati-Parameshwara-sangwada (—dia-logue) (quoted by Narayana in his commentary on the mantra 10 of Hangsopanishad), it has been stated that the colour is of gold.

On the petals are the letters from ba to la with bindu (that is, nada-bindu—the matrika-letters) (—Shatchakranirupana, Verse 14, and in all Tantras and Pouranika accounts). The matrika-letters are arranged from right to left. The colour of the matrika-letters is like that of lightning (—Shatchakranirupana, Verse 14). It has also been stated that the colour is diamond-like white (—Gandharwatantra, ch. 5, p. 27; Rudrayamala, Part 2, 27. 56–57; Goutamiya-tantra, 34. 43–44); white (—Bhutashuddhi-tantra, ch. 1, p. 2); and vermilion-red (—Koula-walitantra, ch. 22, p. 80). It has been stated in the Pouranika accounts that the matrika-letters are of a diamond-white colour.

There are six specific qualities (writtis) on the six petals of the swadhishthana. They are: affection (or indulgence), pitilessness, feeling of all-destructiveness, delusion, disdain and suspicion (—Adhyatma Wiweka, quoted by Narayana in his commentary on Hangsopanishad, Mantra 7). They are arranged in the above order from right to left. Jaganmohana (Footnote 87, in connection with the verse 104, Maha-nirwanatantra) gives the following order: affec-tion, suspicion, disdain, delusion, feeling of all-destructiveness and pitilessness.

Within the swadhishthana (that is, inside the

pericarp of the swadhi*shth*ana) is the half-moon-shaped 'water'-region of Waru*n*a of white'colour and inside it lies the b*i*ja Wa*ng* which is moon-white and seated on a m*a*kara (kind of alligator) (—*Shat*chakranirupana, Verse 15). It has been stated that in the pericarp of the swadhi*shth*ana is situated (Deity) Waru*n*a (—Ka*n*kalamalini-t*a*ntra, ch. 2, p. 5). This means that Waru*n*a, who is in the form of the b*i*ja mantra Wa*ng*, lies in the 'water'-region which is situated in the pericarp of the swadhi*shth*ana. That the watery Waru*n*a-b*i*ja (Wa*ng*) is within this chakra has been stated in the Sammohanatantra, Part 2, ch. 2, p. 2. The Waru*n*a-b*i*ja which is within the Waru*n*a-region has four arms and is seated on makara (—Mri*d*anitantra, quoted in Amara-sanggraha MS). The Waru*n*a-b*i*ja has the pasha (noose) in its hand (—the passage quoted by Kal*i*charana). That the semilunar 'water'-region is within the pericarp of the swadhi*shth*ana has been stated in the Wa*i*dika accounts (—Yoga-shikhopani*sh*a*d*, 1. 176; 5.13). In the Poura*n*ika accounts, it has been stated that the 'water'-region is half-moon-shaped and white and en-closes the b*i*ja Wa*ng* (—De*v*ibhag*a*wata, 11.8.4).

The b*i*ja aspect of Wa*ng* is Deity Waru*n*a, that is, from the b*i*ja wa arises Waru*n*a. There is no distinction between the b*i*ja and the form. Waru*n*a is in the form of Wa*ng* as well as in divine form. The concentration form of Waru*n*a is as follows:

Waru*n*a is white in colour; he has four arms and is seated on m*a*kara; he holds the pasha (noose) in one of his hands.

Wi*shn*u

In the lap of the b*i*ja Wa*ng* (that is in the lap of Deity Waru*n*a who is in the form of Wa*ng*) is Hari (a name of Wi*shn*u—Sh*a*bdakalp*a*drum*ah* and Wach*a*spatyam), who is bright dark-blue (or black) (n*i*la), graceful, youthful and pleasing; he has four arms and is dressed in yellow raiment; he wears shri*w*atsa (a mark on the chest of Wi*shn*u) and koustubha (the celebrated gem worn by Wi*shn*u on his chest) (—*Shat*chakra-nirupana, Verse 16).

Kal*i*charana explains 'in the lap' (a*n*ke) to mean within the bindu which is on the top of the b*i*ja. As Brahma arises from the bindu of

Lang, so Wi*shn*u appears from the bindu of Wang in deep concentration. It has been stated that above the Waru*n*a-b*i*ja (that is, Wa) is the great li*ng*a in the form of Wi*shn*u (—Sam-mohanatantra, Part 2, ch. 2, p. 2). This indicates that Wi*shn*u in the li*ng*a-form is within the bindu of the Wang and emerges from the bindu as Wi*shn*u in deep concentration. The presence of Wi*shn*u has also been mentioned in Rudraya-m*a*la, Part 2, 22.4; Sharadatilakatantra, 5.132; Mri*d*anitantra, quoted in Amarasanggraha MS; Mantramahodadhi, 4.20; To*d*alatantra, ch. 7, p. 14; and *Sh*adamnayatantra, 5. 262–3. Wi*shn*u has been described as the presiding Deity of the swadhi*shth*ana (—Yogashikhopani*sh*ad, 1.176; 5.13).

Kal*i*charana quotes a verse from another T*a*ntra in which it has been stated that Hari (Wi*shn*u), who is in the lap of him who holds the noose in his hand (that is, Waru*n*a), is dark-blue (or black) (shyam*a*) and dressed in yellow raiment and has four arms, and holds a sha*n*kha (conch), chakra (wheel), g*a*da (mace) and padma (lotus) in his hands. The Nirwa*n*atantra (ch. 5, p. 7) says that Wi*shn*u is four-armed, dressed in yellow raiment, adorned with w*a*na-mala (a large garland of flowers of all seasons) and tranquil in appearance.

In the form of Naraya*n*a (an epithet of Wi*shn*u —Wach*a*spatyam, Shabdakalpadrumah, Apte) for concentration, he has been described as holding a conch, wheel and mace (—Atma-prabodhopani*sh*ad, 1.2).

In the commentary on this m*a*ntra, Ganga-charana (Ga*n*gacharana Bhattacharya Wedanta-widyasagara, the commentator of this Upani*sh*ad) quotes a verse from Wi*shn*usanghita which says: Wi*shn*u wears a crown, jewelled ear-rings, shri*w*atsa (a curl)-mark on his chest, and a large garland of flowers of all seasons (w*a*na-mala), he is pleasing in appearance and holds (in his hands) a conch, a wheel, a mace and a lotus, and the world is at his feet.

The dhyana-form of Naraya*n*a as Kri*sh*na is as follows: he is in the fully blown eight-petalled h*ri*t-lotus; his feet are marked with the divine ensign and umbrella, and the shri*w*atsa mark is on his chest, the koustubh*a*-gem on his breast; he wears armlets, a garland (w*a*namala), a crown, bracelets and makara-shaped earrings; he has four arms and holds a conch, a wheel, the sharnga-bow, a lotus and a mace; he is of golden colour, serene, and makes his devotees free from fear. Or concentration can be done on Krishna holding a flute and a horn (that is two-armed) (—Gopalatapinyupanishad, Part 2, 46–9). It is stated that Wishnu as Krishna has two arms and holds the flute (—Nirwanatantra, ch. 5, p. 7). Bhutashuddhitantra (ch. 9, p. 8) says that Hari (Wishnu) is dark-blue (or black) in colour, dressed in yellow raiment, wears the wanamala, the crown, earrings, the shriwatsa-mark, the koustubha-gem, a necklace of jewels and anklets; he has long arms, bright eyes and a kindly disposed face and grants boons.

From the above accounts, the concentration form of Wishnu emerges as follows.

Wishnu is shining dark-blue (or black) in colour, graceful, youthful and serene; he has four arms, and holds in his hands a conch, wheel, mace and lotus, and also the sharnga-bow; he is dressed in yellow raiment and wears shriwatsa-mark and the koustubha-gem on his breast and wanamala on his neck; he is ornamented with the crown, jewelled earrings, anklets; he has bright eyes and is kindly disposed, and he grants boons.

The colour of Wishnu has been generally accepted as dark-blue or black (—Shatchakranirupana, Verse 16; Bhutashuddhitantra, ch. 9, p. 8). In the Waidika form of concentration, Wishnu has been described as of dark-blue or black colour (—Waidika Sandhya-widhi). The colour of Wishnu is also golden (—Gopalatapinyupanishad, Part 2, 49), crystal-white (—Garudapurana, Part 1, 30.11), moon-white (—ibid., Part 1, 31.10; Skandapurana, 1.1.1.1; Mahabharata, 12.332.66); and white (—Mahabharata, 12.272, 28). It has been stated that the colour of Wishnu changes according to yuga (an age of the world—Apte). In the Satya-age, Wishnu is white, in the Treta-age he is red, in the Dwapara-age he is yellow, and in the Kali-age he is black (—Warahapurana, 3.18). A Waidika dhyana form of Narayana (Wishnu) is as follows: He is four-armed, has the colour of pure crystal, wears a crown and is dressed in yellow raiment (—Yoga-

tattwopanishad, 89–90).

Kalicharana says that we should think of Wishnu as seated on garuda, as we have seen that Brahma is seated on the hangsah in the muladhara. It is not necessary to infer this as we find in the Waidika concentration-form that Wishnu is seated on garuda (—Waidika Sandhya-widhi).

It has been stated that it is the Power of Wishnu that maintains, but not Wishnu, so he is as if a corpse (—Kubjikatantra, 1. 26–7). This indicates that the power of Wishnu is Wishnu himself, and therefore the form of his power is the form of Wishnu. So it has been stated that Sawitri (as Power of Wishnu) has the same form as Wishnu (—Rigweda Sandhya-process), and Sawitri is in the form of Wishnu (—Samaweda Sandhya-process). The concentration-form of Sawitri is as follows: Sawitri is of black colour, four-armed, three-eyed, holding a conch, wheel, mace and lotus, youthful, seated on the garuda, the Power of Wishnu and in the form of Wishnu (—Yayurweda Sandhya-process). From this form we have to infer that Wishnu also has three eyes. (For the concentration-form of Wishnu, see Plate 5, left top figure.)

Rakini

Rakini, who is always in the swadhishthana, is of the colour of a blue lotus (that is, dark blue) and holds various instruments in her four hands; she is dressed in splendid raiment and adorned with ornaments, beautiful and delightful (—Shatchakranirupana, Verse 17).

The presence of Rakini in the swadhishthana has been mentioned in the Kankalamalinitantra, ch. 2, p. 5; Shiwasanghita, 5.106; Rudrayamala, Part 2, 22.4; Mantramahodadhi, 4.20; and Todalatantra, ch. 7, p. 14. Rakini is Kundali (—Rudrayamala, Part 2, 42.1). This means that Rakini is one of the forms of Kundali, and consequently, other Powers, situated in different chakras, are also forms of Kundalini. It has also been stated that Power Rakini is the door-keeper of the Swadhishthana (—Sammohanatantra, Part 2, ch. 2, p. 2).

Other concentration-forms of Rakini are as follows.

Rakini who is red in colour, two-armed and

fawn-eyed is shining with the vermilion-red-mark on her forehead, her eyes are gracefully painted with collyrium, she is dressed in white raiment and adorned with various ornaments, and her face is as beautiful as the moon (—Kankalamalinitantra, ch. 5, p. 23).

Divine Rakini is dark-blue (or black) in colour and adorned with various ornaments, and holds a sword and a shield (—Kularnawa, ch. 10, p. 53).

Rakini is dark-blue (or black) in colour, and holds in her hands a spear (or trident), the wajra (thunderbolt), a lotus and a drum (—Koulawalitantra, ch. 22, p. 80).

Rakini is dark-blue (or black) in colour, holds in her hands a spear (or trident), a lotus, a drum and a sharp chisel (or axe); she is power-ful and has three red eyes and prominent teeth; the great, lustrous, divine Rakini is seated on a double lotus (—the verse quoted by Kalicharana).

Kalicharana says that it is to be understood, by seeing Rakini seated on a lotus here, that all six Powers everywhere are seated on red lotuses. (For concentration-form of Rakini, see Plate 5, right top figure.)

Explanation

The petaline processes of the swadhishthana are the processes of the radiations of energies from the central aspect of the chakra into the ida-pingala power-flows. The colour of the swadhishthana-petals is generally vermilion-red. This indicates that there is a mixture of red-radiations of apana with the golden-radiations of wyana. It also indicates that apana radiates in a more concentrated form, while wyana-radiations are less concentrative and slower in character. When the petals become red and deep red, it indicates greater concentration of apana-radiations. The wyana-radiations pre-dominate when the petals are of a golden colour. The whitish-red colour of the petals indicates the white-radiations of samana in combination with the red-radiations of apana.

The matrika-letters are the measures of the power-concentration in the petals. There are six petals as there are six main radiations from the central aspect of the swadhishthana. The matrika-letters are bang, bhang, mang, yang, rang and lang. Their colour is white. They are indicators of the basic ap-mahabhuta power lying within the swadhishthana. The original colour-radiation of bang is moon-white, of bhang and mang shining red, of yang smoke colour, of rang red-lightning colour, and of lang yellow-lightning colour. The original colours of the matrika-letters, except bang, have been changed into white in the swadhishthana-petals. They are influenced by the ap-mahabhuta power.

Petaline Concentration
The six-lettered mantra bang-bhang-mang-yang-rang-lang, with gaps between, will be transform-ed by japa in combination with thought-con-centration into a gapless conjoint mantra which is a swadhishthana-concentration-unit. At this stage the petaline concentration is in the form of a circular ring of vermilion-red colour with the diamond-white conjoint matrika-mantra. When this is successfully done, the power-radiation outwards ceases in concentration.

Mahabhuta-concentration
The first stage is the thought-concentration on ap-mahabhuta in the form of the half-moon-shaped region of white colour. When concentra-tion is very deep this 'water'-region is 'seen' as a white half-moon.

Tanmatra-concentration
When concentration becomes still deeper the white half-moon is reduced to an infinitesimal point which is rasa-tanmatra and is represented by the germ-mantra Wang of white colour.

Dewata-concentration
When concentration on Wang is very deep, Deity Waruna emerges from the bija aspect. Waruna is 'seen' seated on a makara, white in colour, and is holding the pasha (noose). Makara represents immense power operable in the watery medium. In the body, the makara-power operates to maintain circulation at the action and inaction levels in a most efficient manner. Therefore, it plays a most important role in circulatory

development and maintains general health and efficiency of the body in action, relaxation and mental concentration.

Makara also represents sexual vigour, essentially based on endocrine development. The gonadal development is brought about by general and local blood-movements induced by the makara-process. The process comprises general muscular movements, pelvic muscular movements, voluntary muscular relaxation and inactivity, blood purification and mental control of the sex urge. The purificatory and control aspects are indicated by the white colour of the makara.

From the spiritual viewpoint the makara is reducible to the matrika-unit tang. The five prana-powers are aroused and controlled to effect better functioning of the various organs of the body which are controlled by these powers. The circulatory function is improved by wyana-control and the sexual function is developed by apana-control. The dewata aspect of the matrika-unit is aroused in the form of Deity Waruna in yellow-lightning-like radiation.

Waruna, Consciousness-Power in a divine form (dewata), has full control over the 'water'-principle (ap-mahabhuta and rasa-tanmatra), the medium through which the five prana-forces exhibit their functional activities. This subtle 'water' in its essence is amrita—the deathless substance, and in its gross form is blood and various external and internal secretions. So, it is the life-substance, and its controlling power is Waruna. The full creative energy of the life-substance has been imparted to gonadal secretions. The sex impulse and gonadal activities are intertwined with the affective impulse. The uncontrolled expression of sex and associated affective impulses is due to the functioning of the life-force when it is without the spiritual basis. Under this condition, the spiritual nature of a living being remains unroused and Waruna's pasha (noose) becomes operative. The pasha is the primary bondage causing the mind to be fettered by unspiritual pasha-qualities—disgust, bashfulness, fear, sleepiness (or sorrow, or anger), slander, certain family characteristics and the notion and distinction of the race and class. The release from the bondage is only possible by concentra-

tion on Waruna, which finally transmutes the pasha into the form of matrika-unit ang.

Ang is white in colour. By concentration, the control over the five prana-forces is increased through the release of Kundali-power, and consequently pranayama develops. Then Deity Wishnu, associated with this bija, begins to be awakened. However, at this stage, concentration is directed to Wang, and when it becomes very deep, Wishnu is roused from the bindu aspect of Wang.

In deep concentration Wishnu is 'seen' as the shining dark blue (or black) divine form with four arms, holding a conch, wheel, mace and lotus, and seated on the garuda. Wishnu is the Supreme Being into whom all dewas (divine beings in form) enter (—Atharwashikhopanishad, 2.2). This means all divine beings and everything else are absorbed into Wishnu, and only he remains, and nothing else. When the universe and all beings are not absorbed, all are pervaded by Wishnu (—Nrisinghatapanyupanishad, 2.5.2). The word Wishnu is derived from wisha, and which means pervasion (—Wachaspatyam). Wishnu is endowed with the essence of all powers (wirya) (—Nrisinghatapanyupanishad, 2.5.9). By his power, the universe is maintained. He is also the source of the highest spiritual power.

The dark blue (or black) colour of Wishnu indicates that in concentration all forms are absorbed into Wishnu and only he remains, and he appears vast. When Wishnu is 'seen' through the original colour of Wang, he is shining like lightning in yellow colour; his white colour is from Wang as the bija of the 'water'-principle in the swadhishthana. When wyana-force predominates, he is of golden colour and when samana-force and sattwa-quality predominates he is of white colour. In the specific Tantrika forms of concentration, Wishnu's colour has been described as of molten gold, and also of many suns rising at the same time, that is, shining red (—Tantrasara, ch. 2, p. 155). Apana-force and rajas-quality predominate in Wishnu when he is red in colour. When Wishnu is seen as crystal white, he is in the form of purest sattwa, and from this state he becomes formless.

The shankha (conch), chakra (wheel), gada (mace) and padma (lotus) held by Wishnu indicate that he is the supporter of the universe. The shankha is the principle of 'void' (akasha) with which sound is intrinsically related. The chakra is the principle of 'air', gada is the principle of 'fire', padma of 'water', and the 'earth'-principle is in his feet. So Wishnu maintains all the cosmic principles. From the specific viewpoint, the shankha indicates the creative I-ness of five cosmic principles, and each principle is expressed by its bija-mantra—Hang ('void'-principle), Yang ('air'-principle), Rang ('fire'-principle), Wang ('water'-principle), and Lang ('earth'-principle). The shankha of Wishnu is called panchajanya, because it expresses the five cosmic principles by their appropriate mantra-sounds. Shankha in a general way expresses happiness. The chakra indicates the most powerful mind which is fully controlled by Wishnu. More technically, chakra is consciousness. The immense power of consciousness, when uncontrolled, is constantly radiating like spokes which support the rim—the range of diversified consciousness. When the radiated spokes are concentrated to the nave, consciousness is single-pointed and in a state of concentration where God as Wishnu endowed with yoga-power, religion, glory, wealth, passionlessness and knowledge is held and 'seen'. It is the 'seeing' of what is worthy to be seen. So, Wishnu's chakra is called sudarshana.

Gada (mace) is the spiritual knowledge based on the matrika-sounds arising from Kundali-power. Gada is also spiritualized intelligence having immense power. Wishnu's gada is called koumodaki, because he is the source of happiness due to his power of maintaining the world. It is also called koumodi. However, gada destroys unspirituality by spiritual knowledge. Padma (lotus) is the heart-lotus, by concentration made living and in full bloom, in which lies the Supreme Being in divine form. Padma also indicates the universe supported by Wishnu; and the practitioner acquires the true knowledge of the world through deep concentration on it. The sharnga-dhanu (bow) of Wishnu indicates the process of concentration. The koustubha-gem of Wishnu is Atman, pure without qualities and beyond mind-matter which is the real being of Wishnu. The shriwatsa-mark indicates

primus, supported by Wishnu. The wanamala (a garland of flowers of all seasons) is the maya-power which shows the diversified universe. Maya controls all beings, but it is fully controlled by Wishnu and is held round his neck as the garland. All these phenomena are experienced by a practitioner in deep concentration on Wishnu.

Garuda (name of the king of birds) is the concentrated wayu-power developed from the highest form of kumbhaka (breath-suspension) which is under full control of Wishnu. The garuda-process is the pranayamic process which develops the power of suspension to the highest point when the body levitates. So the garuda stage is the highest stage of kumbhaka. It indicates two forms of practice; one is the development of concentration through kumbhaka, adopted in hathayoga; the other is the achievement of natural kumbhaka through concentration, adopted in layayoga. Either concentration-on-Wishnu can be developed by the garuda-process; or deep concentration-on-Wishnu effects natural kumbhaka. There are also two practices which have been developed from the garuda-process: the uddiyana-control which is an important factor in pranayama, and garudasana, a posture for developing the power of maintaining physical stillness in concentration.

From the mantra viewpoint, shankha (conch) is reducible to the matrika-sound shang, chakra (wheel) to ing or lang, gada (mace) to bang, padma (lotus) to ing, thang and garuda to khang or the bija kshing.

Concentration on Rakini

For spiritual purification and increased power of concentration, concentration should be done on Power Rakini. The most suitable colour for increasing internal calmness and concentration is darkblue which is the colour of Rakini. More concentration should be done on her face which is very beautiful and shining. If, in concentration, one-pointedness deviates owing to other thoughts, her three eyes become red, teeth are shown and she appears as frightful. She should be realized in her beauty and power. Her red eyes indicate the sun which is the knowledge by which the outer objects are known. Her face is like the moon. The moon is mind. When the mind is in concentration the sun is separated from the moon due to the absorption of the worldly knowledge. Her beautiful moon-like face is the expression of the highest power of concentration. If the practitioner deviates while concentrating on her face, he is spiritually not quite purified.

Her trident indicates three forms of control— control of prana-forces by pranayama, control of senses by pratyahara, and control of mind by dharana. These control exercises are absolutely necessary for deep concentration. The lotus is the hrit-lotus opened by deep concentration. The drum (damaru) signifies the nada (the silent suprasound) through which Shabdabrahman manifests. The sound of the drum is heard in deconcentration. The chisel (tanka) removes the deeply seated unspiritual qualities. Rakini is 'seen' in concentration in the enlivened hrit-lotus.

Rakini is reducible to the mantra-form Eng. The bija-mantra of Rakini is Rang. The trishula (trident) can be reduced to Oung, abja (lotus) to Sang, Aing, and Drang, damaru (drum) to Khang, and tanka (chisel) to Tang.

3 Manipura

The manipura is the third chakra, above the swadhishthana, and lies in the chitrini nadi.

Terminology

The following are the Tantrika terms of the third chakra.

1 Manipura, mentioned in the Todalatantra, ch. 7, p. 14; ch. 9, p. 17; Matrikabhedatantra, ch. 2, p. 2; Kamadhenutantra, ch. 13, p. 16; Gandharwatantra, ch. 5, p. 27; Kubjikatantra, 5.267; 6. 294; Bhutashuddhitantra, ch. 1, p. 2; ch. 2, p. 2; ch. 3, p. 3; ch. 4, p. 4; ch. 5, pp. 4,5; ch. 6, p. 6; ch. 8, p. 8; ch. 10, p. 9; ch. 14, p. 12; Sammohanatantra, Part 2, ch. 2, p. 2; Wishwasaratantra, ch. 1, p. 10; Mundamalatantra, ch. 6,

p. 9; Koulawalitantra, ch. 22, p. 80; Shaktanandatarangini, 4.30,34; Rudrayamala, Part 2, 25.55; 27.59, 60; 44.20, 24, 26, 58, 67, 69; 45. 7, 10, 11, 13, 16, 18, 19; 46. 35; 56.2; Purashcharyarnawa, ch. 2, p. 90; Shadamnayatantra, 4.64; 5.245, 424; Mridanitantra, quoted in Amarasanggraha MS; Goutamiyatantra, 34.45.

2 Manipuraka, mentioned in the Kankalamalinitantra, ch. 2, p. 5; Mantramahodadhi, 4.22; Tripurasarasamuchchaya, 5.18; Sammohanatantra, Part 2, ch. 2, p. 2; Shaktanandatarangini, 4.11; Rudrayamala, Part 2, 44.61; Tantrarajatantra, 21.82; Purashcharyarnawa, ch. 6. p. 490; Shiwasanghita, 5.111, 113.

3 Dashapatra (ten-petalled lotus), mentioned in the Todalatantra, ch. 9, p. 16; Tararahasya, ch. 4, p. 23; Sammohanatantra, Part 2, ch. 4, p. 4.

4 Dashadala Padma (the lotus with ten petals), mentioned in the Shaktanandatarangini, 4.29; 9.16; Rudrayamala, Part 2, 22.6; Shadamnayatantra, 4.62; 5.265.

5 Dashapatrambuja (the lotus with ten petals), mentioned in the Shaktanandatarangini, 7.14; Gandharwatantra, ch. 8, p. 39.

6 Dashachchada (the lotus with ten petals), mentioned in the Rudrayamala, Part 2, 60.29.

7 Nabhipadma (the navel lotus), mentioned in the Gandharwatantra, ch. 29, p. 112; Shatchakranirupana, Verse 21.

8 Nabhipangkaja (the navel lotus), mentioned in the Sharadatilakatantra, 5.132; Purashcharyarnawa, ch. 5, p. 387.

Position

The manipura is situated in the navel region, that is, that part of the vertebral column which corresponds to the navel region. Technically, the manipura is also called nabhi (the navel) (—Nilatantra, ch. 5, p. 9; Kularnawa, ch. 4, p. 19; Wishwasaratantra, ch. 1, pp. 8, 10; Koulawalitantra, ch. 3, p. 8; Mahanirwanatantra, 5.114). So, the location of the manipura is in the navel region (—Gandharwatantra, ch. 5, p. 27; ch. 8, p. 39; Sammohanatantra, Part 2, ch. 2, p. 2; Koulawalitantra, ch. 22, p. 80; Rudrayamala, Part 2, 22.6; 27.49; Shiwasanghita, 5.111; Goutamiyatantra, 34.45;

Mridanitantra, quoted in *Amarasanggraha* MS; Purashcharyarnawa, ch. 6, p. 490; Shaktananda-tarangini, 4.11,29; 7.14; 9.16; Tripurasara-samuchchaya, 5.18; Mantramahodadhi, 4.22; *Shatchakranirupana*, Verse 19).

In the Waidika accounts, the manipura has also been termed nabhi chakra (—Soubhagya-lakshmyupanishad, 3.3; Yogarajopanishad, Mantra 9). It has also been stated that the manipura is situated in the navel region (—Yogachuda-manyupanishad, Mantras 5, 9; Yogashikhopa-nishad, 1.172; 5.9). Also in the Pouranika accounts it has been stated that the manipura is situated in the navel region(—Dewibhagawata, 7.35.37; 11.1.43).

Description

The manipura (Plate 7) has ten petals. This is supported by the Tantrika as well as by the Waidika and Pouranika accounts. The colour of the petals is like dense rain-clouds (purna-megha-prakasha) (—*Shatchakranirupana*, Verse 19). The commentator Kalicharana interprets purnamegha-prakasha as krishna-warna (= kala-warna—Wachaspatyam and Shabdakalpa-drumah; krishna-warna, kala-warna = black colour—Apte). Bhuwanamohana explains it as follows: purna is gadha (= dense—Apte), the colour like dense clouds, that is, a deep black colour. Let us see what other Tantras say about it.

That the colour of the petals is black (krishna-warna) has been clearly stated in the Bhuta-shuddhitantra, ch. 2, p. 2. It has also been stated that the colour is like rain clouds (—Rudraya-mala, Part 2, 27.59; Goutamiyatantra, 34.46). Here, the black colour has been indirectly indicated. It may also mean the smoke colour (dhumra-warna), as it has been stated that the petals are smoke-coloured (—Goutamiyatantra, 34.47). Dhumra is a mixture of red and black colours (—Wachaspatyam, Shabdakalpadrumah, and Apte). It has also been said that the colour of the petals is nila (—Kankalamalinitantra, ch. 2, p. 5; Sammohanatantra, Part 2, ch. 2, p. 2; Koulawalitantra, ch. 22, p. 80; Tripurasara-samuchchaya, 5.18; Purashcharyarnawa, ch. 6,

p. 490; Mridanitantra, quoted in *Amarasang-graha* MS). The commentator Wishwanatha (in his *Shatchakrawiwriti*) accepts the nila-colour as the colour of the petals, and quotes a passage from the Dakshinamurti in which it is stated that the manipuraka is very nila and the letters *da* to pha are quite nila. Narayana, in commenting on Hangsopanishad, Mantra 10, quotes passages from Parwatiparameshwarasangwada in which the colour of the manipuraka and the letters is said to be blue. Nila is the shyama colour (—Wachaspatyam). Shyama is the black or green colour (—Wachaspatyam and Shabda-kalpadrumah). The following indicate that they are of the colour of nila: shaiwala (a kind of aquatic plant), durwa (a kind of grass), young grass, the shoot of a bamboo, and emerald (marakata) and a sapphire (—Shabdakalpa-drumah). Nila, here, indicates dark green and dark blue. But nila is also the colour black. So, nila indicates three colours: black, dark green and dark blue. It has been said that the petals are the colour of nila like rain clouds in the sky (—Nirwanatantra, ch. 6, p. 8). Here nila is black.

The colour of the petals is also said to be golden (—Gandharwatantra, ch. 5, p. 27; Shiwasan-ghita, 5.111), and red (—Shaktanandatarangini, 4.11). So the petals of the manipura have the following colours: (a) black, (b) dark green or dark blue, (c) golden and (d) red, and of these the black colour has been generally accepted.

On the petals of the manipura are the letters *da*, *dha*, *na*, *ta*, *tha*, *da*, *dha*, *na*, *pa*, *pha*. This has been accepted in all Tantras. The letters are with the nada and bindu (—*Shatchakranirupana*, Verse 19; Nirwanatantra, ch. 6, p. 8; Bhuta-shuddhitantra, ch. 2, p. 2; Tripurasara-samuchchaya, 5.18). This indicates that the letters are matrika-units. The colour of the matrika letters (from *da* to pha) is like the colour of the nila lotus (—*Shatchakranirupana*, Verse 19). Nila means dark-blue here. The colour of the letters is also said to be black (—Bhutashuddhi-tantra, ch. 2, p. 2), and lightning-like (—Kankalamalinitantra, ch. 2, p. 5; Gandharwa-tantra, ch. 5, p. 27; Rudrayamala, Part 2, 27.59; Goutamiyatantra, 34.46; Koulawali-tantra, ch. 22, p. 80). So the colour of the letters is dark-blue, black or lightning-like. The

207

matrika-letters are arranged from the right to the left.

On the petals of the manipura, there are 10 specific qualities (writtis). They are: spiritual ignorance, thirst, jealousy, treachery, shame, fear, disgust, delusion, foolishness and sadness (—Adhyatma Wiweka, quoted by Narayana in his commentary on Hangsopanishad, Mantra 7). They are arranged in the above order from the right to the left. Jaganmohana differs a little and gives the following order: shame, treachery, jealousy, thirst, spiritual ignorance, sadness, passion, delusion, disgust and fear (—Footnote 87, in connection with the verse 5.104, Mahanirwanatantra).

'Fire'-region

In the pericarp of the manipura, lies the 'fire'-region which is triangular in form and the colour is like the rising sun (that is, a red colour); within is situated the bija of wahni (—Shatchakranirupana, Verse 19). Wishwanatha quotes a verse from Mayatantra in which it is stated that the 'fire'-region lying in the pericarp of the ten-petalled lotus is triangular in form and blood-red in colour.

There is in the pericarp of the manipura the 'fire'-region (—Kankalamalinitantra, ch. 2, p. 5; Koulawalitantra, ch. 22, p. 80), which is triangular in form (—Sammohanatantra, Part 2, ch. 2, p. 2; Mridanitantra, quoted in Amarasanggraha, MS) and red in colour (—Nirwanatantra, ch. 6, pp. 8–9) where lies the wahni-bija (fire-germ mantra) (—Sammohanatantra, Part 2, ch. 2, p. 2; Mridanitantra MS). In the Waidika accounts, it has been stated that the 'fire'-region is a triangle (—Yogachudamanyupanishad, Mantra 10; Yogashikhopanishad, 1.177; 5.14) which is red in colour (—Yogatattwopanishad, Mantra 92). Also in the Pouranika accounts, the 'fire'-region has been mentioned as triangular in form and red in colour (—Dewibhagawata, 11.8.5).

Kalicharana says that the wahni-bija is Rang. Agni-bija is Rang (—Warnabijakosha). Agni and wahni are synonyms (—Wachaspatyam; Shabdakalpadrumah). Also, wahni-bija is Rang (—Wachaspatyam; Shabdakalpadrumah). It has been clearly stated that the reta (that is, the letter ra—Wachaspatyam; Shabdakalpadrumah; Apte) is in the red triangle of fire (—Yogatattwopanishad, Mantra 93), and still more clearly, in the red triangular 'fire'-region lies the bija Rang (—Dewibhagawata, 11.8.5).

The matrika-unit rang is red-lightning-like in colour, and there are always the five Deities and five pranas and three forms of power. In the manipura, rang becomes the bija of the 'fire'-principle, and its red-lightning-like colour is retained. From the bija aspect of Rang appears Deity Wahni in deep concentration. The dhyana-form of the bija aspect of Rang is as follows.

The bija or Wahni is seated on a ram, red like the morning sun and four-armed (—Shatchakranirupana, Verse 20). The form of the wahni-bija is Deity Wahni seated on a ram (—Nirwanatantra, ch. 6, p. 9). Also, the form of wahni-bija is four-armed and seated on a ram (—Mridanitantra MS). Kalicharana cites a passage in which the dhyana-form of Wahni is as follows: 'seated on a ram, aksha-sutra (a rudraksha rosary) in one hand, and shakti (a spear) in his other'. He adds that the other two hands are to be thought of as in the attitudes of granting boons and of dispelling fear as is seen in other dhyana-forms. So the dhyana-form of Wahni is as follows: he is shining red, seated on a ram, four-armed, and holds a rudraksha rosary and a spear, and shows the gestures of granting boons and dispelling fear.

Rudra

There lies Deity Rudra in the lap of the wahni-bija (—Shatchakranirupana, Verse 20; Mridanitantra MS). The presence of Rudra in the fire-triangle has been mentioned in the Kankalamalinitantra, ch. 2, p. 5; Nirwanatantra, ch. 6, pp. 8–9; Shiwasanghita, 5.112; Rudrayamala, Part 2, 22.7; Mantramahodadhi, 4.21; Sharadatilakatantra, 5.133; Yogashikhopanishad, 1.177; 5.14; and Yogatattwopanishad, Mantra 93. In the lap of the wahni-bija means in the bindu of Rang. Rudra appears from the bindu of Rang in deep concentration.

A Tantrika dhyana-form of Rudra is as follows.

Rudra is red like pure vermilion colour, appearing whitish because of his body being smeared with ashes; he has three eyes; he is in the attitude of granting boons and of dispelling fear, and he has attained his full growth (—*Shatchakranirupana*, Verse 20). According to Kalicharana Rudra should be concentrated upon as seated on a bull (*wrisha*). This has been supported in the dhyana-form in the Sandhya-process.

During the expiratory phase (rechaka) of pranayama in the sandhya-process, concentration is done on Shambhu (Rudra). The Samaweda form of Shambhu is as follows: he is of white colour, two-armed, holding a trident and a drum, adorned with the crescent moon, three-eyed and seated on a bull. The Yajurweda and the Rigweda forms are the same. In some Rigweda form, Shambhu is dressed in tiger's skin. However, the main differences from the Tantrika form are these: the colour of the body is white instead of red; he holds a trident and a drum instead of showing the attitude of granting boons and of dispelling fear; and he is seated on a bull.

There is a Waidika form of dhyana which is similar to the Tantrika form. It is as follows.

Rudra is three-eyed, his colour is like the morning sun (that is, red), his body is smeared with ashes; he is showing the gesture of granting boons and being kindly disposed (—Yogatattwopanishad, Mantra 93).

It has been stated that a Shiwa-linga, in colour like a black (nila) cloud, is situated in the manipura (in the triangular 'fire'-region) (—Bhutashuddhitantra, ch. 2, p. 2). This Shiwa-linga is the Rudra-linga with six faces lying in the manipura (—Sammohanatantra, Part 2, ch. 2, p. 2). This linga has also been called Siddha (endowed with great yoga-power) Rudra (the Siddha-linga named Rudra—Jaganmohana) (—Shiwasanghita, 5.112). So Rudra has two aspects, the linga- and the dewata-form. In the linga-form, he is black in colour. In the dewata-form he is either red or white. Moreover, the linga-form may remain in substance in the bindu of the bija Rang, from which Rudra-in-form emerges. It has also been stated that Wishnu is in the manipura (—Gandharwatantra, ch. 5, p. 27). This is a special process of concentration. (For the concentration form of Rudra see Plate 8, left top figure.)

Lakini

Power Lakini is situated in the manipura (—*Shatchakranirupana*, Verse 21; Kankalamalinitantra, ch. 2, p. 5; Todalatantra, ch. 7, p. 14; Sammohanatantra, Part 2, ch. 2, p. 2; Shiwasanghita, 5.112; Rudrayamala, Part 2, 22. 7; Mantramahodadhi, 4.21; Koulawalitantra, ch. 22, p. 80; Mridanitantra MS). Lakini has been called the door-keeper (—Sammohanatantra, Part 2, ch. 2, p. 2), because concentration on her makes things easier in the manipura. Also, concentration on Rudra with Lakini is necessary for the attainment of success in yoga (—Rudrayamala, Part 2, 22.7). Lakini has also been called Bhadrakali (—Nirwanatantra, ch. 6, p. 9).

A dhyana-form of Lakini is as follows.

Lakini is four-armed, of shining black (or dark-blue) (shyama) colour, dressed in yellow raiment, adorned with various ornaments, and in deep concentration (—*Shatchakranirupana*, Verse 21). The commentator Ramawallabha interprets 'shyama' as 'the golden colour'. Jaganmohana says that Lakini is of the colour of tapta-gold (Footnote 87, in connection with the verse 104, Mahanirwanatantra). The word tapta is vague. It may mean heated or red-hot. So tapta-gold means red-hot gold, that is, shining red, rather than gold-coloured.

Kalicharana quotes a verse in which the dhyana-form of Lakini is given as follows.

Divine Lakini is nila (black or dark-blue), and has three faces, each having three eyes, with large teeth, and is powerful; she holds in her right hands wajra (a thunderbolt) and a spear (shakti), and her left hands are in the gestures of dispelling fear and of granting boons. This dhyana-form is similar to what has been stated in the Jamala, quoted in the Yogakalpalatika MS. Even the wordings are almost similar.

Other dhyana-forms of Lakini are the following.

Lakini is of the colour of vermilion-red and two-armed; she shines with the vermilion-mark on her forehead; her face is as beautiful as the moon and her eyes are bright and painted beautifully with collyrium; she is clad in white raiment and adorned with various ornaments (—Kankalamalinitantra, ch. 5, p. 23).

Lakini is of a pale red colour, holds a noose and a goad, wears a garland of skulls and is adorned with various ornaments (—Kularnawa, ch. 10, p. 53).

The power of Rudra (Lakini) is blood-red in colour, three-eyed, with large teeth, and powerful, and she assumes the attitudes of granting boons and of dispelling fear (—Gandharwatantra, ch. 9, p. 42). (For the concentration-form of Lakini see Plate 8, right top figure.)

Explanation

The central power of the manipura chakra, designated by Rang, has ten radiations which are also named by the matrika-letters dang, dhang, nang, tang, thang, dang, dhang, nang, pang, phang. The matrika-letters indicate the nature of the radiations. Rang with the ten matrika-letters is the tejas-mahabhuta power in operation. The prana-forces are also being operated along with the mahabhuta power. The tejas-mahabhuta is seen in deep concentration as a red triangle. When the radiations are withdrawn into the central Rang by pratyaharic concentration only the bija Rang remains. It is the rupa-tanmatra power. At this stage all other forces cease to operate.

The colour of the petals is black. It indicates that the prana-force is predominating in the radiations, though there is some samanic radiation. When the petals are smoke-coloured, udana-radiation predominates. When they are dark green or dark blue, prana predominates; when golden, wyana; and when red, prana and apana predominate.

The colour of the matrika-letters in the petals of the manipura is black, dark green or dark blue, golden or red. When they are black, dark green or dark blue they are radiating mainly prana. When they are golden, they radiate wyana, and when red, they radiate both prana and apana. The original colour of dang is like yellow-lightning; that of dhang is like red-lightning; of nang and tang like yellow-lightning; the colour of thang is red; of dang and nang it is like red-lightning; of dhang like yellow-lightning; of pang moon-white; and of phang like red-

lightning. In yellow-lightning, wyana radiates predominantly; in red-lightning prana and apana radiations occur; and in white samana radiation. These individual radiations are modified in the manipura, where each of them radiates the same force conjointly to heighten the effects.

The following are the forms of concentration.

1 Petaline Concentration. The mantra 'dang-phang' should be taken as the unit of manipura-concentration in japa and thought-concentration, and gradually the petals will be changed into a black circular ring without any interruption.

2 Mahabhuta-concentration. In this concentration, consciousness assumes the form of a triangle of the red colour with Rang inside it. The first stage is thought-concentration which is finally developed into real concentration when the red triangle along with Rang is actually 'seen'.

3 Tanmatra-concentration. Now the red triangle disappears and only Rang of red colour remains. This is the rupa-tanmatra.

4 Wahni-concentration. Deep concentration on Rang causes the emergence of Deity Wahni (Agni) from the bija aspect of Rang. Wahni is 'seen' on a ram; he is red in colour, and holds a rudraksha rosary and a spear.

Mesha (ram) is the basic power-in-concentration which supports the central energy as fire (wahni)-energy in the form of Rang. Mesha has four mantra-forms represented by ang, ring, nang and hang. The mesha form is essentially due to nang in which lie the sun-energy and the divine energy of Shiwa. The energy of creativity (as Brahma-energy) and the reduction of energy to consciousness (as Wishnu-energy) are mainly derived from ang. The prana-energy comes from hang. An aspect of creative energy is released as the great and prolongable sexual vigour. But this vigour also remains under control. The mesha-process is the process of full development of the sexual vigour based on the fully energized body, and to harness it by anti-ejaculatory control and to transform the desire into elements constituting concentration. It is an advanced method of gonadal control in which the highly developed sexual vigour is utilized in arousing the whole energy system of the organism, and the roused energies are radiated to the conscious field through desire in concentration, and the energy-desire becomes energy as concentration and supports and increases concentration. For the attainment of Rudra-consciousness-concentration, this process is invaluable and it becomes most effective through the influence of *ring*.

Now a practitioner becomes fit for Wahni-concentration. In Wahni all forms of heat-light-energy are concentrated as pra*na* and are transformed into a conscious form which constitutes Rudra-consciousness. This indicates that pra*naya*ma is an important factor in Rudra-concentration. Wahni-concentration develops into Rudra-concentration. The red colour of Rudra indicates that the ra*jas* force, which is in great concentration and in which both pra*na* and apa*na* form important parts, is spiritualized to form Rudra-consciousness. The Shakti (spear) is the power of concentrating all forms of energy and transforming them into concentration-energy. Akshasutra (a rudra*ksha* rosary) is the *sutra* (thread) or basic power, called Ku*nda*li*ni*, from which arise *ang* force which draws all desires into it, and k*shang* force which absorbs all creative principles. The sh*a*kti and ak*sha*sutra are spiritual powers which create divine consciousness and transform all energies into concentration.

5 Rudra-concentration. When a practitioner is fully prepared by energizing his body and mind, through the practice of pra*naya*ma and Wahni-concentration, he is able to rouse Rudra from the bindu aspect of R*ang* in deep concentration.

Rudra as Supreme Being (Br*a*hman) is one and without a second. This is realized in supreme samadhi. When he manifests his supreme power, he is *I*shwara and is the creator, maintainer and destroyer of the universe. Rudra also appears in a specific divine form—a spiritual, calm and pure form and absorbs all cosmic principles by which an individual is bound to worldliness, when his devotee is spiritually prepared. The word Rudra is derived from 'ruda' which means crying (—Wach*a*spatyam). It is owing to his destructive power, he causes the embodied beings to weep. But actually his destructive power is the power of absorption of all that causes diverseness of consciousness, that is, all anti-samadhi influences. According to K*a*ru*na*maya (Acharya K*a*ru*na*maya Bhattacharya Saraswat*i*, the celebrated Sanskrit scholar of Calcutta, India), Rudra is he who causes the disappearance of 'rut', that is, sorrow, or who bestows 'rut', that is, knowledge. This knowledge is the Br*a*hman knowledge, arising in samadhi.

Rudra is seated on a wr*i*sha (bull). A wr*i*sha which emits power or bestows knowledge. So it has been said that wr*i*sha is knowledge (Weda) and spirituality (dharma). Wr*i*sha is vitality and virility. Rudra is established on spiritual knowledge and power. K*a*ru*na*maya says that Shiwa (Rudra) is the guru of knowledge; wr*i*sha who is in the form of knowledge supports the guru Shiwa who is all knowledge. Rudra is in the attitudes of granting boons and dispelling fear. The bestowing of spiritual knowledge is the best boon, and one can really be free from fear when unspirituality is removed. The mantra-forms of wr*i*sha are u*ng*, sh*ang* and *shang*.

6 Lakin*i*-concentration. To be really prepared for successful concentration in the ma*ni*pura, and especially on Rudra, it is absolutely necessary to concentrate on Lakin*i*. This is why Lakin*i* has been called the door-keeper. Unless a practitioner is able to penetrate inside the ma*ni*pura without any obstruction, he cannot do much. All obstacles are removed by concentration on Lakin*i*, moreover without rousing Lakin*i* it is not possible to rouse Rudra, as the power aspect of Rudra is Lakin*i* without whom he is like a corpse.

The colour of Lakin*i* is black. The colour indicates that she is in ta*mas* form in which she absorbs all creative principles. 'La' of Lakin*i* means to take; she who takes or absorbs all which is cosmic to make her devotee free from the bondage is Lakin*i*. When she appears in red colour, she has been identical with Rudra. Her three heads indicate that the three primary attributes (gu*nas*) are so spiritually controlled that ta*mas* is utilized to make the body inert and sense-consciousness functionless, ra*jas* to develop concentration, and sattwa to maintain divine consciousness. The wajra (thunderbolt) indicates adamantine control and shakti (spear) is the power to transform all forms of energy into concentration-energy.

The mantra forms of Lakini are lang and aing; those of shakti are eng, ah, ang, ing, ring, lring, aing, kang, khang, tang, sang, kling, hring and hsouh; and those of wajra are mang and lang.

4 Hrit

The hrit chakra has not been included in the regular six chakras which are muladhara, swadhishthana, manipura, anahata, wishuddha and ajña. The point is this: Is hrit an independent chakra or a name of the anahata chakra? Let us investigate the matter.

It has been stated that concentration should be done on the astra-bija (the mantra Hung) in the hridaya, that is, the chakra situated in the heart region (—Nilatantra, ch. 5, p. 9). It has been mentioned along with the swadhishthana and navel (manipura), so the chakra in the heart region is anahata. Hridaya (heart) has also been mentioned as from the navel (manipura) to the heart, and from the heart to the throat (wishuddha) (—Todalatantra, ch. 7, p. 14). Here also it is anahata. Concentration should be done on Goddess Mahamaya in the twelve-petalled hrit lotus (chakra) (—Kamadhenutantra, ch. 12, p. 15). Here, the hrit lotus is clearly anahata. Also, concentration should be done on the bija-mantra of Ishtadewata in the luminous hrit lotus having twelve petals (—Kamadhenutantra, ch. 13, p. 15). It is anahata which has twelve petals. The anahata has been clearly indicated in the following two statements: concentration should be done on one's own Shakti mantra in the twelve-petalled hrit lotus (—ibid, ch. 15, p. 19); Concentrating on Kamini (Power) in the pericarp of the twelve-petalled hrit lotus (—ibid, ch. 17, p. 23). It is not quite clear in the statement (Kamadhenutantra, ch. 18, p. 24) 'First concentrating on Kamini in the hrit lotus'; but here the hrit lotus may be the anahata because of the previous statement (ibid., ch. 17, p. 23). In the statement 'Concentrating on the

hutashana ("fire")-bija in the "fire"-region lying inside the hrit lotus' (—Kamadhenutantra, ch. 13, p. 16), it is difficult to determine whether the lotus is hrit or anahata. The 'fire'-region indicates that it is hrit.

The hritpatra and hrit padma indicate the anahata chakra in the following verses: concentrate on Shakti in the hritpatra; the hrit lotus is a great region, it is the place of Brahman and jiwa; the hrit lotus has twelve petals and is luminous; here concentration should be done on God Shiwa (—Brihannilatantra, ch. 8, p. 65). The nyasa (a mantra process) should be done in the heart with concentration on Kakini (—Kularnawa, ch. 4, p. 19); here the heart stands for the anahata. In the following verses anahata is indicated: The twelve-petalled hrit lotus (—Gandharwatantra, ch. 8, p. 39); do concentration on Kundalini who is in the form of mantra, along with luminous Bana-linga, situated in the triangle of hrit (—ibid, ch. 29, p. 109); the luminous Hring (a bija-mantra of Power) is in the hrit lotus (—ibid., ch. 29, p. 112); the nyasa should be done in the hridaya (—Mantramahodadhi, 4.28); hrit padma (—Tararahasya, ch. 1, p. 2); the all pure hrit lotus (—Bhutashuddhitantra, ch. 2, p. 2); hrit lotus (—ibid., ch. 4, p. 4; ch. 6, p. 6); 'seeing' Brahman in the hrit lotus (—ibid., ch. 5, p. 4); Goddess Mangala and others are in the hrit lotus (—ibid., ch. 5, p. 5); hrit lotus is yoga lotus (—ibid., ch. 10, p. 9); concentration on Ishtadewata first in the muladhara, then in the swadhishthana, then in the manipura, then in the hrit lotus, and thereafter in the wishuddha chakra (—ibid., ch. 14, p. 12); the flame-like jiwa is to be brought from the hridayambhoja (hrit lotus) into the muladhara where it should be united with Kundalini; the hridayambuja (hrit lotus) with twelve petals in which are the letters from ka to tha where lies Deity Ishwara (—Sammohanatantra, Part 2, ch. 4, p. 4); hridayasarasija (= hrit lotus) (—Wishwasaratantra, ch. 1, p. 8); the twelve-petalled hridayasarasija (—Koulawalitantra, ch. 3, p. 8); the twelve-petalled hridayambuja (= hrit lotus) decorated with the twelve letters from ka to tha where lies Deity Isha (—Sharadatilakatantra, 5.133); Bana-linga is in the hrit lotus (—Shaktan-

andatarangini, 4.34); the twelve-petalled h*ri*t lotus with the 12 letters from *ka* (—*ibid*., 7.14).

The terms hr*i*dayambhoja (= hr*i*t lotus) (—Rudrayamala, Part 2, 57. 1,3,33,47; 59.23); hr*i*dambhoja (= hr*i*t lotus) (—*ibid*., 57.12,14), hr*i*tpankeruha (= hr*i*t lotus) (—*ibid*., 57.14), hr*i*tpadma (= hr*i*t lotus) (—*ibid*., 57. 19,42); hr*i*dayabja (= hr*i*t lotus) (—*ibid*., 59.24); hr*i*dayakamala (= hr*i*t lotus) (—*ibid*., 59.27); hr*i*dayambuja (= hr*i*t lotus) (—*ibid*., 59.28; 60.9); hr*i*dabja (= hr*i*t lotus) (—*ibid*., 60.10); and hr*i*dambuja (= hr*i*t lotus) (—Shadamnaya-tantra, 4.144)—all stand for the *anahata*.

Anahata is also indicated in the following verses: there is a ten-petalled lotus, then the hr*i*t lotus, and then a sixteen-petalled lotus (—Rudrayamala, Part 2, 60.29). Here the hr*i*t lotus is clearly the *anahata*. The letters *ka-tha* are placed in the hr*i*dambuja (= hr*i*t lotus) (—Mahanirwanatantra, 5.114). Here also, the hr*i*t lotus stands for the *anahata*. Hr*i*tsaroruha (= hr*i*t lotus) is decorated with the letters *ka-tha* and here is situated Deity *I*shwara (—Purash-charyarnawa, ch. 5, p. 387). Here, the hr*i*t lotus stands for the *anahata*.

The numerous evidences from the Tantras show that the hr*i*t lotus in its various names stands for the *anahata*. It is supported by the W*a*idika accounts. It has been stated that hr*i*daya (the lotus situated in the heart region) has twelve petals (—Yogachudamanyupani-shad, Mantra 5). Here the lotus in the heart stands for the *anahata*. In the heart, pra*na* wayu should be held (—Darshanopanishad, 7.12). The heart means the lotus situated in the heart region, and this lotus here is *anahata*. It has been stated that the fourth chakra, lying with its face downwards, is situated in the heart (—Yogarajopanishad, Mantra 10). This chakra is the *anahata*.

In the Pouranika accounts, we also find that the hr*i*t lotus stands for the *anahata*. The order of the chakras as given here is: adhara (mula-dhara), manipura, hr*i*daya (hr*i*t lotus), wishuddhi and ajña (—Shiwapura*na*, 3.3.28). Here the swadhi*sh*thana has not been mentioned. But it is stated that hr*i*daya, that is hr*i*t lotus, stands between the manipura and wishuddhi. This hr*i*t lotus is clearly *anahata*. Further, jiwatman

which is situated in the hr*i*daya (the padma in the heart region) is to be brought through the brahma na*di* to the sahasrara which is above the twelve-petalled lotus (guru chakra) (—Shiwa-pura*na*, 3.5.52,53). This hr*i*t padma is the *anahata*. Concentration should be done on the sun-coloured (red) lotus, with 12 petals which are decorated with the 12 letters from *ka* to *tha*, and is inside the heart (that is the hr*i*t lotus) (—*ibid*., 5b.29. 136,137). This lotus is clearly *anahata*.

In the following verses, the hr*i*t lotus stands for the *anahata*: concentration is to be done on the letter '*a*' lying in the heart (hr*i*t lotus) (—Brahmapura*na*, 61.4); Shiwa is situated in the sahasrara, the eyebrow region (ajña), the palatine region (talu chakra), the throat region (wishuddha chakra) and the heart region (hr*i*t chakra) (—Lingapura*na*, 2.21.28); The nyasa of the mantra H*a*ng should be done in the muladhara, of R*a*ng in the hr*i*daya (heart lotus), of *I*ng in the eyebrow region (ajña chakra), and Hr*i*ng in the head region (sahasrara chakra) (—Dewibhagawata, 7.40.7). In this order—anal region, genital region, navel region, heart region (—Dewibhagawata, 11.1.43), the hr*i*t lotus in the heart region is *anahata*.

We have to investigate farther to know whether the hr*i*t is an independent chakra. It has been stated that mental worship should be done on Power situated in the hr*i*tpundarika (hr*i*t lotus) (—Gandharwatantra, ch. 11, p. 48). Here the hr*i*tpundarika is hr*i*t padma (hr*i*t chakra). Con-centration on Goddess Durga, who is in the hr*i*t padma (hr*i*t lotus), is to be done (—Maya-tantra, ch. 8, p. 7). Most probably, here hr*i*t chakra has been indicated. Hr*i*t padma men-tioned in the Wishwasaratantra, ch. 3, p. 39, may also be hr*i*t chakra. Concentration should be done on Shiwa and Power in the hr*i*t padma (—Mundamalatantra, ch. 6, p. 10), and on the Goddess Kalika in hr*i*dayambhoja (hr*i*t padma) (—*ibid*., ch. 6, p. 12). Here the hr*i*t padma and hr*i*dayambhoja may be hr*i*t chakra. It has been stated that hr*i*t padma should be given as a seat to the Goddess Kalika (in mental worship) (—Mahanirwanatantra, 5.143). Jagan-mohana interprets the eight-petalled lotus in the heart as the seat. In this case it is the hr*i*t lotus. But it can be interpreted as the *anahata* chakra. The term hridayambhuja (—*ibid.*, 5.130) has been interpreted as hrit padma by the commentator Hariharananda, and hridaya padma by Jaganmohana. In both cases it means hrit chakra.

It has been stated more clearly in the Shrikrama (quoted in the Yogakalpalatika MS) that the hrit padma (lotus) has eight petals. More details have been given in the Gitasara in which it has been stated that the hrit padma has eight petals on which are situated eight deities, Indra and others; inside it (that is, inside the pericarp) is the sun, inside the sun is the moon, and inside the moon is the fire; inside the fire is radiance where a seat is located which is ornamented with jewels, and which is very bright; on this seat God Narayana is sitting (—Gitasara, 290–293, quoted in the Yogakalpalatika MS). It has been stated that in the heart region is the fourth lotus *anahata* with twelve petals, and the bright eight-petalled lotus with its face upwards lies in the interior of the *anahata* (—Yogaswarodaya, quoted in the Amarasanggraha MS). That the eight-petalled lotus (that is, hrit lotus) with its face downwards is within the shining fourth lotus with twelve petals (i.e., *anahata*) is also stated in the Tattwayogabindu MS. The eight-petalled lotus (i.e., the hrit chakra) which is within the *anahata* is of golden colour, and there is the celestial wishing-tree (kalpataru) shining red in the pericarp, and at the base of the tree is a gemmed seat (—Mridanitantra, quoted in the Amarasanggraha MS).

The existence of the hrit chakra has been mentioned in the Waidika accounts. It has been stated that Atman is within the golden lotus (hemapundarika) (—Atmaprabodhopanishad, 1.3). This golden lotus is eight-petalled, subtle, stainless and untouched by physical impurities (—Taittiriya Aranyaka, 10.12). The lotus-like hridaya (that is, hrit-lotus) with its face downwards is situated both under (*anahata*) and above the navel (*manipura*), and at its boundary is a subtle hole (sushumna), within which all lies (the whole chakra system) (—Narayanopanishad, Mantras 50, 51). This means that the hrit chakra is situated above the *manipura* and below the

anahata, and within the sushumna where all the other chakras lie. In fact, this hrit chakra belongs to the *anahata* and forms its lower part. The lotus-like hridaya in the sushumna also lies with its face downwards (—Brahmopanishad, Mantra 34). It is the hrit chakra. It has been stated that the lotus-like hridaya with its face downwards should be raised upwards by sitkara (pranayama); within the hridaya is superlight and within it lies the most subtle fire-flame and within that again is Purusha, who is the Supreme Being (—Mahopanishad, 1. 12–14). The hridaya is the hrit chakra, which remains usually with its face downwards. Its face should be turned upwards by special pranayama. In the pericarp of the raised hrit chakra is 'seen' the fire-flame-like Kundalini from which is radiated superlight. In deeper concentration Purusha—Supreme Consciousness—is revealed within Kundalini.

In the following mantras, the hrit chakra has been indicated: fully opened eight-petalled hrit (—Gopalatapinyupanishad, Part 2, Mantra 60); concentration on Supreme Being within the hritpundarika (hrit lotus) (—Maitreyyupanishad, 1.12); concentration on the universal form of God situated in the hridaya-amburuha (hrit lotus) (—Trishikhibrahmanopanishad, Mantra Section, 153); The imperishable Brahman light is within the hritpundarika (hrit lotus) (—*ibid.*, Mantra Section 156); the divine existence in the hridayakamala (hrit lotus) as the internal sign (—Mandalabrahmanopanishad, 2.4.4); the lotus which is situated in the heart region (i.e., the hrit lotus) lies with its face downward (—Yogatattwopanishad, Mantra 137).

In the Pouranika accounts, hrit padma has also been accepted as a separate chakra. Krishna says: 'Controlling the mind in the hridaya (heart)' (—Bhagawadgita, 8.12), and 'Ishwara (God) is situated in the hrit desha (heart region)' (—*ibid.*, 18.61). Here, both 'hridaya' and 'hrit desha' possibly indicate hrit chakra. In the statements—the manifestation of lightning-like splendorous form of Supreme Being in the hritpadmakosha (—Bhagawata, 4.9.2) and the practice of concentration by Dhruwa by fixing the mind in the hridaya (—*ibid.*, 4.8.77), the hrit chakra has been indicated.

In 'the eight-petalled hritpundarika' (—Shiwapurana, 3.3.59), the hrit chakra has also been indicated. Moreover, it shows that the hrit chakra has eight petals. More description of the hrit chakra has been given here: The excellent hritpankaja (hrit lotus), situated in the hridaya (the heart region) should be opened by prana-yama with mantra; in the pericarp of the lotus, concentration should be done on the sun, moon and fire; a gemmed seat should be thought of in the pericarp; the lotus should be thought of as a delicate, beautiful, red like morning sun, in the form of the mantra-letters and with eight forms of superpower in its petals; concentration on God Wishnu should be done in this lotus (—Skandapurana, 2.5.4.21–4). Here, the hrit chakra has been described as having 8 petals of red colour, in which are situated the eight forms of superpower; in its pericarp are the sun, moon and fire, and a gemmed seat; it is an excellent lotus for concentration.

It has been stated in its further exposition that the eight-petalled lotus lying with its face downwards is within the lotus which forms its outer aspect; 'in its pericarp is the (circular) sun region within which lies Shiwa in his most subtle aspect' (—Skandapurana, 6.29. 153–4). The hrit lotus may have one thousand petals according to the mode of concentration. It has been stated that concentration on Ishta-dewata is made in the hrit padma (hrit chakra) which is bright, white and with one thousand petals (—Brahmawaiwartapurana, 1.26.8). The thousand-petalled hritsaroruha (= hrit padma, i.e. hrit chakra) has also been mentioned in the Brahmawaiwartapurana, 4.37.10. The hrit chakra has also been described as having sixteen petals. It has been stated that 'the three nadis (sushum-na, ida and pingala) have been united in the heart where lies a sixteen-petalled chakra which is the seat for concentration and mantra-japa; as this chakra arises in the hridaya (that is, lying in the heart region) it is called the original sixteen-petalled chakra' (—Kalikapurana, 55. 32–4).

In another description, it has been stated that 'the pundarika in the hridaya (the heart region) is above the navel (manipura) which is in the nature of spiritual knowledge, and its pericarp is untouched by passion; this lotus has eight petals having superpowers, and is white, and the prana wayus are also there' (—Linga-purana, 1.86.62–4). The order of the different chakras as given in the verse (—Skandapurana, 1.2.55.44) is as follows: in the navel (i.e., mani-pura), in the heart (i.e., hrit lotus), in the lungs lies the lotus with twelve petals (i.e., anahata). In this order the hrit lotus stands between the manipura and the anahata; it has been accepted as an individual chakra.

In the following passages, the hrit chakra has been indicated: the God Shiwa is situated in the hritpundarika (hrit padma) (—Shiwa-purana, 1.71.70); concentration on Shiwa and Shakti (Power) situated in the hritpankaja (hrit padma) (—ibid., 3.3.54); the worship of Shiwa and Shakti on the seat within hrit padma by dhyana-yajña (concentration) (—ibid., 5b. 29.131); after concentrating on the shining bija-mantra Kshoung lying within the hrit-pankaja (hrit padma) burn all impurities by the directed flames of the bija radiating in all directions (—Agnipurana, 23.3); worship splendorous Atman situated in the hridabja (hrit padma) (—Garudapurana, 1.18.13); con-centration on Deity Brahma situated in the pericarp of the hrit padma (—Padmapurana, 1.15.188); concentration on all-pervading attri-buteless Supreme Being situated in the hollow of the hrit padma (—Brahmapurana, 235.20); Brahma saw Krishna exteriorly in the same form in which he had 'seen' him in the hridayambhoja (hrit padma) (—Brahmawaiwartapurana, 4.20. 18); concentration on Supreme Power in the hridaya (hrit padma) (—Kalikapurana, 55.26); Shiwa is situated in the hritpundarika (hrit padma) (—Sourapurana, 41.81; Lingapurana, 1.98.96); concentration on Supreme Power in the hridambhoja (hrit padma) opened by prana-yama (—Dewibhagawata, 7.40.9).

All the above statements indicate the existence of hrit padma as a separate chakra. Now our findings about the hrit chakra may be summariz-ed as follows.

The hrit chakra, though not included in the six-chakra group, is the fourth chakra, above the manipura, and lies in the chitrini nadi.

Terminology

The following are the Tantrika terms for the hrit chakra:

1 Hrit padma, mentioned in the Mayatantra, ch. 8, p. 7; Wishwasaratantra, ch. 3, p. 39; Mundamalatantra, ch. 6, p. 10; Mahanirwanatantra, 5.143; Shrikramasanghita, quoted in the Yogakalpalatika MS; Gitasara, quoted in the Yogakalpalatika MS.
2 Hritpundarika, mentioned in the Gandharwatantra, ch. 11, p. 48.
3 Hridayambhoja, mentioned in the Mundamalatantra, ch. 6, p. 12.
4 Eight-petalled padma, mentioned in the Yogaswarodaya, quoted in the Amarasanggraha MS; Mridanitantra, quoted in the Amarasanggraha MS.
5 Eight-petalled Kamala, mentioned in the Tattwayogabindu MS.
6 Sixteen-petalled padma, mentioned in the Tararahasya, ch. 4, p. 22.

Waidika terms:

1 Hridaya chakra, mentioned in the Soubhagyalakshmyupanishad, 3.4.
2 Hrit padma, mentioned in the Gopalatapinyupanishad, Part 2, Mantra 60.
3 Hridaya padma, mentioned in the Yogatattwopanishad, Mantras 137–8.
4 Hridaya kamala, mentioned in the Mandalabrahmanopanishad, 2.4.4.
5 Hridaya-amburuha, mentioned in the Trishikhibrahmanopanishad, Mantra Section, Mantra 153.
6 Hridaya padmakosha, mentioned in the Narayanopanishad, Mantra 50; Brahmopanishad, Mantra 34; Mahopanishad, 1.12.
7 Hritpundarika, mentioned in the Maitreyyupanishad, 1.12; Trishikhibrahmanopanishad, Mantra Section, Mantra 156.
8 Hemapundarika, mentioned in the Atmaprabodhopanishad, 1.3.

Pouranika terms:

1 Hrit padma, mentioned in the Shiwapurana, 5b.29.131; Padmapurana, 1.15. 188; 3.31.41; Brahmapurana, 235.20; Brahmawaiwartapurana, 1.26.8; Kalikapurana, 18.76; Garudapurana, 1.23.35.
2 Hritpadmakosha, mentioned in the Bhagawata, 4.9.2.
3 Hritpundarika, mentioned in the Shiwapurana, 1.71.70; 3.3.59; Sourapurana, 34.59; 41.81; Lingapurana, 1.98.96.
4 Hritpankaja, mentioned in the Shiwapurana, 3.3.54; Agnipurana, 23.3; Skandapurana, 2.5.4.21.
5 Hritsaroruha, mentioned in the Brahmawaiwartapurana, 4.37.10.
6 Hridabja, mentioned in the Garudapurana, 1.18.13.
7 Hridambuja, mentioned in the Brahmawaiwartapurana, 4.20.30.
8 Hridambhoja, mentioned in the Dewibhagawata, 7.40.9.
9 Hridayambhoja, mentioned in the Brahmawaiwartapurana, 4.20.18; 4.20.32.
10 Hridaya Kamala, mentioned in the Lingapurana, 2.18.36.
11 Hridaya pundarika, mentioned in the Lingapurana, 1.86.63.
12 Hridaya (lotus in the heart region), mentioned in the Bhagawadgita, 8.12; Bhagawata, 4.8.77; Skandapurana, 1.2.55. 44; Brahmawaiwartapurana, 4.20.38; Kalikapurana, 55.26.
13 Hrit desha (lotus in the heart region), mentioned in the Bhagawadgita, 18.61.
14 Ashta-patra (lotus with 8 petals), mentioned in the Skandapurana, 6.29.153.
15 Adi shodasha chakra (Primary sixteen-petalled chakra), mentioned in the Kalikapurana, 55.33.

Position

The hrit chakra is situated in the heart region above the manipura and just below the anahata, which is also in the heart region. The hrit chakra is, in fact, a part of the anahata, forming its inferior aspect. But the hrit chakra should be considered as an individual chakra.

The hrit chakra lies in the chitrini which is within the sushumna, and the sushumna within the vertebral column. It is that part of the vertebral column which corresponds to the heart region.

Description

The hrit chakra (Plate 10) has eight petals (—Shrikrama and Gitasara, quoted in the Yogakalpalatika MS; Yogaswarodaya and Mridanitantra, quoted in the Amarasanggraha MS; Tattwayogabindu MS; Soubhagyalakshmyupanishad; 3.4; Gopalatapinyupanishad; Shiwapurana, 3.3.59; Skandapurana, 2.5. 4.23; Lingapurana, 1.86.64). It has also been described as having sixteen petals (—Tararahasya, ch. 4, p. 22; Kalikapurana, 55.33), and 1000 petals (—Brahmawaiwartapurana, 1.26. 8; 4.37.10). Usually there are eight petals. In special concentration, the sixteen and 1000 petals are thought of.

Ordinarily, the hrit chakra lies with its face downward (—Tattwayogabindu, MS; Narayanopanishad, Mantra 50; Brahmopanishad, Mantra 34; Soubhagyalakshmyupanishad, 3.4; Yogatattwopanishad, Mantra 137). When the hrit chakra lies in a downward position it is closely connected with the anahata, as if by a stalk (—Yogatattwopanishad, Mantra 138). Its face should be raised upwards for concentration (—Dewibhagawata, 7.40.9). This is done by special pranayama, such as sitkara (—Mahopanishad, 1.12). When it is done the hrit lotus stands with its face upwards (—Yogaswarodaya, quoted in the Amarasanggraha MS; Gopalatapinyupanishad, Part 2, Mantra 60).

The colour of the eight petals of the hrit chakra is golden (—Mridanitantra, quoted in Amarasanggraha MS); also white (—Lingapurana, 1.86.64), and red (—verses quoted by Kalicharana) according to the form of concentration. When the hrit chakra is thought of as having sixteen or 1000 petals, the colour of the petals is white (—Tararahasya, ch. 4, p. 22; Brahmawaiwartapurana, 1.26.8). On the eight petals are situated eight forms of superpower and the mantra-letters of shining red (—Skandapurana, 2.5.4.23). According to Swami Sachchidananda the colour of the petals is shining reddish yellow (—Pujapradipa).

Inside the pericarp of the hrit chakra, is the circular region of the sun (—Skandapurana, 6.29.153; Gitasara, quoted in the Yogakalpalatika MS), and within it the (circular) region of the moon and inside that is the (circular) region of the fire (—Gitasara, quoted in the Yogakalpalatika MS). The colour of the sun-region is vermilion, of the moon-region white, and of the fire-region deep red. Inside it (the fire-region) is the celestial wishing-tree of shining red colour and at the base of it is a gemmed seat (—Mridanitantra, quoted in the Amarasanggraha MS).

Explanation

The hrit chakra is specially suitable for the practice of concentration, mental worship and mantra-japa. The chakra should be raised up and opened by pranayama and thought-concentration when japa, worship and concentration are to be made here. It is a special seat for concentration on Ishtadewata and also other deities.

5 Anahata

In the regular six-chakra group, the anahata is the fourth chakra, but numerically it is the fifth centre. It lies in the chitrini nadi.

Terminology

The following are the Tantrika terms of the anahata.

1 Anahata, mentioned in the Todalatantra, ch. 7, p. 14; ch. 9, p. 17; Kankalamalinitantra, ch. 2, p. 5; Gandharwatantra, ch. 5, p. 27, 28; Mantramahodadhi, 4.23; Kubjikatantra, 5.262; 6.300; Tripurasarasamuchchaya, 5.20; Bhutashuddhitantra, ch. 4, p. 4; Sammohanatantra, Part 2, ch. 2, p. 2; Wishwasaratantra, ch. 1, p. 3,10; Mundamalatantra, ch. 6, p. 9; Koulawalitantra, ch. 22, p. 80; Shaktanandatarangini,

4.12; Rudrayamala, Part 2, 25.26; 27.62; Tantra-rajatantra, 21.83; Purashcharyarnawa, ch. 2, p. 90; ch. 6, p. 490; Shadamnayatantra, 5.266, 425; Shiwasanghita, 5.116; Goutamiyatantra, 34.49; Shatchakranirupana, Verse 22; Yoga-swarodaya, quoted in Amarasanggraha MS; Mridanitantra, quoted in Amarasanggraha MS.

2 Anahata-puri (-abode), mentioned in the Bhutashuddhitantra, ch. 2, p. 2.

3 Padma-sundara (beautiful lotus), mentioned in the Nirwanatantra, ch. 7, p. 9.

4 Dwadasha (the twelve), mentioned in the Todalatantra, ch. 9, p. 16.

5 Dwadashadala (the twelve-petalled), mentioned in the Shaktanandatarangini, 4.29; Rudrayamala, Part 2, 22.8.

6 Suryasangkhyadala (the twelve-petalled), mentioned in the Shaktanandatarangini, 9.16.

7 Hrit padma (heart lotus), mentioned in the Kamadhenutantra, ch. 12, p. 15; ch. 13, pp. 15, 16; ch. 15, p. 19; ch. 17, p. 23; ch. 18, p. 24; Brihannilatantra, ch. 8, p. 65, 66; Gandharwatantra, ch. 8, p. 39; ch. 29, p. 112; Tararahasya, ch. 1, p. 2; ch. 3, p. 18; Bhutashuddhitantra, ch. 2, p. 2; ch. 4, p. 4; ch. 5, p. 4, 5; ch. 6, p. 6; ch. 10, p. 9; ch. 14, p. 12; Shaktanandatarangini, 4.34; 7.14; Rudrayamala, Part 2, 57, 19, 42; 60.29.

8 Hritpatra (heart petal = heart lotus), mentioned in the Brihannilatantra, ch. 8, p. 65.

9 Hritpankeruha (heart lotus), mentioned in the Rudrayamala, Part 2, 57.14.

10 Hritsaroruha (heart lotus), mentioned in the Purashcharyarnawa, ch. 5, p. 387.

11 Hridambhoja (heart lotus), mentioned in the Rudrayamala, Part 2, 57.12, 14.

12 Hridambuja (heart lotus), mentioned in the Mahanirwanatantra, 5.114; Kamadhenu-tantra, ch. 18, p. 24; Shadamnayatantra, 4.144.

13 Hridabja (heart lotus), mentioned in the Rudrayamala, Part 2, 60.10.

14 Hridaya (heart = heart lotus), mentioned in the Nilatantra, ch. 5, p. 9; Todalatantra, ch. 7, p. 14; Kamadhenutantra, ch. 13, p. 16; ch. 18, p. 24; Kularnawa, ch. 4, p. 19; Gandharwatantra, ch. 29, p. 109; Mantramahodadhi, 4.28; Shaktanandatarangini, 4.30.

15 Hridayambhoja (heart lotus), mentioned in the Sammohanatantra, Part 2, ch. 4, p. 4; Rudrayamala, Part 2, 57.1, 3, 33, 47; 59.23.

16 Hridayambuja (heart lotus), mentioned in the Sammohanatantra, Part 2, ch. 4, p. 4; Sharadatilakatantra, 5.133; Rudrayamala, Part 2, 59.28; 60.9.

17 Hridayasarasija (heart lotus), mentioned in the Wishwasaratantra, ch. 1, p. 8; Koulawali-tantra, ch. 3. p. 8.

18 Hridayabja (heart lotus), mentioned in the Rudrayamala, Part 2, 59.24.

19 Hridaya Kamala (heart lotus), mentioned in the Rudrayamala, Part 2, 59.27.

20 Hritpankaja (heart lotus), mentioned in the Shatchakranirupana, Verse 26.

Position

The anahata is situated in the heart region (—Mantramahodadhi, 4.23; Tripurasara-samuchchaya, 5.20; Sammohanatantra, Part 2, ch. 2, p. 2; Wishwasaratantra, ch. 1, p. 3; Koulawalitantra, ch. 22, p. 80; Shaktananda-tarangini, 4.12, 29; 9.16; Rudrayamala, Part 2, 27.62; Purashcharyarnawa, ch. 6, p. 490; Shiwa-sanghita, 5.116; Yogaswarodaya and Mridani-tantra, quoted in Amarasanggraha MS; Tattwa-yogabindu MS). The anahata is called the heart lotus because of its location in the heart region.

In the Waidika accounts, the anahata has also been termed hridaya (heart) (—Narayanopa-nishad, Mantra 50; Brahmopanishad, Mantra 34; Mahopanishad, 1.12), because it is situated in the heart region (—Yogakundalyupanishad, 3.11; Yogashikhopanishad, 1.173; 5.9; Yogarajopa-nishad, Mantra 10). In the Pouranika accounts, the anahata has been described as being situated in the heart region (—Dewibhagawata, 11.1.43).

The actual location of the anahata is not directly in the heart region, but within the vertebral column corresponding to the heart region.

Description

There is a beautiful lotus, situated above the manipura and in the heart region, of the colour of the bandhuka flower (Pentapetes Phoenicea—Monier-Williams) and bright, which possesses the twelve (matrika-) letters from ka (to *tha*) of vermilion colour (on its petals); it is termed *anahata* (—*Shat*chakranirupana, Verse 22). This means that the *anahata chakra* (Plate 11) has twelve petals of deep red colour, and on the petals are the matrika-letters kang, khang, gang, ghang, ṅang, chang, chang, jang, jhang, ñang, tang and *thang* of vermilion colour. The colour of the bandhuka flower is white, vermilion and deep red (—Shaligramanighantubhushana, pushpawarga (flower group). Here, the deep red colour should be taken. The colour should be like the shona flower (Bauhinia Variegata—Monier-Williams) which is deep red (—Waidyakashabdasindhu).

That the *anahata* has twelve petals has been stated in the Kaṅkalamalinitantra, ch. 2, p. 5; Nirwanatantra, ch. 7, p. 9; Gandharwatantra, ch. 5, p. 28; ch. 8, p. 39; Bhutashuddhitantra, ch. 2, p. 2; Sammohanatantra, Part 2, ch. 2, p. 2; ch. 4, p. 4; Shiwasanghita, 5.116; Rudrayamala, Part 2, 22.8; 27.63; Goutamiyatantra, 34.49; Mantramahodadhi, 4.23; Koulawalitantra, ch. 3, p. 8; ch. 22, p. 80; Shaktanandatarangini, 4.12, 29; 7.14; Kamadhenutantra, ch. 12, p. 15; ch. 13, p. 15; ch. 15, p. 19; ch. 17, p. 23; Brihannilatantra, ch. 8, p. 65; Mundamalatantra, ch. 6, p. 9; Sharadatilakatantra, 5.133; Shadamnayatantra, 5.266; Yogaswarodaya and Mridanitantra, quoted in *Amarasanggraha* MS; and Tattwayogabindu MS. There are exceptions. The *anahata* has been described as the pure white sixteen-petalled lotus in the heart region (—Tararahasya, ch. 4, p. 22). The *anahata* has also been called hridaya chakra with eight petals (—Soubhagyalakshmyupanishad, 3.4).

In the Waidika accounts, the *anahata* has been described as having twelve petals (—Yogachudamanyupanishad, Mantras 5,13; Yogashikhopanishad, 1.173; 5.9). That the *anahata* has twelve petals has also been stated in the Pouranika accounts (—Shiwapurana, 5b. 29.136; Lingapurana, 1.8.97; 1.75.35; Dewibhagawata, 7.35.40; 11.1.43).

It has been stated that the colour of the petals of the *anahata* is deep red (—Kaṅkalamalinitantra, ch. 2, p. 5; Shiwasanghita, 5.116; Rudrayamala, Part 2, 22.8; Mridanitantra, quot-

ed in *Amarasanggraha* MS); Mayatantra, quoted by Wishwanatha in his *Shatchakrawiwriti*). The colour of the petals is also stated to be red like the rising sun (—Gandharwatantra, ch. 5, p. 27; Rudrayamala, Part 2, 27.62; Goutamiyatantra, 34,49), like red-hot gold (that is, shining red) (—Shaktanandatarangini, 4.12), shining red (—Brihannilatantra, ch. 8, p. 65), shining vermilion (—Tripurasarasamuchchaya, 5.20; Nirwanatantra, ch. 7, p. 9); a mixture of dark blue and yellow (—Dakshinamurti and Jñanarnawa, quoted in Yogakalpalatika MS; Koulawalitantra, ch. 22, p. 80), yellow (—Sammohanatantra, Part 2, ch. 2, p. 2), and white (—Bhutashuddhitantra, ch. 2, p. 2). In the Pouranika accounts, the colour of the petals of the *anahata* has been stated as red like the sun (—Shiwapurana, 5b. 29.137) and red like the rising sun (—Dewibhagawata, 7.35.39).

The above statements indicate that the colour of the petals of the *anahata* is deep red, shining red, shining vermilion, yellow, dark blue-yellow, and white. The differences in colour are due to the nature of power-radiations and modes of concentration. But the generally accepted colour by the practitioners is deep red.

It has been accepted in the Tantras that the twelve matrika-letters from kang to *thang* are on the petals of the *anahata chakra*. The colour of the matrika-letters has been stated to be vermilion (—*Shat*chakranirupana, Verse 22), deep red (—Nirwanatantra, ch. 6, p. 9); molten gold (that is, shining red) (—Koulawalitantra, ch. 22, p. 80), red (—Rudrayamala, Part 2, 57.19), shining (—Kaṅkalamalinitantra, ch. 2, p. 5), and white (—Bhutashuddhitantra, ch. 2, p. 2).

The matrika-letters are arranged from right to left.

There are twelve specific qualities (writtis) on the petals of the *anahata*, arranged from right to left in the following order: (1) lustfulness, (2) fraudulence, (3) indecision, (4) repentance, (5) hope, (6) anxiety, (7) longing, (8) impartiality, (9) arrogance, (10) incompetency, (11) discrimination, and (12) an attitude of defiance (—Adhyatma Wiweka, quoted by the commentator Narayana in his commentary on Hangsopanishad, Mantra 7). Jaganmohana assigns the qualities and their order as follows: (1) hope, (2) anxiety, (3) endeavour, (4) 'mineness,' (5) arrogance, (6) incompetency, (7) discrimination, (8) egoism, (9) lustfulness, (10) fraudulence, (11) indecision, and (12) repentance (—Footnote 87, in connection with the verse 5.104, Mahanirwanatantra).

Wayu-mandala ('Air'-region)

Here (that is, in the pericarp of the lotus—Kalicharana) is the 'air'-region which is hexagonal (arranged by interlacing two triangles) and smoke-coloured (—Shatchakranirupana, Verse 22). It has been stated that the wayu ('air') (-region) is in the pericarp (of the anahata) (—Kankalamalinitantra, ch. 2, p. 5; Shaktanandatarangini, 4.30; Shadamnayatantra, 5.266). The 'air'-region is six-cornered (hexagonal) (—Nirwanatantra, ch. 7, p. 9; Mridanitantra, quoted in Amarasanggraha MS; Yogatattwopanishad, Mantra 95; Yogashikhopanishad, 1.177; 5.14). The 'air'-region has also been described as circular with six points in the Dewibhagawata, 11.8.6, and Rudrayamala, Part 2, 57.33. This six-cornered region is smoke-coloured (a mixture of black and red colours) (—Mridanitantra, quoted in Amarasanggraha MS; Mayatantra, quoted by Wishwanatha; Dewibhagawata, 11.8.6). It has also been stated as being black in colour (—Yogatattwopanishad, Mantra 95).

Within it (within the 'air'-region—Kalicharana) is the pawana-akshara (that is, the matrika-akshara—matrika-letter, of pawana, which is the 'air'-germ mantra Yang; pawanabija is Yang—Warnabijakosha and Bijabhidhana; pawana-akshara is Yang bija—Kalicharana; pawana-akshara is Yang—Wishwanatha) which is smoke-coloured and with four arms and seated on a black antelope (—Shatchakranirupana, Verse 23). Pawana-akshara is wayu-bija which is Yang. The word akshara means bija (—Commentator Shankara). It has been stated that wayu-bija (Yang) is inside the six-cornered region of 'air' (—Nirwanatantra, ch. 7, p. 9; Sammohanatantra, Part 2, ch. 2, p. 2; Shiwasanghita, 5.116; Mridanitantra, quoted in Amarasanggraha MS; Yogatattwopanishad, Mantra 95; Dewibhagawata, 11.8.6). Wayu-bija is seated on a black antelope (—Mridanitantra, quoted in Amarasanggraha MS). So the form of Yang-bija is smoke-coloured, four-armed and seated on a black antelope. This is the form of Deity Wayu. According to Kalicharana, there should be an ankusha (goad) in the hand of Wayu, as Waruna holds in his hand a pasha (noose). The concentration form of Deity Wayu is as follows.

Wayu is smoke-coloured, four-armed, holding in one of his hands an ankusha, and seated on a black antelope.

It has been stated that there is the circular region of Wayu within which lies the smoke-coloured 'air'-letter (Yang); within it (the circular region) is a six-cornered region which is the seat of the Deity and here one should concentrate on one's own Ishtadewata. Concentration on Wayu should also be made here (in the six-cornered region). Wayu is extremely subtle; he is Supreme Brahman when without form, and when with form, he is in the nature of sound; ... his seat is on the black antelope; he grants boons to the three worlds, is very kind and wears a crown; he is life himself (—Rudrayamala, Part 2, 57.33–8).

Isha

Within it (within wayu-bija—Kalicharana; that is within the bindu of Yang) is Isha who is all mercy, bright and like hangsah, and with his two hands shows the mudras of dispelling fear and granting boons to the three worlds (—Shatchakranirupana, Verse 23).

The expression, 'like hangsah' (hangsabha) requires explanation. Kalicharana has not explained it, but quoted a passage saying that the desired One is splendorous like ten million moons. It indicates that he is like the moon, that is, he is possessed of the colour of shining white. Shankara and Wishwanatha interpret 'hangsabha' to be the colour of the sun, that is, red. On the other hand, the commentators Ramawallabha and Bhuwanamohana translate it as white colour.

Isha is one of the six Shiwas. Isha has also been called Ishwara. So Ishwara is one of the Shiwas (—Rudrayamala, Part 2, 25.53). The presence of Ishwara in the six-cornered 'air'-region has been mentioned in the Tantras (—Nirwanatantra, ch. 7, p. 9; Rudrayamala, Part 2, 22.8; Mantramahodadhi, 4.22; Sharadatilakatantra, 5.133; Purashcharyarnawa, ch. 5, p. 387). In the Waidika accounts, also Ishwara has been stated to be in the 'air'-region (—Yogatattwopanishad, Mantra 96; Yogashikhopanishad, 1.177). Ishwara has been called Hara (—Todalatantra, ch. 7, p. 14) and Shiwa (—Brihannilatantra, ch. 8, p. 65). Ishwara has also been described as Bana-linga (—Sammohanatantra, Part 2, ch. 2, p. 2). It has been clearly stated that Ishwara is in the lap of wayu-bija (—Mridanitantra, quoted in Amarasanggraha MS).

In the anahata, concentration should be done on Ishwara (—Rudrayamala, Part 2, 57.41). His concentration-form is as follows: Ishwara is in the form of (matrika-) letters, four-armed, shining white in colour, and wears a crown and a red garland; he does good to the three worlds and is the lord of the yogis (—ibid., 57, 41–2). Here it has been clearly said that Ishwara is white in colour. Here is another concentration-form:

Shiwa, the conqueror of death, resembles pure crystal (in colour); he is five-faced and of great lustre, with lotus-like beautiful and smiling face and ten long arms; his breast is ornamented with a garland of rudraksha and his head with the matted and twisted hair; and he wears a crown, an earring, an armlet, a bracelet, and is clad in tiger's skin (—Brihannilatantra, ch. 8, p. 65). As Shiwa has been described as having three eyes in all his forms, so here he should be thought of as having three eyes in each of his faces. Kalicharana also says that Shiwa has been described everywhere as having three eyes, hence Isha is also three-eyed. He also quotes a passage saying that one should concentrate on him as wearing a necklace, an armlet, a chain of pearls and an anklet, and clad in silken raiment.

In concentration, the forms of Isha or Ishwara have been described as follows:

(a) One-faced; five-faced.
(b) Two-armed; four-armed; ten-armed.
(c) Colour: pure crystal; shining white.
(d) Three-eyed.
(e) Making the gestures of dispelling fear and granting boons.
(f) Wearing a crown, earrings, armlets, a necklace, anklets and a garland of rudraksha.
(g) Clad in tiger's skin; silken raiment. (See Plate 12, left top figure.)

Kakini

Here (in the pericarp—Kalicharana) is Kakini (Power Kakini—Kalicharana) who is new lightning-like yellow (that is, shining yellow in colour), three-eyed, adorned with all kinds of ornaments and holds in her two hands a pasha (noose) and a kapala (human skull), while the other two hands are in the wara and abhaya mudras (that is, the gestures of granting boons and dispelling fear); she wears a necklace of bones; she is auspicious and joyous and the benefactress of all; and she is fully absorbed in supreme blissfulness in death-conquering union (—Shatchakranirupana, Verse 24). (See Plate 12, right top figure.)

The presence of Power Kakini in the pericarp of the anahata has been mentioned in the Kankalamalinitantra, ch. 2, p. 5; Shiwasanghita, 5.118; Mantramahodadhi, 4.22; Rudrayamala, Part 2, 22.8; Tripurasarasamuchchaya, 5.21; Todalatantra, ch. 7, p. 14; Shadamnayatantra, 5.266; Mridanitantra, quoted in Amarasanggraha MS. Kakini has been described as doorkeeper (—Sammohanatantra, Part 2, ch. 2, p. 2). Power Bhuwaneshwari (the mother of the universe) has been mentioned in the Nirwanatantra, ch. 7, p. 9. It has also been said that Power Lakini is in the anahata (—Tararahasya, ch. 4, p. 22). But these forms are for special concentration.

A concentration-form of Kakini is as follows.

Kakini is white in colour and two-armed, and shines with the vermilion-mark on her forehead, and her eyes are beautifully painted with collyrium, and she is clad in white raiment and adorned with various ornaments, and her face is as beautiful as the moon; concentration should be made on Kakini for the attainment of success in the mantra (—Kankalamalinitantra, ch. 5, p. 23).

Kalicharana quotes a two-lined verse which is exactly the third and fourth lines of the four-lined verse of the Kankalamalinitantra quoted above, except the first word of the first line quoted by him which is 'Krishnambarapari-dhanang', meaning, clad in black clothing, but in the Kankalamalini text the first word of the third line is 'shuklambaraparidhanang', which means clad in white clothing.

In another form, Kakini has been described as having three beautiful faces, which are shining red in colour and very graceful; she is wearing a necklace of skulls and granting success (—Kularnawa, ch. 10, p. 53).

Kakini, in another of her concentration-forms is yellow in colour, with highly developed breasts, carries a trident, a drum, and a noose, and shows the gesture of dispelling fear; she is fully absorbed (in concentration) (mahamatta), and worshipped by the great sages (—Gandharwatantra, ch. 9, p. 42–3). Wishwanatha quotes a verse from a Tantra in which it is stated that Kakini is yellow in colour and holds in her hands a noose, a trident, a skull, and a drum.

Other concentration-forms of Kakini.

'Kakini is as beautiful and splendorous as millions of moons; she is pure and holds the Weda in her hand; her grandeur is that of the celestial trees; her necklace is like the rays of the sun; she appears agitated (with power)' (—Rudrayamala, Part 2, 59.27).

'Kakini has six faces and three eyes (in each face); she is yellow in colour, and holds in her hands a trident, a bow and a skull and makes the gesture of granting boons' (—Jamala, quoted in Yogakalpalatika MS).

'The great Divine Mother Kakini who is worshipped in the three worlds is subtle as well as in form; she has four arms and holds a skull and a trident, and makes the gestures of granting boons and dispelling fear; she is like ten million lightnings (that is, she is shining yellow in colour), and clad in yellow raiment; she wears various ornaments of gold and jewels; she is delighted with the drinking of sudha (amrita—deathless substance) and is fully absorbed (in concentration)' (—Rudrayamala, Part 2, 57, 43–6).

The following are the forms of Kakini in concentration:

(a) One face; three faces; six faces.
(b) Face is beautiful.
(c) Three-eyed.
(d) Colour: shining yellow; yellow; shining red; moon-white; white.
(e) Four-armed; two-armed.
(f) Holding a noose and a skull; a trident, a drum, and a noose; a noose, a trident, a skull and a drum; the Weda; a skull, and a trident; a trident, a bow, and a skull.
(g) Making the gestures of granting boons and dispelling fear; the gesture of dispelling fear; the gesture of granting boons.
(h) Clad in white raiment; black raiment; yellow raiment.
(i) Wearing various ornaments of gold and jewels.
(j) Graceful.
(k) Fully absorbed (in concentration).

Bana-linga

'In the pericarp of this lotus (anahata), there is Power as a triangle (that is, triangular in form—Kalicharana) and her delicate body is like ten million lightnings (that is, she is splendorous); within that (that is, the triangular Power) is the Shiwa-linga (that is, Supreme Being in a specific concentration form) called Bana (that is, Bana-linga) who is gold-like luminous (that is, shining yellow in colour); there is a subtle void (that is, the bindu) on his head as that in a gem and there is the abode in him of the roused superpower of yoga (Lakshmi)' (—Shatchakranirupana, Verse 25).

It should be noted here that the Power is in the form of a triangle, so there is no distinction between the Power and the triangle. The triangle is to be considered as the body of the Power. Because of this, the triangle is the yoni, and so its apex is downward. This also has been expressed by Kalicharana. Kalicharana farther says that this triangle is situated below the wayu-bija ('air'-germ mantra). He quotes a passage in which it is stated that in the lap of the wayu-bija is Isha and below him is the triangle where lies Bana-linga.

The triangle is of lightning-like colour, that is, shining red, or shining yellow in colour. Bana-linga is within the triangle. This means he is within the Power who is triangular in form. This Power supports or holds a dewata in a centre. So it is the holding-power by which an appropriate dewata is maintained in a particular centre or seat. This Power has been termed Pitha-shakti—the holding-power which is the power of concentration. It has been stated that the Pitha-shakti (situated in the anahata) in her dhyana-form is in the form of a triangle, golden in colour, shining like ten million lightnings at the same time (that is, shining yellow colour), and adorned with all kinds of ornaments (—Rudrayamala, Part 2, 57.48–9). In concentration, the Pitha-shakti is in form. This form is not the triangular form, but a specific form of concentration lying in the triangle which is her form of support. So it has been stated that concentration should be done on Bana-linga who is situated by the right side of the Pitha-shakti (—ibid., 57.50).

The triangle in the anahata is called the yoni where lies Bana-linga (—Kankalamalinitantra, ch. 2, p. 5). Therefore, the triangle is situated with its base upward and apex downward. That Bana-linga is situated within the triangle has been stated in the Sammohanatantra, Part 2, ch. 2, p. 2; Gandharwatantra, ch. 29, p. 109; Mridanitantra, quoted in Amarasanggraha MS). About the colour of Bana-linga, it has been stated that he is gold-like luminous (—Shatchakranirupana, Verse 25). The text reads: Kanakakarangaragojjwalah to mean gold-like (kanaka-akara) luminous (ujjwala) colour of the body (anga-raga). The usual meaning of kanaka is gold. Bhuwanamohana has translated it as gold-like luminous colour. Ramawallabha has translated kanaka-akara as gold-colour. But Wishwanatha translates the word kanaka as being similar to the flower of bandhuka, and quotes a passage to support this. The colour of the bandhuka-flower is white, deep red and vermilion. What colour should apply here? Usually, the deep red colour is taken. Jaganmohana says that Bana-linga is blood-red (—Footnote 87, in connection with the verse 5.104, Mahanirwanatantra).

Let us see what other tantras say about the colour of Bana-linga. Bana-linga is as lustrous as the ten thousand suns (indicating that the colour is shining red) (—Gandharwatantra, ch. 5, p. 28; Rudrayamala, Part 2, 27.63; Goutamiyatantra, 34.50; Shaktanandatarangini, 4.12; Dewibhagawata, 7.35, 40); and like pure gold (—Rudrayamala, Part 2, 57.50); and also highly luminous (—Shiwasanghita, 5.117). So the colour of Bana-linga is shining red or gold or shining yellow.

There is a subtle void on the head of Bana-linga. Kalicharana says that there are on the head of the Shiwa-linga the half-moon (ardhachandra) and bindu (point) and within the bindu is a hole which is void. To support it he quotes a verse which says that Bana-linga who is within the triangle is adorned with golden ornaments and with the half-moon on his head. We would put it in this way: the void on the head of Bana-linga is bindu isolated from the body by the half-moon. It indicates that concentration on the form is finally developed into formless Divine Consciousness indicated by bindu.

Jiwatman

There is in the lotus (in the pericarp of the lotus—Kalicharana) in the heart region (this lotus is anahata—Ramawallabha and Bhuwanamohana) hangsah (jiwatman—Kalicharana, Wishwanatha, Ramawallabha and Bhuwanamohana) who is like the flame of a lamp in a windless place (that is, hangsah is luminous and motionless); there is also (in the pericarp of this lotus—Kalicharana) the region of the sun by which the filaments in the pericarp are illuminated (—Shatchakranirupana, Verse 26).

It has been clearly stated in the Kankalamalinitantra, ch. 2, p. 5, that in the pericarp of the anahata are the seats of Wayu and jiwa. In the Bhutashuddhitantra, ch. 2, p. 2, it has been also said that jiwa is always situated in the anahata; and also in the Tararahasya, ch. 4, p. 22; Tripurasarasamuchchaya, 5.21; Goutamiyatantra, 34.51; Soubhagyalakshmyupanishad, 3.4; Yogachudamanyupanishad, Mantra 14; Yogarajopanishad, Mantra 11; Shiwapurana, 3.5.52; Dewibhagawata, 7.35.41).

About the form for concentration of jiwatman, it has been mentioned that he is like the flame of a lamp, the nature of which is Brahman; he is of golden colour (—Bhutashuddhitantra, ch. 2, p. 2); also, jiwa as hangsah is shining like the flame of a lamp (—Sammohanatantra, Part 2, ch. 2, p. 2); hangsakala (jiwatman) is luminous and like the flame of a lamp (lingakara) (—Soubhagyalakshmyupanishad, 3.4); hangsah (jiwatman) is luminous (—Yogarajopanishad, Mantra 11). So the dhyana-form of jiwatman is that he is in the form of linga and like the flame of a lamp. The linga-form here means that his form is like the still flame of a lamp which tapers upward. Hangsah is also shining like gold, or shining gold colour.

The existence of the sun-region has also been mentioned in the Rudrayamala, Part 2, 57.54, and this is mainly for concentration in which also the sun-illuminated filaments of the lotus should be included.

Explanation

The central powers of the anahata, mainly consisting of wayu-power, radiate as petaline force-radiations, twelve in number, and are designated by the matrika-letters kang, khang, gang, ghang, nang, chang, chang, jang, jhang, ñang, tang and thang. The nature of power-radiations is indicated by the colours of the petals and the matrika-letters. The deep red indicates the predominance of prana in combination with apana, the shining red that of prana and udana, the shining vermilion that of prana, udana and wyana; the dark-blue-yellow that of prana and wyana; yellow is essentially wyana and white is mainly samana.

The original colour of kang is vermilion; of khang, chang and tang white; of gang and ghang red like the rising sun; of nang smoke; of chang and thang shining yellow; of jang moon-white; and of jhang and ñang shining red. The original colours of the matrika-letters are changed into vermilion, red, shining red, deep red and white in the anahata-petals. The vermilion indicates the concentration of prana, udana and wyana; the red and deep red that of prana and apana; the shining red that of prana and udana; and the white that of samana. The purpose of this colour-change is to intensify

particular anahata radiations.

The following are the forms of concentration in the anahata.

1 Petaline concentration. The twelve matrika-letters from kang to thang should be made into mantra-form which ultimately will become the unit of the anahata-concentration by japa and thought-concentration. The separate petals will finally become a circular wheel of deep red colour when the externalized radiations will stop.

2 Mahabhuta-concentration. There are two main stages of concentration. The first is thought-concentration in which the six-cornered smoke-coloured wayu-region with the wayu-bija Yang, also of smoke colour, is thought of. Finally, it reaches the second stage when the hexagonal region and Yang are 'seen' in deep concentration.

3 Tanmatra-concentration. When concentration becomes deeper, the hexagonal region gradually disappears, and only the smoke-coloured wayu-bija remains. It is indicative of sparsha (touch) tanmatra.

4 Wayu-concentration. Deep concentration on Yang causes the appearance of Deity Wayu form the bija aspect (ya). Wayu is seen on a black antelope, and is smoke-coloured, four-armed, holding an ankusha (goad).

The krishnasara (black antelope) is the carrier of Deity Wayu. It is a kind of mriga (deer, antelope—Apte). The antelope is very swift. The prana-force becomes metamorphosed into energy as speed through the muscles at the physical level. The krishnasara is the supporter of the activities of prana-forces which have been centralized in Wayu. The pranic activities are the expression of life in the body with which are associated the organic and muscular activities and the senso-intellectual activities and diversiform consciousness. Wayu as mahabhuta-tanmatra is the central energy which can be manifested with tejas-ap-prithiwi ('fire-water-earth') energies and then its motion is modified; when it manifests by itself its motional force is almost boundless and cannot operate in the material field, and, consequently, it creates its own field—the power-field where it operates in conjunction with pranic forces. Prana in the wayu (or power)-field, becomes wayus or motional forces when it is in operation. The principal wayus are five:

prana, apana, samana, udana and wyana.

Prana has another aspect. In that aspect it is what is called daiwa prana (—Brihadaranyakopanishad, 1.5.20), that is, supernormal prana. It exhibits the extraordinary function—cessation of motions, in addition to its motional function. In both states, daiwa prana is free from all disturbances and there is no dissipation. In other words, prana as daiwa prana functions normally and most efficiently in all its motions, and also undergoes a non-throbbing state when kumbhaka becomes natural. Daiwa prana is the basis on which daiwa manas (supernormal mind) (—Brihadaranyakopanishad, 1.5.19) is aroused. It is that aspect of the mind which is above all sorrows and exhibits concentration power by which samadhi becomes the natural mode of consciousness.

Through a process of internalization prana is transformed into daiwa prana. This process is the process of control, indicated by the ankusha (goad) held by Deity Wayu. This control is based on spiritual knowledge, represented by the letter ang. It requires great physical endurance and strong will to withstand, which is represented by the letter ku, for its development to a high degree; and when control becomes natural it gives happiness which is represented by the letter shang. Wayu is of daiwa prana. In him the prana is supercontrolled into daiwa prana. The process of control of prana is pranayama. To make pranayama successful, it is necessary to purify and normalize the pranic activities supported by krishnasara-mriga. From it a process called mriga-process has been evolved for the cardiopulmonary vitalization and development and internal purification. The vitalizing exercise consists of swift running, slow running, long walking, and swimming. The purificatory exercise comprises bhastrika and sahita breathing and shodhana.

From the mantra viewpoint, wayu is in the form of bija-mantra yang from which Deity Wayu is aroused. There are other matrika-letters for wayu. They are kang, khang, ghang, nang, chang, jhang, tang, dhang and sang. The bija-mantra of ankusha is Krong. The other matrika-letters standing for it are jhang, tang and shang. Mriga is represented by hang and ung.

5 Isha-concentration. In deep concentration, Deity Isha emerges from the bindu of the bija-mantra Yang. Isha is Supreme Being endowed with supreme yoga-power. Isha and Ishwara are the same. In his power aspect, Isha is omniscient and omnipotent, whereas the embodied beings have limited knowledge and power; Isha is infinite; he is beyond the universe and also he is within it; he is also hidden within all beings (—Shwetashwataropanishad, 1.9; 3.7).

Isha also assumes divine forms. One of these, the form of Isha, arises at the level of wayu-principle, that is, in the anahata chakra. The colour of Isha is white. It indicates he is all sattwa (of sentience and purity). When his form is roused in the anahata in deep concentration, the practitioner experiences that power emanates from Isha which dispels all fear arising from unspirituality, and strengthens concentration which is the greatest boon to him. The third eye of Isha is the samadhi-knowledge which is always with him. The other two eyes indicate that Isha is also conscious of his worshippers who are in his consciousness in concentration, and in thoughts when in the post-concentration stage. Isha is in the lotus posture, not seated on a carrier, but on the air. This levitation indicates the highest stage of pranayama which is natural to Isha. The anahata is the special centre of prana-wayu, and here pranayama can be developed to its highest level through Deity Wayu. Pranayama becomes firmly established in a disciple devoted to Isha. The mantra forms of Isha are represented by ung, eng, ring, hring, gang, nang, sang, soung, and hang.

6 Kakini-concentration. Kakini is the doorkeeper of the anahata. Concentration on Kakini prepares a disciple to remove all obstacles and develops the power of control. Concentration on Kakini develops enough power to be able successfully to do concentration on Isha. The power aspect of Isha is Kakini. The power which develops in concentration leading to the realization of Supreme Shakti (power) is Power Kakini. The control-power which effects the motionlessness of the prana wayus becomes stabilized in the anahata by Kakini.

The shining yellow colour of Kakini indicates that her power maintains the divine form of consciousness. Her shining red colour indicates that her power is being utilized in the control of prana wayus. When she is white, she is Isha-consciousness. She holds in her hands pasha (noose) and kapala (skull). The kapala is that which preserves 'kang', that is, 'sukhang'. Sukhang is 'su' meaning excellent, and khang which is knowledge. So kapala indicates spiritual knowledge. Pasha is 'pang', meaning the knowledge of atman, and 'asha', meaning desire. That is, one who desires to attain atman-knowledge is indicated by pasha. The bija-mantra of Kakini is Kang.

7 Concentration on Bana-linga. Concentration on Bana-linga consists of three stages. (a) Concentration on the triangular power: the triangular power is the power of holding in concentration expressed by consciousness when it is a triangle. The triangle is that form of consciousness when it is not deviated from one aspect to another of the usual three aspects of the sensory objects. The holding-power should be developed by doing concentration on the subtle lightning-like triangular-shape power. (b) Concentration on the linga-form: the form of Bana-linga is broad at the bottom and tapers gradually to a point in its head. The colour of the Bana-linga is of gold or shining red. One of the two colours should be taken. Concentration should start at the broad aspect, and as concentration becomes deeper, it will move towards the tapering. The process of concentration is this: at first the conscious field of concentration is broader, then gradually the field becomes narrow, and, finally, it is a point, as concentration develops deeper. So the Shiwa-linga form is actually the process of concentration. (c) Concentration on Bindu: 'the Shiwa-linga concentration finally becomes the bindu concentration. When the Shiwa-linga-body concentration develops to its highest point, which is indicated by the crescent, it is transformed into form-less bindu concentration.

8 Concentration on Jiwatman. Concentration on jiwatman is an important factor in the bhutashuddhi process. Jiwatman is the spiritually purified and illuminated embodied being, situated within the power-triangle and below Bana-linga. In the pericarp of the anahata is the

hexagonal wayu-region in which is situated Yang. The power-triangle is below Yang. Bana-linga is within the power-triangle, and jiwatman is inside the triangle, but below Bana-linga.

The form of jiwatman is like the steady flame of a lamp and luminous. Concentration should be done on the motionless flame-like jiwatman with a view to making the I-consciousness as steady as the jiwatman and gradually, in concentration, it should be dissolved into the steady flame-like consciousness.

6 Wishuddha

The wishuddha is the fifth in the six-chakra group, but serially it is the sixth chakra. It is situated within the chitrini nadi.

Terminology

The following are the Tantrika terms of the wishuddha.

1 Wishuddha, mentioned in the Todalatantra, ch. 7, p. 14; ch. 9, p. 17; Kamadhenutantra, ch. 13, p. 16; Kankalamalinitantra, ch. 2, p. 5; Gandharwatantra, ch. 5, p. 28; Mantramahodadhi, 4.24; Kubjikatantra, 6.304; Tripurasarasamuchchaya, 5.23; Bhutashuddhitantra, ch. 2, p. 2; ch. 3, p. 3; ch. 5, p. 5; ch. 8, p. 8; ch. 10, p. 9; ch. 14, p. 12; Sammohanatantra, Part 2, ch. 2, p. 2; Wishwasaratantra, ch. 1, p. 10; Koulawalitantra, ch. 22, p. 81; Shaktanandatarangini, 4.13; Rudrayamala, Part 2, 22.10; 25.56; 27.65.67; Tantrarajatantra, 21.83; Purascharyarnawa, ch. 2, p. 91; ch. 6, pp. 490,492; Shadamnayatantra, 5.267,426; Shiwasanghita, 5.124,126; Goutamiyatantra, 34.52; Shatchakranirupana, Verse 28; Dakshinamurti, Jñanarnawa and Jñanachudamani, quoted in Yogakalpalatika MS; Yogaswarodaya and Mridanitantra, quoted in Amarasanggraha MS.

2 Wishuddhi, mentioned in the Shaktanandatarangini, 4.30.34.

3 Kantha (the neck; it means the wishuddha,

as it is situated in the neck region), mentioned in the Todalatantra, ch. 7, p. 14; Kularnawa, ch. 4, p. 21; Bhutashuddhitantra, ch. 4, p. 4; Mahanirwanatantra, 5.113.

4 Kanthadesha (the neck region, that is, wishuddha), mentioned in the Mantramahodadhi, 4.28; Sammohanatantra, Part 2, ch. 2, p. 2; Wishwasaratantra, ch. 1, pp. 8,10; Koulawalitantra, ch. 3, p. 8; Shadamnayatantra, 4.145.

5 Kantha-padma (the lotus in the neck region), mentioned in the Kankalamalinitantra, ch. 2, p. 5; Purashcharyarnawa, ch. 5, p. 387.

6 Kanthapankaja (the lotus in the neck region) mentioned in the Sammohanatantra, Part 2, ch. 4, p. 4; Sharadatilakatantra, 5.134.

7 Kanthambuja (the lotus in the neck region that is, wishuddha), mentioned in the Rudrayamala, Part 2, 60.52.

8 Kanthambhoja (the lotus in the neck region, that is, wishuddha), mentioned in the Rudrayamala, Part 2, 61.1.

9 Shodasha (the sixteen, that is, wishuddha), mentioned in the Todalatantra, ch. 9, p. 16.

10 Shodasha-dala (the sixteen-petalled, that is, wishuddha), mentioned in the Mundamalatantra, ch. 6, p. 9; Shaktanandatarangini, 4.29; 9.16.

11 Shodashara (the sixteen-petalled, that is, wishuddha), mentioned in the Wishwasaratantra, ch. 1, p. 8; Koulawalitantra, ch. 3, p. 8; Rudrayamala, Part 2, 60.29; Shadamnayatantra, 4.60.

12 Nirmala-padma (the bright, or pure lotus), mentioned in the Nirwanatantra, ch. 8, p. 10.

13 Dwyashtapatrambuja (the sixteen-petalled lotus), mentioned in the Gandharwatantra, ch. 8, p. 39; Shaktanandatarangini, 7.14.

14 Akasha (akasha-lotus, that is, the lotus containing the akasha principle = wishuddha), mentioned in the Bhutashuddhitantra, ch. 5, p. 4; Gandharwatantra, ch. 5, p. 28; Shaktanandatarangini, 4.13.

15 Shodashollasa-dala (the splendorous sixteen-petalled, that is, wishuddha), mentioned in the Rudrayamala, Part 2, 22.9.

16 Shodasha-patra (the sixteen-petalled), mentioned in the Rudrayamala, Part 2, 22.13.

Position

The wishuddha is situated in the neck-region (—Shatchakranirupana, Verse 28; Gandharwatantra, ch. 8, p. 39; Mantramahodadhi, 4.24; Tripurasarasamuchchaya, 5.23; Sammohanatantra, Part 2, ch. 2, p. 2; Koulawalitantra, ch. 22, p. 81; Shaktanandatarangini, 4.13,29; 7.14; 9.16; Rudrayamala, Part 2, 22.9; Purashcharyarnawa, ch. 6, p. 490; Shiwasanghita, 5.124; Yogaswarodaya and Mridanitantra, quoted in the Amarasanggraha MS). The same position has been accepted in the Waidika accounts (—Yogashikhopanishad, 1.174; 5.10) as well as in the Pouranika accounts (—Shiwapurana, 5b, 29.131; Dewibhagawata, 11.1.43). The neck region means that part of the vertebral column (that is, the cervical part of the spinal column) which corresponds to the region of the neck.

Description

The lotus called wishuddha (Plate 14), situated in the neck region, is of the shining smoke colour; and the petals are adorned with all the vowels (that is, the sixteen matrika-letters from ang to ah) of deep red colour which are 'seen' by him whose consciousness is illumined by the concentration-light (diptabuddhi); there is the void-region (nabhomandala) (in the pericarp of the wishuddha) which is like the full moon (that is, shining white—Bhuwanamohana) and circular in shape; (within this region) there lies the form (tanu, that is, the bija) of Ambara (= akasha-bija) which is white and seated on a snow-white elephant (—Shatchakranirupana, Verse 28).

In this verse, there is no clear mention of the petals of the wishuddha. But it has been stated that all the vowels are on its petals. This means that as the number of the vowels is sixteen, so, by implication, the number of the petals is sixteen. Each matrika-letter is on one petal. Kalicharana also says the same. In support of which he quotes a verse which states that above it (anahata) is the smoke-coloured sixteen-petalled lotus; on the petals are sixteen vowels with bindu (that is, the first sixteen matrika-units) which are deep red in colour; its filaments are red and there is the void-region (in its pericarp).

It has been clearly stated that the wishuddha has sixteen petals (—Nirwanatantra, ch. 8, p. 10; Gandharwatantra, ch. 5, p. 28; Mantramahodadhi, 4.24; Sammohanatantra, Part 2, ch. 2, p. 2; Koulawalitantra, ch. 22, p. 81; Sharadatilakatantra, 5.134; Shaktanandatarangini, 4.13; Rudrayamala, Part 2, 27.65; Purashcharyarnawa, ch. 5, p. 387; ch. 6, p. 490; Shiwasanghita, 5.124; Goutamiyatantra, 34.52; Jñanachudamani, quoted in the Yogakalpalatika MS), and its petals are smoke-coloured (—Kankalamalinitantra, ch. 2, p. 5; Tripurasarasamuchchaya, 5.23; Bhutashuddhitantra, ch. 2, p. 2; Sammohanatantra, Part 2, ch. 2, p. 2; Koulawalitantra, ch. 22, p. 81; Shaktanandatarangini, 4.13; Puraschcharyarnawa, ch. 6, p. 490; Shiwasanghita, 5.124; Dakshinamurti, Jñanarnawa and Jñanachudamani, quoted in the Yogakalpalatika MS; Mridanitantra, quoted in the Amarasanggraha MS), or the shining smoke colour (—Gandharwatantra, ch. 5, p. 28; Rudrayamala, Part 2, 22.10; 27.66.

There are vowels (the first sixteen matrika-letters) on the petals of the wishuddha (Wishwasaratantra, ch. 1, p. 8; Koulawalitantra, ch. 3, p. 8; Sharadatilakatantra, 5.134; Purashcharyarnawa, ch. 5, p. 387; Shiwasanghita, 5.124), and these vowels are 16 in number (—Kankalamalinitantra, ch. 2, p. 5; Gandharwatantra, ch. 5, p. 28; Mantramahodadhi, 4.23; Tripurasarasamuchchaya, 5.23; Bhutashuddhitantra, ch. 2, p. 2; Sammohanatantra, Part 2, ch. 2, p. 2; Shaktanandatarangini, 4.13; 7.14; Rudrayamala, Part 2, 27.66; Mahanirwanatantra, 5.113; Shadamnayatantra, 5.267; Jñanachudamani, quoted in the Yogakalpalatika MS; Mridanitantra, quoted in the Amarasanggraha MS). The colour of the vowels is red (—Koulawalitantra, ch. 22, p. 81; Dakshinamurti and Jñanarnawa, quoted in the Yogakalpalatika MS) and also golden (—Mridanitantra, quoted in the Amarasanggraha MS). The sixteen vowels or the matrika-letters are: ang, ang, ing, ing, ung, ung, ring, ring, lring, lring, eng, aing, ong, oung, ang, ah.

There are sixteen specific qualities (writtis) on the sixteen petals of the wishuddha chakra. They are arranged from the right to the left as the petal arrangement, and in the following order: (1) Pranawa (the mantra Ong), (2) Udgitha (the Sama-mantras), (3) Hung (a mantra), (4) Phat (a mantra), (5) Washat (a mantra), (6) Swadha (a mantra), (7) Swaha (a mantra), (8) Namah (a mantra), (9) amrita (deathlessness), and the seven (musical) tones, viz, Shadja and others (—Adhyatma Wiweka, quoted by the commentator Narayana in his commentary on Hangsopanishad, Mantra 7). Jaganmohana gives the names and their order as follows: The seven tones—(1) Nishada, (2) Rishabha, (3) Gandhara, (4) Shadja, (5) Madhyama, (6) Dhaiwata, and (7) Panchama; (8) poison, (9) Hung, (10) Phat, (11) Woushat, (12) Washat, (13) Swadha, (14) Swaha, (15) Namah (these seven mantras), and (16) amrita (—Footnote 87, in connection with the verse of the Mahanirwanatantra, 5.104).

Akasha-region

There is the akasha (void)-region in the pericarp of the wishuddha (—Kankalamalinitantra, ch. 2, p. 5; Bhutashuddhitantra, ch. 2, p. 2; ch. 8, p. 8; ch. 14, p. 12; Koulawalitantra, ch. 22, p. 81; Shaktanandatarangini, 4.30). The akasha is the void-principle (shunyatattwa) (—Bhutashuddhitantra, ch. 4, p. 4), and is in the nature of power (—ibid., ch. 2, p. 2); it is Deity Sadashiwa himself (—Sammohanatantra, Part 2, ch. 2, p. 2). There are five different aspects of akasha, namely, abhrakasha (atmospheric void), jalakasha (void in water), ghatakasha (void within a jar), patakasha (void in relation to a surface), and mahakasha (supreme void) (—Mahamuktitantra, quoted in the Yogakalpalatika MS). The five aspects of akasha have also been stated in the Waidika accounts. They are as follows: gunarahita akasha (attributeless void), parakasha (supervoid), mahakasha (supreme void), tattwakasha (bright void), and suryakasha (sun void) (—Mandalabrahmanopanishad, 1.2.13).

The shape of akasha (void)-region is circular (—Mantramaharnawa, ch. 4, p. 41). It has been stated that there is the moon-region in the pericarp of the lotus (wishuddha); there is also a six-cornered diagram where are situated Sadashiwa and Gouri (—Nirwanatantra, ch. 8, p. 10). It has also been stated that there is a beautiful triangle (in the wishuddha) where the filaments are (that is, in the pericarp), and here (in the triangle) is Sadashiwa (—Sammohanatantra, Part 2, ch. 2, p. 2). It has been stated clearly that there (in the pericarp of the wishuddha) is the akasha-region which is triangular in shape and of smoke colour (—Mridanitantra, quoted in the Amarasanggraha MS). So the akasha-region is circular or triangular. In the Waidika accounts, it has been stated that the akasha-region is circular (—Yogatattwopanishad, Mantra 98; Yogashikhopanishad, 1.178; 5.15). That the akasha-region is circular has also been stated in the Pouranika accounts (—Dewibhagawata, 11.8.7).

The colour of the akasha-region is implied as moon-white (—Shatchakranirupana, Verse 28; Nirwanatantra, ch. 8, p. 10). But the colour has been clearly mentioned as white or crystal-like transparent (swachcha) in the Mantramaharnawa, ch. 4, p. 41. It has also been stated that the colour is ·smoke (—Mridanitantra, quoted in the Amarasanggraha MS). That the colour of the akasha-region is smoke has also been stated in the Waidika accounts (—Yogatattwopanishad, Mantra 98). But the Pouranika account supports the white (or transparent) colour of the region (—Dewibhagawata, 11.8.7). So the akasha-region is white, transparent, or smoke in colour.

The form (tanu) of ambara (mentioned in the Shatchakranirupana, Verse 28) means the bija of Deity Ambara, that is, akasha-bija which is Hang. Ambara is akasha (void) (—Wachaspatyam; Shabdakalpadrumah). Tanu is body or form. Here, it is the mantra-form of akasha. The mantra-forms of ambara and akasha are ang and hang (—Warnabijakoshah). In the wishuddha chakra, the bija-mantra of akasha (or ambara) is Hang. It has been stated that kha-bija is inside the akasha-region (—Mridanitantra, quoted in the Amarasanggraha MS). Kha is akasha (—Wachaspatyam; Shabdakalpadrumah). The mantra-forms of kha are lring and hang (—Warnabijakoshah). So the kha-

bija is akasha-bija which is Hang. It has been clearly stated in the Mantramaharnawa, ch. 4, p. 41, that the bija Hang is in the akasha-region. It has been supported by the Waidika account in which it has been stated that there is the ha-letter (that is, the matrika-letter hang as the bija) in the circular akasha (—Yogatattwopanishad, Mantra 98). That the ha-letter is the Hang-bija has been stated in the Pouranika account which says that concentration should be done on the akasha-region where lies the Hang-bija (—Dewibhagawata, 11.8.7). The Hang-bija is white (—Bhutashuddhi, quoted by Kalicharana).

The akasha-bija Hang is seated on an elephant (—Mridanitantra, quoted in the Amarasanggraha MS; Kankalamalinitantra, ch. 2, p. 5), and the colour of the elephant is white (—Nigamalata; Bhutashuddhi, quoted by Kalicharana).

More about the forms of the Hang-bija

The bija (as Deity Ambara or Akasha) holds the pasha (noose) and ankusha (goad) and makes the gestures of granting boons and dispelling fear; in the lap of the mantra (that is, Hang-bija), there always is he who is known as Deity Sadashiwa; he is white in colour and three-eyed, and has five faces and ten arms, clad in a tiger's skin; his body is united with that of Girija (Power of Shiwa) (—Shatchakranirupana, Verse 29).

The bija-aspect of Hang assumes the ·divine form of Deity Ambara who is white and seated on a white elephant. He has four arms (—Mridanitantra, quoted in the Amarasanggraha MS) and holds a noose and a goad, and makes the gestures of granting boons and dispelling fear (—Nigamalata). This is the concentration form of Ambara.

Sadashiwa

Deity Sadashiwa lies in the lap of Hang-bija (—Mridanitantra, quoted in the Amarasanggraha MS; Nigamalata). In the lap of the Hang-bija means that Sadashiwa is always in the bindu of the bija and manifests himself in form in concentration. The manifested form of Sadashiwa is as follows: he is white in colour (—Shatchakranirupana, Verse 29); he has five faces and three eyes (to each face) (—Nirwanatantra, ch. 8, p. 10; Mridanitantra MS), and ten arms (—Mahanirwanatantra, 14.35; Nigamalata), and is clad in tiger's skin (—Mahanirwanatantra, 14.33; Nirwanatantra, ch. 8, p. 10). The presence of Sadashiwa in the wishuddha chakra has been generally recognized (—Todalatantra, ch. 7, p. 14; Mantramahodadhi, 4.23; Sammohanatantra, Part 2, ch. 2, p. 2; Sharadatilakatantra, 5.135; Rudrayamala, Part 2, 22.9; Puraschcharyarnawa, ch. 5, p. 387; Mantramaharnawa, ch. 4, p. 42; Shadamnayatantra, 5.267).

In the text (Shatchakranirupana, Verse 29), it has been stated that Sadashiwa's body is not different from Girija, that is, Sadashiwa and Girija have the same body. This means that Sadashiwa is in the form of Ardhanarishwara in which the Supreme Power, who is the Mother of the universe in the form of Gouri, is the half of the body of Shambhu (Shiwa) (—Nirwanatantra, ch. 8, p. 10). Kalicharana also interprets it as Ardhanarishwara (half male and half female form). Ardhanarishwara is a form of Shiwa in which the female (that is Shakti—Power) forms the half part of Ishwara (Shiwa) (—Wachaspatyam). It cannot be translated by the word androgyne or hermaphrodite. It is a form in which Supreme Consciousness-Power manifests both the Shiwa and Shakti (Power) aspects distinctly but also in union. The right part is Shiwa and the left part is Shakti. Kalicharana says that Ardhanarishwara is of golden colour on his left half of the body, and white on his right half. He cites a verse in which it is stated that there (in the wishuddha) is Deity Sadashiwa who is clad in white raiment and half of his body is the same as that of Girija, his body being of both silver (white) and gold (yellow) colour. The Ardhanarishwara form is also called Hara(Shiwa)-Gouri(Shakti)-murti (form) (—the commentator Shankara) and Uma (Shakti)-Maheshwara(Shiwa) (—Shabdakalpadrumah).

Sadashiwa as Ardhanarishwara is on the bull, half of whose body is that of the great lion (that is, the half-bull-half-lion) (—Nirwanatantra, ch. 8, p. 10). The carrier (wahana) of Shiwa is the bull, and that of Shakti is the great lion (mahasingha). As the right part is Shiwa and the left part is Shakti (ibid., ch. 8, p. 10), so the bull part is on the right side and the lion part on the left side.

Sadashiwa has ten arms. But in the text (—Shatchakranirupana, Verse 29), there is no mention of the implements which are in his hands. Kalicharana quotes a verse in which the implements carried by Sadashiwa have been mentioned. They are as follows: the shula (trident), the tanka (axe, or chisel), the kripana (sword), the wajra (thunderbolt), dahana (fire), the nagendra (the great serpent), the ghanta (bell), the ankusha (goad), and the pasha (noose), and a hand in abhaya-mudra (the gesture of dispelling fear).

So the concentration-form of Sadashiwa as Ardhanarishwara is as follows.

The right half of the body of Ardhanarishwara is white and the left half is of golden colour; he is on the bull-lion; he has five faces and each face has three eyes; he is clad in tiger's skin; he has ten arms and carries in his hands a trident, a chisel (or an axe), a sword, the thunderbolt, fire, the great snake, a bell, a goad and a noose, and makes the gesture of dispelling fear. (See Plate 15, left top figure.)

Sadashiwa has another form (not as Ardhanarishwara), described as follows. 'He is calm and as bright as ten million moons, and clad in a tiger's skin; his sacred thread is the serpent and his body is smeared with ashes and ornamented with snakes; he has five faces of the smoke, yellow, vermilion, white and deep red colour, and three eyes to each face; his head is covered with matted hair and he holds Ganga (the sacred river by that name); he is adorned with the moon (in crescent form) on his forehead; he has 10 arms, holding in his left hands the kapala (skull), pawaka (fire), the pasha (noose) the pinaka (Shiwa's bow) and the parashu (axe), and in his right hands the shula (trident), the wajra (thunderbolt), the ankusha (goad) and the shara (arrow), and shows wara (-mudra with one of his right hands) (the gesture of granting boons); he is white as snow, the kunda flower, or the moon, and seated on a bull' (—Mahanirwanatantra, 14.32-7). This is also the concentration-form of Sadashiwa.

There is a Waidika concentration-form of Sadashiwa as Ardhanarishwara which is as follows. 'Sadashiwa is like pure crystal (that is, colourless transparent, or pure white) and holds the crescent on his forehead; he has five beautiful faces, three eyes (to each face), and ten arms; he holds all implements and is adorned with all kinds of ornaments, he shows the gesture of granting boons; and one half of his body is of Uma (Power of Shiwa)' (—Yogatattwopanishad, Mantras 100–1).

Power Shakini

In this lotus (that is, in the pericarp of the wishuddha chakra—Kalicharana), is Shakini (the Power named Shakini—Kalicharana) who is white like the ocean of nectar (—Kalicharana) (or whiter than the ocean of nectar—Bhuwanamohana), clad in yellow raiment, and the shara (arrow), the chapa (bow), the pasha (noose) and the srini (goad) are held in her four beautiful hands (—Shatchakranirupana, Verse 30). (See Plate 15, right top figure.)

The presence of Power Shakini in the wishuddha chakra has been generally recognized in the Tantras (—Todalatantra, ch. 7, p. 14; Mantramahodadhi, 4.23; Tripurasarasamuchchaya, 5.23; Rudrayamala, Part 2, 22.9; Shadamnayatantra, 5.267; Jñanachudamani, quoted in the Yogakalpalatika MS). Shakini has been called the doorkeeper (—Sammohanatantra, Part 2, ch. 2, p. 2). It has been said that Shakini and Sadashiwa are the same (—Rudrayamala, Part 2, 61.2). Shakini is the presiding Deity (of the wishuddha) (—Shiwasanghita, 5.125). Shakini has four arms (—Mridanitantra, quoted in the Amarasanggraha MS).

Kalicharana quotes a verse in which the concentration-form of Shakini has been described. The verse states: Deity Shakini is in the form of light; she has five beautiful faces and three eyes to each face; she holds a noose, a goad, and a book in her lotus hands and makes jñanamudra (an attitude of the right hand in which the tip of the first finger touches the tip of the thumb).

The commentator Wishwanatha also quotes a verse from a Tantra in which the concentration-form of Shakini has been stated as follows.

The divine Shakini is splendorous, having five faces with three eyes each, and beautiful teeth, and holding in her lotus hands a bow, a trident, a book, and showing jñanamudra.

He adds that the arrow, the noose, the book and the jñanamudra (in the hands of Shakini) have also been mentioned in another Tantra.

Other concentration forms of Shakini are as follows.

1 Shakini is shining white in colour; she has two arms, and a charming face with beautiful eyes, painted with collyrium; she shines with the vermilion-mark on her forehead, and is clad in black raiment and adorned with various ornaments (—Kankalamalinitantra, ch. 5, p. 23).

2 Shakini has a red face with a sweet smile, and her eyes are painted with collyrium; she is beautifully ornamented and holds the thunderbolt and a staff (—Kularnawa, ch. 10, p. 53).

3 Shakini has five faces, three eyes (to each face), and four arms, holding a noose, a goad, and a book, and making the jñanamudra; she is powerful and has prominent teeth (—Koulawalitantra, ch. 22, p. 81).

4 The amiable Shakini, who gives blessings to the three worlds, is clad in yellow raiment, and beautiful and delighted; she is splendorous; she is beyond the Weda (Wedadya; from the mantra viewpoint, it is the mantra Ong) and she is the source of the Weda (Wedamata; from the mantra viewpoint, the bijas ing, ing, and thang, and the mantra Swaha); her body is moistened by the flowing streams of pure nectar; she has the most charming and smiling face with the three lotus-like beautiful eyes, well-developed breasts and matted hair and is adorned with all ornaments; she has four arms, and carries a lotus and an implement, and makes the gestures of dispelling fear and granting boons; she is also terrific when she is Goddess Shyama (—Rudrayamala, Part 2, 61.3–4).

5 Shakini is both without and with form; she is the mantra-knowledge; she is yellow in colour, three-eyed, four-armed and adorned with all ornaments; she has a smiling face; as Gouri she is united with Sadashiwa; she holds with her lotus hands the skull and the white lotus, and makes the gestures of granting boons and dispelling fear (—Rudrayamala, Part 2, 62. 32–3).

6 Divine Shakini is yellow in colour; she has

five faces and three eyes to each face, and beautiful teeth; she holds with her lotus hands a noose, a trident and a book, and shows jñana-mudra (the symbol of knowledge, done by a particular position of the hand) (—Jamala, quoted in the Yogakalpalatika MS).

The differences in the forms and implements are due to the mode and object of concentration.

Moon-region

There is in the pericarp of the wishuddha the spotless circular lunar region (—Shatchakra-nirupana, Verse 30). Kalicharana says that Divine Shakini is in the moon-region which lies in the pericarp of the wishuddha and he quotes a passage from the Premayogatarangini as his support, which says that there is Power Shakini in the shining lunar region.

Kalicharana says that there is at first the akasha-region in the pericarp of the wishuddha, and inside it is a triangle, within the triangle is the lunar region and within it the akasha-bija and others. This is supported by a verse he quotes which states that concentration should be done on the full moon (that is, the circular lunar region) which is in the triangle situated in the pericarp (of the wishuddha); there (in the lunar region) concentrate on white Akasha (as Deity), clad in white raiment and seated on an elephant; there is Deity Sadashiwa.

The presence of the lunar region in the pericarp of the wishuddha chakra has been mentioned in the Nirwanatantra, ch. 8, p. 10. The Nirwanatantra says that there is the very beautiful Jana-world where the great spiritual darkness ends; outside it (but inside the pericarp) is the lunar region ... in the pericarp lies the gemmed region where is a six-cornered diagram; inside the diagram is the half-bull-half-lion on which is seated (Power) Gouri united with Sadashiwa on her right side. This seems to indicate that there is the lunar region in the pericarp; within it the gemmed region; within the latter is a hexagon, inside which is the Deity in Ardhanarishwara-form.

It has been stated that in the region where the filaments of the wishuddha lotus are (that is, the region surrounded by the filaments; this is

the pericarp) there is a beautiful sky-blue triangle where lies Sadashiwa (—Sammohana-tantra, Part 2, ch. 2, p. 2). The triangle has been farther explained in the Mridanitantra, which says that there (in the pericarp of the wishuddha) is the akasha-region which is a triangle and of smoke colour; inside it is the akasha-bija (Hang) who is four-armed and seated on an elephant; in his lap is the four-faced, three-eyed Sadashiwa; here also is situated Power Shakini who has four arms.

The whole thing may be summarized as follows.

In the pericarp of the wishuddha chakra there is the akasha-region which is circular in shape and white in colour (—Shatchakranirupana, Verse 28). The triangle (mentioned in the Sammohanatantra, Part 2, ch. 2, p. 2) is not to be considered as situated directly in the pericarp, but inside the akasha-region which is in the pericarp. The triangle is the essential part of the circular akasha-region, and, therefore, it has also been termed the triangular akasha-region (—Mridanitantra). The triangle is either sky-blue (—Sammohanatantra, Part 2) or smoke (—Mridanitantra) in colour. Inside this triangle is the circular lunar region (—the verse quoted by Kalicharana). Akasha (in the bija-form) lies inside the lunar region (—ibid.). According to some other authorities, there appears to be a gemmed region inside the lunar region, and inside the gemmed region is a hexagon, and inside it is Ardhanarishwara (—Nirwanatantra, ch. 8, p. 10). As Sadashiwa in the form of Ardha-narishwara, is in the hexagon, so the akasha-bija in whose lap Sadashiwa is (—Mridani-tantra) must be in the hexagon.

According to some authorities the jiwatman (the embodied being) is situated in the wishu-ddha chakra (—Jnanarnawa, quoted in the Yogakalpalatika MS) and concentration should be done on him (—Purashcharyarnawa, ch. 6, p. 492). The wishuddha chakra is the centre for udana-wayu (—Amritanadopanishad, Mantra 34; Dewibhagawata, 7.32,40). According to some other authorities the centre of prana-wayu is in the wishuddha (—Mantramaharnawa, ch. 4, p. 42). The wishuddha is also the centre of the principles of hearing and speech (—Kankalamalinitantra, ch. 2, p. 5; Mantramaharnawa, ch. 4, p. 42).

Explanation

The akasha-power and udana-wayu radiate through the sixteen petaline processes of the wishuddha chakra into the ida-pingala field. The petaline power phenomenon consists of 16 radiations designated by the first sixteen matrika-units from *ang* to *ah*. The colours of the petals and the matrika-letters indicate the nature of the radiations. The smoke colour of the petals indicates the concentration of udana-wayu.

The original colours of the matrika-letters form *ang* to *ah* are as follows: *ang*, *ang*, *ing*, *ung*, *lring*, *aing* are white; *ing*, *ung*, *ring*, *lring*, *ang* are yellow; *ring*, *eng*, *ong*, *oung*, *ah* are red. These matrika-letters become red in the wishuddha. It indicates the concentration of prana-wayu. When the matrika-letters become golden, the concentration of wyana-wayu is indicated. Through the processes of *japa* of the matrika-letters as mantra and thought-concentration the petals are transformed into a circle of smoke colour when all powers shall be internalized. This mantra-form is the unit of concentration at the wishuddha level.

Akasha-principle

The central force of the wishuddha chakra is the akasha-principle which is seen first as a round white form in concentration, and as the depth of concentration increases, a triangle of the colour of sky-blue appears inside it. Then a moon-white circular form, termed the lunar region, appears within the triangle, and finally the akasha-bija Hang is seen in the lunar region.

The Ha aspect (which is the real bija aspect of Hang) develops in concentration as Deity Akasha (Ambara) white in colour, four-armed and seated on a white elephant; he holds a noose and a goad, and makes the gestures of granting boons and dispelling fear. The power imbedded in the bija aspect of Hang is fully roused when it assumes a divine form. The basic aspect of the power is the greatest development of physical power arising from the purity of the body; this is represented ·by the white elephant.

Associated with the physical power is the power of control being exercised on the body and mind; it is represented by the goad (ankusha). Under this condition, the disciple begins to be free from bondage, which is represented by the noose (pasha). The gesture of granting boons (wara-mudra) and that of dispelling fear (abhaya-mudra) are indicative of imparting spiritual knowledge and removing all obstacles in the spiritual path. The mantra-forms of hasti (elephant) are shang, krang and prang; of ankusha (goad) are jhang, tang, shang and krong; and of pasha (noose) is ang.

At the next stage of concentration, Deity Sadashiwa emerges from the bindu of Hang. He is usually seen in the form of Ardhanarishwara (half male-form and half female-form). The right half is Sadashiwa who is white in colour, has five faces and three eyes in each face; he has ten arms and holds a trident, a chisel, a sword, the thunderbolt, fire, the great snake, a bell, a goad and a noose and shows the gesture of dispelling fear; he is clad in a tiger's skin and is seated on the bull side of the bull-lion.

The white colour indicates that the Sadashiwa's form is of pure sattwa (sentience), expressing divine knowledge. His five faces indicate the concentration-knowledge of the five principles represented by the mantras Lang, Wang, Rang, Yang and Hang. In each face there are three eyes. When the two eyes do not see the world, because of their being absorbed in concentration, the third eye opens and expresses samadhi-prajña (true knowledge arising from superconcentration). The trident (shula) indicates the power of absorption of the primus (prakriti) consisting of three primary attributes. The chisel (tanka) indicates that living spiritual strength which removes all unspirituality. The sword (kripana) indicates the destruction of all forms which apparently limit the infinite form-less Being. The thunderbolt (wajra) is the adamantine control of apana-function. The fire (dahana) is the Kundalini-fire of absorption of all cosmic principles. The great serpent (nagendra) is the roused Kundali-power. The bell (ghanta) indicates the silent sound of mantra. The clothed tiger's skin indicates that all power has been controlled and spiritualized for the attainment of samadhi, or liberation.

Ardhanarishwara indicates the union of Shakti (Power) with Shiwa (Supreme Consciousness) as one and the same. The full realization of this occurs at the level of Parama Shiwa (Supreme Consciousness). Below the level of Sadashiwa, Shiwa and Shakti remain separate, but oneness is experienced in concentration. At the material level, both the male and the female forms are of Shakti, and consciousness-in-concentration is the experience of Shiwa in relation to Shakti as Kundalini. But these forms constitute different entities. This causes a differentiation in the pranic force in its life-creating aspect and effects a bifurcation as red-energy (rajas) and white-energy (shukra). The red-energy operates fully and freely in the female form and develops essential feminine qualities which maintain femininity. On the other hand, the white-energy does the same thing in the male. God Brahma as Ardhanarishwara made half part of his body male and the other half female, and they were separated for creative purposes. Owing to the natural affinity of the two forms of energy, man and woman are attracted to each other; each tries to get in contact as much as possible, but there is an inescapable power-limitation when the energy-flow begins to ebb. This only serves a part of our purpose. Unless one is able to ingest the essence of the substance-energy from each other during multi-levelled contacts by exercising control and by applying well-mastered motions, adequately and controllingly, the inner instability will continue and the mental diversiform will not cease. The Ardhanarishwara form of Sadashiwa is the form in which the female process has been united with the male process to manifest the full power phenomena, leading to full union of Shakti in Shiwa. The power aspect of Sadashiwa is Gouri—the eternal Power. When in form, She is of golden colour and three-eyed. The golden colour indicates that the all-directing wyana-force has been centralized in her to effect the motionlessness of the prana-wayus.

When the Power of Sadashiwa is taken as a separate form, she is Power Shakini. As a distinct power-form, Shakini is the presiding Deity of the wishuddha chakra and its door-keeper. This means that the worship and concentration of Shakini are absolutely necessary to acquire competence to be able to do spiritual practices in the wishuddha chakra, and for the removal of all obstacles.

Shakini is white like Sadashiwa. She has also five faces and three eyes to each face like Sadashiwa. She holds in her four hands a bow, an arrow, a noose and a goad. The bow (chapa) and the arrow (shara) indicate the concentration power developed to its deepest form. Her yellow raiment indicates the full control of the prana-wayus through the centralization of wyana-wayu. She is on the lion part of the bull-lion. It indicates that all power-manifestation is under her full control. The mantra-forms of chapa (bow) are ung, kang and ghang, and that of shara (arrow) is phat (—Warna-bijakoshah).

7 Talu

The talu chakra is not included in the six-chakra group. It is the seventh chakra numerically, counting from the muladhara. It is not the chakra which is stated to be situated in the talumula (—Wishwasaratantra, ch. 1, p. 8; Koulawalitantra, ch. 3, p. 8; Dewibhagawata, 11.1.43). The word 'talumula' has been technically used here to mean the lowest part or the base of the palatine region—the neck. The reputed commentator Nilakantha has also interpreted the word as kantha = neck or throat (—Commentary on Dewibhagawata, 11.1.43). So, the chakra situated in the talumula is the wishuddha.

The talu chakra has been mentioned in the Waidika accounts. The term talu chakra has been used in the Soubhagyalakshmyupanishad, 3.6. It is above the kantha chakra (wishuddha) and below the bhru chakra (ajña) (—ibid., 3.5–7). Another Waidika term of the talu chakra is the taluka chakra which has been called the sixth chakra, the fifth being the kantha chakra (wishuddha), and the seventh being the bhru chakra (ajña) (—Yogarajopanishad, Mantras 12, 13, 15). Here it is very clear that the taluka (or talu) chakra is above the wishuddha and below the ajña. The talu chakra has been indirectly mentioned in the Darshanopanishad, 7.12.

In the Pouranika accounts the talu chakra has been mentioned. In connection with the pranayamika-dharana, prana is held in the four-petalled lotus (muladhara), the six-petalled lotus (swadhishthana), the navel region (manipura), the twelve-petalled lotus in the heart region (anahata), the sixteen-petalled lotus (wishuddha), in the palatine region (talu chakra), and finally the brahmarandhra (brahmarandhra or nirwana chakra) (—Skandapurana, 1.2.55. 44–5). Here the talu chakra has been indirectly mentioned. It has been stated that concentration should be done on the hrit lotus, in the anal region (muladhara), navel region (manipura), throat region (wishuddha), palatine region (talu chakra), the eyebrow-space (ajña) in the forehead and dwadashanta (the brahmarandhra or nirwana chakra) in the top part of the brain (Shiwapurana, 5b. 29. 131–2). Here also the talu chakra has been indirectly mentioned. The talu (palate) region as a place for concentration has been mentioned in the Lingapurana, 2.21.28. The talu region indicates the talu chakra which is situated in the palatine region.

The talu chakra has not been dealt with in the general Tantrika texts. It is a special chakra about which a disciple should learn directly from his guru. However, the subject has been briefly treated in certain Tantrika manuscripts. The talu chakra has been mentioned in the Amarasanggraha MS, Brahmasiddhantapaddhati MS and Tattwayogabindu MS. It has been stated in the Tattwayogabindu that the wishuddha chakra is situated in the region of the neck, then the sixth is the talu chakra, and then the ajña chakra is in the eyebrow region. It has been clearly indicated here that the talu chakra is above the wishuddha and below the ajña.

According to Jaganmohana Tarkalankara, a great authority on the Tantras, there is a secret chakra named lalana chakra which is above the wishuddha, and is in the palatine region

(—Footnote 87, in connection with the verse of the Mahanirwanatantra, 5.104, dealing with the chakras). He further says that thereafter (after leaving the wishuddha chakra) Kundalini will pass through the secret chakra lalana and reach the ajña (ibid.). So the lalana chakra and the talu chakra are the same.

Swami Sachchidananda Saraswati says that there is the secret lalana chakra lying within the sushumna which is in the vertebral column, in the region behind the uvula; it is situated above the wishuddha chakra and in the upper part of the neck (—Pujapradipa (by Swami Sachchidananda Saraswati), Part 2, ch. 4, p. 78).

He farther says that there is the very secret lalana chakra, situated between the fifth (the wishuddha) and the sixth (the ajña) chakra, and is taught by the gurus successively ... The seat of the lalana chakra is in the palatine region, above the wishuddha chakra (—Gurupradipa (by Swami Sachchidananda Saraswati), ch. 6, p. 262). He also says that the generally unknown and the secret lalana is situated above the wishuddha and below the ajña chakra, that is, in the upper part of the cervical spinal column, near the uvular region, and inside the sushumna (—Gitapradipa by Swami Sachchidananda Saraswati, p. 121).

The lalana chakra has been mentioned here: then (that is, after passing through the wishuddha chakra) a yoga disciple shall make Kundalini pass, through the secret chakra named lalana by using the mantra 'Hangsah', to the ajña chakra (—Atma-tattwa-darshana, edited by Jaganmohana Tarkalankara, and collected and published by Nilamani Mukhopadhyaya), ch. 2, p. 201).

Terminology

The following are the terms for this chakra.

1 Talu, mentioned in the Soubhagyalakshmyupanishad, 3.6; Brahmasiddhantapaddhati MS; Amarasanggraha MS; Tattwayogabindu MS. It has been indirectly mentioned in the Darshanopanishad, 7.12; Skandapurana, 1.2.55. 44; Shiwapurana, 5b.29.131; Lingapurana, 2.21.28.

2 Taluka, mentioned in the Yogarajopanishad, Mantra 13.

3 Lalana, kept secret by the gurus who
usually instruct their disciples directly.

Position

The talu chakra is situated in the palatine
region within the chitrini nadi. It is above the
wishuddha and below the ajña.

Description

The talu chakra has 12 petals (—Soubhagyalakshmyupanishad, 3.6; Jaganmohana Tarkalankara's Note No 87, in connection with his
translation of the Mahanirwanatantra, 5.104;
Gurupradipa (by Swami Sachchidananda Saraswati), ch. 6, p. 262). According to some other
Tantras, the talu chakra has 64 petals (—Brahmasiddhantapaddhati MS; Amarasanggraha MS;
Tattwayogabindu MS; Gurupradipa (by Swami
Sachchidananda Saraswati), ch. 6, p. 262).

The colour of the petals, when the chakra
is twelve-petalled, is red (—Jaganmohana's Note
87; Gurupradipa (by Swami Sachchidananda
Saraswati), ch. 6, p. 262). When the chakra has
sixty-four petals, the petals are shining white
in colour (—Tattwayogabindu MS).

There is a circular region (karnika) of red
colour, termed ghantika (because of its intimate
relation to the uvular region) in the pericarp of the
lotus, and inside it is a region (bhumi) where lies
the moon's power (chandra-kala) which oozes
nectar (amrita) (—Tattwayogabindu MS). This
region (bhumi) is called the region of nectar
(amritasthali) which shines like a million moons
(that is, shining white in colour), and full of
nectar; within it lies the nectar-oozing moon's
power (—Amarasanggraha MS). The region
of nectar is the reservoir of nectar (amritadhara)
(—Brahmasiddhantapaddhati MS). This is why
it has been stated that the talu chakra is the
centre where the nectar-stream flows (—Soubhagyalakshmyupanishad, 3.6).

In the exterior aspect of the talu chakra is an
interstice which leads to the uvular 'point'
(ghantika-linga wiwara), technically called the
'tenth' (—Soubhagyalakshmyupanishad, 3.6).
This 'point' in the uvular region is also called
the ghantika-lingamula-randhra (uvular 'point')
which leads to the reservoir of nectar in the
chakra (—Brahmasiddhantapaddhati MS).

There are twelve specific qualities (writtis)
on the twelve petals of the talu chakra (when it
is considered as a twelve-petalled lotus), arranged
from the right to the left in the following order:
(1) respect, (2) contentment, (3) offence, (4)
self-control, (5) pride, (6) affection, (7) sorrow,
(8) depression, (9) purity, (10) dissatisfaction,
(11) honour, (12) anxiety (—Jaganmohana's
footnote, No. 87 in his translation of the Mahanirwanatantra, 5.104).

Explanation

The talu chakra is a very important centre for
concentration. There are two main forms of
concentration which are practised here: concentration on the moon-power (chandra-kala),
and the void-concentration (shunya-dhyana).

1 Moon-concentration. Concentrate on the
circular nectar-region of shining white colour
and on the moon-power lying inside it, from
which nectar (white in colour) is oozing constantly. There are two important practices in
connection with this form of concentration:
irradiation and tenth-point-process. The whole
body should be irradiated with nectar in concentration. The tenth-point-process (dashama-
dwara-marga—Yogarajopanishad, Mantra 14)
is the process of tongue-lock consisting of the
pressing with the elongated and retroverted
tongue the tenth 'point' in the uvular region.
During this concentration, it is desirable to
execute the tongue-lock which enhances its
value. This mode of concentration develops the
power to make concentration deeper, prevents
mental diversification, increases energy and
causes well-being. It is always desirable that a
disciple should be in the talu chakra for some
time when making concentration on the chakras.
Whenever there is some lack of power of concentration, concentration should be made here.

2 Void-concentration. The void-concentration is a difficult form of concentration in which

the absorptive concentration power is developed to transform the sense-consciousness into super-consciousness. This process is for advanced disciples and should be learned from a guru.

8 Ajña

The ajña chakra is the sixth of the six-chakra group, but, numerically, it is the eighth chakra. It is situated within the chitrini nadi.

Terminology

The following are the Tantrika terms of the ajña chakra.

1 Ajña, mentioned in the Todalatantra, ch. 7, p. 14; ch. 9, p. 17; Kamadhenutantra, ch. 13, p. 16; Kularnawa, ch. 4, pp. 19, 22; Gandharwatantra, ch. 5, p. 28; Mantramahodadhi, 4.24; Kubjikatantra, 6.308; Tripurasarasamuchchaya, 5.27; Bhutashuddhitantra, ch. 3, p. 3; ch. 5, pp. 4,5; ch. 8, p. 8; ch. 14, p. 12; Sammohanatantra, Part 2, ch. 2, p. 2; Wishwasaratantra, ch. 1, p. 10; Mundamalatantra, ch. 6, p. 9; Shaktanandatarangini, 4.14, 30,34; Rudrayamala, Part 2, 16.22,23,27; 15.37,38; 18.2; 19.25, 36; 20.6,40,42; 21.27; 22.14; 25.56; 27.68; Tantrarajatantra, 21.83; Purashcharyarnawa, ch. 2, p. 91; ch. 6, pp. 490,492; Shiwasanghita, 5.131,148,150; Goutamiyatantra, 34.52; Jñanarnawa, quoted in Yogakalpalatika MS; Yogaswarodaya and Mridanitantra, quoted in Amarasanggraha MS; Tattwayogabindu MS.

2 Ajñapatra (the ajña with petals = ajña lotus), mentioned in the Kankalamalinitantra, ch. 2, p. 5.

3 Ajña-pura (ajña-centre), mentioned in the Bhutashuddhitantra, ch. 2, p. 2; ch. 14, p. 12.

4 Ajña-puri (ajña-centre), mentioned in the Bhutashuddhitantra, ch. 2, p. 2, ch. 10, p. 9.

5 Ajñambuja (ajña-lotus), mentioned in the Rudrayamala, Part 2, 15.66; Shatchakranirupana, Verse 32.

6 Ajña-pankaja (-lotus), mentioned in the Shiwasanghita, 5.141, 147.

7 Jñana-padma (knowledge-bestowing lotus .

mentioned in the Nirwanatantra, ch. 9, p. 11.

8 Dwidala (the two-petalled), mentioned in the Wishwasaratantra, ch. 1, p. 10; Koulawalitantra, ch. 22, p. 80; Shaktanandatarangini, 4.29; 7.14; 9.16; Rudrayamala, Part 2, 16.15; 15.64; 22.11; 60.30; Purashcharyarnawa, ch. 5, p. 387; Shadamnayatantra, 4.59, 60, 169; 5.268; Gandharwatantra, ch. 8, p. 39.

9 Dwidalambuja (the two-petalled lotus), mentioned in the Rudrayamala, Part 2, 16.4,6.

10 Dwidala-kamala (the two-petalled lotus), mentioned in the Brahmasiddhantapaddhati MS.

11 Dwipatra (the two-petalled), mentioned in the Wishwasaratantra, ch. 1, p. 8; Koulawalitantra, ch. 3, p. 8.

12 Bhrusaroruha (the lotus in the eyebrow region), mentioned in the Sammohanatantra, Part 2, ch. 4, p. 4; Sharadatilakatantra, 5.135.

13 Triweni-kamala (the lotus where the three nadis have joined together), mentioned in the Mahamuktitantra, quoted in the Yogakalpalatika MS.

14 Netra-padma (the two-petalled lotus), mentioned in the Kankalamalinitantra, ch. 2, p. 5.

15 Netra-patra (the two-petalled), mentioned in the Tararahasya, ch. 4, p. 23.

16 Bhru-mandala (the eyebrow-chakra), mentioned in the Kularnawa, ch. 4, p. 21.

17 Bhru-madhya (the space between the eyebrows, that is, the lotus situated in the eyebrow space), mentioned in the Mantramahodadhi, 4.28.

18 Bhru-madhyaga-padma (the lotus situated in the space between the eyebrows), mentioned in the Mahanirwanatantra, 5.113.

19 Bhru-madhya-chakra (the chakra situated in the space between the eyebrows), mentioned in the Brahmasiddhantapaddhati MS.

20 Bhru-mula (the eyebrow-root, that is, the lotus in the eyebrow region), mentioned in the Shadamnayatantra, 4.145.

21 Shiwa-padma (-lotus), mentioned in the Shadamnayatantra, 4.144.

Position

The ajña chakra is situated in the space between the eyebrows (—Gandharwatantra, ch. 8, p. 39;

Mantramahodadhi, 4.25; Tripurasarasamuchchaya, 5.27; Sammohanatantra, Part 2, ch. 2, p. 2; Wishwasaratantra, ch. 1, p. 10; Koulawalitantra, ch. 22, p. 80; Shaktanandatarangini, 4.14,29; 7.14; 9.16; Rudrayamala, Part 2, 16.4,27; 22.11; Purashcharyarnawa, ch. 5, p. 387; ch. 6, p. 490; Shiwasanghita, 5.131; Yogaswarodaya and Mridanitantra, quoted in Amarasanggraha MS; Tattwayogabindu MS). It has also been stated that the ajña is in the lalata (the forehead) (—Tararahasya, ch. 4, p. 23; Wishwasaratantra, ch. 1, p. 8; Koulawalitantra, ch. 3, p. 8). Here, the word lalata, which usually means the forehead, has been used technically. Here, it indicates the lowest part of the forehead which is connected with the eyebrow-region. The word lalata has also been used in the Dewibhagawata, 11.1.43. The great commentator Nilakantha interprets lalata as the eyebrow space (bhrumadhya) here. It is to be noted that both Wishwasaratantra and Koulawalitantra have used lalata (—Wishwasaratantra, ch. 1, p. 8; Koulawalitantra, ch. 3, p. 8) as well as bhrumadhya (the eyebrow-space) (—Wishwasaratantra, ch. 1, p. 10; Koulawalitantra, ch. 22, p. 80) to indicate the position of the ajña. This means that lalata here is the eyebrow-space, not the actual forehead as has been interpreted by Nilakantha.

According to the Waidika accounts the ajña is situated in the eyebrow-space (—Yogachudamanyupanishad, Mantra 5; Yogashikhopanishad, 1.175; 5.11; Yogarajopanishad, Mantra 15). As the ajña is situated in the space between the eyebrows, so it has the Waidika terms bhruchakra (—Soubhagyalakshmyupanishad, 3.7; Yogarajopanishad, Mantra 15) and bhru-madhya (the eyebrow-space) (—Yogakundalyupanishad, 1.69). Many Tantrika terms of the ajña are due to its location in the eyebrow-region (see terms Nos 16–21 above). In the Pouranika accounts, the position of the ajña is the eyebrow-space (—Shiwapurana, 5b.29.134; Kalikapurana, 55.30).

So the position of the ajña chakra is in the eyebrow-space. This does not mean that it is situated directly there. It means that the ajña is inside the sushumna at the point where it passes through a part of the brain, lying at the level of the midpoint of the space between the eyebrows.

Description

Shatchakranirupana says: the lotus termed ajña which is like the moon and becomes manifested by the concentration-light has two petals of an intense white colour on which are the matrika-letters hang and kshang; inside it (that is, inside the pericarp of the lotus) is (Power) Hakini who is white like the moon and has six faces and holds the widya (a book), kapala (a skull), damaru (a drum) and japawati (a rudraksha-rosary) and shows mudras (the gestures of granting boons and of dispelling fear); her whole consciousness is Supreme Consciousness (—Verse 32). (See Plate 17.)

Kalicharana interprets 'like the moon' to mean moon-like white colour. He adds that it may also mean that as the moon has nectarous cool rays, so the ajña chakra is cool-rayed. According to the commentator Ramawallabha, it is like the colour of the moon, and Bhuwanamohana has clearly stated that it is white in colour. Wishwanatha explains that it causes moisture (from nectar) like the moon. However, 'like the moon' cannot be interpreted only by white like the moon. To indicate the whiteness of the chakra the word 'sushubhra' (very white) has been used in the text. It has been stated that in the hollow of the ajña chakra is an excellent fluid (that is, the nectar) (—Rudrayamala, Part 2, 18.2). So there is nectar in the ajña as there is in the 'moon'.

The ajña has two petals (—Kankalamalinitantra, ch. 2, p. 5; Nirwanatantra ch. 9, p. 11; Gandharwatantra, ch. 5, p. 28; Tripurasarasamuchchaya, 5.27; Bhutashuddhitantra, ch. 2, p. 2; Sammohanatantra, Part 2, ch. 2, p. 2; ch. 4, p. 4; Wishwasaratantra, ch. 1, pp. 8, 10; Koulawalitantra, ch. 3, p. 8; ch. 22, p. 80; Sharadatilakatantra, 5.135; Shaktanandatarangini, 4. 14; Rudrayamala, Part 2, 15. 65; 16.4,6, 15; 22.11; 60.30; Purashcharyarnawa, ch. 6, p. 490; Shadamnayatantra, 4.144; 5.268; Shiwasanghita, 5.131; Brahmasiddhantapaddhati MS; Jñanarnawa and Mahamuktitantra, quoted in

Yogakalpalatika MS; Yogaswarodaya, quoted in *Amarasanggraha* MS; *Tattwayogabindu* MS; also, Yogachudamanyupanishad, Mantra 5; Yoga-shikhopanishad, 1.175; 5.11; Dewibhagawata, 7.35.45; 11.1.43; Shiwapurana, 5b. 29.135); and the colour of the petals is white (—Kankala-malinitantra, ch. 2, p. 5; Tripurasarasamuchchaya, 5.27; Bhutashuddhitantra, ch. 2, p. 2; Sammohanatantra, Part 2, ch. 2, p. 2; Rudraya-mala, Part 2, 22.11; Purashcharyarnawa, ch. 6, p. 490; Shiwasanghita, 5.131; Mayatantra, quoted by Wishwanatha), or lightning-like colour (—Koulawalitantra, ch. 22, p. 80; Jñanarnawa, quoted in the Yogakalpalatika MS; also, Shiwapurana, 5b. 29.135). On its two petals are the two matrika-letters *hang* and *kshang* (—Kankalamalinitantra, ch. 2, p. 5; Gandharwatantra, ch. 5, p. 28; Tripurasara-samuchchaya, 5.27; Sammohanatantra, Part 2, ch. 2, p. 2; Wishwasaratantra, ch. 1, p. 10; Koulawalitantra, ch. 3, p. 8; Sharadatilaka-tantra 5.135; Shaktanandatarangini, 4.14; 7.14; Mahanirwanatantra, 5.113; Purashcharyarnawa, ch. 5, p. 387; ch. 6, p. 490; Shadamnayatantra, 5.268; Shiwasanghita, 5.131; Jñanarnawa, quot-ed in the Yogakalpalatika MS; Mridanitantra, quoted in the *Amarasanggraha* MS; also, Dewi-bhagawata, 7.35.45; 11.1.43; Shiwapurana, 5b. 29.135), and the colour of the letters is white (—Jñanarnawa, quoted in the Yogakalpalatika MS; Dakshinamurti, quoted by Wishwanatha), golden (—Bhutashuddhitantra, ch. 2, p. 2), variegated (—Sammohanatantra, Part 2, ch. 2, p. 2), or shining (—Koulawalitantra, ch. 22, p. 80). The shining colour may mean bright white.

It has also been stated that the matrika-letters on the petals of the ajña are *lang* (the second la which is pronounced as *da*) and *kshang*, and shine like ten million moons (that is, shining white) (—Rudrayamala, Part 2, 22.13). Accord-ing to Jaganmohana (—Note 87 on the Maha-nirwanatantra, 5.104) the matrika-letters *hang* and *kshang* are red in colour. He further says that *lang* (= *dang*) is hidden in the pericarp (—*ibid.*). Sachchidananda says the same (—Gurupradipa (by Swami Sachchidananda Saraswati), ch. 6, p. 263).

It has been stated that the borders of the three nadis (that is, the ida, pingala and sushumna) are situated in the space between the eyebrows, termed the tripatha-sthana (the junc-tion of the three power-lines) which is six-cornered and (can be magnified) to four-fingers' breadth, and red in colour; this is what is called the ajña chakra by the yogis (—Kali-kapurana, 55.30). It means that in the ajña chakra, situated in the eyebrow space, are the ends of the ida and pingala which form a junction in combination with the sushumna, and this junction is called the tripatha-sthana, which is in the form of a six-cornered region and red in colour. The Waidika term is the trikuta (—Brahmawidyopanishad, Mantra 73) where the ida, pingala and sushumna have been united, that is, in ajña. So, the ajña has a red, six-cornered region in its pericarp. The ajña has also been called the trirasra (the triangle) (—Linga-purana, 1.75.39), because it contains the triangular process in its pericarp.

The ajña chakra has been described as having within it the beautiful kama chakra; inside the kama chakra is the very subtle prashna chakra, and inside that the phala chakra (—Rudraya-mala, Part 2, 20.6–7). These special chakras are for the practice of special concentration.

Hakini

Power Hakini is situated in the pericarp of the ajña (—Todalatantra, ch. 7, p. 14; Kankala-malinitantra, ch. 2, p. 5; Kularnawa, ch. 4, p. 19; Mantramahodadhi, 4.24; Tripurasarasam-uchchaya, 5.27; Koulawalitantra, ch. 22, p. 80; Shadamnayatantra, 5.268; Shiwasanghita, 5.131; Mridanitantra, quoted in *Amarasanggraha* MS). The various concentration-forms of Hakini are as follows.

1 Hakini is moon-white in colour, six-faced and six-armed; she holds a book, a skull, a drum, and a rudraksha-rosary, and makes the gestures of granting boons and of dispelling fear (—Shatchakranirupana, Verse 32).

2 Hakini is white in colour; she has six faces of red colour, each with three eyes; she holds in her hands the drum, the rudraksha-rosary, the skull and the book, and makes the gestures of granting boons and dispelling fear; and she is seated on a white lotus (—A verse quoted by

Kalicharana in his commentary on Verse 32). (See Plate 18.)

3 The colour of Hakini is a mixture of white-black-red; she is two-armed and her face is moon-like beautiful with rolling eyes, like a moving black bee; she shines with the vermilion-mark on her forehead and her eyes are beautifully painted with collyrium; she has curled hair and is clad in red raiment and her upper garment is white (—Kankalamalinitantra, ch. 5, p. 23).

4 Hakini is like the dark-blue cloud (that is, her colour is dark-blue) and has one, two, three, four, five or six faces (according to the type of concentration) which glitter like stars; she holds the skull, the spear, and the shield, and she makes the gesture of dispelling fear (—Kularnawa, ch. 10, p. 53).

5 Hakini is white in colour; she has three eyes and holds the rudraksha-rosary, the drum, the skull, the book and the bow, and shows the mudra (either the gesture of granting boons or that of dispelling fear) (—Koulawalitantra, ch. 22, p. 80).

6 Hakini is red in colour; she has six faces and three eyes to each face; she holds a drum, a rudraksha-rosary, a skull and a book and shows mudras (that is, the gestures of granting boons and of dispelling fear) (—Jamala, quoted in the Yogakalpalatika MS).

7 Hakini is pure white (or) like a blue lotus (that is, dark-blue in colour), and has six faces (—Mridanitantra, quoted in the Amarasanggraha MS).

Itara-linga

Shatchakranirupana says: it is well known that the seat of the subtle (sukshmarupa) manas (sense-mind) is at an intermediate point (antarala) of this lotus (ajña); inside the pericarp of this (ajña) is a triangle (yoni) which is the seat (pada) of Itara-Shiwa (Shiwa endowed with the power of full control over desires) who is revealed in his linga-form (absorptive concentration-form) (lingachihnaprakasha); here is also the seat (pada) (which is triangular in shape) of the Supreme Power as Kundalini (paramakula), like the streaks of lightning flashes, causing the rousing of the brahma nadi (brahma-sutra-prabodha), and manifesting as the first

bija (primary source) of the Wedas (that is, the first mantra Ong); a practitioner, being calm mentally, should do thought-concentration according to the order (prescribed by the guru) (—Verse 33).

The 'subtle manas' indicates that the manas has a specific centre of operation which is beyond the centres of the operation of the senses which are situated in the lower five chakras. The term 'antarala' (an intermediate point) indicates that there is a subcentre within the ajña where the seat of the manas is.

Kalicharana has interpreted 'lingachihnaprakasha' to mean shining in the linga-form. It means that Itara-Shiwa is in the linga-form. But the linga-form should never be translated here as phallic form. The linga is the central point within the triangle.

About the order, Kalicharana says that the order as given in the text should not be taken, but the arrangements of words according to their import is to be adopted. He gives the following order: First, Power Hakini in the pericarp; next, Itara-linga within the triangle which is above Hakini; then, above him (Itara-linga), is the pranawa (Ong) in the triangle; and lastly, manas which is above pranawa. This is the right order of thought-concentration.

The meaning of brahma-sutra, as given by Kalicharana, is chitrini nadi. But Ramawallabha, Wishwanatha, Bhuwanamohana and Shankara give its meaning as brahma nadi. The brahma-sutra is the brahma nadi.

The presence of Itara-linga in the ajña has been mentioned in the other Tantras. It has been stated that Itara-linga is situated in the ajña (—Sammohanatantra, Part 2, ch. 2, p. 2) inside the triangle lying in its pericarp (—Kankalamalinitantra, ch. 2, p. 5), and the triangle is called yoni, and Itara-linga is like the rising sun (that is, red in colour) (—Koulawalitantra, ch. 22, p. 80). The colour of Itara-linga has also been stated as golden (—Shaktanandatarangini, 4.14), or like the moon (shining white) (—Yoginihridaya, quoted by Wishwanatha).

Pranawa

More has been said about pranawa in the text. Within that (the triangle before mentioned—

Kalicharana), in this chakra (the ajña) is the seat of splendorous (pradipabhajyotis), pure (shuddha), aroused (buddha) inner consciousness (antaratman) (that is, the divine conscious power Kundalini) who is manifest (from her subtle form) through the (first) sounds (warna) which form the pranawa; above it (the bija aspect of the pranawa, that is, O letter) is the half moon (called nada) and above that (half moon) is the ma letter in the bindu form (thus, O with nada-bindu becomes Ong); above this (that is, Ong) is the nada (which is not the nada of Ong) which is shining white in colour (—Shat-chakranirupana, Verse 35).

About the pranawa, it has been stated that in this chakra (ajña) there is the bija in akshara-form (akshara-bija) (that is, the first bija-mantra Ong) which is moon-white; it is splendorous (—Shiwasanghita, 5.132–3). In this chakra, there is splendorous consciousness like light on which concentration should be done (—Soubhagyalakshmyupanishad, 3.7). This is the lustre of Kundalini. Here (in ajña) is the circular light for concentration (—Yogarajopanishad, Mantra 15). The circular light indicates the luminous coils of Kundalini.

Explanation

The name 'ajña' for this chakra is due to the fact, when stated literally, that the transference of Guru's ajña (order) occurs in this chakra. But it has deeper meaning. Ajña is the power in 'Ou'-form, which means the Kundali-power. Guru is the first divine form of the formless Supreme Being, centered in the guru chakra. From Guru Kundali-power radiates as Oung to the ajña chakra to rouse Ong residing in the triangle there when consciousness begins to be of Kundalini. In the ajña chakra, Kundalini is in the form of Ong, that is, in the pashyanti-form. When the aroused Kundalini is conducted from the muladhara to the ajña, Ong is absorbed into Kundalini and consciousness becomes of Kundalini. In the ajña there is another possibility of making consciousness of Kundalini. It is the rousing and transforming of Ong by the radiated Oung-power from Guru into Kundalini when

consciousness becomes of Kundalini.

The Petals

The ajña has two petals of shining white colour. The two petals are the two radiations of power, one passing downwards through the lower five chakras, and the other passing upwards through the upper chakras. The radiations are white, sentient and powerful. The two radiations are the hang and kshang radiations. In hang and kshang radiations are five wayus, five divine powers and Kundali-power. The original colour of hang is shining red, and of kshang is moon-white. In the ajña, hang becomes moon-white, and kshang retains its original colour. The shining white colour indicates the greater concentration of udana-wayu. The udana-wayu arouses the sense and sentient principles in the five lower chakras and sense-consciousness, intelligence and attention in the upper three chakras. When hang and kshang are united in concentration, the lower radiation stops and the power becomes united with the upper radiation. Now, the forceful upper radiation is not received in the centres of sense-consciousness and intellection but passes directly to the centre of dhi which effects samadhi.

Concentration on Hakini

Concentration on Power Hakini is the basic concentration of the ajña chakra. The practitioner gets all the necessary powers and qualities to be able to work in the ajña through the concentration on Hakini.

The six faces of Hakini indicate the five principles centered in the five lower chakras and the manas in the ajña system. The third eye in the centre is the concentration-light, and the other eyes indicate the perceptual knowledge and thoughts. She is said to have one, two, three, four, five or six faces. One face indicates concentration in which I-ness has been dissolved; two faces indicate concentration in which I-ness still remains; three faces—the three primary attributes; four faces—gross sensory knowledge, supersensory knowledge, presensory knowledge and nonsensory knowledge; five faces—the knowledge of five principles in the lower five chakras; and six faces—perceptual knowledge, thoughts, attention, and concentration-knowledge of three forms—dharana, dhyana and samadhi. It indicates Kundalini-knowledge when her faces are red in colour.

The white colour of her body indicates her highly rarefied form of sattwa (sentience). The dark-blue colour of her body indicates the sattwa-form which is ready to proceed to a formless state. The red colour of her body indicates the fully aroused Kundalini in form. It indicates the harmonious actions of the three primary attributes when her body colour is a mixture of white, red and black.

Hakini holds in her hands widya (book), kapala (skull), damaru (drum) and japawati (rudraksha-rosary), and shows the wara (granting boons) and abhaya (dispelling fear) mudras (by special positions of the hands). The widya is the spiritual knowledge of samadhi transformed into communicable word-forms represented in a book. The kapala indicates the existence of consciousness without the material instrumentation; or the functioning of consciousness when it is disjoined from the body. This consciousness is spiritual consciousness and develops from deep concentration. Damaru indicates the silent sounds of mantras developed from the waikhari form. The japawati indicates the spiritual practice of awakening the mantra. The wara is the imparting of spiritual knowledge and the abhaya is the removal of all obstacles to concentration.

The bija-mantra of Hakini is hang. The mantra-forms of widya are ang, ing, ung, ring, gang and chang; of kapala—kang, lring; of damaru—khang; of aksha (rudraksha)—ung, bring; of wara—thang, dang, shang.

Concentration on Itara-linga

The linga is the specific form of formless Shiwa (Supreme Consciousness) which is held in consciousness in concentration. It is not a detailed form but a basic form most suitable for the practice of concentration. It is a tapering form on which concentration starts from its thick starting end, and as concentration goes deeper, it becomes slender and smaller and, finally, it is a point when concentration is still deeper. This point is also reached in concentration when it is applied on shalagrama (sacred stone) of Wishnu (Supreme Being). There are many forms of shalagrama of which the round or the oval are the most important for concentration. In concentration on the shalagrama, the reduction of form is from the circumference to its central point.

The linga is subtle, that is, it is a form in consciousness created in the process of concentration in which are involved three factors: the holding-power of concentration, its application on an appropriate form in an appropriate bright colour, and the absorptive power which develops step by step to transform the line-linga into a point-linga. These three factors associated with concentration are represented by the three power-lines constituting the triangle in which the linga is formed. The reduction of the linga to a point is the process of absorptive concentration. Those who are unable to create a clear conscious form of the linga in concentration, are advised to practise with an appropriate gross form to establish thought-form.

CHAPTER 11
Exposition of the Chakras (continued)

The chakra system can be grouped into three main forms: first, the six-chakra system, consisting of the six main chakras—muladhara, swadhishthana, manipura, anahata, wishuddha and ajña, with two supplementary chakras, hrit and talu, to which is added the sahasrara. Secondly, the ajña system which consists of the ajña, manas, indu, nirwana and sahasrara. The guru chakra, sahasrara, Supreme Bindu, Supreme Nada, Shakti principle, Shiwa principle and Parama Shiwa constitute the third, the sahasrara system.

Ajña System

The ajña proper (Plate 19) consists of the following factors, which are arranged in this order: first, Power Hakini in the pericarp of the ajña; second, above Hakini, is Itara-linga, situated within a triangle; and third, above Itara-linga, is the pranawa in a triangle (this triangle is above the triangle where lies Itara-linga). The pranawa is constituted of the bija 'O', joined with nada and bindu, that is Ong.

Above this is nada (—Shatchakranirupana, Verse 35). 'Above this' means above the pranawa, that is, above the bindu of Ong. In other words, the second nada is not to be confused with the nada of Ong. This second nada is above the bindu of Ong, and, consequently, above the triangle in which is situated the pranawa.

At an intermediate point or position of the ajña is the subtle manas (—Shatchakranirupana, Verse 33). This point or position is between the bindu of Ong and the second nada which is above the pranawa. So the order is this: Ong, manas (which is above Ong); and nada (second). The qualifying word 'subtle' has been used here in a technical sense. The manas is not itself a sense like smell-sense or sight-sense, but plays an important role in making the senses operative. It is more rarefied and powerful than the senses. The senses are under its control. To signify its special characteristics, it has been qualified by the word subtle. The sense-principles are connected with the lower five chakras. The manas is situated above them in the ajña. The sense-operation requires the instrumentation of the body, but manas may operate independently of the body, so it is subtle. This manas can be termed sense-mind, because of its connection with the senses. The manas receives sensory radiations and then conducts them to the second nada.

It has been stated that manas is always shining in the two-petalled lotus (ajña) (—Kankala-malinitantra, ch. 2, p. 5). This manas is sense-mind. Manas is intimately related to ahang (I-ness) (which includes chitta-consciousness), buddhi (intellective mind) and prakriti (menti-matter principle) (—ibid., ch. 2, p. 5). Here the whole mind has been referred to, the whole of which manas is a part. Farther, the seat of manas is always in the ajña chakra (—Bhuta-shuddhitantra, ch. 2, p. 2; ch. 8, p. 8; Koulawali-tantra, ch. 22, p. 80; Shaktanandatarangini, 4.16, 30; Sammohanatantra, Part 2, ch. 2, p. 2).

It has been stated that the manas tattwa (principle) is above the void (shunya) principle which is situated in the throat region (that is, the wishuddha chakra) (—Bhutashuddhitantra, ch. 4, p. 4). The manas principle is the whole mind termed antahmanas or antahkarana. It is situated above the wishuddha chakra, that is, in the ajña system. Mind in a functioning state manifests its different aspects. The general characteristics of mind are: thinking power (wibhutwa) and nonspatiality (wyapakatwa) (—ibid., ch. 4, p. 4). Mind has the power to reach everywhere; it is the source of all knowledge; here lies the 'I-ness' which sees everything (—ibid., ch. 4, p. 4). It is clear that the seat of mind is in the ajña system, and its aspect as sense-mind is in ajña proper. Other aspects of mind are above it.

Now, what is the second nada (the nada above Ong), mentioned in the Shatchakranirupana, Verse 35? This nada has been mentioned in the Sharadatilakatantra, 5.136; Shadamnayatantra, 5.268; Shiwasanghita, 5.149; Koulawalitantra, ch. 22, p. 81; and Shrikrama, quoted in Yogakalpalatika MS. It has been stated that manas mandala (chakra), situated in the space between the eyebrows (that is, ajña), is in the form of nada (—Yogashikhopanishad, 1.178; 5.15). From this it is clear that the second nada is the manas chakra. It has also been termed surya mandala (—Kankalamalinitantra, ch. 2, p. 5). It has been stated that dwipashikhakara jñananetra (knowledge-light) is in the ajña (—Soubhagyalakshmyupanishad, 3.7). The jñananetra is indicative of manas chakra. The manas chakra is situated above sense-mind (which we may term manas 2).

It has been stated that here (that is, the position above the manas mandala) is the shambhawa sthana (the position belonging to Shiwa, that is, shambhawa chakra) (—Yogashikhopanishad, 5.16). The shambhawa chakra is also termed shitangshu mandala. The shitangshu mandala (chakra) is above the space between the eyebrows (that is, ajña) and it is called the anahata chakra having 16 petals (—Yogakundalyupanishad, 1.69). We have already seen that there is a chakra named anahata as the fourth chakra below the wishuddha

chakra, belonging to the six-chakra group. Here, the shitangshu chakra has a special Waidika name—anahata which is unrelated to the anahata of the six-chakras group. This chakra may be termed anahata 2. The shitangshu has also been called indu chakra (ibid., 1.71). We can say it is the moon chakra. The words shitangshu and indu are synonyms, and mean the moon.

Another Tantrika term for the indu chakra is chandra (moon) mandala (chakra). It has been stated that beyond the nada (nadanta, that is, above the manas chakra) is chandra mandala where lies Shiwa (Wrishabhadhwaja) with his Power (Shakti) (—Koulawalitantra, ch. 22, p. 81; also in the Kankalamalinitantra, ch. 2, p. 5; Nirwanatantra, ch. 9, p. 11). The indu chakra has also been indicated by the term nadanta (that is, the chakra beyond the nada—manas chakra) (—Koulawalitantra, ch. 22, p. 81; Sharadatilakatantra, 5.136; Shrikrama, quoted in the Yogakalpalatika MS).

It has been stated that there are three pithas (literally seats, but technically chakras) named bindu, nada and shakti as the lotuses in the forehead (—Shiwasanghita, 5.149). Here, the nada lotus is the manas chakra, and the shakti lotus seems to be the indu chakra. The Pouranika term 'shakti' (—Shiwapurana, 3.3.28) which is above the ajña also appears to stand for the indu chakra. The bindu pitha (chakra) (—Shiwasanghita, 5.149) which is situated below the nada lotus appears to be the seat of manas 2 (sense-mind). The bindu pitha appears to be above but in close relation to the bindu of Ong in the ajña. The indu chakra has also been termed kailasa chakra (—Gandharwatantra, ch. 5, p. 28; Shaktanandatarangini, 4.14; Rudrayamala, Part 2, 27.69; Goutamiyatantra, 34.53; Mridanitantra, quoted in Amarasanggraha MS; Dewibhagawata, 7.35.46).

Above the indu chakra is the nirwana chakra (—Soubhagyalakshmyupanishad, 3.8; Brahmasiddhantapaddhati MS). The nirwana chakra is also called parabrahma chakra (—Soubhagyalakshmyupanishad, 3.8); brahmarandhra chakra (—Yogarajopanishad, Mantra 16; Kankalamalinitantra, ch. 2, p. 5; Kularnawa, ch. 4, p. 22; Shiwapurana, 3.3.68; Agnipurana, 74, 13;

Skandapurana, 1.2.55.45); bodhini chakra (—Gandharwatantra, ch. 5, p. 28; Shakta-nandatarangini, 4.14; Rudrayamala, Part 2, 60. 30; Goutamiyatantra, 34.53); rodhini chakra (—Mridanitantra, quoted in Amarasanggraha MS; Dewibhagawata, 7.35.46); bodhana chakra (—Rudrayamala, Part 2, 27.69); chitkala-shakti (—Shadamnayatantra, 5.269); shatapatra (hundred-petalled) chakra (—Tattwayogabindu MS); kala chakra (—ibid.) dwadashanta chakra (—Shiwapurana, 2.11.40; 5b.29.132; Garuda-purana, Part 1, 23.48); shanta (—Shiwapurana, 3.3.28); shantipada (shanti padma or chakra) (—Shiwapurana, 5a.7.4); dwadashantapada (dwadashanta padma or chakra) (—Agnipurana, 74.10).

The nirwana is the last chakra in the chitrini nadi. The chitrini is inside the wajra and wajra inside the sushumna. This means that the sushumna is the outermost nadi containing within it the wajra as the second internal nadi, and within the wajra is the chitrini nadi as the third internal nadi. All the chakras are in the chitrini. Inside the chitrini lies the brahma nadi. The brahma nadi is also called brahmarandhra. It is extremely subtle and usually remains only potentially. It becomes actual when Kundalini passes through it.

The sushumna arises from the central aspect of the kanda-mula which is situated just below the muladhara. It then goes upward centrally within the vertebral column and the head and ends at the terminal part of what is called brahma-randhra. The wajra arises from the kanda-mula at the same starting point as that of the sushumna, and, passing through it, ends where the brahmarandhra and the sushumna terminate. The chitrini extends from the starting point of the wajra, goes upward within the wajra and ends where the sushumna and wajra terminate, that is, the end point of the brahmarandhra. The innermost brahma nadi starts from the orifice of the Swayambhu-linga in the muladhara and extends through the chitrini and ends where the sushumna, wajra and chitrini terminate.

The starting points of the sushumna, wajra and the chitrini are from the kanda-mula and that of the brahma nadi is from the Swayambhu-linga in the muladhara. This is clear. But the

terminal points of these nadis need more clari-fication. Confusion arises with the term brahma-randhra. The brahmarandhra is also intimately related to the brahma nadi. The brahma-randhra appears to have two aspects: brahma-randhra as brahma nadi and as the brahma-randhra region in the head.

Kundalini being aroused and uncoiled passes through the hollow into the brahma nadi (—Yogakundalyupanishad, 1.46). This indicates the presence of the brahma nadi in the mula-dhara. The roused Kundalini extends herself into the sushumna (—ibid., 1.66) and becomes connected with the brahmarandhra (—ibid., 1.83). This means that the roused Kundalini in the muladhara chakra enters the brahma nadi or brahmarandhra through the sushumna. So, the brahma nadi and brahmarandhra are the same and are in the muladhara, which is appro-ached by Kundalini through the sushumna. The brahma nadi or the brahmarandhra is within the sushumna. So it has been stated that the brahma nadi is seen inside the sushumna when 'cut' into halves (—Yogashikhopanishad, 5.17), and the sushumna is in the form of brahma, that is, it possesses the brahma nadi within (—ibid., 6.5). It has been more clearly stated that there is a subtle vacuity inside the sushumna, and it is called brahma nadi (—ibid., 6.9). Also, Kundali has kept closed the brahmarandhra lying within the sushumna (—Warahopanishad, 5.23); Kundalini lies (in the muladhara) by enclosing the brahmarandhra (—Shandilyopa-nishad, 1.4.8). All these are clear indications that brahma nadi or brahmarandhra is in the muladhara and inside the sushumna.

The brahma nadi is inside the chitrini (—Toda-latantra, ch. 8, p. 15; Tararahasya, ch. 1, p. 2; ch. 4, p. 22; Koulawalitantra, ch. 22, p. 80; Shaktanandatarangini, 4.8; Rudrayamala, Part 2, 29.41). The brahmarandhra is also inside the chitrini (—Shiwasanghita, 2.18; Tripurasara-samuchchaya, ch. 3, p. 8; Sammohanatantra, Part 2, ch. 2, p. 2; Sharadatilakatantra, 25.32). From this it appears that the brahma nadi and brahmarandhra are the same. But according to some authorities the brahmarandhra is within the brahma nadi (—Koulawalitantra, ch. 22, p. 80; Shaktanandatarangini, 4.8). This means that the central aspect of the brahma nadi—the real vacuity—is the brahmarandhra, the immediate external aspect of which is brahma nadi; and all these are situated inside the chitrini. Practically, both are the same.

The chitrini is inside the wajra and the wajra is inside the sushumna (—Tararahasya, ch. 4, p. 22; Koulawalitantra, ch. 22, p. 80; Rudrayamala, Part 2, 25.51–52; Tantrarajatantra, 27.44).

The brahma nadi is called brahma-marga (-path), as Kundalini passes through it to reach the sahasrara (—Todalatantra, ch. 8, p. 16). The brahma nadi leads to spiritual success; it is stimulated by Kundalini, the mother of yoga who passes through it when going to be united with Shiwa (in the sahasrara) (—Shadamnaya-tantra, 4.177). All cosmic principles are absorbed by Kundalini when passing through the brahma nadi, so it is said that it devours all principles (—Yogashikhopanishad, 1.125). Kundali-power is established in the great path brahmarandhra (ibid., 6.47).

About the course of the sushumna, it has been stated that it passes from the kanda-mula (or muladhara) to the brahmarandhra (—Gandharwatantra, ch. 5, p. 27; Tripurasarasamuchchaya, ch. 3, p. 8; Bhutashuddhitantra, ch. 6, p. 5; Shaktanandatarangini, 4.8; Mandalabrahmanopanishad, 1.2.6; Dewibhagawata, 11.8. 1–2). The brahmarandhra mentioned here is not the brahma nadi but a region where the sushumna ends. It can also be the brahmarandhra chakra. It is situated in the head. It is clear from the statement that the sushumna extends to the head, and it is called the brahmarandhra (—Shandilyopanishad, 1.4.10). The brahmarandhra region or chakra lies in the topmost part of the head where the sushumna ends. About the origin and the end of the sushumna, it has been stated that it arises from the central part of the kanda and extends to the head (—Koulawalitantra, ch. 22, p. 80). The brahmarandhra is situated in the head (—Skandapurana, 1.2.55.45; 3.1.13.39).

The brahmarandhra as the nadi as well as the region (or chakra) has been clearly stated here: the sushumna extends to the brahmarandhra (here it is the region or chakra); the extremely subtle brahmarandhra (here it is the nadi) is inside the chitrini (—Tripurasara-

samuchchaya, ch. 3, p. 8). There are other expressions which indicate that the brahmarandhra is a region or chakra, viz.—from muladhara to brahmarandhra (—Nilatantra, ch. 5, p. 9); in a nyasa process (a mantra process), the order is ajña, forehead (indu chakra), brahmarandhra (—Kularnawa, ch. 4, pp. 19–20); concentration on the pranawa which extends from the muladhara to the brahmarandhra should be made (—Shiwapurana, 3.3. 68); the nada (sound) which arises from the muladhara and goes to the brahmarandhra after piercing the twelve knots is to be uttered and concentrated upon (—ibid., 3.6.41); the order from the hrit (anahata) is throat (wishuddha), talu (-chakra), eyebrow-space (ajña) and brahmarandhra (-chakra) (—ibid., 5a.28.46; Agnipurana, 74.13); after passing through the six chakras, it should be brought to the brahmarandhra (—Brahmawaiwartapurana, 4.20.29). That the brahmarandhra is a chakra has been clearly stated in the Soubhagyalakshmy-upanishad, 3.8; Yogarajopanishad, Mantra 16; and Brahmawaiwartapurana, 1.26.5.

Another term 'dwadashanta' has been used for brahmarandhra as a region or chakra. It has been stated that the light-like jiwa (embodied being) is to be brought by the instrumentation of pranawa to the dwadashanta (—Bhutashuddhitantra, ch. 5, p. 4). The dwadashanta indicates brahmarandhra. 'From the muladhara to the dwadashanta' (—Shiwapurana, 2.11.40); here the dwadashanta indicates the brahmarandhra. It is still clearer here: the jiwa-consciousness which is in the hrit (anahata) is to be brought through the path of the brahma nadi to the white sahasrara lotus situated above dwadashanta (that is, brahmarandhra) (—ibid., 3.5.52–53); also, 'Next to indu (-chakra) is dwadashanta (brahmarandhra), and thereafter is the white lotus (guru chakra)' (—ibid., 5a. 28.49). The order of the chakras has been given as—eyebrow-region (ajña), forehead (indu chakra), and dwadashanta (brahmarandhra) in the head (—ibid., 5b. 29.132). The exact location of the dwadashanta has been indicated in this mantra: 'The short pranawa is in the bindu, the long is in the brahmarandhra, and the protracted in the dwadashanta' (—Warahopanishad, 5.70). Here, both brahmarandhra and dwadashanta have been used. The well-known commentator Upanishadbrahmayogi interprets dwadashanta as the upper part of the brahmarandhra. This indicates that the region is brahmarandhra and its upper part is dwadashanta. However, as the dwadashanta is also a lotus (—Garudapurana, 1.23.48), like the brahmarandhra, there cannot be two chakras in the region. Above the indu chakra is the nirwana chakra which is the last chakra in the chitrini. This nirwana chakra has been termed brahmarandhra and also dwadashanta chakra.

It has been stated that at the talu-mula (the upper end of the palatine region) lies the upper end of the sushumna with its inner vacuity (that is, brahmarandhra, and consequently, it includes the wajra and chitrini) and from where the sushumna goes downward to the end of the triangle situated in the muladhara; in the proximity of (the upper border of) the talu-sthana (palatine region) is a lotus (belonging to) the sahasrara, in the pericarp of which (that is, the pericarp of the guru chakra) is a triangle, facing posteriorly, where the end-point of the sushumna with its vacuity is situated; it is called the brahmarandhra, and extends from here to the muladhara (—Shiwasanghita, 5.161–4).

The talu-sthana is a region which is externally related to the palate, so it is the palatine region. Technically, it is that part of the sushumna which passes from the talu chakra upwards to its end-point termed the sushumna-mula (upper extremity of the sushumna), and this end-point is in the talu-mula (upper border of the palatine region). So, the upper extremity of the sushumna lies in the upper border of the palatine region and from this point the sushumna goes downward to the end of the muladhara-triangle. This means that the sushumna starts from the lowest point of the muladhara (that is, mula-kanda) and goes upward and terminates at the end-point of the palatine region, called the talu-mula. This endpoint is also called the brahmarandhra. The brahmarandhra as a nadi extends from the talu-mula to the muladhara. In other words, the brahmarandhra which is inside the chitrini (—Shiwasanghita, 2.18) passes from the muladhara as a nadi and ends at the point where the sushumna ends. The end of the sushumna lies in the talu-mula, which is also called brahmarandhra and dwadashanta. At this end-point is the nirwana chakra which is also called the brahmarandhra chakra and dwadashanta chakra. However, the sushumna is neither continuous with nor proceeds into the guru chakra belonging to the sahasrara, but ends in the proximity of the chakra.

The above study indicates that the term brahmarandhra has been used in two senses: one, as a nadi or vacuity within the chitrini nadi which runs from the muladhara to the head where the sushumna ends; the other, as the region or point where the sushumna-mula is situated, that is, the upper terminal point of the sushumna. This region or point has been variously termed the talu-mula, brahmarandhra, and dwadashanta. It may also be called the sushumna-mula. This terminal point is marked by the presence of the nirwana chakra. This chakra is also called the brahmarandhra chakra and dwadashanta chakra.

Here is still another important point which needs to be discussed. Does the brahmarandhra extend into the sahasrara? According to the commentary of Kalicharana on the first verse of the Padukapanchaka the 'brahmarandhra-sarasiruha' has been rendered as 'that lotus called the thousand-petalled in which is the brahmarandhra'. It can simply be translated 'brahmarandhra lotus'. The translation of the verse can be done as follows: at the higher position (udare) of the brahmarandhra lotus, and always in contact with it, is the wonderful white twelve-petalled lotus which lies as a crown of the kundaliwiwarakanda (that is, the chitrini nadi); I adore it. This twelve-lettered (petalled) lotus is the guru chakra. So, the guru chakra is above the chitrini (and, consequently, the sushumna).

In the Gandharwatantra (ch. 5, p. 23), we find a passage which reads that concentration should be made on the guru lying in the circular region of the moon in the lotus with 1000 petals which is situated in the brahmarandhra. Apparently, it indicates that the sahasrara is in the brahmarandhra. This means the extension of the brahmarandhra beyond the head, and beyond the terminal point of the sushumna and the nirwana chakra. It is contrary to most of the documents cited above. It also conflicts with the passage in the Gandharwatantra (ch. 5, p. 27) itself, which says that the sushumna extends through the vertebral column from the mula-kanda to the brahmarandhra. This brahmarandhra-point is situated in the head where the sushumna ends (—Shandilyopanishad, 1.4.10). The sahasrara is situated above this (that is, the brahmarandhra—Jaganmohana—the commentator) and outside the body (that is, outside the cranium which is the topmost part of the body) (—Shiwasanghita, 5.198). Therefore, the brahmarandhra is the end point of the cranium where the sushumna, and consequently, wajra and chitrini, terminate. This terminal point is within the cranium. But the sahasrara is situated extra-cranially; so, the sushumna and all nadis inside it cannot proceed to the sahasrara. Hence, the literal meaning of 'situated in the brahmarandhra' should be changed to the technical meaning—'situated in the proximity of the brahmarandhra'. In a similar manner the expression 'In the sahasrara, lying in the brahmarandhra, the God Sadashiwa is situated' (—Bhutashuddhitantra, ch. 3, p. 3) should be changed (that is, lying in the proximity of the brahmarandhra).

It has been stated that Kundalini passes through the ajña situated in the forehead (eyebrow-space) to the sahasrara lying face downwards, and above the topmost point of the sushumna nadi which is inside the vertebral column (—Tararahasya, ch. 4, p. 23). Here it is stated that the sahasrara is above the terminal point of the sushumna, that is, above the head. It has also been stated that the twelve-petalled lotus (that is, guru chakra) is situated at the end-points of the three nadis (that is, sushumna, wajra and chitrini) (—ibid., ch. 4, p. 23). It is clear that the guru chakra is situated above the terminal point of the sushumna in the head. So, the guru chakra is above the cranium.

It has been clearly stated that at the end of the Kundalirandhrakanda (sushumna), situated in the dwadashanta (= brahmarandhra), is the twelve-petalled, shining, white lotus. The face of this lotus is turned upwards; it is the seat of guru, and outside it (guru chakra) is the lotus with 1000 petals—with a moon-like, shining, white colour (—Sammohanatantra, Part 2, ch. 2, p. 2). So, the guru chakra is above the brahmarandhra and situated extra-cranially, and its top is covered by the sahasrara.

The exact position of the brahmarandhra has been mentioned in the Kankalamalinitantra (ch. 2, p. 5). But the literal translation of the text will give an incongruous meaning. So, it should be explained from the technical viewpoint. The literal translation of the text is: the imperishable sahasrara lotus is white in colour and lies with its face downwards; it is decorated with the shining letters from a to ksha; in its pericarp is antaratman (jiwatman; but here Supreme Spirit), and then the guru, and the surya-mandala and the chandra-mandala, then mahanada-wayu followed by brahmarandhra. If the first, italicized 'then' before the guru means 'above', then the meaning would be that the guru is above antaratman which is absurd. If 'above' is used for 'then' in all places, the meaning would be: above antaratman is the guru, and above him is the surya-mandala, above it is the chandra-mandala, above it mahanada-wayu, and above it brahmarandhra. The arrangement of things like this does not exist in the sahasrara. Of course, there is the chandra-mandala in the sahasrara. The guru is situated below the pericarp of the sahasrara, that is, in the guru chakra which is the lower aspect of the sahasrara. So, the italicized 'then' (before the guru) would indicate 'below' antaratman; 'and the surya-mandala and the chandra-mandala' would be below the guru (-chakra) (and above the ajña). The surya-mandala indicates the manas chakra; above it is the chandra-mandala to indicate the indu chakra; above it mahanada-wayu; and above it the brahmarandhra.

The following passages from the Kankalamalinitantra (ch. 2, p. 5) read thus: 'In that randhra (that is, brahmarandhra) lies wisarga; above it (it means not only above wisarga, but also above the sahasrara) is divine Shankhini; below Shankhini is the chandra-mandala (within the sahasrara) where lies a triangle; kailasa

(the abode of Shiwa) is situated in the triangle;
... here lies the perpetual and unchanging
amakala.'

The wisarga is the power-bridge through
which Kundalini passes from the brahmarandhra
to the guru chakra and sahasrara. We get the
following order: ajña, surya-mandala (manas
chakra), chandra-mandala (indu chakra), mahanada-wayu, brahmarandhra (here lies the nirwana chakra), wisarga (which connects brahmarandhra with the), guru chakra, sahasrara,
Shankhini. Shankhini is Supreme Kundalini in
the spiral form lying above the sahasrara.
Kundalini becomes Shankhini after passing
through the sahasrara.

The three forms of specific orders of the chakras
and associated power aspects have been given
in the Sammohanatantra, Part 2.

Form 1 (ch. 2, p. 2). The order is this: ajña,
indu, half-moon-shaped nada, plough-shaped
mahanada, power añji, unmani, twelve-petalled
chakra (guru chakra), sahasrara where lies the
chandra-mandala, wisarga, dhruwa-mandala
(infinite region).

Form 2 (ch. 2, p. 2). Order: muladhara,
swadhishthana, manipura, anahata, wishuddha,
ajña, bindu, kalapada, nirodhika, indu, nada,
nadanta, unmani, wishnuwaktra (-mouth),
dhruwamandalika Shiwa (Infinite Consciousness).

Form 3 (ch. 4, p. 4). Order: muladhara to
ajña, bindu, kala-nada, nadanta, unmani,
wishnuwaktra, guruwaktra, Parama Shiwa
(Supreme Consciousness).

From the above three forms we get the following order:

Muladhara to ajña chakras
Bindu
Kala
Nirodhika
Indu
Nada (half-moon-shaped)
Mahanada (plough-shaped)
Añji kala
Unmani
Twelve-petalled lotus (guru chakra)
Circular region of the moon (sahasrara)
Wishnuwaktra

Guruwaktra
Wisarga
Dhruwamandala, or Parama Shiwa

This order presents stages through which
Kundalini passes from the muladhara to Parama
Shiwa. The first stages are from the muladhara
to the ajña. In the ajña Power Hakini, Itara-
linga and pranawa are absorbed in this order
into Kundalini. Then comes bindu. This bindu
may be supposed to be the second bindu closely
related to the bindu of pranawa, and is the seat
of manas 2 (sense-mind). Associated with the
second bindu are three forms of power, namely
kala, nirodhika and indu. The sense-mind
ordinarily functions in relation to the senses
by kala. By the power nirodhika, the sensory
function of the sense-mind is controlled, and
then it is able to receive outer objects directly;
this power is indu. Here indu is not the indu
chakra. Kundalini absorbs all these.

Then is the half-moon-shaped nada. It is the
same as the second nada, and is the seat of the
manas chakra where lies chitta (sense-consciousness). Above it is plough-shaped mahanada,
also called nadanta. Here there is no clear
indication where the indu chakra is situated.
It has been stated in the Kankalamalinitantra,
ch. 2, p. 5, that the chandra mandala (indu
chakra) is below the mahanada. Also, in the
Shatchakranirupana, Verse 39, the position of
the plough-shaped mahanada is above the seat
of Bhagawan (indu chakra). So, the indu
chakra is to be placed above the half-moon-
shaped nada and below the plough-shaped
mahanada. Above it is the nirwana (or brahmarandhra) chakra. Here two forms of power are
situated—añji and unmani. This chakra is the
seat of dhi (concentrative mind). By the power
of añji dhi functions as attention, in conjunction
with the intellective mind. When añji is controlled by unmani concentration develops. In
this chakra lies I-ness. Kundalini absorbs all
these and then passes through the power-bridge
(wisarga) into the guru chakra and sahasrara.
Wishnuwaktra and guruwaktra are in the sahasrara. Wishnuwaktra is the final stage of the
samprajñata samadhi. It is dissolved into guru-
waktra which is the entrance to the Supreme

Bindu where *asamprajñata* samadhi starts. The final stage is dhruwa-mandala—the infinity of *Parama Shiwa*. There is the wisarga (second) which separates sahasrara proper from Supreme Bindu.

For the passing of Kundalini from the ajña another order has been given, using different technical terms: after piercing the ajña, Kundalini passes into the bodhini chakra, then through kataha to parnashaila; then through dyumani to ghatadhara where absorption of mind takes place; above it is the brahma-chakra where calmness prevails; above it the brahmadanda, and above that is only water (that is, void) where the lustrous sahasrara is seen; next comes the karnikasthana (pericarp); above it is the siddhakhadga; then there is the matrika-mandala containing all bijas (germ-mantras); above it are nectarous pretabija (= Hsouh) where concentration should be made on Supreme Power (—Rudrayamala, Part 2, 60. 30-4).

Now, the description of the chakras situated in the ajña system has to be made in the right order.

9 Manas

The manas chakra, numerically from the muladhara, is the ninth. It is situated within the chitrini nadi.

Terminology

1 Manas mandala (chakra), mentioned in the Yogashikhopanishad, 1.178; 5.15.

2 Manas chakra, mentioned by Jaganmohana Tarkalankara in Foot-note 87 on the Mahanirwanatantra, 5. 104; by Swami Sachchidananda Saraswati in the Gurupradipa, p. 275; Pujapradipa, Part 2, p. 79; Jñanapradipa, Part 1, p. 173.

3 Nada, mentioned in the Shatchakranirupana, Verse 35; Sharadatilakatantra, 5. 136; Shadamnayatantra, 5. 268; Shiwasanghita, 5. 149; Koulawalitantra, ch. 22, p. 81; Sammohanatantra, Part 2, ch. 2, p. 2; ch. 4, p. 4; Shrikrama,

quoted in the Yogakalpalatika MS.

4 Surya mandala, mentioned in the Kankalamalinitantra, ch. 2, p. 5.

5 Jñananetra (knowledge-light), mentioned in the Soubhagyalakshmyupanishad, 3.7.

Position

The manas chakra is situated above the second bindu which is just above the bindu of pranawa in the ajña (—Sammohanatantra, Part 2, ch. 2, p. 2; ch. 4, p. 4). The second bindu has not been mentioned in the Shatchakranirupana Verse 35, where it was simply stated that the nada (manas chakra) is above the bindu of pranawa in the ajña chakra. The Shiwasanghita (5.149) mentions the second bindu as bindu pitha (or bindu chakra), and gives the order as follows: bindu pitha, nada pitha, shakti pitha. So, the nada pitha (chakra), which is the manas chakra, is above the bindu pitha and is situated above the ajña chakra. Here, the second bindu has been termed as bindu pitha, that is, bindu chakra.

So, the position of the manas chakra is above the bindu chakra, situated above the pranawa-bindu in the ajña.

Description

The manas chakra is white (—Shatchakranirupana, Verse 35; Koulawalitantra, ch. 22, p. 81). It has six petals, and these are connected with the senses of smell, taste, form, touch and sound, and sleep. The petals assume the sense colours, that is, the petal connected with smell becomes yellow. Those connected with taste, form, touch, and sound, are white, red, ash, and white respectively. The petal representing sleep is black.

Explanation

The manas chakra is the seat of chitta (sense-consciousness). Here, the absorption of chitta takes place. It has been stated that the nada (manas chakra) which is the abode of all bliss is the place or position for the absorption of chitta by the niralamba-pura (-mudra) (the process of sense-control), the secret of which can be learnt from the parama-guru (a guru who has been given the secret which has been handed down in regular succession from the gurus); by the practice of this yoga-process, the yogi 'sees', in deep concentration, the subtle fire (that is, the sushumna which is subtle and fiery), and then inside it the shining forms (that is, inside the sushumna is seen the chitrini where lie the chakras) (—Shatchakranirupana, Verse 36). The absorption of chitta occurs when Kundalini passes through the manas chakra.

In waking (and not in deep concentration), chitta is constantly receiving sensory radiations through manas 2 (sense-mind). From the sensory area of the the brain, the sensory impulses of smell, taste, sight, touch and sound, on being reduced to non-material wayu-forms, pass through the ida nadi to the appropriate chakras, and proceed from there to the sense-mind. Smell in wayu-form passes to the muladhara, taste to the swadhishthana, form-colour to the manipura, touch to the anahata and sound to the wishuddha. The senses get their own characteristic qualities in the chakras, and are radiated through the petaline processes of the chakras to the ida and are carried to the sense-mind, by this nadi. The sense-mind sends the senso-mental radiations to chitta where the senso-mental patterns are changed into conscious forms, and the I-ness recognizes them as smell, taste, sight, touch and sound. In this manner, consciousness is being undulated and is assuming different sensory forms, and becomes tinged with characteristic sense-colours. Smell gets its yellow colour, taste its white, sight its red, touch its ash colour and sound its white when they pass through the appropriate chakras.

When the senso-mental radiations are stopped or obstructed by the predominance of the tamas quality in chitta, consciousness is masked, and a state of nonconsciousness is induced. The induced nonconsciousness in the normal state is sleep. But there is always a permanent area of unconsciousness connected with chitta where all post-conscious and unconscious impressions (sangskaras) are stored. Pleasurable impressions are conveyed to chitta by memory as a notion (bodha), which becomes a feeling (bhawa), and the feeling develops as love (raga), which becomes mixed with desire (kama) arising from thought and perception. Desire, being mixed with will (manasyana), develops as volition (chikirsha) and then as conation (kriti). Conation, as conative impulse (kratu), passes to the appropriate chakra (one of the five lower chakras), and emerges as a pre-motor impulse, and is carried to the brain by the pingala.

Consciousness is the phenomenon in which sentiency is manifested, derived from the sattwa attribute of primus, which presents two forms: dichotomous and unitary. In the dichotomous form there is a constant and changeless individualized entity endowed with the power of being aware of what is happening in the other aspect. This individualized entity gives rise to the I-feeling in relation to the objective aspect of consciousness. In fact, consciousness is no consciousness unless a union takes place between the 'I' and what the 'I' knows. As this knowing or consciousness is conjugated in character, it is called sangjñana, that is, united knowledge or consciousness. What the 'I' knows are the contents of consciousness radiated into it sensorially from the outer world. This consciousness is termed chitta—sense-consciousness. Radiations from buddhi (intellective mind) also penetrate into chitta. When the senso-mental radiations are controlled by pratyahara, thoughts and intellection are also controlled, and now chitta is transformed into dhi (superconsciousness). The emptying of the sensory objects and the elimination of thoughts do not make consciousness vacant. In superconsciousness, the contents are subtle objects. The subtle objects come into being naturally in superconsciousness as the gross objects are naturally contents of sense-consciousness. The 'I' as an experiencer remains the same here too. The dichotomous consciousness is transformed into a unitary form only at a higher stage of samprajñata samadhi when the individualized I-ness is absorbed into all-I, all-dewata, or Kundalini consciousness. The individualized 'I'-consciousness remains an indispensable aspect of chitta and dhi up to the levels of dhyana and the first three stages of samadhi. Thereafter, the stage of

I-lessness develops. The seat of the 'I' is in the nirwana chakra.

10 Indu

The indu chakra, numerically from the muladhara, is the tenth. It is situated within the chitrini nadi.

Terminology

1 Indu (moon) chakra, mentioned in the Yogakundalyupanishad, 1.71.

2 Shitangshu (moon) mandala (chakra), mentioned in the Yogakundalyupanishad, 1.69.

3 Sixteen-petalled Anahata, mentioned in the Yogakundalyupanishad, 1.69.

4 Shambhawa (belonging to Shiwa) Sthana (chakra), mentioned in the Yogashikhopanishad, 5.16.

5 Chandra (moon) mandala (chakra), mentioned in the Kankalamalinitantra, ch. 2, p. 5; Nirwanatantra, ch. 9, p. 11; Koulawalitantra, ch. 22, p. 81.

6 Chandra (= Chandra mandala—Jaganmohana), mentioned in the Shiwasanghita, 5.188.

7 Kailasa (an abode of Shiwa), mentioned in the Gandharwatantra, ch. 5, p. 28; Shaktanandatarangini, 4.14; Rudrayamala, Part 2, 27.69; Goutamiyatantra, 34.53; Mridanitantra, quoted in Amarasanggraha MS; Dewibhagawata, 7.35. 46.

8 Shakti (power), mentioned in the Shiwapurana, 2.11.40; Shiwasanghita, 5.149.

9 Widya-pada (-chakra), mentioned in the Shiwapurana, 5a. 7.4.

10 Nadanta, mentioned in the Koulawalitantra, ch. 22, p. 81; Sharadatilakatantra, 5.136.

11 Soma, mentioned by Jaganmohana in his note No. 87 in connection with the explanation of the Mahanirwanatantra, 5.104, and note No. 42 in relation to his explanation of the Shiwasanghita, 5.188; and by Swami Sachchidananda in his works Jñanapradipa, ch. 3, p. 152, Pujapradipa, Part 2, ch. 4, p. 48, 80, and Gurupradipa, ch. 6, p. 279.

Position

The indu chakra is situated above the manas chakra (—Kankalamalinitantra, ch. 2, p. 5; Koulawalitantra, ch. 22, p. 81; Shiwasanghita, 5.149; Shrikrama, quoted in the Yogakalpalatika MS.

Description

The indu chakra (Plate 20) is moon-white in colour, as its name indicates. It has sixteen petals (—Yogakundalyupanishad, 1.69). According to Jaganmohana this chakra has sixteen petals. Swami Sachchidananda quotes a passage from the Tantra in which it is stated that the ninth is the brahma chakra which is decorated with sixteen petals (—Jñanapradipa, Part 1, ch. 3, p. 153). He identifies brahma chakra with soma chakra. The colour of the petals is also moon-white.

On the petals are the following specific qualities (writtis) which are arranged from right to left: (1) mercy; (2) gentleness; (3) patience; (4) non-attachment; (5) control; (6) excellent qualities; (7) joyous mood; (8) deep spiritual love; (9) humility; (10) reflection; (11) restfulness; (12) seriousness; (13) effort; (14) controlled emotion; (15) magnanimity; (16) concentration.

It has been stated that there is the purna chandra mandala (full moon region, that is, chandra or moon chakra) in the ajña (system); in its pericarp, there is a nine-cornered region where lies the manidwipa (the isle of gems); in the isle of gems is the Shambhu-bija (that is, the germ-mantra of the God Shiwa—Hang) which (with sah which denotes Shakti—Power) is in the form of hangsah (swan); hangsah (as mantra in its power as consciousness) is Supreme Brahman, and (in its power-in-sound-form) is Shiwa in divine form; the beak of the swan is the pranawa, the wings are the Agama and Nigama (two forms of the Tantra), the feet are Consciousness-Power, the three eyes are the three bindus, and he is in a golden lotus; in the lap of the hangsah (that is, in the bindu of the Hang bija) is Deity Parashiwa with Power Siddhakali on his left, who is eternal bliss (Nirwa*na*tantra, ch. 9, p. 11).

It has been stated that above the nad*a* (that is, in the chandra mand*ala*) is W*ri*shabhadhwa*ja* (an epithet of Shiw*a*) with his Power (—Koula-wa*li*tantra, ch. 22, p. 81). The concentration form of W*ri*shabhadhwa*ja* is as follows: He is like crystal-white in colour, with braided hair and adorned with (crescent-) moon (in his forehead), and decked in tigerskin (*ibid.*). The concentration form of his Power is: she is yellow in colour, and holds in her beautiful hands a drum, a trident, a noose, and makes an attitude of dispelling fear; she is beautiful and adorned with various ornaments (—*ibid.*). It has also been stated that Parashiw*a* is with Power Hakin*i* in the ajña (system) (—Mantrama-hodadhi, 4.24).

The presence of Deity Parashiw*a* has been mentioned in the *Shad*amnayatantra, 5.268. Parashiw*a* has also been mentioned as Sadashiw*a* in the form of a swan situated in a chakra (indu chakra) above the ajña (—*Shad*amnayatantra, 3.76). He has been mentioned as Mahadew*a* (Shiw*a*) and W*ri*shabhadhwa*ja* who is like crystal white (—Shr*i*krama, quoted in the Yoga*kalpa*-latika MS). He has also been called Bhagawan (God) as immutable and Supreme Being, endow-ed with supreme yoga-power (—*Shat*chakra-nir*upa*na, Verse 37).

Explanation

The indu chakra is the seat of buddhi (intellective mind). This is indicated by the term 'widya pada' (widya chakra) given to the indu chakra. It has been stated that first Shakti (Power) becomes manifested from Shiwa who is in union with Shakti; from Shakti shantya*tita* pada (sahasrar*a* chakra), and then shanti pada (nirwa*na* chakra), and thereafter widya pada (indu chakra) (—Shiwapurana, 5A. 7.4). The word 'widya' is derived from wid*a*, meaning jñana (knowledge). The word 'buddhi' is derived from buddh*a* to mean also jñana. Jñan*a* means buddhi-w*ri*tti (Wach*a*spatyam), that is, intel-lection. P*a*da means a place or position (—Apte), here a chakra. This chakra is the seat of buddhi the general function of which is intellection. So, buddhi is the intellective mind.

There is a difference between sense-knowledge (sangjñan*a*) and intellection, which is technically termed wijñan*a*. Though some rudimentary intellection is involved in sense-knowledge, yet intellection is specific in character and exclusive to buddhi. Sense-knowledge, of course, plays a great role in the functioning of buddhi. The main functions of the buddhi are: man*i*sha (higher intellection), m*a*ti (thought), man*a*na (intellection), d*ri*sh*ti* (insight), and medha (reten-tive power). On the one hand, buddhi functions in relation to perception, and, on the other, it can be abstracted into a field which is outside the perceptual field. When K*u*nd*a*lin*i* passes through this chakra, buddhi becomes absorbed into her.

In the indu chakra is situated Parashiw*a*, the sixth Shiw*a*. Concentration is made on him in this chakra.

11 Nirwa*na*

The nirwa*na* chakra, which is numerically the eleventh from the m*u*ladhara, is situated within the chitri*ni* nad*i*.

Terminology

1 Nirwa*na*, mentioned in the Soubhagya-lak*sh*myupanishad, 3.8; Brahmasiddhanta-paddhati MS.

2 Brahma*ra*ndhra (chakra), mentioned in the Yogarajopanishad, Mantra 16; Yogashikhopa-nishad, 6.47; Trishikhibrahma*n*opanishad, Man-tra Section, Mantra 151; Shand*i*lyopanishad, 1.4.10; Adwayatarakopanishad, Mantra 5; N*i*la-tantra, ch. 5, p. 9; Kankalamalin*i*tantra, ch. 2, p. 5; Kular*n*awa, ch. 4, pp. 20, 22; Mantra-mahodadhi, 4.28; Agnipurana 72.31; 74.13; 88.43; Skandapurana, 1.2.55.45; 3.1.13.39; Gandharwatantra, ch. 5, p. 27; Bh*u*tashuddhi-

tantra, ch. 6, p. 5; Brahmawaiwartapurana, 1.13.17; 1.16.67; 4.20.29; Dewibhagawatapurana, 11.1.48.

3 Parabrahma chakra, mentioned in the Soubhagyalakshmyupanishad, 3.8.

4 Bodhini (chakra), mentioned in the Gandharwatantra, ch. 5, p. 28; Shaktanandatarangini, 4.14; Goutamiyatantra, 34.53; Rudrayamala, Part 2, 60.30.

5 Bodhana, mentioned in the Rudrayamala, Part 2, 27.69.

6 Rodhini, mentioned in the Mridanitantra, quoted in the ·Amarasanggraha MS; Dewibhagawatapurana, 7.35.46.

7 Chitkalashakti (chakra), mentioned in the Shadamnayatantra, 5.269.

8 Shanta (chakra), mentioned in the Shiwapurana, 3.3.28.

9 Shantipada (chakra), mentioned in the Shiwapurana, 5a, 7.4.

10 Shatapatra (hundred-petalled) chakra, mentioned in the Amarasanggraha MS.

11 Shatadala (hundred-petalled) chakra, mentioned in the Tattwayogabindu MS.

12 Kala chakra, mentioned in the Tattwayogabindu MS.

13 Dwadashanta (chakra), mentioned in the Shiwapurana, 2.11.40; 3.5.53;

14 Dwadashanta pada (chakra), mentioned in the Agnipurana, 74.10.

15 Dwadashanta Sarasija (= lotus), mentioned in the Garudapurana, Part 1, 23.48.

16 Brahmarandhra Pankaja (lotus), mentioned in the Brahmawaiwartapurana, 1.26.5.

17 Shirshantargata (being in the interior of the cranium) mandala (chakra), mentioned in the Mandalabrahmanopanishad, 1.4.1.

Position

The nirwana is the last chakra within the chitrini nadi, the first being muladhara. At the end point of the nirwana, chitrini ends and, consequently, the wajra and sushumna also terminate. This terminal point is within the cranium, and there is nothing intracranially beyond this terminal point. The brahmarandhra or brahma nadi also ends at this terminal point, but a non-nadi connection between the intracranial brahma nadi and the extracranial guru chakra is maintained by the wisarga (power-bridge).

So, the position of the nirwana chakra is at the upper terminal point of the chitrini nadi within the cranium at its topmost end.

Description

The nirwana chakra (Plate 21) is shining white (—Amarasanggraha MS). It has 100 petals (—Brahmasiddhantapaddhati MS; Amarasanggraha MS; Tattwayogabindu MS). The petals are also lustrous white. Inside the chakra (that is, in the pericarp) is Shiwa in shining smoke-colour and concentration should be made on him (—Soubhagyalakshmyupanishad, 3.8; Brahmasiddhantapaddhati MS).

In the (pericarp of the) chakra lies jalandharapitha (-seat) which leads to liberation (—Soubhagyalakshmyupanishad, 3.8; Brahmasiddhantapaddhati MS). It is consciousness, shining in blue light (—Yogarajopanishad, Mantra 17).

Inside this chakra is situated Supreme Consciousness-Power (—Yogashikhopanishad, 6.47). That is, Kundalini as Divine Consciousness-Power is realized in concentration here.

Explanation

The nirwana chakra is the centre of dhi (concentrative mind) as well as ahang (I-ness). Chitta (sense-consciousness) exhibits multi-objectivity in relation to which buddhi (intellective mind) functions in a general manner. But when a particular sense-object is singled out from many sense-objects, buddhi exercises its specific function and as a result clear thought and intellection and greater retentive power (medha) are exhibited. The selection of a single object, or a group of objects from many, and focusing it in consciousness are the functions of dhi as awadhana (attention). Attention also exercises a tremendous influence on buddhi by which deep thought and intellection are aroused and finally become higher and deeper thought-intellection (manisha). Attention is the secondary function of dhi.

The principal function of dhi is concentration. Concentration is a mental mechanism or process effecting the centralization of consciousness by eliminating all its contents except one, which becomes identified with consciousness in its contraction or condensation to bindu—the point. In this process the mental control power is roused to the highest degree, which functions at three levels: first, the centralization of consciousness by the elimination of its contents by holding a single object in consciousness without interruption; second, the identification of consciousness with the held object in non-perception and non-thought-non-intellective concentration; and third, raising the depth of concentration to its highest point when I-consciousness becomes the submerged factor, and consciousness is in its highest concentration and in full identification with the object held. The first level is called dharana—holding-concentration; the second level is dhyana—objects-absorptive concentration; and the third is samprajñata samadhi—superconscious concentration.

Samprajñata samadhi has four stages. At the first stage, objective elimination is effected by holding a sensory object. At the second stage, the holding is of subtle objects (mahabhutas and tanmatras); at the third, the holding is done on lustrous conscious forms (dewatas); and at the fourth, consciousness is all-dewata, or all-I-ness, or all-Kundalini. So, samprajñata samadhi consists of (1) sensorial superconscious concentration; (2) non-sensorial superconscious concentration; (3) dewata concentration; and (4) formless concentration. Formless concentration consists of (a) all-dewata concentration; (b) all-I concentration; and (c) all-Kundalini concentration.

Consciousness exhibiting sensory phenomena does not terminate when these phenomena cease to occur there, but continues as superconsciousness when subtle phenomena take place. In other words, chitta as sense-consciousness is transformed into dhi as concentrative consciousness—the sangjñana-wijñana into prajñana.

In the nirwana chakra, concentration is done on lustrous Shiwa and on jalandhara of shining blue in colour. From the mantra viewpoint,

jalandhara indicates the bija 'Gang'. Gang is the spiritual knowledge developed in concentration.

When Kundalini passes through the nirwana chakra, I-ness is absorbed into her.

Sahasrara System

The sahasrara system (Plate 22) starts with the guru-chakra which is the lower aspect of the sahasrara itself. The first question is where the sahasrara lies. To determine the location of the sahasrara is a problem, because it has been described in the texts in different ways. It has been stated that the sahasrara lies in the great brahmarandhra path (—Yogachudamanyupanishad, Mantra 6; Shaktanandatarangini, 4.29; 9.16). If the sahasrara is included in the brahmarandhra, then the location would be incorrect. The right interpretation is that the brahmarandhra is not isolated from the sahasrara but is in contact with it through the power-bridge (wisarga); however, it is not within the brahmarandhra.

There are other similar expressions which also should be technically explained. 'The sahasrara lying in the head' (—Kularnawa, ch. 4, p. 22; Guptasadhanatantra, ch. 2, p. 2; Bhutashuddhitantra, ch. 3, p. 3; Shaktanandatarangini, 4.1; 4.25; Shyamarahasya, ch. 1, p. 3; Shiwapurana, 3.3.63; 4.40.26) and 'The sahasrara lying in the brahmarandhra' (—Gandharwatantra, ch. 5, pp. 23, 24; Bhutashuddhitantra, ch. 3, p. 3; Purashcharanarasollasa, ch. 9, p. 9; Jñanarnawa, quoted in Shyamarahasya, ch. 1, p. 3; Shiwasanghita, 5.138; Brahmawaiwartapurana, 1.26.5); here, 'in the head' or 'in the brahmarandhra' is to be interpreted 'in the void in contact with the head or brahmarandhra', otherwise these statements will go against other statements and the fact. It has been stated that the roused divine Kundalini passes into the region of void through the sushumna-path, and comes back to her abode (in the muladhara) (—Phetkarinitantra, ch. 14, p. 39). The region of void is where the sahasrara lies. It is a well-known fact that Kundalini passes into the sahasrara where union takes place with Parama Shiwa. It has been stated that the mantra becomes living when Kundalini is roused by Hangsah mantra and conducted into the great lotus sahasrara for the union with Parama Shiwa in the form of Bindu (—Todalatantra, ch. 6, p. 12); also, the roused Kundalini, eager to be in the sahasrara (for the union) passes through the brahma-path (that is, brahma nadi) into the sahasrara (—ibid., ch. 8, p. 16). So, this void is the sahasrara or where the sahasrara lies. This is why the sahasrara has been termed akasha (void) chakra (—Soubhagya-lakshmyupanishad, 3.9; Brahmasiddhantapaddhati MS; Tattwayogabindu MS), wyoma (void) chakra (—Yogarajopanishad, Mantra 17), wyomambuja (—Yogashikhopanishad, 6.48), and wyomambhoja (—Tripurasarasamuchchaya, 4.12). It has been clearly stated that the sahasrara is in the void (—Mundamalatantra, ch. 2, p. 5), and so the akasha (void) chakra is the thousand-petalled lotus (sahasrara) (—Brahmasiddhantapaddhati MS).

About the location of the sahasrara, the Shatchakranirupana (Verse 40) says, above that (tadurdhwe), in the region of void, which is at the end of (that is, above) where shankhini is, and below wisarga, is the lotus of a thousand petals.

The commentator Kalicharana interprets 'above that' (tadurdhwe) as above all that has been said before. It is vague. Shankara and Bhuwanamohana say 'above the mahanada'. This is also not precise. According to the Shatchakranirupana, the order of 'forms' above pranawa in the ajña system is as follows: subtle manas (in the second bindu)—nada (second nada = manas chakra)—seat of Bhagawan (Parashiwa in the indu chakra)—plough-shaped mahanada—shankhini—void region where lies the lotus of 1000 petals. We have seen that above mahanada is brahmarandhra (—Kankalamalinitantra, ch. 2, p. 5). In this text there is no mention of the brahmarandhra, but instead of that, shankhini.

What is shankhini? Kalicharana, Wishwanatha, Ramawallabha and Bhuwanamohana say that shankhini is a nadi by that name. It has been stated that the nadi termed shankhini goes up through the cavity of the throat to the head where it remains with its face downwards; it carries nutrients and becomes the source of nourishment (to the brain) (—Yogashikhopanishad, 5.25). Shankhini is a subtle nadi which lies within the cranial cavity. Its gross replica is the internal carotid artery (arteria carotis interna) through which the brain receives its main blood supply. The term shankhini seems to indicate the highest point within the cranial cavity, which is above mahanada. Beyond shankhini lies a void region. In the text, the word 'shikhara' (of shankhini) has been used. Kalicharana interprets it as 'mastaka' (= the head or top of anything—Apte); Wishwanatha as 'agra' (= the foremost or topmost point—Apte); and Ramawallabha and Bhuwanamohana as 'agrabhaga' (= fore-part, tip—Apte). It gives a clearer meaning if it is interpreted as antamatra (—Wachaspatyam) = the end-point. This means that at the end-point of shankhini lies a void-region. So shankhini appears to be synonymous with the nirwana chakra, that is, the topmost part of shankhini which is above mahanada is nirwana chakra.

Beyond the upper border of shankhini, but in contact with it, is a void. This void is outside the cranium (—Shiwasanghita, 5.198). Kalicharana interprets 'void' as 'the place where there are no nadis, and it indicates that it (the void) is above where the sushumna ends'. So, the void is outside the head and where there are no nadis—shankhini, sushumna, wajra, chitrini and brahma nadis, and consequently, these nadis end intracranially. It has been stated that Kundalini passes from the bodhini (= nirwana) chakra by piercing the skull (kataha) to enter certain intermediate forms and reaching an all-water (void) region where the lustrous sahasrara is seen (—Rudrayamala, Part 2, 60. 30-2). This clearly shows that the sahasrara is in the void which is outside the skull, and to reach the sahasrara the head has to be pierced. The sahasrara has a Waidika term kapalasamputa, that is, it is a shining sheath-like hemispherical formation over the skull. This indicates that the sahasrara is, like an umbrella, above the head.

In the brahmarandhra lies wisarga (—Kankala-malinitantra, ch. 2, p. 5) which like a bridge connects the nirwana chakra with the sahasrara. Therefore, to reach the sahasrara from the nirwana chakra the head has to be pierced and the wisarga passed through. This wisarga should not be confused with the wisarga which is above the sahasrara. Also, the shankhini nadi which is in the head and below the void region is not the same as divine Shankhini (—Kankalamalini-tantra, ch. 2, p. 5), who is Supreme Kundalini in a spiral form and is above the sahasrara.

The void region, situated above the topmost point of shankhini nadi, has been termed mahashunya (great void) chakra (—Amara-sanggraha MS; Tattwayogabindu MS). There is nothing above it. It is the sahasrara system. It consists mainly of the sahasrara and Supreme Bindu. The sahasrara can be considered as having three aspects: lower aspect, which is the guru chakra as the lower part of the sahasrara; the middle aspect, which is the sahasrara proper; and the higher aspect which leads to Supreme Bindu. It is more convenient to study the sahasrara system in three parts: guru chakra and sahasrara in its middle and higher aspects.

12 Guru

It has been stated that concentration should be on Guru who is in the sahasrara (—Nila-tantra, ch. 1, p. 1; Todalatantra, ch. 3, p. 4; Matrikabhedatantra, ch. 7, p. 10; Brihannila-tantra, ch. 6, p. 31; Kankalamalinitantra, ch. 3, p. 7; Kularnawa, ch. 4, p. 22; Guptasadhana tantra, ch. 2, p. 2; Gandharwatantra, ch. 5, p. 24; Shaktakrama, ch. 1, p. 1; Tararahasya, ch. 1, p. 2; Purashcharanarasollasa, ch. 8, p. 8; Shaktanandatarangini, 4.1; 4.25; Shyamara-hasya, ch. 1, p. 3; Shiwapurana, 3.3.63; Brahma-waiwartapurana, 1.26. 5–6). This comprehensive statement indicates that Guru's place is within the sahasrara; and this place has a specific name and is a part of the sahasrara.

The statement 'Concentrating with all efforts on the lotus at the feet of Guru, which lies in the sahasrara' clearly indicates that there is a lotus at the feet of Guru within the sahasrara as its part. The lotus within the sahasrara has also been described as 'In the lotus, adorned with thousand petals, is a circular moon region where lies Guru and concentration should be done on him' (—Gandharwatantra, ch. 5, p. 23). This means that there is a lotus on which the sahasrara stands as an umbrella, that is, this lotus is the lower part of the sahasrara. 'The lotus at the feet of Guru' means the lotus where Guru lies. The lotus at the feet of Guru has also been called guru-pura (Guru's abode) (—Sammohanatantra, Part 2, ch. 4, p. 4), guru-sthana (Guru's place) (—Purash-charanarasollasa, ch. 9, p. 9) and guru-pada (Guru's feet or place) (—Shadamnayatantra, 5.99). The words pura, sthana and pada techni-cally signify a chakra, so guru-pura, guru-sthana and guru-pada stand for guru chakra. The guru chakra has also been termed dwada-sharna (twelve-lettered) lotus (—Tararahasya, ch. 1, p. 1; Sammohanatantra, Part 2, ch. 2, p. 2; Shaktanandatarangini, 4.31; Padukapan-chaka, Verse 1), dwadashadala (twelve-petalled) padma (lotus) (—Shaktanandatarangini, 4.31), urdhwamukha padma (lotus with its face up-wards) (—Bhutashuddhitantra, ch. 8, p. 8; Shaktanandatarangini, 4.30) and shukla abja (white lotus) (—Tararahasya, ch. 1, p. 2; Mahanirwanatantra, 5.26).

That the guru chakra is a part of the sahasrara is indicated by the following statements: 'There (in the sahasrara) is a twelve-lettered twelve-petalled (lotus)' (—Mridanitantra, quoted in Amarasanggraha MS); 'There is a twelve-petalled lotus connected with the pericarp of the sahasrara' (—Gherandasanghita, 6.9); 'The sahasrara is vast and is associated with the twelve-petalled (lotus) (that is, the guru chakra belongs to the sahasrara)' (—Shadamnayatantra, 5.99); 'Above the pericarp of the twelve-lettered lotus lies the thousand-petalled lotus' (—Tara-rahasya, ch. 1, p. 1); 'Concentration should be done on Guru who is in the face-up twelve-petalled lotus, situated in the lower part of the face-down thousand-petalled lotus' (—Shak-tanandatarangini, 4.31).

In connection with the above passage (from

the Shaktanandatarangini), Brahmananda quotes a verse from the Yamala and explains it himself. This verse is exactly the same as verse 1 of the Padukapañchaka which has also been interpreted by Kalicharana. 'I adore the twelve-lettered, that is, twelve-petalled, lotus. What is the distinctive character of the lotus? It is like a head-ornament of the stalk which supports the passage of Kundali, running from the muladhara lotus to the God Sadashiwa in the form of Bindu situated in the pericarp of the thousand-petalled lotus, that is, the chitrini nadi. As the twelve-lettered lotus stands on the head of the chitrini nadi, so the word ornament (bhushana) has been used. What more? It is inseparably connected with the pericarp of the brahmarandhra lotus, that is, it is situated at the lower part of the pericarp of the sahasrara lotus with inseparable connection' (—Brahmananda: Shaktanandatarangini, 4.32).

There are two most important points in this verse which need to be carefully considered. First, a connection of this lotus with what has been termed 'Kundali-wiwara-kanda' (= the support of the passage of Kundali). The passage of Kundali means the brahma nadi. It is supported by the chitrini nadi. The chitrini is within the wajra, and the wajra within the sushumna. So, the essence is that the sushumna, with all its internal nadis, has a connection with the twelve-lettered lotus. To indicate the connection the word 'mandita' has been used. Brahmananda explains it by head-ornament. Kalicharana interprets 'adorned by chitrini'. However, there is no vital difference between them. Kalicharana makes it clear by saying: 'As a lotus stands on its stalk, so the twelve-lettered lotus is adorned by the stalk in the form of the chitrini nadi.' This means, the twelve-lettered lotus stands on the chitrini nadi. The implication is that the chitrini and brahma nadis are in contact with the twelve-lettered lotus, but not continuous with it. So, the sushumna-wajra-chitrini-brahma nadis end at the proximity of the twelve-lettered lotus. It has been supported by the Sammohanatantra, Part 2, ch. 2, p. 2, which says: 'The twelve-lettered lotus is situated at the top of the end-point of the chitrini nadi which contains in it brahmarandhra (Kundalirandhrakandanta).

It is the abode of Guru who is lustrous white. This lotus stands always with its face upwards. There is a lotus with a thousand petals which lies outside the face-upwards lotus (as an umbrella).'

Second, there is a constant relation between the twelve-lettered lotus and the brahmarandhra lotus. Both Brahmananda and Kalicharana explain brahmarandhra lotus as sahasrara. But the author thinks it unnecessary to regard brahmarandhra as sahasrara. It has been clearly stated that the brahmarandhra chakra is the nirwana chakra (—Soubhagyalakshmyupanishad, 3.8), not the sahasrara. Numerous statements have been quoted to show that brahmarandhra ends either as a nadi or a region intracranially, and beyond this is a void region where there are no nadis and there it is situated extracranially, and in this void lies the sahasrara. Kalicharana has explained in this way—the brahmarandhra lotus, that is, the lotus—the thousand-petalled lotus—in which is the brahmarandhra. The brahmarandhra lotus is the nirwana chakra at the end point of the chitrini nadi. The twelve-lettered lotus is in constant connection with the pericarp of the brahmarandhra (nirwana) lotus.

A question was raised by Dewi (Parwati): the great lotus sahasrara stands always with its face downwards; how is it possible for Guru to be there? Mahadewa's reply: the lotus (sahasrara) lies always with its face downwards, but it contains a pericarp which has its face always upwards (—Purashcharanarasollasa, ch. 8, p. 8). Mahadewa gives a further explanation. He says: 'The chitrini nadi containing lotuses is in the form of Power. It extends from the muladhara and all the chakras are in this nadi. Chitrini is an aspect of Kundali-chitrini is Kundali, and therefore, it is, as Kundalini, in three and a half coils, residing always in the triangular process of the lotus (muladhara). Where there is the upper end of the chitrini nadi, there lies the face-upwards (chakra = guru chakra), in constant contact with the topmost point of the chitrini, the pericarp of which is in the nature of power going upwards. ... The pericarp with the upwardly power has the Kundali-coils in it and therefore it is bright. ... This pericarp (that is, the pericarp of the twelve-petalled lotus, imbedded in the sahasrara) is in contact with the upper end of the chitrini. Concentration should be done (on Guru situated) in the pericarp. This is why the pericarp (of the twelve-petalled lotus) is with its face upwards and with the power directed upwards' (—ibid., ch.9, p. 9).

From the above it is clear that the sahasrara which stands with its face downwards contains a lotus as its part with its face upwards and, consequently, its pericarp is upward. That this upwardly directed pericarp of the twelve-petalled lotus is within the sahasrara has been made clear by Mahadewa himself. He says: In the lower deep hollow part (gahwara) of the sahasrara lies the pericarp which stands always with its face upward (—Purashcharanarasollasa, ch. 8, p. 8). This upwardly faced lotus in its lower edge is in contact with the upper end of the chitrini nadi.

Terminology

1 Dwadasharna (twelve-lettered) Sarasiruha (lotus), or Padma (lotus), mentioned in the Padukapanchaka, Verse 1; Tararahasya, ch. 1, p. 1; Shaktanandatarangini, 4.31,32; Sammohanatantra, Part 2, ch. 2, p. 2.

2 Dwadashadala (twelve-petalled) Saroja (lotus), or Padma (lotus), mentioned in the Tararahasya, ch. 4, p. 23; Shaktanandatarangini, 4.31,32; Gherandasanghita, 6.9.

3 Dwadashapatraka (twelve-petalled), mentioned in the Mridanitantra, quoted in Amarasanggraha MS.

4 Urdhwamukha (upward-face) padma (lotus), mentioned in the Bhutashuddhitantra, ch. 8, p. 8; Sammohanatantra, Part 2, ch. 2, p. 2; Shaktanandatarangini, 4.30.

5 Shukla (white) Abja (lotus), mentioned in the Tararahasya, ch. 1, p. 2; Mahanirwanatantra, 5.26.

6 Gurupada padma (lotus with Guru's feet), mentioned in the Kamadhenutantra, ch. 17, p. 23.

7 Gurupura (Guru chakra), mentioned in the Sammohanatantra, Part 2, ch. 4, p. 4.

8 Gurusthana (Guru chakra), mentioned in the Purashcharanarasollasa, ch. 9, p. 9.

9 Gurupada (Guru's place = guru chakra), mentioned in the Shadamnayatantra, 5.99.

10 Brahma Chakra, mentioned in the Rudrayamala, Part 2, 60.31.

11 Somamandala (-chakra), mentioned in the Purashcharyarnawa, ch. 2, p. 91.

Position

The guru chakra is situated in the void-region as the lower part of the sahasrara; it is situated at the top of the upper end of the sushumna.

Description

The guru chakra (Plate 23) is white (—Padukapanchaka, Verse 1; Sammohanatantra, Part 2, ch. 2, p. 2; Gherandasanghita, 6.10), and it is therefore called shukla abja (white lotus) (-Mahanirwanatantra, 5.26; Tararahasya, ch. 1, p. 2). It has twelve petals (—Padukapanchaka, Verse 1; Tararahasya, ch. 1, p. 1; ch. 4, p. 23; Sammohanatantra, Part 2, ch. 2, p. 2; Shaktanandatarangini, 4.31,32; Shadamnayatantra, 5.99; Mridanitantra, quoted in Amarasanggraha MS; Gherandasanghita, 6.9). The colour of the petals is white, as the lotus is white. On the twelve petals are twelve letters, so the lotus is called the dwadasharna (twelve-lettered). The letters are Ha, Sa, Kha, Freng, Ha, Sa, Ksha, Ma, La, Wa, Ra, Yung (—Gherandasanghita, 6.10) which constitute the Guru-mantra, and are arranged from right to left. The colour of the mantra-letters has not been mentioned. As Guru is white in colour, so the mantra-letters would also be white, as the form and the mantra of Guru are identical.

The pericarp of the lotus is always with its face upward (—Purashcharanarasollasa, ch. 8, p. 8; ch. 9, p. 9), so it is called urdhwamukha padma (upward-face lotus). The top of this lotus is adorned with the thousand petals (like an umbrella) (—Gandharwatantra, ch. 5, p. 23); as the thousand-petalled lotus stands above the pericarp of the twelve-petalled lotus

259

(—Tararahasya, ch. 1, p. 1), and on the outside (—Sammohanatantra, Part 2, ch. 2, p. 2). The pericarp of the twelve-petalled lotus is like a circular moon region (—Gandharwatantra, ch. 5, p. 23), consequently, it is moon-like, lustrous and nectarous (—Purashcharanarasollasa, ch. 8, p. 8). It is the place where concentration on Guru should be done. For this, the detailed knowledge of the pericarp is necessary.

It has been stated: 'Inside the open pericarp of the (twelve-petalled) lotus is a triangular region (abalalaya), formed by the lines beginning with A, Ka and Tha; in the corners of the triangle are the letters Ha, La and Ksha, and all these form a diagram; I adore it' (Padukapañchaka, Verse 2; here, the text interpreted by Kalicharana has not been strictly followed; a manuscript text in possession of the author's guru has been used).

The three lines which constitute the triangle are A-line, consisting of sixteen letters from a to ah; Ka-line, consisting of sixteen letters from ka to ta; and Tha-line, consisting of sixteen letters from tha to sa. The letters on the lines and in the three corners within the triangle are together fifty-one matrika-units. The triangle is situated with its apex downward. The A-line starts from the apex and forms the left side of the triangle. On this line are sixteen letters from a to ah. The A-line is called wama, Brahma or rajas line.

The Ka-line starts from the top of the left side and forms the base of the triangle. On this line are sixteen letters from ka to ta. The Ka-line is called the jyeshtha, Wishnu or sattwa line. The Tha-line starts from the right end of the base line and goes down to meet the apex, thus forming the right side of the triangle. On this line are sixteen letters from tha to sa. The Tha-line is also called the roudri, Shiwa or tamas line. The letter ha is at the apex, la at the left corner and ksha at the right corner, inside the triangle. These lines and letters form the Power-yantra—the triangular process of Kundalini, called abalalaya.

It has been stated that there are three gunas (as three lines) in the pericarp of the twelve-petalled lotus, and (the lines) are in the nature of Brahma, Wishnu and Shiwa (—Purashcha-

ranarasollasa, ch. 9, p. 9). This means that there is a triangle in the pericarp, which is formed by the Brahma, Wishnu and Shiwa lines, that is, the A-Ka-Tha triangle. So it has been said that the splendorous Kundalini-coils are in the pericarp (—ibid., ch. 9, p. 9), that is, inside the triangle in the pericarp. More clearly, the pericarp contains a triangle in which lies Kundali, so it is said to be in the form of three and a half coils (—ibid., ch. 8, p. 8). Because of the presence of Kundalini, the triangle is called abalalaya.

The triangle in the pericarp is formed by the lines beginning with A, Ka and Tha (—Mridanitantra, quoted in Amarasanggraha MS; Sammohanatantra, Part 2, ch. 2, p. 2; Gherandasanghita, 6.11), and within the triangle in its corners are the letters ha, la and ksha (—Gherandasanghita, 6.11; Sammohanatantra, Part 2, ch. 2 p. 2). The triangle is in the nature of Brahma, Wishnu and Shiwa (—Tararahasya, ch. 4, p. 29).

It has been stated: 'Inside that triangle is the region of the jewelled altar (manipithamandala); the whitish-red lustre of the gems in the altar, seems to challenge the brilliance of the bluish-yellow (pingala) lightning flash; nada-bindu as an aspect of the altar is connected with Supreme Consciousness embodied as Wagbhawa-bija (chinmaya wapu) (—Padukapañchaka, Verse 3).

The jewelled altar shines so brightly that it appears more splendorous than the brilliance of a lightning flash. The compound word nadabindumanipithamandala may be interpreted as manipithamandala with nada and bindu; or nada and bindu and manipithamandala; or manipithamandala in the form of nada and bindu. The commentator Kalicharana has rejected the third alternative because of the dissimilarity of their colours. He says that as nada is white and bindu is red, they can never be whitish-red which is the colour of the altar. But this is not a strong argument. The white and red when mixed together produce the patala (pale red) colour. He explains that nada is below, bindu is above, and the region of the jewelled altar is in between the two. He states that 'chinmaya wapu' is the body of nada, bindu and manipithamandala in the form of knowledge.

He does not accept that 'chinmaya wapu' stands for wagbhawa-bija because, as Guru is white, his bija is also white, and the attribute of whitish-red lustre to the bija does not fit.

But the words in this verse should be translated technically, as they indicate the modes of concentration to be practised. When concentration is done on Guru in form, he is thought of as white in colour and is on the jewelled altar of whitish-red lustre. But concentration is also done on the mantra-form of Guru. Chinmaya wapu means Chit or Supreme Consciousness embodied as Wagbhawa-bija, that is Aing which is the Guru-mantra. Nada-bindu is an aspect of the jewelled altar. The jewelled altar becomes absorbed in the nada-bindu of the bija Ai to form Guru-bija-mantra. In concentration on the mantra-form, the jewelled altar is not thought of, but only the bija Ai with nada-bindu, that is, Aing.

The manipitha (jewelled altar) has simply been called pitha (altar) which is with nada-bindu and is beautiful (—Gherandasanghita, 6.12). The manipitha has also been called bright singhasana (throne) in the Kankalamalinitantra, ch. 3, p. 7. There, it has been stated that splendorous Antaratman (Brahman) is in the thousand-petalled lotus; in addition to it, there is (within the twelve-petalled lotus which is the lower aspect of the sahasrara) the bright throne between nada and bindu on which Guru is seated, who is to be contemplated on. On, and in connection with, nada is a lustrous position to be thought of as the jewelled altar or bright throne in gross form of concentration, above which is bindu.

Above it is hangsah-pitha (seat). It has been stated: 'Above it, there is the primordial Hangsah who is the centre of splendour, growing like a flame, and who manifests himself as the destroyer of the universe by his great power of destruction; I do concentration on him' (—Padukapanchaka, Verse 4). Above it means above the space which is above nada, that is, manipitha. Above manipitha is bindu, and within the bindu is Hangsah. So, the bindu is the hangsah-seat. Hangsah is Shiwa and Shakti. Hangsah is splendorous. This means that Shiwa is in union with Kundalini. Hangsah is the destroyer of the universe, that is, the aroused Kundalini exhibits

her great power of absorption, being in Shiwa, by which all cosmic principles are absorbed into her. Hangsah represents a pair: Hang is Shiwa and Sah is Power as Kundalini.

It has been stated that concentration should be done on Guru in Hangsah (—Kularnawa, ch. 4, p. 22; Nilatantra, ch. 1, p. 1); also, concentration is done on Guru in hangsah-seat (—Shyamarahasya, ch. 1, p. 3). Hangsah is above the altar (—Gherandasanghita, 6.12), that is in bindu, which is above the jewelled altar. So, bindu is Hangsah, that is, Kundalini united with Shiwa. And from a mantra viewpoint, Hangsah is in the bindu of the Guru-bija-mantra Aing.

It has been stated: 'There, that is, in the Hangsah-seat, are the lotus-feet of Guru from which the saffron-like red-coloured and honey-imbibed nectar flows, and which are cool like nectar of the moon (or the rays of the moon) and the place of all good; my mind contemplates them' (—Padukapanchaka, Verse 5).

Guru's feet are actually the source from which the streams of life-substance of red colour containing the essence of vitality (makaranda) constantly flow; and concentration on that causes revivification of the mind and revitalization of the body.

'The lotus-feet of Guru are in the hangsah-seat, as it has been stated that the footstools (paduka) of Guru are in Hangsah' (—Gherandasanghita, 6.12). 'Where the footstool is, there is Guru, and concentration on Guru should be done there' (—ibid., 6.13). The footstool is the spiritual symbol of Guru, indicating the presence of Guru.

It has been stated: 'I adore the lotus feet of Guru, situated in the lotus lying in contact with the head; the lotus feet are on the jewelled footstools and all unspirituality disappears when one comes in contact with them; they are red like young leaves; their nails are as bright as the moon; they are moistened with nectar and as beautiful as the lotuses in the lake' (—Padukapanchaka, Verse 6).

Guru's lotus feet are on the jewelled footstool. This jewelled footstool is not the jewelled altar situated above nada and below bindu. The footstool is on the Hangsah-seat and the

Hangsah-seat is in bindu. Guru's feet are always on the bright footstools in Hangsah, and, in fact, they indicate that Guru, in form, is lying in Hangsah, where concentration should be done.

The following are the concentration-forms of Guru.

1 Guru is moon-like white with smiling face and bright eyes and his body has odour of purity; he wears the garment of flowers, holds a lotus in his hand and makes gestures of granting boons and of dispelling fear; he is all dewatas (—Nilatantra, ch. 1, p. 1).

2 Guru is like a mountain of silver, that is, white and motionless; he is seated in wirasana (hero posture), adorned with all ornaments, wearing a white garland and dressed in white raiment; he makes the gestures of granting boons and of dispelling fear; his Power (as Divine Mother) is seated on his left thigh, holds with her right hand the divine body of Guru, and with her left hand a blue lotus, and is adorned with red-coloured ornaments; Guru's look is kind, and he is with knowledge and in bliss (—Kankalamalinitantra, ch. 3, p. 7).

3 Guru is like a mountain of silver (white and motionless), he is with his Power who has a divine face and is self-luminous (—Nirwana-tantra, ch. 10, p. 13).

4 Guru, who is Shiwa, is moon-white, holding in his hand a lotus, and making the gestures of granting boons and of dispelling fear; he wears a fragrant garland of white flowers; his face is smiling and his eyes are bright; he is all dewatas (—Kularnawa, ch. 4, p. 22).

5 Guru is splendorous like the autumnal moon, that is, shining white in colour, with lotus-eyes, moon-like beautiful and smiling face, he wears a garland of divine flowers and is dressed in divine raiment, and his body is anointed with a fragrant substance of divine character; on his left side is his beautiful Power of deep red colour; he holds in his hand a lotus and his hands are in the gestures of granting boons and dispelling fear (—Guptasadhana-tantra, ch. 2, p. 2).

6 Guru is like pure crystal (in colour), adorned with white-coloured ornaments, wearing a garland of white flowers, seated in padma-sana (lotus posture), and established in yoga; he is two-eyed, calm (in samadhi) and very kind; his hands are in wara (granting boons) and abhaya (dispelling fear) mudras; his Power, who is red in colour, is seated on his left thigh and holds his body with her right hand while holding a blue lotus with her left hand; his eyes are red and his face smiling; he is all bliss and, as God (Ishwara), he should be very respectfully saluted (—Gandharwatantra, ch. 5, p. 23).

7 Guru is like pure crystal (in colour), anointed with a fragrant substance, calm and smiling; he makes the gestures of granting boons and dispelling fear and his look is very kind; he is with his Power, who is seated on his left thigh, adorned with white coloured ornaments; he is in full bliss (—Shaktakrama, ch. 1, p. 1).

8 Guru is white in colour, adorned with various ornaments, three-eyed, and seated in swastikasana (auspicious posture); he is glad to see the lotus-face with ruddy lips of his Power of red colour by his left side (—Tararahasya, ch. 1, pp. 1–2).

9 Guru is white-coloured, two-armed, calm and has a pleased countenance (—Sammohana-tantra, Part 2, ch. 4, p. 4).

10 Guru is like ten thousand moons, that is, intensely shining white in colour; his hands show the gestures of granting boons and dispelling fear; he is dressed in white raiment, wears a garland of white flowers, and his body is anointed with white sandal paste; he is with his Power, who is red, seated on his left thigh; he is divine, imperishable; he is Shiwa and Supreme Guru (—Shaktanandatarangini, 4.2).

11 Guru is like pure crystal (in colour), dressed in silken cloth; smeared with a fragrant substance and adorned with white-coloured ornaments; he is calm and smiling and his look is kind; he makes the gestures of granting boons and dispelling fear and holds a lotus; he is with his Power, who is red in colour and is seated on his left thigh; she holds his beautiful body with her right hand and a blue lotus with her left hand and all this makes a lovely picture; Guru's lotus-eyes are full of supreme bliss (—Shyamarahasya, 1.10).

12 Guru is two-eyed, two-armed, and dressed with white raiment; he wears a garland of white

flowers and his body is anointed with the white sandal paste; one of his hands shows wara-mudra (the gesture of granting boons), and the other makes abhaya-mudra (the gesture of dispelling fear); he is calm and very kind; his Power (Shakti) embraces him (by her right arm, lying on his left side) and holds with her left hand a blue lotus; he is gracious-looking and smiling and grants the desires of his worshippers (—Mahanirwanatantra, 5.26–28).

13 Guru is divine, three-eyed, two-armed, and dressed in white raiment; he wears a garland of white flowers and his body is anointed with the white sandal paste; he is with his Power, who is red in colour (—Gherandasanghita, 6.13–14).

14 Guru is like pure crystal (in colour) and two-eyed; he makes the gestures of granting boons and dispelling fear; he is Shiwa and very beautiful (—Shiwapurana, 3.3.64).

15 Guru holds in his hand a book (wyakhya-mudra; it can also be translated as: Guru holds a book and makes the gesture of granting boons); he is delighted, smiling, tranquil, contented and kind; he is Brahman (—Brahmawaiwartapurana, 1. 26. 6–7).

From the above descriptions, the form of Guru for concentration is as follows:

1 Guru is either moon-white or like pure crystal in colour.
2 He has two eyes. He may also be thought of as three-eyed. His eyes are bright.
3 He has two arms. He makes the gestures of granting boons and dispelling fear; or holding a book in one of his hands, and showing wara mudra (granting boons) with the other hand.
4 His face is lustrous, calm, contented, delighted, kind and smiling.
5 He is dressed in white raiment; he wears a garland of fragrant white flowers, and is adorned with ornaments of white colour; his body is smeared with the white sandal paste.
6 Guru assumes padmasana (lotus posture), swastikasana (auspicious posture), or wirasana (hero posture).
7 His Shakti (Power) is seated on his left thigh, holds his body with her right hand

and a blue lotus with her left hand. The Power is red in colour and has a face as beautiful as a lotus.

Explanation

The twelve-petalled lotus is a great centre of concentration. Here, dhyana is perfected and developed to its highest level, and transformed in sahasrara into samprajñata samadhi. Two main forms of dhyana are practised here: first, dhyana on form; and finally, dhyana on luminosity. Dhyana on Guru is the concentration on form, and dhyana on Kundalini is the concentration on luminosity.

From the mantra viewpoint, Guru is derived from the matrika-letters Gang, Ung, Rang and Ung. Gang exhibits attributes and is also beyond attributes; it contains five dewas and powers, and five prana-wayus; there is Kundali in it; it is like the morning sun (vermilion) in colour. Ung contains five dewas and five prana-wayus; Kundalini lies in it; it is yellow in colour. Rang contains five dewas, five prana-wayus, three Powers; in it lies Kundali; it is like red-lightning (shining red in colour). So, the basic power of Guru is Kundalini and there are five Shiwas and Powers in a latent form in him.

The ga-aspect is the highest spiritual knowledge arising from samadhi. It has been stated that Guru removes darkness arising from unspirituality, designated by 'gu', by control, designated by 'ru' (—Dwayopanishad, Mantra 4). But the meanings of 'gu' and 'ru' as stated here are secondary. In the Yamala, it has been stated that 'gu' means which gives success, and 'ra' is what burns impurities, and 'u' is Shiwa, so Guru is in the nature of these three (—Shaktanandatarangini, 2.8). This is also the secondary meaning.

The U-aspect is Shiwa. So it has been stated that Guru is Shiwa (—Kularnawa, ch. 4, p. 22; Purashcharanarasollasa, ch. 8, p. 8; Shaktanandatarangini, 4.2; 4.5; Shiwapurana, 3.3.64); Guru is Brahman (—Gandharwatantra, ch. 5, p. 24; Tararahasya, ch. 1, p. 2; Brahmawaiwartapurana, 1.26.7). But Shiwa or Brahman has two aspects; as Supreme Consciousness without the limitation of mind, and as Power-Consciousness manifesting mind in the form of samadhi-consciousness. Supreme Consciousness is full, infinite and static in which Supreme Power remains in Shiwa as Shiwa. Here, Shiwa is Parama Shiwa, Brahman is without attributes. At this stage, Shiwa-consciousness is not limited by the mind, so it is non-mental, and supreme and infinite. This is the asamprajñata-samadhi-consciousness. This aspect is in Guru in latent form. The aspect which becomes manifest in Guru is Power-Consciousness appearing in form. In this aspect, Guru is Ishwara (—Gandharwa-tantra, ch. 5, p. 23), that is, he is endowed with omnipotency and omnisciency. He is divine (dewa) (—Gherandasanghita, 6.13). He assumes a mental form (—Purashcharanarasollasa, ch. 9, p. 9), that is, Parama Shiwa appears in subtle form as Guru in dhyana. Consciousness in dhyana is in the form of Shiwa when concentration is done on Guru.

Guru as Shiwa is beyond the six Shiwas—Brahma, Wishnu, Rudra, Isha, Sadashiwa and Parashiwa, and, therefore, he is the seventh Shiwa who is Parama Shiwa, appearing in form. So, Guru is Parama Shiwa in form. Guru is with his Shakti (Power). But his Power is beyond the six Powers lying with six Shiwas. In Parama Shiwa, Supreme Power becomes one and the same with Shiwa. In Guru, the Power is manifested. Guru and his Power are the replica of Shiwa-Shakti principle. His Shakti is Kundalini in form. The ra-aspect of Guru is Shakti and the u-aspect indicates her union with Shiwa. So, in concentration-form she is seated on Guru's left thigh and in embrace. It has been stated that Guru's Power is called unmani (—Purashcharanarasollasa, ch. 9, p. 9). Unmani is that power by which consciousness becomes free from all objects, and is established in Shiwa-form. This is the highest state of samprajñata samadhi. This power arises from Kundalini, and Kundalini in form is Guru's Power.

When dhyana on Guru develops to its highest point, one is able to go beyond form and dhyana is transformed into a luminous type. This means that now it is possible to make dhyana directly and without thought, on the splendour of Kundalini. Now, the form aspects of Guru and his Power are absorbed into Kundalini and she appears as splendorous. On the accomplishment of dhyana-on-splendour, the practitioner is able to pass into the sahasrara proper and attains samprajñata samadhi in which his whole consciousness becomes splendorous Kundalini.

Concentration on Guru consists of the following stages.

1 Thought-concentration on: the white twelve-petalled lotus on which is twelve-lettered Guru-mantra of white colour; the pericarp of the lotus is moon-white.

2 Thought-concentration on: the a-ka-tha triangle, red in colour, situated within the pericarp, with its apex downward, and with all letters which are on the three lines—starting from the left line, then the base line and finally the right line, and the letters ha, la, ksha in the corners.

3 Thought-concentration on: nada of white colour, situated above the triangle; above nada is the jewelled altar of very bright whitish-red colour; and above it is bindu of red colour.

4 Thought-concentration on: Guru-bija mantra Aing of white colour, lying within the triangle.

5 Thought-concentration on: luminous Hangsah, lying within the bindu of the bija-mantra Aing. Note. Hangsah is Shiwa in union with Kundalini, and by deep concentration Shiwa-Kundalini should be aroused as Guru and his Shakti in form.

6 Thought-concentration: within the pericarp of moon-white colour of the white twelve-petalled lotus is the red triangle and above it is white nada, and above that is the shining whitish-red jewelled altar, and above the altar is red bindu, and within bindu is Guru of moon-like white with his Shakti of red colour. From the Guru's feet the saffron-like red life-substance is continuously being irradiated. Above the head of Guru, there is the down-faced white thousand-petalled lotus, covering him like an umbrella.

7 Dhyana on Guru and his Shakti in form.

8 Dhyana on splendorous Kundalini.

Now we come to the sahasrara proper.

13 Sahasrara

The sahasrara is the last chakra in the chakra system. It is the thirteenth chakra, numerically from the muladhara. The sahasrara and its lower part, guru chakra, are not situated within the chitrini nadi, as this nadi ends intracranially, and the sahasrara, including guru chakra, lies in the void region, where there are no nadis.

Terminology

1 Sahasrara (Thousand-petalled), mentioned in the Adwayatarakopanishad, Mantra 13; Mandalabrahmanopanishad, 1.41; Goutamiyatantra, 35.54; Todalatantra, ch. 3, p. 4; ch. 8, p. 16; ch. 9, p. 17; Gayatritantra, 2.3; Matrikabhedatantra, ch. 2, p. 2; ch. 3, p. 3; ch. 7, p. 10; Gandharwatantra, ch. 5, p. 24; Kamadhenutantra, ch. 17, p. 23; Shaktakrama, ch. 1, p. 1; Kubjikatantra, 5.263; Tararahasya, ch. 4, p. 23; Bhutashuddhitantra, ch. 2, p. 2; ch. 3, p. 3; ch. 10, p. 9; ch. 14, p. 12; ch. 15, p. 13; Mayatantra, ch. 6, p. 5; Purashcharanarasollasa, ch. 2, p. 2; ch. 8, p. 8; ch. 10, p. 11; Wishwasaratantra, ch. 2, pp. 11, 23; Mundamalatantra, ch. 2, p. 5; Koulawalitantra, ch. 3, p. 7; Shaktanandatarangini, 4.1; 4.16; 4.21; 4.34; Shyamarahasya, ch. 1, p. 3; Rudrayamala, Part 2, 22.16; 60.32; Mahanirwanatantra, 5. 143; Purashcharyarnawa, ch. 6, p. 491; Shadamnayatantra, 3.75; 4.54, 73, 140, 141; 5.99, 103, 243, 389; Shiwasanghita, 5.138, 161, 163; Mridanitantra, quoted in Amarasanggraha MS; Shiwapurana, 3.3.63; 3.5.53; Dewibhagawata, 7.35.47; Kankalamalinitantra, ch. 2, p. 5.

(a) Sahasrara Padma (Thousand-petalled lotus), mentioned in the Shaktakrama, ch. 1, p. 1; Tripurasarasamuchchaya, 5.41; Bhutashuddhitantra, ch. 3, p. 3; Sammohanatantra, Part 2, ch. 4, p. 4; Koulawalitantra, ch. 22, p. 81; Shaktanandatarangini, 4.25; Mahanirwanatantra, 5.86; Shiwasanghita, 5.190.

(b) Sahasrara Mahapadma (the great thousand-petalled lotus), mentioned in the

Todalatantra, ch. 2, p. 2; ch. 6, p. 12; ch. 7, p. 14; ch. 9, p. 17; Kankalamalinitantra, ch. 2, p. 5; Nirwanatantra, ch. 3, p. 5; Guptasadhanatantra, ch. 2, p. 2; Shaktakrama, ch. 1, p. 1; Tararahasya, ch. 1, p. 2; Mayatantra, ch. 6, p. 5; Purashcharanarasollasa, ch. 2, p. 2; ch. 8, p. 8; ch. 9, p. 9; Wishwasaratantra, ch.1, p.10; Shaktanandatarangini, 4.15; Purashcharyarnawa, ch. 6, p. 490; Gherandasanghita, 6.9.

(c) Sahasrara Ambuja (thousand-petalled lotus), mentioned in the Gandharwatantra, ch. 5, p. 28; Rudrayamala, Part 2, 27.70; Mridanitantra, quoted in Amarasanggraha MS.

(d) Sahasrara Saroruha (thousand-petalled lotus), mentioned in the Shaktanandatarangini, 4.29; Shiwasanghita, 5.188, 198.

2 Sahasraradala (thousand-petalled), mentioned in the Kubjikatantra, 5.265; 6.312.

3 Sahasradala (with or without Padma, Pankaja, Kamala) (lotus with one thousand petals), mentioned in the Yogachudamanyupanishad, Mantra 6; Nilatantra, ch. 1, p. 1; Kamadhenutantra, ch. 15, p. 19; Kankalamalinitantra, ch. 3, p. 7; Nirwanatantra, ch. 10, pp. 12,14; Radhatantra, 5.11; 6.7; 11.9,23; 14.1; Gandharwatantra, ch. 29, p. 112; Kubjikatantra, 6.314; Tararahasya, ch. 1, p. 1; Bhutashuddhitantra, ch. 1, p. 1; ch. 3, p. 3; Wishwasaratantra, ch. 2, p. 11; Koulawalitantra, ch. 3, p. 7; Shaktanandatarangini, 4.24, 29,31; 9.16; Shyamarahasya, ch. 1, pp. 3,15; ch. 4, p. 79; Brahmasiddhantapaddhati MS; Amarasanggraha MS; Tattwayogabindu MS; Padmapurana, 5.38,73; Brahmawaiwartapurana, 4.21, 174; Dewibhagawata, 9.42.8; Kularnawa, ch. 4, p. 22.

4 Sahasrara Kamala, Pankaja, or Padma (lotus with a thousand petals), mentioned in the Yogakundalyupanishad, 1.86; Brahmawaiwartapurana, 1.26.5.

5 Sahasrachchada Pankaja (thousand-petalled lotus), mentioned in the Sammohanatantra, Part 2, ch. 2, p. 2.

6 Sahasrabja (thousand-petalled lotus), mentioned in the Mundamalatantra, ch. 2, p. 5; ch. 6, p. 9.

7 Sahasrapatra (with or without Kamala) (thousand-petalled lotus), mentioned in the

Purashcharyarnawa, ch. 6, p. 492; Skandapurana, 7.1.31; Mahabharata, 12.331.21.

8 Sahasraparna Padma (thousand-petalled lotus), mentioned in the Padmapurana, 1.39.153; Matsyapurana, 168.15.

9 Sahasradala Adhomukha Padma (thousand-petalled, face-down lotus), mentioned in the Purashcharanarasollasa, ch. 10, p. 11.

10 Adhomukha Mahapadma (the great face-down lotus), mentioned in the Purashcharanarasollasa, ch. 9, p. 9.

11 Sthana (literally, a place; here sahasrara), mentioned in the Yogakundalyupanishad, 1.74.

12 Kapalasamputa (a hemispherical covering over the skull, that is, technically, sahasrara), mentioned in the Yogashikhopanishad, 1.76.

13 Wyomambuja (lotus in void), mentioned in the Yogashikhopanishad, 6.48.

14 Wyomambhoja (lotus in void; void lotus), mentioned in the Tripurasarasamuchchaya, 4.12.

15 Wyoma (with or without chakra and sthala), mentioned in the Yogarajopanishad, Mantra 17; Phetkarinitantra, ch. 14, p. 39; Gandharwatantra, ch. 29, p. 112.

16 Akasha Chakra (chakra in void; void chakra), mentioned in the Soubhagyalakshmyupanishad, 3.9.

17 Shiras Padma (lotus in contact with the head; topmost lotus; highest lotus), mentioned in the Brihannilatantra, ch. 6, p. 31.

18 Amlana Padma, or Pankaja (fresh or bright lotus), mentioned in the Purashcharanarasollasa, ch. 9, p. 9.

19 Dashashatadala Padma (lotus with one-thousand petals; thousand-petalled lotus), mentioned in the Shatchakranirupana, Verse 40.

20 Shuddha Padma (pure, or white lotus), mentioned in the Shatchakranirupana, Verse 52.

21 Shantyatita (Sahasrara), mentioned in the Shiwapurana, 3.3.29; Garudapurana, 1.23.48.

22 Shantyatita Pada (Sahasrara Chakra), mentioned in the Shiwapurana, 5a. 7.3.

23 Parama Shiras (supracranial chakra), mentioned in the Bhagawata, 10.87.18.

Position

The sahasrara lies in the void-region where there are no nadis; it is outside the cranium, but in contact with the top-end of the chitrini nadi, lying intracranially, through wisarga (power-bridge). At the terminal part of the chitrini is the nirwana chakra, which is connected through the wisarga, indirectly with the twelve-petalled lotus, which is the lower aspect of the sahasrara.

Description

The sahasrara has 1000 petals (—Shatchakranirupana, Verse 40; Yogachudamanyupanishad, Mantra 6; Nilatantra, ch. 1, p. 1; Kamadhenutantra, ch. 15, p. 19; Kankalamalinitantra, ch. 3, p. 7; Nirwanatantra, ch. 10, p. 12; Kularnawa, ch. 4, p. 22; Kubjikatantra, 6.314; Bhutashuddhitantra, ch. 3, p. 3; Sammohanatantra, Part 2, ch. 2, p. 2; Purashcharanarasollasa, ch. 8, p. 8; Shaktanandatarangini, 4.29; Shyamarahasya, ch. 1, p. 3); this is why it is called sahasrara, sahasraradala, sahasradala, sahasra kamala, sahasrabja, sahasrapatra and sahasraparna.

The colour of the petals is white (—Shatchakranirupana, Verse 40; Kankalamalinitantra, ch. 2, p. 5; Kubjikatantra, 6. 314; Sammohanatantra, Part 2, ch. 2, p. 2; Shaktanandatarangini, 4.29; Shyamarahasya, ch. 1, p. 3; Mridanitantra, quoted in Amarasanggraha MS; Shiwapurana, 3.3.63); red (—Shaktanandatarangini, 4.25); yellow (—Shiwapurana, 4.40.26) and golden (—Tripurasarasamuchchaya, quoted in Yogakalpalatika MS). The petals are also variegated— white, red, yellow, black and green; now they appear as white, then red, then yellow, again white, then green (—Nirwanatantra, ch. 10, p. 12); also, the petals are white, red, yellow, black and green; now it is white, then black, yellow, red and green; in this manner, the petals acquire different colours (—Purashcharanarasollasa, ch. 9, p. 9).

The petals of the sahasrara are the seat of all powers (—Kubjikatantra, 6.315; Nirwanatantra, ch. 10, p. 12; Purashcharanarasollasa, ch. 9, p. 9), all mantras (—Kubjikatantra, 6.315), and the matrika-letters (—Shaktanandatarangini, 4.29). There are 50 matrika-letters on the petals (—Mridanitantra, quoted in Amarasanggraha MS). The Shatchakranirupana names the matrika-letters which are on the petals. There are two readings of the text. In one, the text reads as 'lakaradyairwarnaih', that is, the letters beginning with la. The la is the second la pronounced rha or da. In this connection Kalicharana says that here it is not meant that the letters are to be read from the end to the beginning (wiloma), but the meaning is to take la, and leave ksha out. The letter-arrangement has been more clearly stated in the Kankala-malinitantra, ch. 2, p. 5. It says that on the petals of the sahasrara are the letters from a to what is the end of ksha (akaradi kshakarantaih). Kali-charana interprets anta (after kshakara) as awa-sana, that is, termination. At the end of ksha is la, so the la is to be taken by leaving ksha out. This is the opinion of Kalicharana. That the arrangement of the letters on the petals should be from the beginning to the end, not the reverse, and from a to la by leaving ksha out has been stated in the Todalatantra, ch. 9, p. 17. It has been declared there that Kundali, being in the sahasrara and seeing Shiwa there, encircles Shiwa-linga in the form of a garland consisting of matrika-letters from a to la (akaradilakaranta) in which ksha is in the mouth, that is, ksha becomes the central letter (meru). This garland of matrika-letters is called panchashika mala (a garland of fifty letters). The string of this garland is Shakti-Shiwa. The matrika-letters strung in the garland are fifty from a to la, and ksha becomes the central letter, and is not counted. The japa is made from a to la (anuloma) and also from la to a (wiloma). However, the arrangement of letters on the petals is from a to la, and without ksha.

The text of the Shatchakranirupana (Verse 40) can be read as 'lalatadyairwarnaih', literally, all letters from lalata. The usual meaning of lalata is the forehead. But it does not apply here. Technically, lalata indicates the letters a, tha and ha (—Warnabijakosha). Here lalata stands for a, so the meaning is, letters from a. The commentator Shankara explains it as fifty letters from a placed in twenty layers. The commentator Wishwanatha says 'all the matrika-letters from a'. Ramawallabha only says 'letters from a'. Bhuwanamohana makes it clearer by saying, from the beginning of a to the end of

ksha (akaradi kshakaranta). Kalicharana makes it still clearer. He says that it is to be understood as meaning that the fifty letters from a to ksha are to be taken by leaving out la.

The petals are arranged in twenty layers, each layer containing fifty petals. In each layer, there are fifty matrika-letters on the fifty petals. So the matrika-letters from a to la (rha) or ksha go round each layer; and each matrika-letter is on one petal. The matrika-letters are arranged on the petals from right to left. The colour of the matrika-letters has not been mentioned in the text. Kalicharana says that as the matrika-letters are white, they should be thought of as white here (on the sahasrara-petals). (See Plate 24.) But the normal colours of the matrika-letters are different; some are white, some yellow, while others are red, smoke-coloured, etc. In the Kankalamalinitantra (ch. 2, p. 5), it has been stated that the matrika-letters are shining. It may mean white, or red, or any colour. However, when the petals are thought to be white, the letters may be taken to be white. When the petals are thought of as having other colours, the letters can be thought of as having the colour of the petals or their normal colours.

The sahasrara stands with its face downward (—Shatchakranirupana, Verse 40; Kankala-malinitantra, ch. 2, p. 5; Nirwanatantra, ch. 10, p. 12; Tararahasya, ch. 4, p. 23; Tripura-sarasamuchchaya, 5.41; Purashcharanarasollasa, ch. 8, p. 8; Koulawalitantra, ch. 22, p. 81; Shaktanandatarangini, 4.29; Shyamarahasya, ch. 1, p. 3; Purashcharyarnawa, ch. 6, p. 490; Brahmasiddhantapaddhati MS), and its fila-ments are red in colour (—Shatchakranirupana, Verse 40; Tripurasarasamuchchaya, 5.41; Sam-mohanatantra, Part 2, ch. 2, p. 2; Shaktan-andatarangini, 4.29; Purashcharyarnawa, ch. 6, 490), and they are also lightning-like splendorous (—Purashcharanarasollasa, ch. 9, p. 9). The arrangement of the petals is such that the sahasrara appears as bell-shaped. (See Plate 25.) The pericarp of the sahasrara is of a golden colour (—Kubjikatantra, 6. 316; Purashcharanarasol-lasa, ch. 9, p. 9), and is endowed with various powers, and within in it lies all knowledge (—Purashcharanarasollasa, ch. 8, p. 8). Here are

267

the seats of Supreme Being (—Bhutashuddhi-tantra, ch. 14, p. 12); Shadamnayatantra, 5.103) and Supreme Power (—Bhutashuddhitantra, ch. 10, p. 9; Shadamnayatantra, 5.243); it is the centre of immortality (—Shadamnayatantra 5. 389). Now we have to study the pericarp in detail.

The Shatchakranirupana says: 'Within the pericarp of the sahasrara is the full moon (that is, the circular moon-region) which is shining brilliantly and without the spots. It radiates abundant light which is nectarous (that is, full of life) and delightful. Inside the circular moon region is the lightning-like luminous triangle (trikona). Inside this triangle is void (shunya) (that is, Supreme Bindu) which lies concealed (that is, realizable only by dhyana) and is worshipped by the yogis' (—Shatchakranirupana, Verse 41).

The presence of the circular region of the moon (chandramandala) in the pericarp of the sahasrara has been mentioned in the Kankala-malinitantra, ch. 2, p. 5; Sammohanatantra, Part 2, ch. 2, p. 2; Mayatantra, ch. 6, p. 5; Purashcaranarasollasa, ch. 2, p. 2; Shyam-arahasya, ch. 1, p. 15; ch. 4, p. 79). Rays are being emitted from the moon-region (—Tripura-sarasamuchchaya, 5.41; Koulawalitantra, ch. 22, p. 81). The moon-region is in the nature of consciousness (—Shiwapurana, 3.5.53). There is a triangle within the moon-region (—Kan-kalamalinitantra, ch. 2, p. 5; Shyamarahasya, ch. 1, p. 15; Amarasanggraha MS; Mridani-tantra, quoted in Amarasanggraha MS; Tattwa-yogabindu MS). This triangle has also been termed trikuta, that is, three-cornered = triangle (—Soubhagyalakshmyupanishad, 3.9; Brahma-siddhantapaddhati MS).

There is the void (shunya) within the triangle which lies inside the circular moon-region. The void has been termed supreme void (para-shunya), which is with the upward-power (Kun-dalini), and dhyana should be done here (—Soubhagyalakshmyupanishad, 3.9). Supreme Power as Kundalini lies concealed here (—Yoga-rajopanishad, Mantra 18). The roused Kundali passes into the sahasrara through the brahma nadi (—Todalatantra, ch. 8, p. 16), so she is called the upward power. She is concealed here,

she is only known by dhyana. The term supreme void has also been accepted in the Tantras. It has been stated that the supreme void (parama-shunya) which is inside the triangle of the sahasrara is with the upward-power (Kundalini), and dhyana should be done on the supreme void (—Brahmasiddhantapaddhati MS). The presence of the void in the triangle of the sahasrara has been mentioned in the Mridani-tantra (quoted in the Amarasanggraha MS). The void has been described as the abode of Parama Shiwa who is infinite and beyond mind-matter (niramaya) (—ibid.). About the void, it has been stated: 'That (that is, void), which is well concealed (in another reading: which is to be kept secret with care) is the main root of abundant and never-ending supreme bliss; it is subtle and its pure form becomes manifest along with nirwana-kala and moon (shashi)-kala, that is, ama-kala, by the long and regular practice of dhyana' (—Shatchakraniru-pana, Verse 42).

In this void is Parama Shiwa. So, it has been stated: 'Here, that is, in the void, the celebrated Dewa (Divine Being) known as Parama Shiwa is situated. He is without form (in another read-ing: he is in his supreme aspect as infinite and formless); he is in union (rasa) (with Kundalini) and is also the one and the same (wirasa) (with Kundalini); like the sun, he destroys the darkness of unspiritualness and delusion' (—Shatchakra-nirupana, Verse 42).

The void is a circular process (writta) consist-ing of Kundali-power around the formless Parama Shiwa. The void has been clearly explained here: Shiwa is in the form of Void and the circumference of the circle (writta) is Supreme Kundali who is splendorous and is in three and a half coils; the Yamala says that the writta is Kundalini Power in whom lies the three primary attributes, and the void aspect (of the writta) is Shiwa, who is the great Ishwara; Kundalini is always there in coils around Shiwa like a snake; Bindu (Supreme Bindu) is in the nature of Shiwa and Shakti (Power) and gives life and liberation; that eternal Divine Power (Kundalini) is the source of all in her Nada (Supreme Nada) aspect (—Shaktanandatarangini, 4.15).

This void (shunya) cannot be represented by

the bijas Ang, Ang, Khang, Thang and Hang. Hang is the germ-mantra of akasha (void) mahabhuta, so this void is beyond akasha. In this void, there is neither akasha nor mind. So it has been termed supreme void (paramashunya). It can only be designated by Bindu. But this bindu is not a point. It is 'non-magnitudinous' and 'non-positional', and still it exists. Because of this it has been termed Parabindu— Supreme Bindu. This Supreme Bindu is the Supreme Void. It has been stated that Bindu signifies void (Shunya) and also quality (guna) (—Todalatantra, ch. 6, p. 13). The void indicates the absence of magnitude and position; therefore, it is without mind and matter. The void is that in which matter-mind and its source primus are absorbed, and what remains is Shiwa in union with his Power (Shakti). Kundalipower finally absorbs into her prakriti (primus) from which arises the phenomenon of mind-matter, and remains in coils in Shiwa. Because of Shiwa and Power (Shakti) the void is in the nature of a writta or circle. The void aspect is Shiwa and the quality aspect indicated by the circumference of the circle is the Power. So it has been said that Parama Shiwa is immutable and supremely subtle and in the form of Bindu (—Todalatantra, ch. 8, p. 15). The subtle and changeless aspect of Bindu is the void which is Shiwa. Shiwa is also with his Power. This Power is in a state of Supreme contraction. This is Supreme Bindu. So Supreme Bindu is both Shiwa and his Power.

Bindu stands in relation to the sahasrara (Goutamiyatantra, 34.54; Dewibhagawata, 7. 35.47). So it has been said that the sahasrara is the centre of Bindu (—Gandharwatantra, ch. 5, p. 28; Mridanitantra, quoted in Amarasanggraha MS). This Bindu is Parabindu. It has been clearly stated that the sahasrara lotus which is all pure is the centre of Parabindu (Supreme Bindu) (—Rudrayamala, Part 2, 27.70).

More has been stated about Parama Shiwa: Bhagawan, that is Shiwa endowed with yoga-power, from whom the nectar (power of eternal life) is continuously and abundantly flowing, imparts to the yogi whose thoughts are purified the real knowledge of Atman (the highest spiritual knowledge arising in samadhi); the Supreme Being (Sarwesha, literally, the Lord of the universe), known by the name of Parama Hangsah (that is, Parama Shiwa) from whom the waves of all happiness are continuously overflowing is situated here (—Shatchakranirupana, Verse 43).

Shaiwas (the worshippers of God Shiwa) call it (the centre where is Parama Shiwa) the abode of Shiwa; the Waishnawas (the worshippers of God Wishnu) call it the abode of Supreme Being (Paramapurusha, that is, Wishnu); others (the worshippers of Harihara) call it the centre of Harihara (a conjoined form of Wishnu and Shiwa); those who are devoted to the lotus feet of Divine Shakti (that is, the worshippers of the Goddess Shakti) call it the centre of Dewi (Shakti); and other great yogis call it the pure place of Prakriti-Purusha (—ibid., Verse 44).

It has been stated: 'Within the pericarp of the sahasrara, there is the nectarous ocean wherein lies the isle of gems, and inside the isle of gems is the wishing tree; there lies a lustrous temple with four doors; inside the temple is an altar consisting of fifty matrika-letters; there is a jewelled throne on the altar, and on the throne is seated Mahakali (Supreme Power) in union with Maharudra (Parama Shiwa). He who is Maharudra (Supreme Rudra or Shiwa) is Mahawishnu (Supreme Wishnu) and Mahabrahma (Supreme Brahma). The three are one, there is only the difference in name' (—Nirwanatantra, ch. 10, pp. 13–14, abridged). It indicates that Parama Shiwa (Supreme Consciousness) is also called Supreme Rudra, Supreme Wishnu and Supreme Brahma. The description of the centre as given here is for the purpose of dhyana.

Parama Shiwa is without form (—Shatchakranirupana, Verse 42); he is Brahman and immutable (—Tararahasya, ch. 4, p. 23); he is only 'being' (or he is in himself), fully quiescent and beyond mind-matter (—Bhutashuddhitantra, ch. 3, p. 3). This supreme aspect of Parama Shiwa is beyond samprajnata samadhi, it is only 'realizable' in asamprajnata samadhi. In a super-concentrated state of consciousness induced by samprajnata samadhi (—Wishwasaratantra, ch. 2, p. 11), a highly rarefied form in white colour (—Tararahasya, ch. 4, p. 23) shines forth. Now, the infinite Supreme Shiwa becomes Sakala Shiwa—Shiwa with manifested Power. Now, the individualization of Shiwa and Power occurs.

Shiwa is always with Power (Shakti). In the supreme state both Shiwa and Shakti are formless and there is no double existence as they are not individualized. So Shiwa and Shakti are in supreme union as one and the same. This is what has been called the state of wirasa. When Shiwa and Shakti are individualized, they are also in union, and this is the state of rasa. So it has been stated that Supreme Shiwa who also assumes a cosmic form and Supreme Kundalini are always in the great lotus sahasrara (—Todalatantra, ch. 7, p. 14); also, in the sahasrara, there is the union between Supreme Shiwa and Kundalini (—Bhutashuddhitantra, ch. 3, p. 3); Supreme Shiwa is with Supreme Kundalini (—ibid., ch. 14, p. 12); Supreme Shiwa is with Shakti (—Wishwasaratantra, ch. 2, p. 11). All these statements indicate that Supreme Shiwa as Sakala Shiwa assumes form in the sahasrara. At first the form is non-specific, vast and luminous. At this stage, the whole consciousness is in a luminous form and in deepest concentration. This is the state of samprajñata samadhi. When concentration becomes less deep, the luminosity changes into distinct form and it is held in consciousness continuously and without interruption. This is the state of dhyana. The dhyana form is transformed at the highest stage of concentration into samadhi form. Both Shiwa and Shakti appear in dhyana and samadhi forms.

A dhyana form of Shiwa in the sahasrara is as follows: 'Shiwa is like pure crystal in colour; he is joyful and smiling; he has three lotus-eyes and eight beautiful arms; he wears a garland of 1000 lotuses; he is adorned with ear-rings, a necklace of pearls, and handsome anklets' (—Bhutashuddhitantra, ch. 9, p. 8).

Ama-kala and nirwana-kala are situated within the triangle of the sahasrara. The Shatchakranirupana (Verse 46) says: 'Here (that is, within the triangle situated in the pericarp of the sahasrara) is the excellent sixteenth power (kala) of the moon (called ama) which is like the morning sun (that is, shining red in colour), pure (that is, samadhi-consciousness is maintained by her); her form is like the hundredth part of a delicate lotus-filament (that is, she is subtle); she is with Kundali-power (para); she is always lightning-like splendorous; she is with her face downward (that is, in one-half coil, crescent); there is the uninterrupted flow of perpetual bliss and she is the source of the abundantly flowing nectarous stream.'

Ama-kala is always in a roused state and not subject to growth or decay (that is, unchanging) (—Kankalamalinitantra, ch. 2, p. 5); she is red like the morning sun and is as subtle as the hundredth part of the tip of a hair (—Tripurasarasamuchchaya, 5.46); this sixteenth kala of the moon (ama-kala) stands with her face downward and is the centre of the constantly flowing nectarous stream (—Koulawalitantra, ch. 22, p. 81).

About nirwana-kala, it has been stated that: Inside it (ama-kala) is the famous nirwana-kala (manifested power of absorption of Kundalini); she is the most excellent; she is like the thousandth part of the end of a hair (that is, extremely subtle); she is endowed with supreme yoga-power (Bhagawati) and is in all beings as Ishtadewata; she is consciousness herself; she is bent like a crescent moon (that is, in one-half coil); and she is as lustrous as the brilliance of all suns shining at one time (that is, extremely shining red in colour) (—Shatchakranirupana, Verse 47).

Nirwana-kala is situated inside ama-kala; she is called the seventeenth kala (manifested power) and is crooked (—Kankalamalinitantra, ch. 2, p. 5); she is bent like a crescent moon (half-coiled) and as subtle as the thousandth part of the tip of a hair (—Tripurasarasamuchchaya, 5.47; Koulawalitantra, ch. 22, p. 81). Nirwana-kala is subtle and in the nature of consciousness (—Mridanitantra, quoted in Amarasanggraha MS). Nirwana-kala is also called the seventeenth nirañjana-kala which is as bright as the lustre of ten million suns and as cool as ten million moons (—Amarasanggraha MS; Tattwayogabindu MS).

There is Nirwana Shakti (all-absorbing Kundali-power) inside nirwana-kala. About Nirwana

Shakti, it has been stated that: inside it (nirwana-kala) is supreme and primordial Nirwana Shakti, splendorous like ten million suns (red and extremely lustrous), the mother of the universe; she is like the ten-millionth part of the end of a hair, and so, extremely subtle; in her is the constantly flowing stream of love (indicating that she is in union in supreme love with Parama Shiwa); she is the life of all beings; she graciously conveys the knowledge of Brahman to the mind of the yogi (—Shatchakranirupana, Verse 48).

The Tripurasarasamuchchaya (5.48) says: Nirwana Shakti is supreme and is situated within nirwana-kala; she is as bright as the radiance of ten million suns and as subtle as the ten millionth part of the end of a hair, so she is concealed; she is matrika, always conscious of Shiwa (nityodita) and pure; here lies the seat of Shiwa; it is here that the vast nectarous stream flows; she is without a support (that is, she is in herself).' Nirwana Shakti is red in colour (—Koulawalitantra, ch. 22, p. 81), very subtle and in the form of consciousness (—Mridanitantra, quoted in Amarasanggraha MS). It has been stated that there is nirodhika (the supreme control power) in the form of fire within nirwana-kala where sound is unmanifest, and there lies splendorous supreme Nirwana Shakti who is the source of the universe (as matrika) (—Kankalamalinitantra, ch. 2, p. 5).

The Shatchakranirupana (Verse 49) says: 'Within her (that is, Nirwana Shakti) is the centre where lies Shiwa (Shiwapada); it is beyond mind-matter (amala), eternal, all love and bliss, of pure consciousness; it is revealed in yoga (asamprajñata samadhi); some wise men call it the place of Wishnu, others call it Hangsah, while the spiritual persons call it the place where the real knowledge of Atman leading to liberation is attained.'

It has been stated: 'In Nirwana Shakti changeless and formless Shiwa (Parama Shiwa) is to be realized; it is here that Kundali-power is in the form of mudra (that is, in the form of ou-letter; or, in love-bliss because of her union with Shiwa) who again goes back to the adhara (muladhara) lotus' (—Kankalamalinitantra, ch. 2, pp. 5–6). There is also the centre in Nirwana Shakti of Shiwa; it is eternal, immeasur-

able, pure, ever-existing, and static; the wise men call it the abode of Wishnu, some call it the place of Brahman, others call it the abode of Hangsah, and others again call it the centre of Supreme Being (nirañjanapada) who is all (niralamba) (—Tripurasarasamuchchaya, 5.49, and Koulawalitantra, ch. 22, p. 81). It has been farther stated that the centre of Nirwana Shakti is above nirwana-kala; the worshippers of Shiwa call it the abode of Shiwa, the worshippers of Wishnu call it the abode of Supreme Purusha (Wishnu), others call it the abode of Hari-Hara, the worshippers of Dewi (Divine Power) call it the abode of Dewi, and the yogis call it the pure place of Prakriti and Purusha (—Shaktanandatarangini, 4.33).

It has been stated that there is a linga (Shiwa-linga) in the pericarp of the sahasrara which is like red-hot gold (that is, shining red in colour); but sometimes the linga becomes white, sometimes black, sometimes yellow and sometimes blue; sometimes the linga is in the form of matrika-letters; it is bright and beyond thought (—Mundamalatantra, ch. 2, p. 5). The presence of Shiwa-linga in the sahasrara has been mentioned in the Todalatantra, which says that Kundali, coming into the sahasrara and seeing Shiwa, encircles the Shiwa-linga in the form of a garland consisting of the matrika-letters (—Todalatantra, ch. 9, p. 17).

Above the circular region of the moon in the pericarp of the sahasrara is wisarga (power-bridge) (—Sammohanatantra, Part 2, ch. 2, p. 2). So it has been stated that the sahasrara is situated below the wisarga (—Shatchakranirupana, Verse 40; Tripurasarasamuchchaya, 5.41; Koulawalitantra, ch. 22, p. 81; Purashcharyarnawa, ch. 6, p. 490). Wisarga is Supreme Kundalini (—Radhatantra, 2.44). Wisarga is the sixteenth matrika-letter associated with a. A is the secondary part. Wisarga is like red-lightning (shining red in colour) in which lie in essence five pranas, five dewatas and all knowledge; it is Kundali (—Kamadhenutantra, 3.16). A (Ang) as the first matrika-letter is the coil of Kundali-power a part of which radiates upwards as a straight line indicating an upward direction of force-motion. The straight force-motion arises from the coiled force-motion and consists of a starting point and an end point, the two points being represented by two perpendicular dots. In the sahasrara, the first point lies just beyond ama-kala and the second point just below Supreme Bindu. So, the two points form a power-bridge through which Kundalini passes from the sahasrara to Supreme Bindu. Wisarga is power (—Tantrabhidhana), an aspect of Kundali-power.

Above wisarga (that is, above the second point of wisarga) is Divine Shankhini (—Kankalamali-nitantra, ch. 2, p. 5). Shankhini is Supreme Kundalini in the spiral form. From the view-point of sahasrara, Shankhini is above the circular moon-region where lies the first point of wisarga. Technically, the first point of wisarga lies just beyond amakala. The second bindu of wisarga lies under Supreme Bindu, and Shankhini is above it.

Above wisarga is dhruwa-mandala (—Sammohanatantra, Part 2, ch. 2, p. 2). Dhruwa-mandala is infinity of Parama Shiwa. Wisarga goes upward from ama-kala and passes through Wishnu-waktra and Guru-waktra to reach dhruwa-mandala. Shankhini as Supreme Kundalini goes beyond wisarga and reaches dhruwa-mandala to be united with Sakala Shiwa, and finally to be absorbed into Parama Shiwa.

Explanation

Aditya (God Shiwa) is Surya (Illumination); he is the possessor of light-power (rashmi), so he is called Harina; the light-power is in the nature of consciousness, so he is Jatawedas; he is the source of vital power (prana), so he is Parayana; he is without a second and splendorous (eka-jyotih); he is with 1000 light-powers (sahasra-rashmi) and exists in 100 forms; he is life in all beings and gives heat; he is in all forms (wishwa-rupa) (—Prashnopanishad, 1.8).

The secret of the sahasrara has been technically expounded by Rishi Pippalada in the above mantra. Aditya—the first God as Shiwa with his aroused Shakti (Power) technically known as Shiwa-Shakti principle, is from Aditi—the infinite Supreme Mother. He is the Sun as he is in the nature of illumination. He is endowed with the light-power having the aspects of illumination and consciousness. He is the one without a second, and splendorous. This indicates that he is with Supreme Kundalini who is all splendour. Shiwa is in spiritual union with the radiant Kundali-power so he is 'Sun'. Kundalini at the Supreme Bindu level is Shabdabrahman where lies parashabda—the principle of sound. At this stage, prana—the living-energy principle of the Supreme Mother in her power aspect—becomes concentrated to the highest point to be able to make parashabda manifest as radiant sound (pashyanti) which is Pranawa (Ong). There is a congregation of 1000 light-powers in pranawa, and there is a summation of 50 sound units which constitute matrika. At the next stage, the radiant sound begins to be transformed into suprasound (madhyama), and in this process 1000 petals are created by the 1000 light-powers which constitute the sahasrara; and the 50 matrika sounds are released from the pranawa sound and become distinct and are combined with the light-powers in twenty-fold strength. Each matrika sound has twenty aspects, viz., Kundali-power, three bindus, three gunas, three specific powers, five dewatas and five pranas, which make twenty. Because of this fact, the petals are arranged in twenty layers, each layer consisting of fifty petals which contain fifty matrika-letters.

The light-power is from Shiwa-Shakti. Shiwa is represented in white colour and Shakti in red colour. The colour of the light-power is a mixture of white and red which produces kamala colour which is pale-red. So the light-power is of kamala colour and its petaline expansion is called kamala (lotus) having 1000 petals. Another name of kamala is sahasrapatra (a thousand petals) (—Shabdakalpadrumah). 'ka' of kamala means Surya ('sun'), endowed with illuminating power; 'mala' of kamala indicates the expression of this power as rashmis—light-powers. So kamala is the thousand-fold manifestation of the illuminating power as light-powers in the form of petals. Also, 'ka' is illumination and is represented by the bija-mantra Wang (—Tantrabhidhana), and 'mala', derived from mrij, which means 'to sound' (—Apte). This indicates that the illuminating power in operation emits sounds. These sounds are the matrika sounds as suprasound phenomenon. The 1000 *rashmis* which are *kamala* and inseparably associated with *matrika* sounds form the *sahasrara*.

The particularized forms of *matrika* develop in the lower six *chakras* from the *ajña* to the *muladhara*. These six *chakras* have fifty petaline processes derived from the light-powers of the *sahasrara* in their specific manifestation. The fifty *matrika*-letters are arranged on the petals of these *chakras*. The fifty *matrika* sounds become 100 when combined with the evolutionary and involutionary modes of practice, that is, working on in both regular and reversed orders. God Surya exists in 100 forms. It has also been stated in the *Akshyupānishad* (Sec. 1) that God Surya ('Sun') is in the form of light (*jyotirupa*) and radiates 1000 light-powers (*sahasrarashmi*), and is in 100 forms. The splendorous *Kundali*-power makes Shiwa also splendorous and he becomes Surya. Kundalini in her *prana* aspect becomes Supreme Nada when *prana* is infused with potential sound-power, and then she becomes Supreme Bindu in which *prana*-power is supremely concentrated and ready to emit the potential *nada*, which is now the principle of sound, as radiant sound which is in the form of *pranawa*. From the radiant sound arises the suprasound which emits 1000 light-powers and along with it fifty *matrika* sounds in twenty strengths, which create the thousand-petalled lotus. From the *sahasrara* arises the hundred-petalled *nirwana chakra*. This is why it has been stated that the God Surya exists in 100 forms.

The Infinite Power, that is, Shakti of Shiwa, has the power to contract infinitely to be Bindu—Immense Potential, which becomes the centre of immense creative energy. This infinitely contracted Bindu is non-magnitudinous and non-positional, but it swells to create around it a finite 'field' termed *sahasrara*. The infinitely condensed power in Bindu is *prana*-energy as a dynamic triangle in which the infused *nada*-power remaining in substance, determines the character of the emission of *prana* necessary for creative evolution. The hidden *nada* assumes $a - u - m$ in trace and in equilibrium represented by the triangle. The pranic concentration at a certain point effects the emission of $a-u-m$ as

radiant sound. It is the first manifested central light-force containing in it 1000 light-powers. When the radiant sound is transformed into suprasound the 1000 light-powers become distinct and assume a petaline form, and the sound aspect emits *matrika*-sounds. This petaline process and its ground elements constitute *sahasrara*.

Bindu is void. Here, Bindu is Supreme Bindu because it is in a state of infinite contraction and so the void is supreme void. Supreme void indicates a state which is beyond mind-matter, without names and objects. This void, consequently, is the void of matter and also mind. It is non-material and non-mental power around Shiwa-consciousness. The power is *Kundali*-power into which mind-matter phenomena have been absorbed, and the supreme void has been created, and this void is *Kundali*-power in its highest spiritual form, lying around Shiwa. This void is the centre of *sahasrara*.

There is a possibility in man of reducing all his experiences into a form in which consciousness becomes *samprajñana* (superconsciousness) of the highest order, which is only attainable in the highest stage of *samprajñata samadhi*, which is able to receive and retain the prototype of *Sakala* Shiwa—Being-Consciousness-Bliss without names and forms. This experience is finally developed into a unique form—the Supreme Spiritual Reality—one and whole, infinite and supreme. Here are neither experiencer nor what is to be experienced but only that Reality, which is there because of his power of beingness. It is being which is also consciousness and bliss. This infinity is reachable when the *samadhi*-consciousness is recoiled into Supreme Power which at the infinite point is nothing else than that Reality—*Parama* Shiwa.

It has been said that *yoga* should be done between Kundalini and Atman—the supreme reality, which is in the nature of illumination and bliss, beyond mental consciousness, beyond the universe but is the essence of it; which is in himself, and is supremely subtle, that is, only 'is'; and the reality is beyond the *sahasrara* (—*Gandharwatantra*, ch. 29, p. 112). Shiwa is illumination itself. It does not require a revealer to know him. But the unchanging persistence of Shiwa, the very beingness of Shiwa indicates his power. The power to exist, to persist is his. Consequently, Shiwa and his Power are not two entities, but one and the same, and is understandable as two aspects of the same entity—Illumination or Shiwa aspect, and Power or Shakti aspect. Even the idea of two aspects of the same entity arises from the mind having dualistic functions. In the intellectual state, illumination and being do not represent one, but two aspects. On the other hand, this mental duality melts away in asamprajñata samadhi, and Shiwa and Shakti are revealed as one and the same, not as two aspects of one thing. Shiwa is revealed as Shakti, and Shakti as Shiwa. Difficulties arise when we subject this real nondualistic revelation to time, and, consequently, it is brought down to the mental level. This Being-Power from a purely power aspect is Becoming-Power which manifests its supreme wibhuti (yoga-power) as nama (ideas) and rupa (form). In supreme yoga, Shiwa and Shakti is one and the same—Shakti manifests in Shiwa as his beingness and Shiwa being in Shakti is illumination.

Shakti as Supreme Power is also able to manifest its power as yoga-power which effects the universe of mind-matter as a finite phenomenon by veiling the Infinite. The supreme state in which Shiwa is Shakti and Shakti is Shiwa is beyond intellectual thoughts. Really it is neither dualistic nor nondualistic, but beyond dualistic and nondualistic. It is the state of asamprajñata samadhi. Asamprajñata samadhi is beyond the sahasrara. In the asamprajñata samadhi state, Supreme Power is Supreme Kundalini and she is one and the same with Parama Shiwa.

Kundalini as Kulakundalini is in the muladhara chakra in yoga-sleep (samadhi) in Shiwa as Swayambhu-linga. She is a non-entity in undulatory consciousness, so she is called as if sleeping. In a living form, she is roused in concentrated consciousness. The roused Kundalini is termed Wahni ('Fire')-Kundalini of deep red colour who extends from the muladhara to the bottom of the anahata. In the anahata, she becomes Surya ('Sun')-Kundalini who is

of very bright vermilion colour and extends to the bottom of the ajña chakra. In the ajña chakra, she becomes Chandra('Moon')-Kundalini of shining moon-colour and is nectarous and extends to the nirwana chakra. In the sahasrara she becomes Turya(samadhi)-Kundalini who is in the nature of pure consciousness and becomes reflected in the consciousness in samprajñata samadhi.

Kundalini is roused in the muladhara and conducted through all chakras into the sahasrara by the Kundalini-yoga process. Dhyana is the fundamental part of this yoga. Dhyana is done stage by stage on Kundalini throughout the chakra system from the muladhara to the nirwana, first on Fire-Kundalini, then on Sun-Kundalini and finally on Moon-Kundalini. The roused Kundalini in dhyana exhibits her absorbing power, and sense-perceptions together with mental factors associated with them are absorbed in the five lower chakras and the ajña and the manas chakras. Intellection and thoughts are absorbed in the indu chakra. Moon-Kundalini then passes from the nirwana chakra through the wisarga (power-bridge) to the power-triangle lying inside the moon-like lustrous and nectarous circular pericarp of the guru chakra. From the power-triangle Kundalini goes into the lightning-like luminous triangle situated inside the shining circular moon-region which is within the pericarp of the sahasrara. Here Moon-Kundalini becomes Turya-Kundalini, that is, the form of Kundalini realizable only in samprajñata samadhi.

Kundalini exhibits her three aspects—while she is in the luminous triangle of the sahasrara. The first is the ama-kala aspect. In this aspect, Kundalini is without form but subtle and shining red and in half-coil. The half-coiled red-power transforms dhyana into samprajñata samadhi. In the first stage of dhyana, there is a complete form of an object in consciousness, and the practitioner becomes fully conscious of the whole form. As dhyana goes deeper, only a part remains in consciousness, and the rest disappears. Then, this part also disappears, and consciousness becomes full with subtle luminosity. This luminous dhyana is the dhyana of Kundalini. This dhyana is first on the fire-form, then on the sun-form, and finally on the moon-form. The moon-form dhyana develops into samprajñata samadhi at the ama-kala point by the roused half-coiled red-power of ama-kala. In samprajñata samadhi, consciousness is in the form of subtle Kundalini in her post-dhyana three-half coiled beingness; consciousness is only of Kundalini and nothing else.

The second aspect of Kundalini is nirwana-kala. When samprajñata samadhi attains its highest point of development, the nirwana-kala aspect begins to be unfolded. It is a stage beyond samprajñata samadhi. Now, Kundalini manifests her great absorptive power by which samadhi-consciousness is absorbed into her. The absorptive power is associated with the nirodhika-wahni (the power of supreme control). When the power of supreme control is fully exercised Kundalini appears in her third aspect—Nirwana Shakti—all-absorbing Kundali-power. Now, Kundalini absorbs prakriti, purusha and maya-principles and passes into the void (supreme void), lying within the luminous triangle, as a circular process. The central aspect of the void is Shiwa and around him lies Kundalini in coils, thus forming the circumference of the circle. The void consists of Shiwa and Shakti in their four aspects beyond which is Parama Shiwa. The first part of the void which is connected with the sahasrara is Supreme Bindu, then Supreme Nada, then Shakti, and then Shiwa. The first coil of Kundalini is around Supreme Bindu, the second coil around Supreme Nada, the third coil around Shakti, and the half-coil around Shiwa. Now the prana-concentration in Supreme Bindu is transformed into Kundali-power concentration in asamprajñata samadhi. Asamprajñata samadhi starts at this point. Kundalini then absorbs into her Supreme Bindu, then Supreme Nada, then Shakti principle; then Kundalini is in union with Shiwa and absorbs him within her; Kundalini is now without coils and is absorbed into Parama Shiwa. This is the final stage of asamprajñata samadhi.

Supreme Bindu in its creative aspect emits prana-energy as radiant sound which makes the shining circular moon-region appear, as if an expansion of Bindu. The Kundali-power activities form a luminous triangle within the moon-region, which becomes a centre where Kundalini manifests her different aspects—ama-kala, nirwana-kala, nirodhika-wahni and Nirwana Shakti, and finally passes into the void which is an integral part of the triangle. Kundalini forms the circumference aspect, and Shiwa lies in the centre of the void. The radiant sound is then transformed into suprasound consisting of 1000 light-powers (rashmis) which terminate in expanded petaline process to form sahasrara. The nada aspect of the suprasound develops into matrika having fifty distinct sound-units. The fifty matrika-units in twentyfold strength are arranged on the petals of the sahasrara. The sahasrara is the general aspect of the sound power.

The petals of the sahasrara present different colours. When the petals are red, the light-powers exhibit specialized creative energy by which a miniature replica of the sahasrara—the nirwana chakra with 100 petals is first formed and it becomes the seat of ahang (I-ness); then indu chakra—the seat of buddhi (intellect); then manas chakra—the seat of chitta (consciousness); then ajña—the seat of manas (sense-mind); then the lower five chakras from wishuddha to muladhara—the seats of the senses, tanmatras, mahabhutas and divinities. The supra-sound power becomes specialized and the matrika sounds also become particularized and are seated on the fifty petals of the lower six chakras from ajña to muladhara.

When the petals of the sahasrara are yellow, it indicates the expression of mahan (supra-I-ness) consciousness. When the petals are white, it indicates samprajñata samadhi; when green, it indicates the absorption of mahan into Kundalini; and when black, Kundalini as Nirwana Shakti passes into the void. The specific colours of the petals of the lower six chakras are due to the specific manifestation of powers associated with them and matrika. The particularized suprasound (madhyama) becomes audible sounds (waikhari) in the sensory field.

The description of the chakras has been summarized in Table 11.1.

Table 11.1 The chakra table

	1 MULADHARA
	Sushumna starts from Kanda-mula, lying just below Muladhara, and goes upward centrally within the vertebral column.
	Wajra starts from the starting point of Sushumna and goes upward, lying within Sushumna.
	Chitrini starts at the starting point of Wajra and goes upward, lying within Wajra.
	Brahma nadi or Brahmarandhra (as nadi) starts from the orifice of Swayambhu-linga in Muladhara and goes upward, lying within Chitrini.
Terminology	
Waidika	muladhara, adhara, mulakanda, brahma
Tantrika	muladhara, adhara, mula chakra or padma, brahma padma or chakra, bhumi chakra, chaturdala, chatuhpatra
Pouranika	muladhara, adhara
Position	externally, perineal region, close to anus
Petals	
number	four; arranged from right to left
colour	blood-red (deep red), shining red, yellow, golden (shining yellow)
Matrika-letters	
on petals	four in number; Wang Shang Shang Sang, arranged from right to left
colour	gold (shining yellow), blood red (deep red)
Writtis	
on petals	four in number; arranged from right to left
name	1 greatest joy; 2 natural pleasure; 3 delight in controlling passion; 4 blissfulness in concentration
In the pericarp	quadrangular 'earth'-region
colour of the ER	yellow, golden (shining yellow)
'Earth'-bija (in ER)	Lang
colour	yellow, shining yellow
Form of 'earth'-bija	deity Indra
Concentration form of Indra	Indra is yellow in colour, four-armed, holding the Wajra and a blue lotus in his hands, mounted on the white elephant Airawata
In the bindu of Lang	deity Brahma
Concentration form of Brahma	Brahma is deep red, young, four-faced, three-eyed, four-armed, holding a staff, a sacred water-pot, and a rosary of rudraksha, and making the gesture of dispelling fear; seated on a swan
Presiding divinity	power Dakini
Concentration of Dakini	Dakini is shining red or shining white in colour; she has beautiful face with three eyes; four-armed, holding a trident, a skulled staff, a swan and a drinking vessel; seated on a red lotus
Triangle	
colour	shining deep red
Swayambhu-linga	inside the triangle
form	broad at the bottom and tapers to a point at the top
colour	shining deep red, black (or green), golden (shining yellow)
Kundalini as Kula-Kundalini	Supremely subtle, lightning-like splendorous; also of shining red, white and black (or dark-green) colour; in three and a half coils around Swayambhu-linga

2 SWADHI*SHTHANA*

Terminology	
Waidika	swadhi*shtha*na, me*dhra*
Tantrika	swadhi*shtha*na, a*dhishtha*na, bh*ima*, *shat*patra, *shad*dala padma, wari-chak*ra*
Poura*nika*	swadhi*shtha*na
Position	externally, genital region
Petals	
number	six, arranged from right to left
colour	vermilion, deep red, shining red, whitish red, lightning-like, golden
Matrika-letters	
on petals	six in number: *Bang Bhang Mang Yang Rang Lang*, arranged from right to left
colour	lightning-like, diamond-white, white, vermilion
Writtis	
on petals	six in number; arranged from right to left
name	1 affection; 2 pitilessness; 3 feeling of all-destructiveness; 4 delusion; 5 disdain; 6 suspicion
In the pericarp	half-moon-shaped 'water'-region
colour of WR	white
'Water'-b*ija* in WR	W*ang*
colour	moon-white
Form of 'water'-b*ija*	deity W*aruna*
Concentration form of W*aruna*	W*aruna* is white in colour, four-armed, holding a noose, and seated on a m*akara*
In the bindu of W*ang*	deity Wi*shnu*
Concentration form of Wi*shnu*	Wi*shnu* is shining dark-blue (or black), golden, crystal-white, moon-white, and white; youthful and graceful; three-eyed, four-armed, holding a conch, wheel, mace and lotus; dressed in yellow raiment; wears shri*watsa*-mark, Koustubha-gem and w*anamala*; seated on g*aruda*
Presiding divinity	power Raki*ni*
Concentration form of Raki*ni*	Raki*ni* is dark-blue (or black), or red in colour; beautiful-faced, vermilion-mark on forehead; three-eyed; dressed in white raiment; two-armed, holding a sword and a shield; or, four-armed, holding a trident, a lotus, a drum and the W*ajra*, or a chisel; seated on a red lotus

3 MA*NI*PU*RA*

Terminology	
Waidika	ma*ni*pura, ma*ni*puraka, nabhi chak*ra*
Tantrika	ma*ni*pura, ma*ni*puraka, dashapatra, dashadala padma, dashapatrambu*ja*, dashach*cha*da, nabhipadma, nabhipa*n*kaja
Poura*nika*	ma*ni*pura, nabhi chak*ra*
Position	externally, navel region
Petals	
number	ten, arranged from right to left
colour	black, dark-green or dark-blue
Matrika-letters	
on petals	ten in number: *Dang Dhang Nang Tang Thang Dang Dhang Nang Pang Ph*ang, arranged from right to left
colour	dark-blue, black, lightning-like

277

3 MA*N*IPU*R*A (continued)

W*r*ittis	
on petals	ten in number, arranged from right to left
name	1 spiritual ignorance; 2 thirst; 3 jealousy; 4 treachery; 5 shame; 6 fear; 7 disgust; 8 delusion; 9 foolishness; 10 sadness
In the pericarp	triangular 'fire'-region
colour of FR	red, deep red
'Fire'-b*ī*ja in FR	R*ang*
colour	red
Form of 'fire'-b*ī*ja	deity W*a*hni
Concentration form of W*a*hni	W*a*hni is shining red; four-armed, holding a rudrak*sha* rosary and a spear, and showing the gestures of granting boons and dispelling fear; seated on a ram
In the bindu of R*ang*	Deity R*u*dr*a*
Concentration form of R*u*dr*a*	R*u*dr*a* is red or white; three-eyed; two-armed, showing the gestures of granting boons and dispelling fear; seated on a bull
Presiding divinity	power L*a*kin*i*
Concentration form of Lakin*i*	Lakin*i* is black or dark-blue, vermilion, pale-red, or deep red in colour; three-eyed, or three-faced with three eyes in each face; four-armed, holding W*a*jr*a* and a spear, and making the gestures of granting boons and dispelling fear; or two-armed, holding a noose and a goad, as showing the gestures of granting boons and dispelling fear; dressed in yellow raiment, or white raiment; seated on a red lotus

4 H*R*IT

Terminology	
W*a*idika	h*r*idaya chakra, h*r*it p*a*dm*a*, h*r*id*a*ya p*a*dm*a*, h*r*id*a*ya kamala, h*r*id*a*ya-amburuha, h*r*id*a*ya p*a*dmakosha, h*r*itpu*n*dar*ī*ka, h*e*mapu*n*dar*ī*ka
Tantrik*a*	h*r*it p*a*dm*a*, h*r*itpu*n*dar*ī*ka, h*r*id*a*yambhoja, eight-p*e*talled p*a*dm*a*, eight-petalled kamala, sixteen-petalled p*a*dm*a*
Poura*n*ika	h*r*it p*a*dm*a*, h*r*itpadmakosha, h*r*itpu*n*dar*ī*ka, h*r*itpa*n*kaja, h*r*itsaroruha, h*r*idabja, h*r*idambuja, h*r*idambhoja, h*r*idayambhoja, h*r*idaya kamala, h*r*id*a*ya pu*n*dar*ī*ka, h*r*id*a*ya, h*r*it desha, *ashta*patra, adi *sho*dasha chakra
Position	externally, heart region
Petals	
number	eight, arranged from right to left
colour	golden, white, red
on petals	eight forms of superpowers, arranged from right to left
In the pericarp	circular sun-region, moon-region (within sun-region); fire-region (within moon-region)
colour	sun-region—vermilion
	moon-region—white
	fire-region—deep red
In the fire-region	red whishing-tree; gummed seat (at the base of the tree)

5 *A*NAH*A*T*A*

Terminology	
W*a*idika	anahata, h*r*idaya chakra, dwadashar*a* chakra, fourth chakra
Tantrik*a*	anahata, anahata-pur*i*, padm*a*-sundar*a*, dwadasha, dwadashadala, suryasangkhyadala, h*r*it p*a*dm*a*, h*r*itpatra, h*r*itpa*n*keruha, h*r*itsaroruha, h*r*idambhoja, h*r*idambuja, h*r*idabja, h*r*idaya, h*r*idayambhoja, h*r*idayambuja, h*r*idayasarasija, h*r*idayabja, h*r*idaya kamala, h*r*itpa*n*kaja

5   *ANAHATA* (continued)

Pouranika	anahata
Position	externally, heart region
Petals	
number	twelve, arranged from right to left
colour	deep red, shining red, shining vermilion, yellow, dark blue-yellow, white
Matrika-letters	
on petals	twelve in number; *Kang Khang Gang Ghang Nang Chang Chang Jang Jhang Ñang Tang Thang*, arranged from right to left
colour	vermilion, deep red, shining red, white
Writtis	
on petals	twelve in number, arranged from right to left
name	1 lustfulness; 2 fraudulence; 3 indecision; 4 repentance; 5 hope; 6 anxiety; 7 longing; 8 impartiality; 9 arrogance; 10 incompetency; 11 discrimination; 12 an attitude of defiance
In the pericarp	hexagonal 'air'-region
colour of AR	smoke-coloured, black
'Air'-bija in AR	Y*ang*
colour	smoke-coloured
Form of 'air'-bija	deity Wayu
Concentration forms of Wayu	Wayu is smoke-coloured; four-armed, holding ankusha; seated on a black antelope
In the bindu of Y*ang*	deity *Isha*
Concentration form of *Isha*	*Isha* is shining white as pure crystal in colour; one-faced, or five-faced, three-eyed; two-armed, four-armed, or ten-armed; making the gestures of granting boons and dispelling fear; clad in tiger's skin or silken raiment
Presiding divinity	power Kakini
Concentration form of Kakini	Kakini is shining yellow, shining red, moon-white or white in colour; one-faced, three-faced or six-faced; three-eyed; four-armed or two-armed; holding a noose and a skull; a trident, a drum, and a noose; a noose, a trident, a skull, and a drum; a skull and a trident; a trident, a bow, and a skull; the Weda; making the gestures of granting boons and dispelling fear; the gesture of dispelling fear; the gesture of granting boons; clad in white raiment, black raiment, or yellow raiment; seated in a red lotus
In the pericarp	a triangle
colour of the triangle	lightning-like, golden
Within the triangle	Bana-linga
colour	golden, shining red
In the pericarp	Jiwatman
Concentration form	motionless flame of a lamp, shining gold colour

6   WISHUDDHA

Terminology	
Waidika	wishuddha, wishuddhi, k*antha* chakra
Tantrika	wishuddha, wishuddhi, k*antha*, k*antha*desha, k*antha*padma, k*antha*pankaja, k*antha*mbhuja, k*antha*mbhoja, *shodasha*, *shodasha*-dala, *shodasha*ra, nirm*ala*-padma, dwy*ashta*patrambuja, akasha, *shodasha*hollas*a*-d*ala*, *shodasha*-patra
Pouranika	wishuddha, wishuddhi
Position	externally, neck-region

6 WISHUDDHA (continued)

Petals	
number	sixteen, arranged from right to left
colour	smoke colour, shining smoke colour
Matrika-letters	
on petals	sixteen in number; *Ang Ang Ing Ing Ung Ung Ring Ring Lring Lring Eng Aing Ong Oung Ang Ah*, arranged from right to left
colour	deep red, red, golden
Writtis	
on petals	sixteen in number, arranged from right to left
name	1 Pranawa (mantra O*ng*); 2 Udgitha (the Sama-mantras); 3 Hu*ng* (a mantra); 4 Pha*t* (a mantra); 5 Washa*t* (a mantra); 6 Swadha (a mantra); 7 Swaha (a mantra); 8 Nama*h* (a mantra); 9 Amrita (nectar) and seven (musical) tones, viz. 1 ni*s*hada; 2 *r*ishabha; 3 gandhara; 4 *s*hadja; 5 madhyama; 6 dhaiwata; 7 pañchama
In the pericarp	circular akasha-region
	a triangle inside the akasha-region
	circular lunar region inside the triangle
colour	akasha-region; white, transparent or smoke
	triangle; sky-blue or smoke
	lunar-region; white
Akasha-bija	H*ang*
	inside lunar region
colour	white
Form of Akasha-bija	deity Ambara (Akasha)
Concentration form of *Ambara*	*Ambara* is white in colour; four-armed, holding a noose and a goad, and making the gestures of granting boons and dispelling fear; seated on a white elephant
In the bindu of H*ang*	deity Sadashiwa
Concentration form of Sadashiwa	Sadashiwa as *A*rdhanarishwara: The right half of the body (the Shiwa aspect) is white, and the left half (the Power aspect) is golden; five-faced, three-eyed; ten-armed, holding a trident, a chisel (or an axe), a sword, the wajra, fire, the great snake, a bell, a goad and a noose, and making the gestures of dispelling fear; clad in tiger's skin
Presiding divinity	power Shakin*i*
Concentration form of Shakin*i*	Shakin*i* is shining white, or yellow in colour; five-faced, three-eyed, four-armed, holding a bow and arrow, noose and goad; or a noose, a goad and a book and making the attitude of jñanamudra; or a bow, a trident and a book and showing jñanamudra; or a noose, a trident, and a book, and showing jñanamudra; or two-armed, holding the Wajra and a staff; clad in yellow raiment or black raiment; seated in a red lotus

7 TALU

Terminology	
Waidika	talu, taluka
Tantrika	talu, lalana
Poura*n*ika	talu
Position	externally, palatine region
Petals	
number	twelve; sixty-four
colour	red (when twelve); shining white (when sixty-four)

7   TALU (continued)

Writtis	
on petals	twelve in number (when the petals are twelve), arranged from right to left
name	1 respect; 2 contentment; 3 offence; 4 self-control; 5 pride; 6 affection; 7 sorrow; 8 depression; 9 purity; 10 dissatisfaction; 11 honour; 12 anxiety
In the pericarp	a circular region (ghantika)
	nectarous region (amritasthali) within the circular region
	moon-power (chandra-kala) within the nectarous region
colour	circular region: red
	nectarous region: shining white

8   AJÑA

Terminology	
Waidika	ajña, bhru chakra, bhruyugamadhyabila, baindawa-sthana, dwidala
Tantrika	ajña, ajña-patra, ajña-pura, ajña-puri, ajñambuja, ajñapankaja, jñana-padma, dwidala, dwidalambuja, dwidala-kamala, dwipatra, bhru-saroruha, triweni-kamala, netra-padma, netra-patra, bhru-mandala, bhru-madhya, bhru-madhyaga-padma, bhru-madhya-chakra, bhru-mula, shiwa-padma
Pouranika	ajña, dwidala, trirasna
Position	externally, eyebrow-region
Petals	
number	two
colour	white, lightning-like
Matrika-letters	
on petals	two in number: Hang Kshang, arranged from right to left
colour	white, golden, variegated, shining
In the pericarp	power Hakini
Concentration form of Hakini	Hakini is moon-white, white, a mixture of white-black-red, dark-blue, or red in colour; she has one, two, three, four, five or six faces; six faces of red colour; three-eyed; six-armed, holding a book, a skull, a drum, and a rudraksha rosary, and making the gestures of granting boons and of dispelling fear; holding a rudraksha rosary, a drum, a skull, a book, and a bow, and showing the mudra; holding a skull, a spear, and a shield, and making the gestures of granting boons and of dispelling fear; two-armed; clad in red raiment with the white upper garment; seated on a white lotus
In the pericarp above Hakini	a triangle
Within the triangle	Itara-linga
colour	moon-white, golden, red
Above Itara-linga	a triangle
	pranawa (Ong) in the triangle
colour	moon-white
Above pranawa-bindu	subtle manas (manas 2) (in bindu pitha)
Above Manas 2	nada (manas chakra)
colour	shining white

9   MANAS

Terminology	
Waidika	manas, mandala, jñananetra
Tantrika	nada, manas, surya mandala
Pouranika	
Position	above bindu pitha which is just above the pranawa-bindu in ajña
Petals	
number	six
colour	normally white, but then assume sense colours (yellow, white, red, ash and white) when senses operate, and become black in sleep
In the pericarp	Chitta

10   INDU

Terminology	
Waidika	indu, shitangshu mandala, sixteen-petalled anahata, shambhawa sthana
Tantrika	chandra (chandra mandala), chandra mandala, kailasa, shakti, nadanta, soma
Pouranika	kailasa, shakti, widya-pada
Position	above manas
Petals	
number	sixteen, arranged from right to left
colour	moon-white
Writtis	
on petals	sixteen in number, arranged from right to left
name	1 mercy; 2 gentleness; 3 patience; 4 non-attachment; 5 control; 6 excellent-qualities; 7 joyous mood; 8 deep spiritual love; 9 humility; 10 reflection; 11 restfulness; 12 seriousness; 13 effort; 14 controlled emotion; 15 magnanimity; 16 concentration
In the pericarp	a circular moon-region
	a nine-cornered region (within the moon-region)
	the isle of gems (within the nine-cornered region)
	Shambhu-bija (Hang) with sah in the form of a swan (within the isle of gems)
	Parashiwa with his power Siddhakali (in the bindu of Hang mantra)
Seat	Buddhi (intellective mind)

11   NIRWANA

Terminology	
Waidika	nirwana, brahmarandhra (chakra), parabrahma chakra, dwadashanta, shirshantargata mandala
Tantrika	nirwana, brahmarandhra (chakra), bodhini (chakra), bodhana, rodhini, chitkalashakti (chakra), shatapatra chakra, shatadala chakra, kala chakra, dwadashanta
Pouranika	brahmarandhra, rodhini, shanta, shantipada, dwadashanta, dwadashanta-pada, dwadashanta sarasija, brahmarandhra pankaja
Position	at the upper terminal point of Chitrini, within the cranium
Petals	
number	100
colour	shining white

11 NIRWA*N*A (continued)

Seat	dh*i* (concentrative mind) and *a*hang (I-ness) Su*sh*um*na* terminates in talu-m*u*la (upper end of palatine region), also called br*a*hm*a*randhr*a* and dwad*a*shanta, which is the topmost point within the cranium. This end-point of su*sh*um*na* is marked by nirw*a*na ch*a*kra, also called br*a*hm*a*randhr*a* and dwad*a*shanta ch*a*kra W*a*jr*a*, Chitri*ni* and Br*a*hm*a* n*a*di also terminate at the upper end of su*sh*um*na*

12 GURU

Terminology Tantrik*a*	dwad*a*shar*na* sarasiruh*a* or p*a*dm*a*, dwad*a*shad*a*la saroj*a* or p*a*dm*a*, dwad*a*shap*a*tr*a*k*a*, *u*rdhw*a*mukh*a* p*a*dm*a*, shukl*a* abj*a*, guru-p*a*d*a* p*a*dm*a*, guru-pur*a*, guru-sth*a*n*a*, guru-p*a*d*a*, br*a*hm*a* ch*a*kra, soma-m*a*nd*a*l*a*
Position	in void-region, situated supracranially
Petals	
number	twelve, arranged from right to left
colour	white
M*a*ntr*a*-letter	
on petals	twelve in number: *Ha Sa Kha Freng Ha Sa Ksha Ma La Wa Ra Yung* (Guru-m*a*ntr*a*), arranged from right to left
colour	white
In the pericarp	a circular moon-region a triangle (within the moon-region) the jewelled altar of whitish-red lustre with nad*a* below and bindu above (inside the triangle) or *A*ing (inside the triangle) hang*sa*h-seat (within the bindu) jewelled footstools (on hang*sa*h-seat) Guru's lotus-like feet (on the jewelled footstools)
Concentration form of Guru	Guru is moon-white, or like pure crystal in colour; two-eyed, or three-eyed; two-armed, making the gestures of granting boons and dispelling fear, or holding a book and showing w*a*ra or abh*a*ya mudra; dressed in white raiment; in lotus, auspicious, or hero posture; his power is seated on his left thigh, and holds with her left hand a blue lotus; she is red in colour

13 S*A*H*A*SR*A*R*A*

Terminology W*a*idik*a*	sahasrar*a*, sahasr*a*d*a*l*a*, sahasrar*a* kamal*a* (pa*n*k*a*j*a*, or p*a*dm*a*), sth*a*n*a*, kap*a*las*a*mp*u*ta, wyom*a*mbuj*a*, wyom*a*, akash*a* ch*a*kra
Tantrik*a*	sahasrar*a*, sahasrar*a* p*a*dm*a*, sahasrar*a* mahap*a*dm*a*, sahasrar*a* ambuj*a*, sahasrar*a* saroruh*a*, sahasr*a*d*a*l*a*, sahasr*a*d*a*l*a* p*a*dm*a*, pa*n*k*a*j*a*, or kamal*a*, sahasr*a*chch*a*d*a* pa*n*k*a*j*a*, sahasr*a*bj*a*, sahasr*a*p*a*tr*a*, sahasr*a*d*a*l*a* adhomukh*a* p*a*dm*a*, adhomukh*a* mahap*a*dm*a*, wyom*a*mbhoj*a*, wyom*a*, shir*a*s p*a*dm*a*, amlan*a* p*a*dm*a* (or pa*n*k*a*j*a*), d*a*shash*a*tad*a*l*a* p*a*dm*a*, shuddh*a* p*a*dm*a*
Poura*ni*k*a*	sahasrar*a*, sahasr*a*d*a*l*a*, sahasrar*a* kamal*a* (pa*n*k*a*j*a*, or p*a*dm*a*), sahasr*a*p*a*tr*a*, sahasr*a*parn*a* p*a*dm*a*, shanty*a*tit*a*, shanty*a*tit*a* p*a*d*a*, par*a*m*a* shir*a*s
Position	in void-region, as the upper part of the guru ch*a*kra

13   SAHASRARA (continued)

Petals	
number	1000, arranged from right to left, in 20 layers, each containing 50, and the arrangement of the petals gives the appearance of the sahasrara as bell-shaped
colour	white, red, yellow, golden, changing colours of white, red, yellow, black and green
Matrika-letters	
on petals	50 in number in each layer: Ang to L(rh)ang or Kshang, arranged from right to left
colour	petal-colour, or normal colour
Pericarp	
colour	golden
In the pericarp	the circular moon-region
	the luminous triangle (inside the moon-region)
	ama-kala (inside the triangle)
	ama-kala is subtle, shining in colour and crescent-shaped (in one-half coil)
	nirwana-kala (inside ama-kala)
	nirwana-kala is very subtle, shining red in colour, and crescent-shaped (in one-half coil)
	nirodhika-fire (within nirwana-kala)
	nirwana shakti (inside nirwana-kala)
	nirwana shakti is extremely subtle, and shining red in colour
	void (inside the triangle)
	void is in the form of a circle and is the centre of Supreme Bindu
	Wisarga; its first point is just beyond ama-kala, and the second point is just below Supreme Bindu
	Divine Shankhini who is above the second point of Wisarga, and extends from Supreme Bindu, passing through Supreme Nada, Shakti principle to Sakala Shiwa in coils, and then is absorbed into Parama Shiwa

CHAPTER 12
Location of the Chakras

The sushumna nadi passes through the interior of the vertebral column. The sushumna is not a nerve, a nerve substance, or a material tubular structure; consequently, it is not visualized on dissecting the vertebral column. It is a subtle nadi. The nadis are not wires, but subtle lines of direction of force caused by, and intrinsically associated with, wayu-energy.

Wayu is an energy in a subtle form; it is completely free from particles; it has no mass, no charge, and no interaction with matter. Therefore, it cannot exist in the material field. This does not mean that it cannot exist at all. Matter-energy is a three-cornered phenomenon, in which particles, radiation and light are component factors. So, it is the triangular tejas-energy with which are connected, as its parts, ap-energy involved in the principle of conservation of energy, and kshiti-energy which maintains mass in matter. When the three-cornered energy pattern is transformed into the six-cornered form, mass becomes zero, electrical character disappears, and it is released from matter; instead, it exhibits non-ceasing energy-radiations which form nadis, vitality is infused into it, and it shows creativity by which the living-matter-organization is evolved. Wayu-nadi operates in the subtle nadi-field with super-velocity and causes the appearance of force-motion-lines which are subtle nadis. The presence of such nadis cannot be detected in matter; though a part of the subtle energy, being externalized, penetrates constantly into organized living matter and makes it function as a living body. Moreover, the nadis appear to be steady because

of their supervelocity, if one sees them from the material field.

The wayu-energy field is the expansion of more concentrated energy as bindu (point). The bindu tends to release its concentrated energy which expands around it to form a field. This is the evolutionary aspect of wayu-energy. Wayu as concentrated energy is in bindu-form, and its expansion is the wayu-nadi-field. This bindu-and-field phenomenon occurs in all planes. In matter, the atoms are like the bindu and what is around them is their field. Atoms are also the fields of the elementary particles. In living matter, a nucleus is the bindu and the cytoplasm around it is its field. In mind, ahang (I-ness) is the bindu which creates chitta (mental consciousness) as its field.

Wayu-energy as chitra-power concentrates and centralizes to form a petaline bindu, termed chakra or lotus. The chakra-formation occurs throughout the course of the chitrini nadi at certain points. The lower chakras are the specific and detailed manifestations of the more central nirwana chakra situated at the upper end of the chitrini nadi. The sahasrara is the original chakra from which emerges first the nirwana chakra. The sahasrara itself is the field of Supreme Bindu, as an atom is a field of particles on the material plane. Wayu-nadi is the field of wayu in the form of the centralized chitra-power as its bindu.

The chitrini is the prana-force-motion-line which is a white radiation. The chitrini-radiation is enveloped by the vermilion wajra-radiation and the wajra by the deep-red sushumna-radiation. There is a void in the central aspect of the chitrini nadi where there is no radiation. This void has been termed brahmarandhra or brahma-void. It is a potential void, but it becomes brahma nadi when Kundali-power passes through it. There is no possibility of seeing with our eyes the sushumna and its internal radiations wajra and chitrini, and the chakras which are in the chitrini (or by the aid of supersensitive instruments), because they exist and function supramaterially. They are 'seen' however in dhyana when consciousness develops the power to reject sensory objects and receive directly subtle objects. The supramaterial field is the deep internal layer which is superimposed by the living-matter substance. In this physical surface layer there are particular positions which correspond approximately to certain vertebral and cranial points. These physical positions are the seats of resonance, caused by the power-radiations from the subtle chakras when they are aroused by thought-concentration done in these positions. The positions of the chakras in the chitrini can only be sensed through the aroused physical positions. But it is not easy to know directly these positions. There is a practical means of approaching these positions through certain vertebral and cranial points with which they are closely related. The determination of the vertebro-cranial points is more easily done through the surface points which approximately correspond to the vertebro-cranial points.

For this purpose, a brief anatomical account of the vertebral column, the cranial cavity and the central nervous system contained therein, may be useful. It may be pointed out here that no attempt has been made to consider the functional significance of the central nervous system, either as a whole or as parts which are disclosed in the anatomical approach. Our object is the linking of the chitrini positions with the physical positions through the vertebro-cranial points as correctly as possible.

The Vertebral Column (Columna vertebralis)

The vertebral column is the central axis of the body, which extends from the base of the skull down to the end of the trunk. It consists of 26 single bones, of which 24 are free vertebrae, and the other 2 are the sacrum and os coccygis. Of the 24 free vertebrae, 7 are in the neck region, and are called the cervical vertebrae; 12 are in the thoracic region, and are called the thoracic vertebrae; and 5 are in the lumbar region, and are called the lumbar vertebrae. The sacrum is composed of 5 fused bones, and the coccyx is formed by the consolidation of 4 or 5 bones. The vertebrae are placed one upon another with discs of fibrocartilage between them, and are held together by ligaments, and strengthened by spinal muscles.

A vertebra consists of an anterior part, termed the body, and a posterior part, termed the vertebral arch. The body and the arch form an opening in a vertebra, termed the vertebral foramen. The foramina, placed one above another, constitute the vertebral canal. The vertebral canal extends from the vertebral foramen of the atlas (the first cervical vertebra) and passes through the cervical, thoracic, and lumbar regions into the sacral canal formed by the vertebral foramina of the sacral vertebrae. The spinal cord is located within the vertebral canal.

The Cranial Cavity

The cranial cavity is formed by the frontal, occipital, temporal, parietal, sphenoid and ethmoid bones, which are firmly and immovably connected with each other. These bones belong to the skull. The brain is lodged within the cranial cavity. The skull is placed on the atlas.

The Spinal Cord (Medulla spinalis)

The central nervous system consists of two parts: the brain, located within the cranial cavity; and the spinal cord, lying within the vertebral canal. The spinal cord extends from the upper border of the atlas to the lower border of the first, or the upper border of the second, lumbar vertebra.

The central portion of the spinal cord is composed of the grey matter, and the peripheral part is made up of the white matter. The grey matter consists of nerve cells, nerve fibres, and neuroglia. The white matter consists chiefly of medullated nerve fibres. The spinal cord is invested by three membranes which are the continuation of those which envelop the brain. The outer membrane is called the dura mater. There is the extradural space between the wall of the vertebral canal and the dura mater, which contains areolar tissue, fat, and veins. The second coat is made up of arachnoid mater. There is a potential space, called the subdural space, between the dura and the arachnoid, which contains a minute quantity of fluid. The third inner membranous sheath which invests the spinal cord is the pia mater. The subarachnoid space, lying between the arachnoid and the pia, contains the cerebrospinal fluid.

The spinal cord, at its caudal end, tapers to a cone-shaped extremity, termed the conus medullaris. A threadlike structure, termed the filum terminale, emerges from the apex of the conus medullaris and goes downwards into the coccyx.

The Filum Terminale

The conus medullaris is usually considered the true end of the spinal cord, occurring at the level of the first or the second lumbar vertebra. At this point, the conus medullaris continues as a delicate filament, termed the filum terminale, which extends downwards through the vertebral canal into the sacral canal, which is the continuation of the former. Then it leaves the canal and passes into the first or second segment of the coccyx, where perhaps the canal exists in a potential form, and, finally, it becomes attached to the dorsal surface of the coccyx (first or second segment). The filum terminale consists of two parts: the upper part, called the filum terminale internum, which is about 15 cm long and descends from the second (or first) lumbar vertebra to the second sacral vertebra; and the lower part, called the filum terminale externum, which is the continuation of the filum terminale internum, about 8 cm long, and attached to the dorsal surface of the first or second segment of the coccyx at its inferior end.

The filum terminale consists of the pia mater, some nerve cells and fibres, and the dural and arachnoidal sheaths. The filum terminale internum is more or less the miniature spinal cord, as all the elements present in the spinal cord are also found there. The central canal which lies within the upper part of the filum terminale internum (a distance of about 5 or 6 cm, superiorly) contains the grey matter around it. However, the neurogenic tissue begins to decrease gradually in the filum terminale, as it descends and there is a gradual shrinking of its tissues.

The Central Canal

There is a very narrow canal, called the central canal (the canalis centralis medullae spinalis), which is situated centrally in the grey matter of the spinal cord. It arises from the fourth ventricle of the hindbrain at the level of about the middle of the medulla oblongata, and descends through the lower half of the medulla oblongata to the upper end of the spinal cord at the level of the upper border of the atlas. From here the canal proceeds downwards to the conus medullaris, where it becomes dilated to form the terminal ventricle. The canal then passes into the filum terminale for about 5 or

6 cm where it ends. It forms the neural part of the filum terminale. It is lined with ciliated ependymal cells and is filled with cerebrospinal fluid.

The Brain (Encephalon)

The brain is divided into three main parts: hindbrain (rhombencephalon), consisting of the medulla oblongata, pons and cerebellum; midbrain (mesencephalon) consisting of the tectum, cerebral peduncles, and tegmentum; and forebrain (prosencephalon), consisting of the endbrain (telencephalon) and interbrain (diencephalon).

The brain stem is formed by the medulla oblongata, pons, and midbrain. In other words, the brain stem comprises practically all the parts, except the cerebellum and cerebrum.

The Medulla Oblongata

The medulla oblongata is a conical body, about 2.5 cm long. It is continuous with the upper end of the spinal cord at the level of the foramen magnum, and extends upwards to the lower margin of the pons. The medulla oblongata is divided into right and left halves by the anterior median fissure. Two bundles of nerve fibres, which arise from the cerebrum, descend through the crura cerebri and the pons to the anterior surface of the medulla oblongata to form the pyramids, lying on each side of the anterior median fissure. Most of the fibres of the pyramids decussate in the inferior part of the medulla oblongata to form the lateral corticospinal tract, and the rest descend without crossing, and form the anterior corticospinal tracts. They are called the pyramidal tracts. These tracts extend to the spinal cord. The communication between the medulla oblongata and the spinal cord with the cerebellum is via two bundles of fibres, termed the interior cerebellar

peduncles, which arise from the medulla oblongata.

The Pons

The pons is the superior part of the hindbrain and is situated in front of the cerebellum. Its lower border is connected with the upper border of the medulla oblongata. It presents a broad convex ridge on its ventral surface, which separates it from the midbrain above, and the medulla oblongata below. The ridge is composed of transverse bundles of nerve fibres, and the pontine nuclei. These nerve-fibre bundles collect posteriorly, on each side, to form the middle cerebellar peduncle, which connects with the cerebellar cortex. This anterior ridge forms the basilar part of the pons. Two large bundles of nerve fibres, termed the crura cerebri, descend from the ventral surface of the midbrain to the basilar part of the pons where they form the longitudinal fascicles. Most of these fibres end in the pontine nuclei, and the rest pass as the pyramids from the lower border of the pons to the medulla oblongata. The dorsal part of the pons is continuous inferiorly with the medulla oblongata, and superiorly with the midbrain.

The cerebellum is situated in the posterior cranial fossa, dorsally to the medulla oblongata and pons. It consists of two hemispheres.

The Midbrain

The midbrain is the short, thick necklike structure which connects the hindbrain on one side, and the forebrain on the other. It consists of the cerebral peduncles, including the tegmentum, and the tectum.

Each half of the ventral part of the midbrain extends superiorly to the corresponding half of the forebrain, and is called the cerebral peduncle. The ventral part of the cerebral peduncle is called the crus cerebri. The crus cerebri is a broad bundle of nerve fibres, which arises in the corresponding cerebral hemisphere, and descends to the pons and medulla oblongata.

The dorsal part of the cerebral peduncle is called the tegmentum. It is composed of grey and of white matter. It is continuous inferiorly with the dorsal part of the pons, and superiorly with the hypothalamus. There is a thin layer of grey matter, called the substantia nigra between the crus cerebri and the tegmentum.

The tectum is that part of the midbrain which is posterior to the aqueduct. It consists of four small swellings, two on each side, the superior and inferior colliculi, which are composed of gray matter. Each superior colliculus is connected with the thalamus. The pineal body is situated between the superior colliculi.

The Interbrain (Diencephalon)

The interbrain is the inferior part of the forebrain, lying above the midbrain. It consists of the thalamus, hypothalamus, metathalamus, and epithalamus. The thalamus forms the greater portion of the diencephalon. Medially, the two thalami are separated by the third ventricle. The thalamus consists of gray matter. It is the great sensory relay station and is interconnected with most parts of the cerebral cortex.

The Cerebrum

The upper part of the forebrain is the endbrain (telencephalon), or the cerebrum. The fundamental part of it is the paired cerebral hemispheres which form the largest part of the brain. There is a small unevaginated part under the large evaginated hemispheres, called the telencephalon medium.

The two cerebral hemispheres are almost separated from each other by the longitudinal cerebral fissure (fissura longitudinalis cerebri)

in which is situated the falx cerebri. The surface of the hemispheres is convoluted. The elevations are called gyri. The gyri are separated from each other by grooves and fissures, called sulci. The interlobar sulci form lobes. There are four lobes in each hemisphere: the frontal lobe (lobus frontalis), parietal lobe (lobus parietalis), temporal lobe (lobus temporalis), and occipital lobe (lobus occipitalis).

The convoluted surface of the hemispheres is covered by a layer of grey matter, consisting of nerve cells which are arranged in six strata. This cover of gray matter is called the cerebral cortex. Under this surface cortex lies the white matter. There is also the subcortical grey matter (basal ganglia) under the white matter. The white matter consists of the nerve fibres which are of three types: association fibres, which interconnect various parts of the same hemisphere; commissural fibres, which connect the parts of one hemisphere with those of the other; and projection fibres, which connect the cerebral cortex with other parts of the central nervous system. Of the commissural fibres, the corpus callosum is the most important. It is a thick, broad, arched body of nerve fibres, situated at the bottom of the longitudinal cerebral fissure. It connects one hemisphere with the other.

The Ventricular System of the Brain

The central canal of the spinal cord extends upwards through the foramen magnum into the inferior half of the medulla oblongata and opens into the fourth ventricle at about the level of the middle of the medulla oblongata. The fourth ventricle (ventriculus quartus) is the cavity of the hindbrain; it extends from the superior border of the pons to the middle of the medulla oblongata, and is situated in front of the cerebellum and behind the medulla oblongata and pons. Its superior end is narrow and is continuous with the cerebral aqueduct.

The cerebral aqueduct (aquaeductus cerebri) is an elongated narrow cavity, lying in the midbrain. It communicates with the third ventricle above. The third ventricle (ventriculus tertius) is a narrow cavity the greater part of which lies in the interbrain between the two thalami, and only a small part of it extends into the telencephalon medium, and the lamina terminalis is its rostral boundary. The third ventricle communicates with the lateral ventricles above through the two interventricular foramina. The lateral ventricles (ventriculi laterales) are two c-shaped cavities, situated one in each cerebral hemisphere, and communicate with the third ventricle.

The ventricles of the brain contain the cerebrospinal fluid through which they are in continuation with the central canal of the spinal cord. The cerebrospinal fluid perhaps circulates around the brain and the spinal cord. The cerebrospinal fluid may serve to remove the metabolic waste products and to cleanse the nerve tissue.

The Blue Line

The blue line passes centrally through the filum terminale, spinal cord, and brain, as if it were the bisecting line, since these structures through which it passes show the bisectional pattern in their forms. The blue line, in reality, is the 'one-dimensional' line, indicating the boundary of the material aspect of the body, and beyond which, and extramaterially, lies the nadi-chakra (the non-material power-field), the central aspect of which is the sushumna nadi. The blue line also serves a practical purpose. It indicates certain borderland positions which have the greatest affinity with the chakras.

The blue line starts centrally within the filum terminale at its inferior end, lying (according to our picture) at the level of the second segment of the coccyx. It then ascends centrally through the filum terminale to reach the caudal end of the central canal, lying about 5 or 6 cm down in the filum terminale internum from its superior end. The blue line then passes into the central canal at this point, and ascends centrally through

the entire length of the central canal to the point where the central canal opens into the fourth ventricle, on a level with the middle of the medulla oblongata.

The blue line now passes centrally through the fourth ventricle, the cerebral aqueduct, and then the third ventricle, lying in the diencephalon. Thereafter the blue line passes through the rostral end of the third ventricle in its telencephalic part, the so-called telencephalon medium, to reach the lamina terminalis. From here it ascends through the anterior commissure, farnix, septum pellucidum, and corpus callosum. Finally, the blue line passes into the longitudinal, cerebral fissure which is situated between the two cerebral hemispheres, and reaches a central point of the cerebral cortex, above which lies the bregma.

The Course of the Sushumna

The blue line indicates indirectly the course of the sushumna nadi. The sushumna rises as the pranic radiation-line of deep red colour from the force-concentration centre, termed the kanda-mula. The kanda-mula is situated extramaterially at a position which corresponds approximately to the point lying just below, but intimately connected with, the inferior end of the filum terminale. The sushumna starts from the central aspect of the kanda-mula. The kanda-mula is situated just below, but closely connected with, the starting point of the blue line. The sushumna ascends, as the blue line does, through the filum terminale, central canal, fourth ventricle, cerebral aqueduct, third ventricle, telencephalon medium, anterior commissure, farnix, septum pellucidum, corpus callosum and longitudinal cerebral fissure, and reaches a central point of the cerebral cortex. This is the superior end point of the sushumna. This terminal point of the sushumna has been technically termed the talu-mula, brahmarandhra, and dwadashanta.

The wajra nadi, which is situated within the sushumna as its second internal nadi, is vermilion red in colour, and arises from the same starting point as the sushumna (remaining within it), following the course of the blue line, and terminates where the sushumna ends. The chitrini is situated within the wajra as the third internal nadi, and is white in colour. It begins at the starting point of the wajra (and, consequently, of the sushumna) and proceeds upward along with the wajra, following the course of the blue line, and ends at the terminal point of the wajra and sushumna. The brahma nadi is situated within the chitrini. It starts from the muladhara, that is, a little above the starting point of the sushumna, or, more precisely, just above the inferior end of the blue line. The brahma nadi ascends along the chitrini (being within the chitrini), following the course of the blue line, and terminates at the superior end points of the chitrini, wajra, and sushumna. Therefore, the terminal points of all the four nadis are the same. These nadis have been clearly shown in the figure, Plate 26.

Ida and Pingala

Kanda-mula is the power station from which the sushumna, ida and pingala have arisen as pranic radiation-lines. The kanda-mula is situated at an extra-material position just below the caudal end of the filum terminale, and under, but in contact with, the muladhara chakra. The sushumna starts from the central aspect of the kanda-mula and rises straight through the filum terminale, central canal and ventricles to the cerebral cortex where it ends. The sushumna, in its upward course, is spiraliform.

The ida originates from the left aspect of the kanda-mula and runs outside the vertebral column, and then ascends, remaining on the left side of it, and reaches the ajña chakra where it joins the sushumna. Similarly, the pingala starts from the right aspect of the kanda-mula, proceeds outside the vertebral column, and extends upward, remaining on the right of the vertebral column, and reaches the ajña when it joins the sushumna. So the

positions of the ida and pingala in relation to the sushumna are: the sushumna assumes a central position and the ida is on its left side, and the pingala on its right side. The upper ends of the ida and pingala are in the ajña where they are in union with the sushumna. But the sushumna does not terminate here. It goes upwards to the cerebral cortex point and ends there.

The ida and pingala assume two positions in their upward courses: bow and half-coil. In the bow position, the ida and pingala, in their upward course, become like a bow, the one end of which is in the kanda-mula, and the other end is in the ajña. In the half-coil position, the ida and pingala, in their upward course, go round the chakras—muladhara, swadhishthana, manipura, anahata and wishuddha—in a semicircular way by alternating their courses from left to right and right to left, and reach the ajña. (See Plate 26.)

Positions in the Chitrini

The positions are normally formed by the chitra-power-centralization at certain points along the course of the chitrini nadi. This centralized and plexiform power arrangement is technically called the chakra or lotus. The positions indicate the locations of the chakras in the chitrini.

It is very difficult for a beginner, practising concentration to form a clear notion of the locations of the chakras in the chitrini. An advanced layayogi 'sees' the chakras in deep concentration, there is no problem for him. To help the beginners, the gurus have introduced a method of sensing the positions in the chitrini by determining certain borderland physical positions which are linked with the chitrini positions. These physical positions are enlivened by thought-concentration and become the centres of receiving the replicas of the chakras. This increases the depth of concentration, and, in proper time, thought-concentration is finally transformed into dhyana.

These physical positions are near, and closely

connected with, certain vertebro-cranial points, which again correspond approximately to certain surface points. The surface points are particular points in the specified external areas or regions of the body. The surface points correspond approximately to certain vertebral and cranial points which are very closely related to the physical positions where the replicas of the chakras appear in thought-concentration. A layayoga guru is able to make his pupil feel the chakras by placing his fingers (the guru's) on the appropriate points of the pupil's back.

To determine the vertebro-cranial points in relation to the surface points, a number of roentgen pictures of some of our pupils were taken. The surface-vertebro-cranial relations, based on these pictures, are shown in the figure, Plate 27.

Surface and Vertebro-cranial Relations (Plate 27)

There are ten surface points:

1 Perineal Point, situated in the perineal region. It corresponds to the vertebral point which lies in the second segment of the coccyx, where the filum terminale ends caudally. This we call the coccygeal point. Very close to the last-named point is also the caudal end of the blue line. At this point of the blue line is situated physical position 1 which indicates approximately the location of the muladhara chakra in the chitrini.

2 Genital Point, situated, in the male, at the root of the penis, and, in the female, in the clitoral region. It corresponds to the vertebral point which lies in the fourth sacral vertebra. This is called the sacral point. The sacral point corresponds to a point in the blue line which is within the filum terminale. At this point in the blue line is situated physical position 2 which indicates approximately the location of the swadhishthana chakra in the chitrini.

3 Navel Point, situated in the abdominal region. It corresponds to the lumbar point, lying in the fourth lumbar vertebra. The lumbar point corresponds to a point in the blue line which is within the filum terminale internum. At this blue-line point lies physical position 3 which indicates approximately the location of the manipura chakra in the chitrini.

4 Thoracic Point, situated in the thoracic region, on a level with the middle of the heart. It corresponds to the thoracic vertebral point, lying in the ninth or tenth thoracic vertebra. The thoracic vertebral point corresponds to a point in the blue line which is situated within the central canal of the spinal cord. In this blue-line point lies physical position 4 which indicates approximately the location of the anahata chakra in the chitrini. Just below the anahata is situated the hrit chakra, also in the chitrini.

5 Cervical Point, situated in the neck region. It corresponds to the cervical vertebral point, lying in the fourth cervical vertebra. The cervical vertebral point corresponds to a point in the blue line, which lies within the central canal of the spinal cord. In this blue-line point lies physical position 5 which indicates approximately the location of the wishuddha chakra in the chitrini.

6 Nasal Point, situated in the nasal region, between the apex and the middle part of the external nose. It is equivalent to the palatine point. The nasal point corresponds to the medullary point, lying in the medulla oblongata. The medullary point corresponds to a point in the blue line which is approximately at the junction between the rostral end of the central canal in the medulla oblongata and the lower part of the fourth ventricle. In this blue-line point lies physical position 6 which indicates approximately the location of the talu chakra in the chitrini.

7 Eyebrow Point, situated in the space between the eyebrows. The eyebrow point corresponds to the ventricular point A,

Table 12.1 Chakra-location Table

Surface Point	Vertebral Point	Cranial Point	Blue-line Point	Location of Chakra in Chitrini
1 Perineal Point in perineal region	Coccygeal Point in segment II of coccyx		Physical Position 1 at caudal end of blue line	1 Muladhara Chakra
2 Genital Point at root of penis	Sacral Point in sacral vertebra IV		Physical Position 2 blue-line point lying within filum terminale	2 Swadhishthana Chakra
3 Navel Point in abdominal region	Lumbar Point in lumbar vertebra IV		Physical Position 3 blue-line point lying within filum terminale internum	3 Manipura Chakra
4 Thoracic Point in thoracic region	Thoracic Vertebral Point in thoracic vertebra IX or X		Physical Position 4 blue-line point lying within central canal of spinal cord	5 Anahata Chakra 4 Hrit Chakra Just below anahata
5 Cervical Point in neck region	Cervical Vertebral Point in cervical vertebra IV		Physical Position 5 blue-line point lying within central canal of spinal cord	6 Wishuddha Chakra
6 Nasal/palatine/ Point in nasal region		Medullary Point in medulla oblongata	Physical Position 6 blue-line point lying at junction of rostral end of central canal and lower part of ventricle IV	7 Talu Chakra
7 Eyebrow Point in space between eyebrows		Ventricular Point A in caudal part of ventricle III	Physical Position 7 blue-line point lying in caudal part of ventricle III	8 Ajña Chakra
8 Forehead Point A in forehead		Ventricular Point B rostral part of ventricle III	Physical Position 8 blue-line point lying in rostral part of ventricle III	9 Manas Chakra
9 Forehead Point B above forehead point A		Telencephalic Point in telencephalon	Physical Position 9 blue-line point lying in telencephalon	10 Indu Chakra
10 Head Point above forehead point B		Cerebral Point in cerebral cortex	Physical Position 10 at upper end of blue line, lying in cerebral cortex	11 Nirwana Chakra

lying in the caudal part of the third
ventricle. The ventricular point A corresponds to a point in the blue line, which
lies in the caudal part of the third ventricle.
In this blue-line point lies physical position
7 which indicates approximately the
location of the ajña *chakra* in the chitri*ni*.

8   Forehead Point A, situated in the forehead.
It corresponds to the ventricular Point B,
lying in the rostral part of the third ventricle
in the telencephalon medium. The ventricular point B corresponds to a point in
the blue line, which lies in the rostral
part of the third ventricle. In this blue-
line point lies physical position 8 which
indicates approximately the location of
the ma*nas chakra* in the chitri*ni*.

9   Forehead Point B, situated in the forehead,
just above the forehead point A. It corresponds to the telencephalic point, lying in
the region where the lamina terminalis
and commissura anterior are situated.
The telencephalic point corresponds to
a point in the blue line in the telencephalic
region where lie the lamina terminalis and
commissura anterior. In this blue-line
point lies physical position 9 which indicates
approximately the location of the indu
chakra in the chitri*ni*.

10   Head Point, situated above the forehead
point B. It corresponds to the cerebral
point, lying in the cerebral cortex. The
cerebral point corresponds to the upper
end-point of the blue line, situated in the
cerebral cortex. In this blue-line point
lies physical position 10 which indicates
the location of the nirwa*na chakra* in the
chitri*ni*. The upper end of the blue line

indicates the terminal points of the
su*sh*um*na*, wa*j*ra, chitri*ni*, and bra*h*ma
na*di*, and at this terminal point of the
chitri*ni* lies the nirwa*na chakra*.

There are two *chakras* which are not located
in the chitri*ni*. These are the guru *chakra*, and
the sa*h*asrara, which is above guru but is in
connection with it. The upper end of the chitri*ni*
lies intracranially, and is marked by the presence
of the nirwa*na chakra*. Beyond the intracranial
end of the chitri*ni* and the nirwa*na chakra* is
the extracranial void-region where lie the guru
chakra and sa*h*asrara. The intracranial end of
the chitri*ni*, and, consequently, the nirwa*na*
chakra are connected to the guru *chakra* by
wis*a*rga (power-bridge). Wis*a*rga consists of
two rings arranged vertically. The lower ring
is placed in close contact with the intracranial
end of the chitri*ni*, and the upper ring lies in
close contact with the guru *chakra*. This means
that the void-region is crossed by the wis*a*rga
from the nirwa*na chakra* to the guru *chakra*.

The location of the *chakras* can be
summarized as shown in Tables 12.1 and 12.2.

Table 12.2   *Chakra*-location table

Region	Location of Chakra
Wis*a*rga bridges the void-region between nirwa*na* and guru	
Void-region 1 lying extracranially	Guru *Chakra*
Void-region 2 lying extracranially	Sa*h*asrara

PART 3

CONCENTRATION
PRACTICES

CHAPTER 13
Physical Purification and Vitalization

It is often ignored that the body plays an important role in the development of mental calmness and concentration. Only a purified and vital body can function efficiently at a certain organic functional level without radiating disturbing influences on the mind.

The brain which is the central organ of the body is connected with the mind. A high order of functional activities of the brain depends very much upon the state of the blood and its adequate circulation through the brain. The blood functions affect the cardiac, respiratory, alimentary, eliminative, endocrine and muscular functions. Physical culture, based on hathayoga, should be adopted for the normalization of the body as a whole.

Normalization of the eliminative functions of the body is an essential factor of blood purification and this creates a very favourable condition in the brain for its more perfect functioning. Some surplus materials tend to accumulate in the body during the course of time which do not contribute to its vital functions. This state is mainly due to a lack of vigorous blood circulation, consumption of foods in excess of the body's needs, and the bacterial unhealthfulness of the colon.

Fasting is a natural means of consumption and elimination of the accumulated materials. So, it is a very important factor in the purification of the body. By fasting, all the organs of the body are rested and become functionally more efficient. Moreover, the cells of the body are reenergized. However, knowledge of how to fast properly is very important.

Blood circulation should be accelerated above the normal resting level by muscular exercise. General muscular exercise serves this purpose. Automatic deep breathing exercise should be a part of the general exercise. Running at slow and moderate speeds, and swimming are excellent automatic deep breathing exercises. In growth-strength exercise, vigorous circulation takes place in the skeletal muscles. In constitutional exercise, circulation is increased in the skeletal muscles as well as in the vital organs.

Pranayamic breathing has special value, so it should be an important part of exercise. In pranayamic breathing, circulation is accelerated through the activities of the respiratory muscles and the big muscles of the body remain inactive. Under this condition, the increased circulation seems to produce better effects on the nervous system and the internal organs, as the muscular avidity for materials from the blood is less. It is our experience that circulation should be accelerated both by muscular exercise and pranayamic breathing in order to develop and maintain a high degree of efficiency of the nervous system and vital strength.

Kumbhaka (breath-suspension) is an essential part of pranayamic breathing. It produces a specific effect on brain functioning. By kumbhaka, a measured compression on the brain can be applied through compression on the ventricles of the brain and the subarachnoid space by causing an increased venous pressure of the brain. This compression arouses the vital activities of the nerve cells. In a prolonged kumbhaka, outwardly directed mental tendencies causing mental disturbances begin to be internalized, and an inner calmness develops. The practical aspect of the purificatory and vitalizing processes of physical culture can be briefly considered under the following five headings: purification, internal cleansing, diet, muscular exercise and pranayamic breathing.

Purification

Undertake a short fast. It cleanses the system, improves the power of digestion and absorption, gives the body a physiological rest and builds vitality. The duration of the fast is three days. The three-day-fast with colon washing will remove all the accumulated contents of the colon and make it clean and healthy.

First day of fasting.

After a normal evacuation of the bowels in the morning, take a glass (about 300–350 ml; 10 or 12 ozs) of lactose drink. This consists of a glass of warm water in which lactose (2 or 3 heaped table-spoons) has been mixed and flavoured with fresh lemon juice. Then rest for 30 minutes. Thereafter, water should be drunk in the following manner:

Drink a cup of warm water with a little lemon juice taken at intervals of 30 or 40 minutes for 3 hours. If there are free evacuations of the bowels during the water-drinking period or immediately afterwards, it is not necessary to cleanse the colon with water. Then take a bath and rest. During the resting period, a cup of cold water can be drunk now and then. But if there is no evacuation of the bowels, or evacuations are not satisfactory, then cleanse the colon thoroughly by autolavage. There should be three or four lavages. Then cleanse the stomach by gastric lavage (only once). Thereafter take a bath and rest. In the evening, take a glass of fresh orange juice.

Second day of fasting.

In the morning, start water-drinking (warm water with fresh lemon juice) for 3 hours as on the first day. Then colonic autolavage, bath and rest as before. Drink a glass of fresh orange juice in the evening.

Third day of fasting.

Same as second day.

On the fourth day, the fast should be broken. In the morning, perform colonic autolavage once. Then take a bath. Thereafter, take 250 ml (8 ozs) of fresh orange juice 4 times a day. Drink cool water as desired.

On the fifth day, take a milk diet, a milk-fruit diet, or a fruit-greens diet with some milk; continue the diet for 7 or 10 days. Thereafter, normal diet should be adopted.

This mode of purification can also be done as a yearly cleansing.

Internal Cleansing

The abridged yogic internal cleansing comprises oral cleansing, gastric autolavage, colonic autolavage, and pharyngonasal water bath. A special colonic exercise has also been described here.

Oral cleansing.

Clean the teeth with a fresh tooth-stick made of the semi-hard twig of some suitable plant, or a good toothbrush and toothpaste. Use a tonguescraper in cleansing the tongue. The thumb should be used in cleansing the palate. Plenty of water should be used in oral cleansing. The mouth should be well-rinsed. Oral cleansing should be done every day in the morning.

Gastric autolavage.

Drink 4 to 6 glasses of water and vomit it out. This gastric cleansing should be done when the stomach is empty. So, the best time for it is the morning, after oral cleansing. It can be done about once or twice a month, and during fasting.

Colonic autolavage.

Assume a squatting posture in a bathtub filled with water about navel-deep, or in a basin with water. Suck water into the colon through the rectum and get it into the caecum. Then evacuate the bowels. The temperature of the water should usually be lukewarm. For a thorough cleansing, suction, from three to four times, should be done in the morning when the stomach is empty. It is done during fasting. Suction is also done in the evening, after exercise and before dinner; this suction is usually done once. Thorough cleansing can be done once a week, or once a fortnight or every month. Evening suction can be done once or twice a week.

Care should be taken not to depend too much on colon washing. Colonic health and efficiency should be developed by exercise and diet. Washing is a supplementary means, but it is also necessary.

There is a special colonic exercise which is helpful in training the colon to evacuate completely. This exercise should be done in the morning when the stomach is empty and, if possible, after a normal evacuation of the bowels. Laxative foods should be added to the diet in varying proportions according to need. The technique is as follows.

First suck water through the rectum to reach only the lower half of the descending colon. Retain the water and then perform the following abdominal exercise in this order: (1) Nouli, from right to left, 15 to 30 times; (2) Nouli, rolling, 15 to 30 times; (3) Downward abdominal wave-motions, 15 to 30 times. Rest.

There may be an evacuation after this exercise; if not, do not worry. Practise this exercise either every day or on alternate days, until colonic efficiency is sufficiently developed.

There is also a suggestion-method which is helpful in making the colon evacuate normally. Suggest to your colon, with concentrated thought and with the belief that it will obey it, that it should function normally and effectively every day. Do it for a few minutes. It can be done any time. Mental calmness is very helpful for the evacuative function of the colon.

Pharyngonasal water bath.

Take a glassful of water. Draw the water through the nostrils and eject it through the mouth. The water should be lukewarm or cold (not too cold). Take about 450 ml (15 ozs) of water. This should be done every day in the morning, preferably after oral cleansing.

Diet

Prana as life-dynamism infuses its ojas (intrinsic force) into a suitable form of matter by which it is transformed into a living body. Ojas operates in the living body, as the basic life-force, and from it three fundamental principles of operation have come into being, by which the body is maintained as living matter, termed protoplasm. Brahmanic physiology does not accept that protoplasm itself is the life-substance but explains that life-force is not a part of matter. It is accepted as a subtle force capable of being infused into matter and making it life-like.

The cells of the body are not life-substance units, or life-minims. If it were so, then there would have been life in the atoms of which the cells are constituted; but there is no trace of life in them. Atreya says that the body and its different structures are composed of innumerable extremely minute and imperceptible constituents, that is, atoms. The atoms are the minima of matter and they maintain the entire material structure. Atoms maintain the material aspect of protoplasm, in which the life-force functions. This physiological dualism was the accepted theory in ancient Indian physiology.

The three principles, by which the body as a living organism is maintained are technically termed wayu, agni or pitta, and soma or kapha. Wayu is the principle of bioenergy. It operates in the body in relation to, and in cooperation with, agni and soma. Agni is the catabolic principle by which substances of the body are broken down to release energy to be utilized in the bodily functions. On the other hand, soma is the anabolic principle by which the broken down parts of the body are reconstructed and also new construction is effected. The anabolic processes require energy to function and this energy is released by the catabolic processes. The catabolic functions also require energy and that is connected with wayu.

Agni is in the nature of fire to which the oblation of substances in the body is naturally and constantly being offered owing to the influence of ojas. Bioenergy which remains latent in the tissues or substances in the body becomes available to the body as energy for motion and heat by the action of *agni*, that is, catabolism. The cellular, nervous and endocrine activities, and all other organic functions are carried out by activated bioenergy. The heat which is thus produced cannot be changed into any other forms of energy. Heat is necessary for the body. It is associated with all functional activities and it maintains the normal body temperature. The excess of heat is eliminated from the body by evaporation, convection and conduction.

The action of *agni*, at a certain point, causes a reaction in bioenergy which then tends to conserve the substances of the body and energy. This activates *soma* which exhibits its 'cooling' function. *Soma* utilizes the energy released by catabolism in its cooling process of synthesizing substances which become parts of the body. It is anabolism. All the processes which are going on in the body—the breaking down of substances and the release of energy on the one hand, and, on the other hand, conservation of substances and energy—are due to pranic *ojas*, and, consequently, they are pranic functions in the body and are technically termed pra*na*na, i.e., what is now known as metabolism.

There are a number of root substances or constituents of the body, which maintain its integrity. These substances are the main sites where the action of *ojas* as the vitalizing principle is more forceful. These substances have been termed dhatus. A dhatu is that which holds, maintains or contains the concentrated *ojas*. Ojas is in all parts of the body, but it is in greater concentration in dhatus. There are seven kinds of dhatus, viz., *rasa* (body-water), *rakta* (blood), mang*sa* (muscle), meda (fat), *asthi* (bone), ma*jja* (marrow) and shukra (gonadal substances). The degree of concentration of *ojas* in all dhatus is not the same. It is lowest in body-water, and highest in gonadal substances.

Dhatus are not exactly the tissues of the body. A tissue is a collection of similar cells and their intercellular substances, having a particular function. It is the basic anatomical and physiological component of the body. The basic tissues of the body have been classified as these: epithelium, connective tissue, skeletal tissue, muscular tissue and nervous tissue. Adipose tissue has been included in the connective tissue. The fluids of the body have not been included here. The fluids are blood, lymph and tissue fluids. Cartilage has been included in the skeletal tissue. The muscle tissue presents three forms: skeletal, cardiac and smooth.

On the other hand, r*asa* (colourless fluid) and blood are enumerated as two separate dhatus; fat has been taken as a dhatu; marrow and gonadal substances have been counted as two kinds of dhatus. It appears that marrow (ma*jja*) has been used here in a broader sense to include not only bone marrow but also marrow-like spinal cord and brain, that is, nerve tissue. So, practically all dhatus, except gonadal substances (shukr*a*), are tissues, and they function like a tissue.

R*asa* is the water content of the body. It is in all parts of the body. The water content is higher than solids. About 60 per cent of the body is water. The entire body water may be divided into two parts: intracellular and extracellular. The intracellular fluid is more than half of the total body water. The rest is the extracellular fluid which comprises interstitial fluid, lymph, plasma water, and fluids in the cartilage and bone (transcellular fluids).

The influence of *ojas* makes body-water a most important element in the body, and without it life-processes cannot function. First of all, substances which are catabolized to release energy, and substances which are anabolized for the conservation of body tissues and energy come from outside the body as foods. The natural foods need to be transformed into their simpler forms for absorption into blood. This is done in the alimentary canal. Digestion requires a certain amount of water in the stomach and small intestine. The main sources of water in the gastrointestinal tract during digestion are water which has been drunk, water-content of foods, and fluids secreted by the salivary and gastric glands, small intestine, pancreas and liver.

Now, purified and fluidiform basic food substances are absorbed through the intestinal mucosa into the blood plasma. In the plasma the blood cells are suspended. Since the plasma and the cells, in the form of a red fluid, are enclosed within the blood vessels, blood has been regarded as a distinct dhatu. Plasma is actually a part of the extracellular fluid. A continuous transference of the nutrients occurs from the blood plasma to the interstitial fluid in the capillaries, and then from the interstitial fluid to the intracellular fluid. This process also removes excretory substances from the cells to the extracellular fluid. So, we see that body-water (rasa) plays a most important role in prana*na* (metabolism). But this transport system is maintained by the blood movement throughout the body. The blood movement is principally maintained by the heart, and is assisted by the vascular smooth-muscle and skeletal muscular movements. Ojas is here in higher concentration. It is the red cells which carry oxygen to the cells.

The next higher dhatu is muscle. Muscle consists of cardiac, smooth and skeletal. Cardiac muscle has an inherent power to exhibit automatic rhythmic contraction which is utilized as a pump to maintain blood circulation. The level of circulation can be increased by muscular exercise. It is the skeletal muscles which can be willed to make movements. Muscular movements have far-reaching effects on the body. The entire organic system, including the nervous system, can be influenced favourably and its functions can be improved by muscular exercise. Muscular exercise comprises posture exercise, contraction-control exercise, growth-strength exercise and speed-endurance exercise. Smooth muscle is widely distributed in different organs. It is found in the alimentary canal, kidney, ureter, bladder, urethra, trachea, bronchus, and female and male sexual organs. The movements of smooth muscle are involuntary, but the skeletal muscular movements exercise a great influence on it. The oj*as* concentration in the muscles is high, and, consequently, muscle exhibits dynamic function by which every part of the body is influenced.

The next is fat. In the body, fat is found in three main forms: neutral fat (triglycerides), phospholipids and cholesterol. Phospholipids and cholesterol are integral parts of the cells. However, large quantities of fat are stored as neutral fat in the adipose tissue—the fat depot.

The fat-absorbing adipose tissue, which is the main part of med*a* dhatu, is able to take up excess fat, store it, and then release it when the body needs it. Another unusual function of fat is to form a thin sheath of subcutaneous fat over the skeletal muscles, which gives them a smooth appearance. Such fat-coated muscles, if rightly developed, are able to exhibit great strength and very strong contractive power, by which they are made to appear as hard as rock. These muscles can also be made to relax voluntarily to such an extent that they seem as soft as butter.

Then comes bone. It gives support and stability to the body and is involved in motion. The next is marrow. As bone marrow, it is the source of the red blood corpuscles. Marrow as brain is the fundamental control centre of the body, and it is the only organ which reacts in response to mental activities. Oj*as* is very active here.

Sexual Dynamism

Shukr*a* is the seventh dhatu, in which the concentration of ojas (life-force) is the greatest. Shukr*a* is, fundamentally, sexual energy, functioning in relation to, and as an essential part of, sexual secretions produced by the sexual glands of the female and male. Sexual secretions are both external and internal. This energy system is sexual dynamism, which creates the sexual urge involving emotions, thoughts and body. The urge is the continuous sexual impulse towards consummation by overcoming all obstructions. So, the desire for enjoyment, and the enjoyment itself, are not artificial but real. The desire is not a graft, but a part of blood-bone-muscle-mind. No amount of moralizing or philosophizing is helpful in nullifying the desire.

It has been suggested that if a large amount of energy is spent by doing heavy or long-continued muscular exercise, the strength of the urge may be decreased until it is almost dormant. There may be a temporary lack of desire due to an accumulation of a very large amount of fatigue-products in the system. But as soon as the body recuperates, sexual desire returns. In many cases even heavy exercise fails to suppress desire. Consequently, it is difficult to get rid of the 'horror of sex'. Prolonged mental work also does not help. Of course, it is possible to lessen its intensity by devotion to certain ideals with great fervour and attention. When the desire is quiescent, this diversion may afford temporary relief, but when it is ardent, the ideal is shattered.

It has been said that unusually intelligent and brilliant persons lead a sexually continent life. A few examples, which include Newton, Kant, Pascal, Carlyle, Leibniz and Beethoven, are given as demonstrations. But it has also been stated that these men were unbalanced and unhealthy. However, there have been also highly intellectual persons and even geniuses who have led a loose sexual life. The author was acquainted with a highly intelligent man who knew more than thirty oriental and occidental languages, but led a loose life and died prematurely. He also knew a talented musician who showed extraordinary ability in vocal music, but had very loose sexual morals. The effects on intelligence of conservation of sexual energy have not been clearly demonstrated, because it is very difficult to find a person with brilliant thoughts, leading a life in which the sex urge has been fully controlled.

Does great muscular strength require complete sexual control? Not a single strong man can be found who has led a life of complete sexual continence. During intensive physical training, some strong men stop entirely all sexual indulgence, as the champion wrestlers of India, or the boxing champions of the West, while others follow moderation. Anyhow, heavy training indicates the necessity of stopping completely or partially sexual wastages. There are also examples of strong men who led a loose sexual life.

Food has a great influence on sexual impulse. A well-balanced nutritious diet maintains sexual desire and vigour at a high level. The effects of milk or meat are practically the same. An exclusive milk diet does not cause a cessation of sexual desire. A lactovegetarian diet, an essentially herbivorous diet or a mixed diet—all have the same effects. A restricted diet does not affect sexual desire very much; in some cases it may be reduced.

An ascetic mode of life, with reduced diet and sleep and endurance of the rigours of the seasons, does not make desire impotent; in certain cases, it may reduce sexual desire. It has been said that a restricted protein diet decreases sexual desire. Evidence shows that a diet comprising rice, vegetables and some fish maintains strong sexual desire. Overeating stimulates sexual desire. Similarly, highly complicated and rich food has the same effect. A short fast does not decrease sexual desire, but a prolonged fast causes a decrease.

What do the yogis say about this question? First of all, let us investigate the mode of life they usually lead. We can classify the yogis into two groups: ordinary practitioners, and yoga masters. The yoga practitioners are advised to restrain sexual desire; and they try to do so as best they can. The net result is that they generally lead a well-controlled sex life in which all excesses have been abandoned, but complete control is rarely attained.

If we investigate the lives of yoga masters, we find that there are two categories: those who have led a partially controlled, and those who have led a completely controlled, sex life. Goutama Buddha, Chaitanya, Bhaskarananda and Ramakrishna were married. Buddha and Bhaskarananda each had one son in the earlier part of their lives, and thereafter led lives of complete control. On the other hand, though Chaitanya and Ramakrishna were married, they had no children, and there is reason to assume that they led a life of complete control.

Shankaracharya, Tailanga Swami, Bamakshepa and Lokanatha were unmarried and led a life of complete sexual control. These are a few examples. But there were, and still are, yogis advanced in yoga some of whom lead (and led) a partially controlled sex life, whereas others lead a fully controlled sex life.

Strict sexual control is necessary when practising advanced kumbhaka (breath-suspension). A pupil, who has prepared himself by undergoing a purificatory process and is mentally clean, experiences an inner reaction during the practice of kumbhaka, if he has had sexual intercourse. The reaction indicates that both cannot go together. There are some persons who are unable to abandon sexual indulgence completely, and, consequently, they have to give up the practice of kumbhaka.

At a lower level of concentration, complete sexual control is not indicated, but there must be moderation, never excess. At a higher level of concentration, full sexual control becomes automatic; it is naturally established.

In yoga, there are two most important processes of gaining voluntary control over the sex urge: wajroli and sahajoli. Wajroli control is extremely difficult, and it is only possible for advanced pupils to undertake it. However, when wajroli is mastered, the full control over orgasm and ejaculation in the male, and over orgasm and fully developed 'receptivity' in female is attained. The whole sexual process is completely under control.

Sahajoli is comparatively easier. A process of sense-withdrawal at different stages of contact, executed both passively and dynamically at exact points, is the fundamental part of sahajoli. A well-restrained indulgence at certain intervals is permitted during the first stages of the practice. The essential part of the process is to sublimate sexual energy in contact-control, in deep concentration. The amaroli process gives a pupil the necessary vigour which is required for the practice of sahajoli. It is essentially a chemical regulation of the body.

Functions of Food

Food is the fuel which keeps the metabolic fire burning in the body. Therefore, its nature and functions should be rightly understood. Food contains substances, the qualities of which are indicated by their specific flavours. Flavour is the expression of the taste quality belonging to ap-energy which becomes linked to the fluid aspect of the material body. So, the flavour which is in the fluid portion of food

is the indicator of the nature and quality of the substance contained in food. All foods can be classified according to their predominant flavours. There can be a mixture of flavours in a food, indicating that that food contains a mixture of substances. Sometimes a flavour may be masked owing to different combinations.

There are six original flavours: sweet, acid, saline, pungent, bitter and astringent. Consequently food can be classified into six groups. Foods belonging to the sweet-flavour group have these main qualities: (1) Bringhana, that is, substances which cause tissue repair and promote tissue growth. In modern terms, these substances are essentially proteins. In growth, fats and carbohydrates may also take part. Phospholipids are constituents of tissues. They are fats and are derived from food fats. Actual tissue growth, especially muscular growth, may accompany the fat accumulation. This accumulated fat is derived from food fats and carbohydrates. Carbohydrates and fats also play a part in growth by supplying enough energy needed by the body in various activities, thus sparing proteins. (2) Balya, that is, substances from which the release of energy for heat and action occurs. These effects are mainly due to the catabolism of carbohydrates and fats. Protein may also take part in the process, especially if sufficient quantities of carbohydrates and fats are not available. (3) Jiwaniya, that is, life-supporting substances. In modern terms they are vitamins. (4) Laxative.

Foods belonging to the acid-flavour group are appetizers, digestants, laxatives, blood-forming and energizers. These qualities indicate that these foods contain mineral elements. Saline-flavour foods have practically the same qualities. Pungent-flavour foods are appetizer, digestant, constipating and stimulating. They are helpful in counteracting obesity. Bitter-flavour foods are digestant. They purify blood and restore the natural relish for food. The astringent quality has many medicinal properties. It causes constipation.

Food Selection

Let us first take two nourishing foods—milk and meat, and make a careful observation of their nutritive qualities. Milk and meat both belong to the sweet-flavour food group. According to modern food science, these two foods are excellent protein foods, containing complete proteins.

Milk contains bringhana substances (proteins) which repair the tissues and promote their growth. Meat has the same qualities. Milk is strengthening (balya); it means that milk not only causes growth, but along with it, it increases power or vitality of the tissues. Milk also effects perfect repair and maintains or enhances vitality in the repaired tissues. This growth-vitality factor may be solely due to proteins or, more probably, proteins combined with sugar, fat, mineral elements and vitamins, or some unknown factors. However, the natural body-building materials of milk are highly effective and can support both growth and vitality. Meat also has the properties of increasing vitality associated with growth. Milk contains jiwaniya substances, that is, vitamins. Milk is very rich in riboflavin. Meat also contains vitamins. It has more thiamine and less riboflavin than milk.

Milk increases sexual vigour. Meat has the same property. So both milk and meat fuel sexual desire. Milk has certain special qualities. It causes an enhancement of ojas (life-force). It has properties which help to maintain youth and develop the natural immunity of the body. It is also laxative. It is specially valuable for children, old people, the sexually promiscuous and persons suffering from emaciation. It also increases mental energy.

On the other hand, meat is very suitable for construction and reconstruction of the body, and is very strengthening. It is also valuable in cases of emaciation. It is highly beneficial for those who do heavy muscular exercise. When the level of growth-impulse of the body is very low, and a rapid rate of growth is desired, milk is more suitable than meat. But when growth is accompanied by an increase in fat, meat is better in counteracting fat accumulation. When milk does not give satisfactory results in growth and development, meat should be tried, and vice versa. The best milk is the milk from young and healthy cows. The best meat is the flesh of the young and healthy goats.

From the above studies, either milk or meat may be taken as basal food in a diet. First, let us consider milk. The question which arises in this connection is: as milk is nutritionally a complete food and there are no other foods which alone can take its place, can it form the sole article in a normal diet, i.e., can milk as a mono-diet be a normal diet? The answer is, that a normal diet, which is a diet for every day should contain foods which have all flavour qualities in their right proportion, as a permanent balanced diet. So, milk alone, though an excellent food by itself, cannot serve this purpose. Milk diet is actually a rebuilding diet, indicated in cases where the level of vitality and functional efficiency of the body have been reduced to a subnormal level. When the growth impulse and vitality of the cells are very low, the alimentary, circulatory, glandular and eliminative functions are lowered, and the body is in a state of sub-health, and in many chronic affections, milk diet is excellent. It has a great therapeutic value. It is also a wonderful natural means of purifying the whole alimentary canal.

The next question is whether fruits added to milk, that is, a milk-fruit diet, can be made a normal diet. Milk-fruit diets are special diets, essentially having corrective and rebuilding effects. A carefully selected milk-fruit diet may be followed for a prolonged period, but still it needs to be supplemented by other suitable foods. Either sweet fruits, acid fruits or both can be used with milk. Ripe mango is essentially a sweet fruit. It is energy-giving, and it increases sexual vigour. It has also laxative effects. Ripe bananas are sweet fruits. They stimulate growth and increase energy and sexual vigour. Sweet grapes are essentially sweet-flavour fruits. They are highly nutritious, prevent physical decay, increase sexual vigour and are laxative. Dates are sweet fruits. They promote growth and strength, and increase sexual vigour. One or more kinds of fruit can be used in a milk-fruit diet; they can be eaten alone as fruit or may form part of a normal diet. It may be noted here that all sweet fruits increase sexual vigour and desire.

Ripe pineapple is a sweet-acid fruit. It gives energy and is laxative. Kamala (a kind of orange) is also a sweet-acid fruit which stimulates digestion and is laxative. Ripe pomegranates are either almost sweet or sweet-acid fruits. They give energy and increase digestive power and sexual vigour. These fruits and other acid fruits can be taken alone, or combined with milk and sweet fruits, or form part of a normal diet. They stimulate sexual vigour.

Milk is an excellent food, the basis of a normal diet. To such a normal diet, either rice or whole-wheat bread can be added. Rice and whole-wheat are sweet-flavour foods. They are nutritious, produce energy and increase sexual vigour. Rice is constipating, but whole-wheat is laxative. Some butter may be added to the cereal foods. Cow butter is the best. It is a sweet-acid-astringent-flavour food. It is strengthening and increases sexual vigour. It is slightly constipating. Various vegetables, including leaves, flowers, fruits, stalks and bulbs, should be added. And finally, both sweet and acid fruits should be added. This will make an ideal normal diet. Milk can sometimes be replaced by whole sour milk.

Meat can also be taken as the basis of a normal diet. In this connection, it can be noted that meat cannot be the sole article in a normal diet. The carnivorous animals live almost wholly on the flesh of other animals. But they not only eat muscle but also blood, organs and bones. This makes a difference. However, a man cannot be transformed into a carnivorous animal, nor is it desirable to make him truly carnivorous like the Eskimos. So, an exclusive meat diet is not a human diet. In a normal diet, meat can be a basic food, to which plenty of vegetables and fruit should be added. Whole sour milk can also be added with great advantage. Such a diet is nutritious and strengthening, and increases sexual vigour. Rice, or whole-wheat bread, and butter can be added to increase the nutritional value of the diet.

There is also a third possibility. Instead of making milk or meat a basic food in a diet, pulses (dal) can be taken as the chief articles. Pulses contain body-building substances (proteins), almost equal to meat, but they are inferior in quality. Therefore, milk or meat should be added to the pulses to raise their nutritional value. The pulses have a high percentage of energy-giving substances (mainly carbohydrate, but also some fat). Some pulses increase sexual vigour. Also, certain pulses are laxative, while others are constipating.

There are many kinds of pulses. The following are commonly used: mudga, or mug (Phaseolus Mungo), masha (Phaseolus Radiatus), chanaka (chick-pea), kalaya (dry pea), masura (lentil), adhaki (Cajanus Indicus Spreng), and triputa (vetch). To make the pulse diet more balanced and nutritious, add some rice or whole-wheat bread, butter, and liberal quantities of vegetables and fruit. Above all, some milk, whole sour milk or meat should be added to the diet to improve the qualities of the proteins.

In cooking pulses and vegetables, some spices can be used. They increase palatability and give a charming colour to the food. But excessive spices should never be used. The commonly used spices are: coriander seed, cummin seed, anis seed, turmeric, ginger, black pepper, fresh green pepper and salt. They are appetizing, digestant and have medicinal properties. Some of them are slightly stimulating. They improve the qualities of food.

Muscular Exercise

According to hathayoga, exercise is a complex muscular process in which the skeletal muscles either function dynamically when the level of bodily activities is raised to a desired, higher level, or statically when the body is statically maintained in a desired posture, or all muscular activities are voluntarily stopped. The dynamic function is purposeful, volitional and conscious, and contraction is graded to the full contraction point. The static function is associated with the development of vital endurance, and also the conservation of energy. It creates a state in which there is a physical submission to mental functions. The dynamic function is executed in a postural manner as well as in a free muscular way. Muscular exercise stimulates the growth and development of the body through the systematized movements of the fundamental musculature.

The following exercises are to be performed in the order indicated below.

1 Relaxation and Breathing. Assume the adamantine posture, that is, sit on the heels with the body erect. Now, relax the body by ceasing all physical efforts and strain, and by making the mind calm and passive. Mental passivity is to be attained slowly and in a calm attitude, avoiding mental strain. Patience is absolutely necessary. When you are fairly re- laxed, perform both nostrils breathing with slow and full inspiration and expiration, being fully conscious of breathing and without mental diversions. Maintain mental calmness through- out. Spend about 10 or 15 minutes doing these exercises.

2 Diaphragm Raise. Sit on heels. Draw inward and lift upward the front abdominal wall in expiratory breath-suspension as much as possible. Maintain it for a short time, then relax the abdomen and inspire. Repeat 50 to 100 times.

3 Quick Squat. Assume standing position. Do squatting with a short forward jump. Do this rapidly. Repeat 30 to 50 times.

4 Serpent Raise. Assume prone-lying posi- tion, with the palms at shoulder-width on the floor. Raise the body from the hips upward and backward as much as possible, inhaling. Lower the body, exhaling. Repeat 10 to 15 times.

5 Snake Raise. Assume prone-lying position with the hands clasped behind the back. Raise the body as high as possible from the hips, inhaling. Lower the body, exhaling. Repeat 10 to 15 times.

6 *Makara* Raise. Assume prone-lying position with the hands clasped behind the head. Raise the body as high as possible from the hips, inhaling. Lower the body, exhaling. Repeat 10 to 15 times.

7 Locust Raise. Assume prone-lying position

with the arms by the sides. Raise the legs from the hips as high as possible, inhaling. Lower the legs, exhaling. Repeat 10 to 15 times.

8 Bow. Assume prone-lying position and hold the ankles with the hands by bending the legs at the knees. Raise the body and thighs as high as possible, inhaling. Lower the body and thighs, exhaling. Repeat 10 to 15 times.

9 Spine-twist. Sit with the left heel set against the perineum, and the right knee vertical. Now, twist the body to the right by grasping the left knee with the left hand and the right ankle with the right hand behind the back. Maintain the position for one or two minutes. Then twist the body in a similar manner to the left side.

10 Lateral Body-bend. Assume standing posi- tion, with the legs far apart, hands clasped be- hind the head. Bend laterally to the right and touch the right knee with the head, exhaling. Go back to the original position, inhaling. Perform the movement on the left side. Repeat 6 to 12 times, each side.

11 Abdominal Raise. Assume supine-lying position, with the hands clasped behind the head. Raise the body slowly to a sitting position, exhaling. Lower the body to the original position, inhaling. Repeat 10 to 15 times.

12 Plough. Assume supine-lying position, with the arms by the sides. Raise the legs and the body to roll overhead to the floor, exhaling. Return to the original position, inhaling. The rolling movement can be done slowly as well as quickly. Repeat 10 to 15 times.

13 Lateral Abdominal Raise. Assume right side-lying position, with the right forearm locked behind the right side of the head. Now raise the head and trunk laterally as high as you can without twisting the body, exhaling. Return to the original position, inhaling. Do this on the left side. Repeat 6 to 12 times, each side.

14 Curling. Assume standing position, with the arms by the sides, the palms forward, the hands clenched. Contract the arm muscles fully and at the same time contract the latissimus muscles on both sides. Now bring the forearms, bending at the elbows, close to the shoulders without moving the upper arms. Then return

to the original position. Inhale when curling the hands and exhale when lowering them. Repeat 10 to 20 times.

15 Body Press. Assume the suspended, prone-lying position, supporting the body on the hands and feet. Press the body to full arms length, inhaling. Return to the original position, exhaling. This exercise can be done fairly slowly as well as quickly. Repeat 30 to 50 times.

16 Relaxation. Assume the supine-lying position, with the arms by the sides. Relax the whole body. Maintain for 5 minutes.

17 Stand-on-head. Make the body inversely perpendicular on the head, with interlocked forearms around the head. Maintain the position for 10 minutes.

The best time for these exercises is the late afternoon, 5 or 6 hours after lunch, and definitely before dinner. After exercise, take a short rest and then take a warm, cleansing bath to be immediately followed by a cold shower or a cold pouring. Then drink a glass of cold water.

Walking, running and swimming should be combined with the above exercises for the best results. The following is the schedule:

Monday	Exercise
Tuesday	Walking and running
Wednesday	Exercise
Thursday	Swimming
Friday	Exercise
Saturday	Long walk
Sunday	Rest

(For fuller details of exercise and associated factors, see the author's *Hathayoga*, published by L.N. Fowler, London, 1959; 2nd edn 1963, reprinted 1974.)

Pranayamic Breathing

The pranayamic breathing consists of five forms of breathing exercise. Their techniques and order are given below.

1 *Mahamudra* Breathing. Sit with the left heel set against the perineum, the right leg stretched forward and the hands placed on the right knee. Make both-nostrils, long-slow inspiration. At the end of the inspiration, suspend breath with chin-lock (by bending the head forward and setting the chin against the top of the sternum). Then bend the body forward along the line of the extended leg, hold the right toes with both hands, and maintain the head position midway. Now, count 6. Then return to the original position, place the hands on the knees and bring the head to its normal position. Now, make both-nostrils, long-slow expiration. Then perform the exercise on the other side, and, finally, with both legs extended forward. Repeat 3 to 5 times each side.

2 *Matsyendrasana* Breathing. Sit in spine-twist posture, with the head up. Make both-nostrils, long-slow inspiration. At the end of inspiration, suspend breath with chin-lock, and count 6. Then raise the head and make both-nostrils, long-slow expiration. Then perform the exercise on the other side. Repeat 3 to 5 times, each side.

3 *Bhujangasana* Breathing. Assume prone-lying position, with the palms on the floor at shoulder-width. Make serpent raise with both-nostrils, long-slow inspiration, suspend breath with chin-lock and count 6. Then return to the original position with both-nostrils long-slow expiration. Repeat 3 to 5 times.

4 *Bhastrika* Breathing. Assume lotus posture. Make short-quick expirations and inspirations, by using mainly the lungs and keeping the abdomen relaxed and motionless. Make 100 expulsions. Immediately after this do ujjayi breathing.

5 *Ujjayi* Breathing. Assume lotus posture. Make both-nostrils, long-slow inspiration, then breath-suspension with chin-lock, and finally, both-nostrils, long-slow expiration. This is one round. The relative measures of inspiration, suspension and expiration are 1–4–2. We are giving here three measures for the convenience of the pupils: 4–16–8, 8–32–16 and 16–64–32. Number of rounds, 3 to 12.

The best time for the practice of pranayamic breathing is the morning after evacuation of the bowels and oral cleansing. Pharyngonasal water bath should be done after oral cleansing and before pranayamic breathing. It is very useful to do pranayamic breathing before the practice of concentration. If concentration is practised both in the morning and evening, then, in the morning practice, do first breathing and then concentration, and in the evening practice do only concentration. Pranayamic breathing should be done once a day.

CHAPTER 14
Mental Purification and Rejuvenation

Mental qualities, though fundamentally mind-born, become involved in physical activities. The mental influence on the body is clearly seen in the ability to execute muscular movements correctly, effectively, and in a well-controlled manner. In the training of the body, intelligence, attention, co-ordination, accuracy, and other mental qualities are brought into play. Learning new and complicated movements and their correct and orderly performance requires attention, control and skill. All this indicates that physical excellence is closely associated with mind, and mind reacts by exhibiting certain of its qualities.

But how far is mind itself developed by physical culture? Mental qualities, which are brought into play by muscular movements, indicate that a certain aspect of the mind is influenced which has practical value in everyday life at the physical level. In the mental field, this physicomental development does not appear to much enhance these qualities, which form the core of mental life. It is true that mental energy which is involved in the development of a high order of mind, functions more effectively when it is supported by a vast amount of nerve energy the source of which is a healthy and vigorous body. So, physical culture has a place in mental development, but it is only a fraction. When mental qualities are released in the mental field by the mental energy function, they are forceful in their expressions, and are able to create mental dynamism which ultimately moulds the pattern of mental life.

Thoughts are replicas in known forms of an unknown mental reality which is the centre of the mental power system. In this power system mental energy flows and tends to be at maximal concentration point. At this point mental consciousness is highly focussed, and thereby the unknown reality is revealed. When it is revealed, it appears to be beyond mind. Thought is a mental function of replicating what has been revealed deep inside, and also all facts which are imaged in sense-consciousness.

In a more practical way, when thought is intimately associated with perception on the physical level, its force is scattered, and consciousness diversified. Now, thought becomes a 'mirror' of everyday life. Unless we are able to bring its force to a focus, thought will remain an open book of our lives. On its way to concentratedness, thought exhibits highly intellectual constructiveness. But as concentration increases its intellectuality is transformed into mono-form thought-consciousness which is very close to concentrated inner mental consciousness, and at a certain point, thought-concentration becomes real conscious concentration of mind.

Those mental qualities, which help to rouse the concentration factor in thought, are concentration qualities. There is a mental antagonism between the concentration qualities and those qualities which tend to decentralize thought-force. The mental practice is first directed towards the control of anticoncentration qualities. This is mental purification. Mental purification creates a mental state in which all qualities which interrupt and weaken concentration are in coil by the emergence of concentration qualities. When mental purity is established, thought-force begins to concenter.

The control process is frequently interrupted by the penetration of diversifying mental qualities. When mental character is sufficiently weakened, mind becomes fully externalized. Now consciousness is the playground of pride, arrogance, anger, harshness and other black qualities around the self which has been over-emphasized and is in a dark cloud of ignorance. Ignorance veils the spiritual light and under such a condition desires, hopes, sadness, fear, disgust, jealousy, disdain and delusion are released. Unless these impurities are cleaned out from the mind, thought-force is without strength, and without developing it to a high degree, concentration is not possible. Thought-force and concentration grow in that mental soil which has been nourished by restfulness, meditativeness, self-control, firmness, patience, magnanimity, mercy, fearlessness, truth, sincerity, cleanliness and energy.

Discipline

The first and foremost step towards mental purification and for the development of thought-force is the practice of tapasya—vigorous disciplining of the body and mind. An aspiring pupil must undertake it. There is no ease-comfort way.

The first step of mental purification is as follows: Be happy when you find that people around you are happy, and be really sorry when you find that they are sorry; that is, make the happiness and sorrow of others your own and feel in the same manner. Similarly, when you find that others are doing good things, be glad for it; but when you find that they are doing the wrong things, just isolate yourself from them. This practice will gradually cleanse your mind.

Start with the practice of disciplining your body and mind. First of all, subject your body to cold, heat, sun and rain; hunger and thirst; and lack of sleep. You have to carry endurance to the pain point. Train the body by vigorous

muscular exercise as well as in motionlessness. Certain appropriate postures can be selected for the practice of motionlessness carried to the pain point.

The most important part of mental control is the control of the sex urge. Sex urge has two main phases: the mental which consists of sexual thoughts and emotions, and the physical which includes all forms of sexual acts. Therefore, control has two parts: thought control and control of orgasm and ejaculation. Physical control is subordinate to mental control, but it is necessary.

The main point in mental control is to prevent sexual thought-emotions leading to action. It is possible and necessary to restrict thought-emotions, however intense they may be, to the mental field, without allowing them to exercise their influence on the sexual organs to the extent that causes volitional acts. The waves of intensified thought-emotions should be mentally endured. To do it in a systematic way practise this thought control process:

Assume either accomplished posture (siddhasana) or lotus posture (padmasana). Keep the whole body absolutely motionless. Now, endure mentally and resolutely the thrusts of intensified sexual desires. Continue this practice until the emotion evaporates. If it becomes very difficult to exercise control, then change the posture to spine-twist posture (matsyendrasana), and practise it as long as it is necessary. If it is still difficult, assume knee-heel posture (watayanasana) and do it. The posture should be continued beyond the pain point, and until the mind becomes calm.

When you have gained sufficient mental strength by the regular practice of enduring sexual desire, then start with the following thought process. It is indicated when very strong sexual desire arises in the mind. The process: Assume accomplished posture. Think deeply that sex-fire is burning in the muladhara. Then rouse apana-force, red in colour, lying in the muladhara, by concentrated thought in conjunction with anal contraction, and then get sex-fire absorbed into apana. Now, raise the apana along with sex energy through the sushumna upward to reach the wishuddha chakra, by deep thinking. Here lies the smoke-coloured udana-force. By deep thinking, transfer sexual energy to udana which will carry it to the indu chakra. Here, transform sexual energy to moon-coloured life-force which is located in the indu chakra. Patiently practise this process.

Mental Rejuvenation

Assume accomplished posture. Think deeply that moon-coloured life-force has been concentrated in the indu chakra. From this concentrated life-force lifeful radiations are being emitted. Then the life-energy gradually becomes condensed to form a perfect body, a body which is vital, vigorous, youthful, internally purified and diseaseless; the senses being calm; and mind shining, but perfectly tranquil.

It is better to practise this process in the morning after pranayamic breathing (see chapter 13). It can also be practised any time if you feel like doing it, omitting pranayamic breathing.

CHAPTER 15
Posture, Breath-control and Sense-withdrawal

The first thing in the practice of concentration is to arrange an appropriate room which is most suitable for the practice. The room should be in a secluded part of the house. It should be neither very big nor very small, nor too high, nor too low. It should be very clean; there must be no furniture or any other things. It should be kept well-ventilated and have free access to natural light. It must be completely free from bad odours. This room should not be used for any other purposes or by other persons.

The seat on which the practitioner will sit for concentration should be comfortable, but not too soft. A soft and thick blanket can be used as a seat, and if necessary it can be folded to get the desired thickness. It should be covered with a piece of washable clean white cloth. Under the blanket, a seat made of kusha grass (Poa cynosuroides) may be placed, if possible. The seat should be large enough for the practice. This seat is exclusively for the practitioner; no one else should be allowed to use it.

Before starting the practice, the room should be thoroughly ventilated by opening the doors and windows. Thereafter they should be closed. The atmosphere in the room must be calm. There must be no smell—good or otherwise—in the room. The practitioner's mouth should be completely tasteless and odourless, and his breath odourless. To keep them in that state, overeating should be strictly avoided, and odoriferous foods, viz., onions, garlics, etc. should be omitted. By making the room dark and by closing the eyes during the practice, sight impressions are eliminated. The room should be neither warm nor cold. This means that the practitioner should feel neither warm nor cold sensation. The neutralization of temperature is very important. There should be no air currents in the room, and the practitioner should not feel any air flow on his body. And above all, there should be no sound heard in the room. This is very difficult. But still an attempt should be made to get the room free from sounds as much as possible.

The Practice

Sit on your seat. Assume accomplished posture (siddhasana). Technique: sit with the left heel against the perineum; place the right leg on the left leg, the right heel pressing the abdomen. Care should be taken not to press the genitals. Place the hands with palms upward, the right on the left, in the lap, above the right foot. Keep the trunk straight. Assuming this posture, say the mantra Ong for a few minutes. Then be silent and calm.

Now, relax the whole body consciously. Any physical effort, or any tendency to make an effort should be abandoned by mental effortlessness—a definite mental passivity. It is difficult, but not impossible. It requires patience and time. 'Hurrying' should be strictly abandoned. To make yourself passive, you should not be active. Passivity should be developed in a strictly passive way. Otherwise, it will defeat its purpose. Try to feel that you are fully passive and in complete silence.

Then make your body as still as a mountain by deep thought. Your whole thought-consciousness will be wholly of 'mountain-like still body'. Continue this thinking sufficiently long. The secret of success lies here; being completely passive and perfectly motionless, think very deeply that your body is becoming as still as a mountain. This thought should go on continuously, without any interruption by any other thoughts even for a moment.

By continual practice, a stage will be reached when, automatically, the normal resting breath rate will begin to decrease to under 10 a minute, and gradually to 5, 4, 3, 2 a minute. After that, and by continued practice, the breath rate may be 1 a minute, or even less. However, somewhere, at the 3–2–1 level, an automatic sense-withdrawal may take place. In this state no sensory impressions are registered in consciousness. If there is difficulty in getting automatic sense-withdrawal even when the breathing goes down to 1 a minute, then practise the special thought-form, sense-withdrawal process which is as follows.

Assume accomplished posture (siddhasana). Now inspire slowly through both nostrils, and at the same time think deeply that extremely subtle lightning-like Kundalini has been roused, in the red triangle of the muladhara. At the end of inspiration, suspend breath with chin-lock, and think that the sense of smell has been absorbed completely into Kundalini; finally, expire slowly through both nostrils and think that you are now without the sense of smell. There is no measure for the breathing. Inspiration and expiration should be done slowly and carried out to the full extent, and suspension should be discontinued when there is a definite feeling of difficulty.

In this manner, the absorption by Kundalini of the sense of taste in swadhishthana, the sense of sight in the manipura, the sense of touch in the anahata, and the sense of hearing in the wishuddha should be made by deep thinking in combination with breathing. An inspiration, suspension and expiration make one round. There will be five rounds in this process. This practice will gradually develop the power of sense-withdrawal.

CHAPTER 16
Practice of Dharana

After automatic sense-withdrawal is established, dharana (holding-concentration) develops by itself in consciousness. When the principles of mahabhutas and tanmatras along with the sensory principles are controlled, a dewata (divine form) appears automatically in consciousness and is held there. But this automatic dharana is extremely difficult to achieve. Therefore, more simple thought-form dharana should first be practised.

The essential point in thought-form dharana is to hold a dewata in his (or her) own form in consciousness by deep thought. The dewata will occupy the whole consciousness, that is, the practitioner's whole consciousness is dewata, and nothing else. The holding power should be so strong that the dewata does not slip from consciousness at any time. The firm holding will make the dewata appear clear, shining, and lively. This stage should be maintained for approximately the same time as breath-suspension. Breath-suspension is the time when on prolongation difficulty is experienced in holding the breath any longer. By practice, the sense of breath-suspension time, without actually doing breath-suspension, is acquired. The breath-suspension time is equal to holding time in dharana. This is one unit of holding.

The Practice

Assume accomplished posture. First come to low breathing points: 4–3–2–1. At this stage,

consciousness is usually almost without sensory impressions. However, at this point commence the practice of dharana. Dharana comprises three forms and each form has several stages.

Dharana, First Form

Stage 1
Hold the deity Brahma in consciousness by deep thought. Think that Brahma is shining deep red in colour, preadolescent in appearance, seated in the lotus posture, having four faces, each with three eyes; four arms, holding a staff with his upper left hand, a sacred waterpot with his lower left hand and a rosary of rudraksha with his lower right hand; and making the gesture of dispelling fear with his upper right hand; he is clothed in the skin of a black antelope, and seated on a white swan. (See Plate 2, left top figure.) Make the picture vivid in consciousness and hold it for one unit of holding time, and then go to stage 2.

Stage 2
Hold the deity Wishnu in consciousness by deep thoughts. Wishnu is shining dark blue in colour, graceful and youthful, and clad in yellow raiment; he has four arms, and holds in his hands a conch, wheel, mace and lotus (flower); he is seated on garuda. (See Plate 5, left top figure.)

Stage 3
Hold the deity Rudra in consciousness by deep

thought. Rudra is vermilion-red in colour, three-eyed, two-armed, and the hands are in the attitudes of granting boons and dispelling fear; he is dressed in a tiger's skin and seated on a bull. (See Plate 8, left top figure.)

Stage 4

Hold the Deity *Isha* in consciousness by deep thought. *Isha* is shining white in colour, three-eyed, two-armed, making the gestures of dispelling fear and granting boons; he is in the lotus posture and clad in silken raiment. (See Plate 12, left top figure.)

Stage 5

Hold the Deity Sadashiwa as *Ardhanarishwara* (right half male and left half female form) in consciousness by deep thought. The right half of the body is male, white in colour, clad in tiger's skin, having five faces, with three eyes in each face; he has ten arms, holding a trident, a chisel, a sword, the thunderbolt, fire, the great snake, a bell, a goad and a noose, and making the gesture of dispelling fear. The left half of the body is female, golden in colour, clad in a beautiful dress. He is seated on the bull-lion. (See Plate 15, left top figure.)

To summarize

First, think deeply of the Deity Brahma (holding time = breath-suspension time).

Then, without thinking of anything else, pass directly from Brahma-thought to thinking about the Deity Wishnu; then the Deity Rudra; then the Deity *Isha*; and finally, the Deity Sadashiwa.

When the first form of dharana is well-established in thought, commence with the second form.

Dharana, Second Form

Stage 1

First think that the Deity Indra is seated on a white elephant. Indra is shining yellow in colour, four-armed, holding a thunderbolt in his upper right hand and making the gesture of dispelling

fear with his upper left hand; his lower two hands are in the concentration attitude. When the Indra-form is vivid in consciousness, hold it during the breath-suspension time.

Then think that young Brahma is seated in the lap of Indra. When the Brahma-form is vivid, hold it in consciousness during the breath-suspension time.

Then think of both Indra and Brahma (seated in Indra's lap) together, and hold them in consciousness during the breath-suspension time.

Next think that Power Dakini is seated in the lap of Brahma. Dakini is in the lotus posture, shining red in colour, three-eyed, four-armed, holding a trident, a sword, a skulled staff, and a drinking vessel; clad in black antelope's skin. Make the Dakini-form vivid and hold it in consciousness during the breath-suspension time.

Finally, all the three forms together should be thought of deeply and held in consciousness during the breath-suspension time. (See Plate 3.)

After this is done, start with stage 2.

Stage 2

Practise the three-levelled thought exactly as in the stage 1. First, think of the Deity Waruna in the lotus posture on a *makara*; he is shining white in colour, four-armed, holding the noose in one of his hands.

Then think of the Deity Wishnu in the lap of Waruna. Next think of the Power Rakini, seated in lotus posture, in the lap of Wishnu. Rakini is dark-blue in colour, three-eyed, four-armed, holding a trident, the thunderbolt, a blue lotus and a drum with her hands. Finally, think of the three forms at the same time. (See Plate 6.)

Stage 3

First think of the Deity Wahni, seated on a ram, fire-like red in colour, four-armed, holding a rudraksha rosary and a spear, and in the attitudes of granting boons and dispelling fear. In the lap of Wahni is seated the Deity Rudra. In the lap of Rudra the Power Lakini is seated in the lotus posture. Lakini is shining dark-blue in colour, dressed in yellow raiment, three-faced with three eyes in each face, four-armed, holding the thunderbolt and a spear, and making the gestures of granting boons and dispelling fear. Finally, think of the three forms together. (See Plate 9.)

Stage 4

First think of the Deity Wayu, seated in the lotus posture on a black antelope. Wayu is smoke-coloured, four-armed, holding a goad and making the gestures of granting boons and dispelling fear. In the lap of Wayu is seated the Deity Isha. In the lap of Isha the Power Kakini is seated in the lotus posture, clad in black raiment, shining yellow in colour, three-eyed, four-armed, holding a noose and a skull, and making the gestures of granting boons and dispelling fear. Finally, think of the three forms together. (See Plate 13.)

Stage 5

First think of the Deity Akasha, shining white in colour, seated in the lotus posture on a white elephant. Akasha is four-armed, holds a noose and a goad, and is making the gestures of granting boons and dispelling fear. In the lap of Akasha is the Deity Sadashiwa as Ardhanarishwara. In the lap of Sadashiwa is the Power Shakini. Shakini is in the lotus posture, dressed in yellow raiment, shining white in colour, five-faced with three eyes in each face, four-armed, holding a bow and arrow, a noose and a goad in her hands. Finally, think of the three forms together. (See Plate 16.)

To summarize

First, think deeply of Indra-Brahma-Dakini; then, Waruna-Wishnu-Rakini; then, Wahni-Rudra-Lakini; then, again, Wayu-Isha-Kakini; and finally, Akasha-Sadashiwa-Shakini.

Dharana, Third Form

When the second form of dharana is well-established in thought, commence the third form.

Stage 1

Think deeply of the Deity Parashiwa alone. Parashiwa is crystal-white in colour, seated in the lotus posture, three-eyed, and making the gestures of granting boons and dispelling fear. Thinking should not be interrupted after breath-suspension time, but all efforts should be made to continue the thought-form un-interruptedly up to 2, 3, 4 or more breath-suspension times. In this way dharana is lengthened. (See Plate 20, male figure.)

When you are fairly established in it, proceed to the second stage.

Stage 2

Think of Power Siddha Kali alone. Siddha Kali is dark blue in colour, three-eyed, four-armed, holding a sword and a head, and assumes the attitudes of dispelling fear and granting boons. (See Plate 20, female figure.)

When this thought-form is clear and prolonged, commence with the third stage.

Stage 3

Think deeply that Power Siddha Kali is being absorbed into the Deity Parashiwa, and finally, they unite in the form of Parashiwa. Think of Parashiwa and his Power as one and the same. Try to prolong this thought without any interruption. This is the process of the prolongation of dharana. When it is sufficiently prolonged, and there is adequate control of the thought, the practitioner is fit for the practice of thought-form dhyana.

CHAPTER 17

Practice of Dhyana

In the practice of thought-form dhyana, thought of Kundalini is the essential point. Kundalini in her real nature is without any form and subtle. When thought is purified and made more powerful and concentrated by the practice of thought-form dharana in which a divine form is held in consciousness, dhyana of subtle Kundalini is possible. Kundalini should be considered as supremely subtle and conscious power by which everything which is non-kundalini is absorbed into her, and in this manner Brahman in its supreme and infinite aspect as Parama Shiwa is revealed. Kundali-power does not create the world, but absorbs the world and reveals Supreme Consciousness which, otherwise, remains hidden in 'cosmicity'. Kundalini herself is Supreme Consciousness when her power aspect is recoiled into That.

To be able to think of formless and subtle Kundalini, it is necessary to think that Kundalini is light-like and ·without a definite form. It is extremely difficult to think of formless, splendorous Kundalini, but it will be possible by constant efforts.

Dhyana Process

Assume accomplished posture and reduce breathing to 4–3–2–1. At this calm moment, think deeply of Kundalini as fire-like in colour and brightness within the red-coloured triangle of the muladhara. Make the thought of Fire-Kundalini as deep as possible by its uninterrupted continuity, without any sense of time. When this thought is well established, then think that Fire-Kundalini is extending upwards through the brahma nadi and enters the swadhishthana. Here, make deep thought of Fire-Kundalini as has been done in the muladhara. Then again think that Fire-Kundalini is extending into the manipura where deep thinking should be done.

From the manipura, Fire-Kundalini extends into the anahata where she is transformed into sun-like splendorous Kundalini, termed Sun-Kundalini. Here, deep thought of Sun-Kundalini should be made.

Then think that Sun-Kundalini is extending upwards into the vishuddha chakra where deep thinking of Sun-Kundalini is to be made. Thereafter, think that Sun-Kundalini is passing upward into the ajña chakra, and there she is transformed into moon-like lustrous Kundalini, known as Moon-Kundalini. Here, deep thinking of Moon-Kundalini should be made. Then think that Moon-Kundalini passes into the nirwana chakra, and there deep thinking should be done.

Finally, think that Moon-Kundalini passes into the sahasrara chakra where she is transformed into spiritual consciousness-power, termed Turya-Kundalini. To be able to apprehend Turya-Kundalini and to form an extremely refined 'imprint' in consciousness, thought should be developed into a highly concentrated stage. Deep thinking of Turya-Kundalini should be made in the sahasrara. Thought should be converted into almost concentration, and gradually thought-form will automatically be transformed into real form in which Kundalini will appear as real Power-Consciousness, and finally as Supreme Consciousness.

If separate practices of thought-form dharana and dhyana appear more difficult, then the bhutashuddhi process can be undertaken. Bhutashuddhi is the special process of layayoga for developing actual concentration. But thought-form dharana and dhyana as pre-bhutashuddhi practices are extremely helpful and contribute much in making bhutashuddhi successful.

CHAPTER 18
Practice of Bhutashuddhi

Bhutashuddhi is a process which is executed by deep thinking. It is not an imaginary mode of thought, but it is an exact replication of events naturally occurring in kundaliniyoga. These events are rousing of Kundalini, the passing of roused Kundalini through the brahma nadi, the absorption of all principles lying within the chakras by Kundalini, and finally, the absorption of Kundalini herself into Supreme Shiwa in supreme yoga—mind-transcendent asamprajñata samadhi, which is attained through the process of samprajñata samadhi, occurring in the sahasrara at the amakala point.

A yogi who has been established in kundaliniyoga has full experiences of what happens in the various phases of this yoga process and is able to replicate all facts, in exact order, which normally take place in this yoga. In fact, bhutashuddhi is the replicated kundaliniyoga in thought. To be able to do kundaliniyoga, concentration in the forms of dharana and dhyana are the prerequisites. With the help of such a concentration Kundali-power is actually roused, and then she exhibits the absorptive power stage by stage when passing through the different chakras. The absorptive power develops absorptive concentration, which is advanced dhyana, culminating in samprajñata samadhi in time.

In the rousing of Kundalini, some hathayoga processes are helpful, especially when concentration has not been developed to a point of effectiveness. The full mobilization of concentrated bioenergy (wayu), subtle 'radiant' energy and subtle sound is absolutely necessary to effect a reaction in Kundali-power. But if there is a

diversion of these subtle energies, then they become less effective in the subtle field. The most concentrated forms of these energies are found in specific subtle sounds (mantras). These sounds are only operable in deep concentration. So, in deep concentration, Kundali-power responds to these sounds. If the depth of concentration is below the threshold, sounds will not produce the full effects.

The effectivity of the subtle sounds lies in the partial withdrawal from the body of the pranic forces by causing a reversed force-motion and making them concentrated to a sound-emitting point. The pranic withdrawal and concentration can be successfully done in deep concentration. Conversely, according to hathayoga, some special musculo-respiratory efforts exert a squeezing effect by which the pranic forces are forced into the subtle realm where they exhibit reversed motions. Apana force is essentially related to Kundali-power in the muladhara. It is more or less in a diffused state, because it is constantly penetrating into the body along with other pranic forces, to play its role in the vital functioning of the body.

The general field of operation of apana is the abdominal region. Specifically, the apanic activities extend to the pelvic and perineal regions. The abdominal, pelvic and perineal muscles and smooth muscles of the alimentary canal and sexual organs are involved in apanic actions. The locking process of hathayoga aims at producing a voluntary functional stasis for the withdrawal of pranic forces into their centres in the chakras. The apana withdrawal is effected by perineal and navel locks. The full actions of these two locks are exhibited when the tongue-lock, neck-lock and chest-lock are executed in conjunction with them, in right order and with right force. It is absolutely necessary to learn the lock process and its application directly from a guru.

The withdrawn apana becomes concentrated in the muladhara as kandarpa-energy which is 'seen' in concentration as a shining deep-red triangle. The kandarpa-energy, when roused by mantra, becomes more concentrated and its desire-enjoyment aspect is under control. If this energy at this point is loosened, then it becomes a strong desire for enjoyment and radiates into the pelvic apparatus to incite sexual functions. Yonimudra is a great help at this stage. Because it helps to arrest the downwardly directed force-motion by perineal lock, and especially, when it is strengthened by navel, chest, neck and tongue locks.

Yonimudra serves three purposes. At the first stage, it helps the withdrawal of apana from the body and its concentration in the muladhara. Second, it helps the mantra in rousing kandarpa-energy. Third, it helps to prevent the downward flow of apana.

A bija-mantra is the pranic force concentrated to a point when its sound-emitting power is exhibited. This is mantra. It operates in the subtle field, but is silent on the material plane. Mantra has replicated gross sound which is operable with right technique at the physical level, and it acts on the subtle mantra. This is called waikhari sound. Through the waikhari mantra the concentrated pranic force can be made to act on Kundali-power. The gross bija-mantra 'Yang' is utilized to rouse kandarpa-energy. By the mantra influence, this energy is roused and concentrated and made to 'knock' on Kundalini with full force. The deviation of the energy is prevented by the mantra and yoni-mudra. The mantra is done in left nostril inspiration to increase its potency.

Kandarpa-energy exhibits its full power when it is strengthened by a subtle radiant energy which is represented by the gross bija-mantra 'Rang'. The mantra is operated by deepened thought while inspiring through the right nostril.

When the mantras 'Yang' and 'Rang' are forcefully executed in concentrated thought, there are reactions in Kundalini. But still more powerful knocking is necessary. This is done by the application of a very powerful gross mantra 'Hung' done with breath-suspension in yonimudra. This mantra (called kurcha bija) causes the rousing of Kundali-power.

The whole process of rousing Kundalini is apanayama (apana-control), a special form of pranayama. It consists of yonimudra, left nostril inspiration with the mantra 'Yang', left nostril expiration without mantra, right nostril inspiration with the mantra 'Rang', right nostril expiration without mantra, both nostrils inspiration without mantra, breath-suspension with the mantra 'Hung', and both nostrils expiration without mantra.

Kundalini is that power which is neither material nor mental but matter-mind-transcendent in character. So, Kundali-power is unmanifested in the energy play at the physical level and in the mentation on the mental plane. So, this power appears as if 'sleeping' in the body and in consciousness when it is in a coiled state. This does not mean that this power is null. When consciousness is concentrated to single-pointedness Kundalini is caught in it. Kundalini then appears as supreme absorptive power by which anything which is not spiritual is withdrawn from consciousness and, finally, mental consciousness is absorbed into it. She appears then as Supreme Consciousness. It indicates that Kundalini is real power solely concerned in developing samadhi; so this power reveals Supreme Consciousness which she is. Kundalini exists supreme-consciously in all the chakras from the muladhara to the sahasrara, and beyond the sahasrara which is the realm of asamprajñata samadhi. Kundalini in the muladhara is within the yoni, termed kula, so she is called Kulakundalini. The yoni is a triangular process formed of kandarpa-energy where there is the possibility of concentrating apana and receiving subtle radiant energy and specific subtle sound power. It is only possible here to combine these forces in gross mantra form with apana and create a formidable effective power to knock at Kundalini.

Kundalini as supreme being in supreme concentration lies in the triangle of the muladhara. Mental consciousness at the sensory and intellective levels is unable to register any impression of Kundalini in such a state, so she appears latent, unmanifested and even nonexistent in our consciousness. But when consciousness is raised to the superconscious level by transforming it to a concentrating consciousness, the infinite and supreme Kundalini is apprehended as supremely subtle and lightning-like splendorous. This finiteness is not a being at the supreme level, but a transitional phenomenon occurring at the mental level. It is the 'seeing' of Kundalini through the mind. The rousing of Kundalini is actually a reflection of supreme Kundalini on the concentrated mental consciousness as an extremely subtle and shining being. This reflection is imaged in concentrated mental consciousness and is held firmly. This is automatic (and real) dharana—holding-concentration. By pranic withdrawal and concentration, consciousness is able to receive the 'light' of Kundalini superconsciously and to hold it firmly.

When the automatic dharana is established, the absorbing power of Kundalini, or the power from Kundalini causing the absorption of cosmic principles, manifests in mental consciousness which is in a state of dharana. The absorptive power manifests as absorptive concentration in mental consciousness.

Absorptive concentration functions in three ways: it causes an absorption of mahabhutas and tanmatras, dewatas and sensory principles, step by step, occurring in the lower five chakras. So, it is a process of pratyahara and dharana combined. Then, the absorption of chitta in which sensory objects are imaged, and buddhi which interprets things which have been perceived, occurs in the manas and indu chakras. Now, the possibilities of mental consciousness to divert from its concentratedness to perceptual and intellective multiformity become remote. Then, dharana is transformed into dhyana when Kundalini is experienced in the nirwana chakra. In other words, dharana develops into dhyana in the nirwana chakra. Thereafter, Kundalini rises up into the sahasrara chakra where dhyana is transformed into samprajñata samadhi (superconscious concentration) at the

ama-kala point. The concentration-light-knowledge develops in samadhi to its highest point, and as a result Kundalini is revealed in her almost supreme aspect. This realization is splendid by itself, and highest on the mental plane. Now, mental consciousness is only Kundalini.

Thereafter, the nirwana-kala point is reached when samadhi consciousness is absorbed and only Kundalini in her supreme form remains. Now, Kundalini becomes nirwana shakti—the power which exists after the complete absorption of everything except Kundalini. Then Kundalini is Supreme Bindu, then Supreme Nada, then Shiwa-shakti, then Sakala Shiwa, and finally Parama Shiwa. These are the stages of mind-transcendent supreme concentration—asamprajñata samadhi. This is the yoga which is attained through Kundalini, so it is called kundaliniyoga.

It takes a long time and hard practice to attain samadhi in the sahasrara. It takes still longer time and harder practice to get samadhi consciousness absorbed and Kundalini shining alone in her supreme aspect. So long as dhyana is not transformed into samadhi, the process in the sahasrara and beyond is to be done through dhyana. In this manner, dhyana gradually will be ripened into samadhi. It cannot be forced. Give enough time for the purification and rarefication of mental consciousness. Continual and regular practice is the secret of success. The Guru's help at this stage is indispensable.

When the withdrawal of apana and its reverse motion and concentration are not actually accomplished, that is, when apanayama is not effective, and mantras used in this connection are not forceful, the actual rousing of Kundalini, and consequently, the attainment of automatic dharana are not possible. All this indicates that yonimudra is weak, pranayama is not forceful, and concentration shallow. Under this condition, apana remains uncontrolled and mantra lifeless. Here, bhutashuddhi is indicated, and by its regular and systematic practice, a practitioner will acquire fitness for the practice of Kundaliniyoga.

The central point of bhutashuddhi is to centralize thought to a very high degree with a view to making it deep and forceful. This is what is called thought-concentration. This process consists in thinking a chosen objective image and trying to see it very clearly; then making the whole thought only of that object, by preventing any other thoughts and without allowing the contemplated thought to slip from consciousness. In other words, the objective image should be the whole thought, and full attention should be focussed on that. No intellectual functioning should participate in the thought. In this way the single thought form should be developed. By maintaining it steadily and unmixed, and by its uninterrupted continuance with the focussing of full attention on it, thought will be vivid and forceful, and by constant practice the monothought will be transformed into real concentration.

Now, let us take up bhutashuddhi. Before undertaking the practice the chakra system should be very carefully studied, memorized and contemplated on. (See Chapters 10–11.)

Another very important thing is to create a condition of the body—an ideal physical condition—for the successful practice of bhutashuddhi. This ideal condition is the physical excellence in which the following signs are manifested:

1 A complete elimination of a coated tongue, bad mouth odour, bad breath and unpleasant body odour.
2 Natural, regular, and complete evacuation of the bowels in two or three motions a day.
3 Good sleep.
4 A feeling of strength and joyousness.

This physical state is the result of regular and uninterrupted practice of right exercise, pranayamic breathing, right diet and internal cleansing.

Bhutashuddhi Process

Bhutashuddhi comprises a series of practices to be done in the right order. The best time for its practice is the morning. But if it is not possible to do it in the morning, the next best time is the evening, before dinner. The following is the order of the practices.

1 After getting up in the morning, do oral cleansing and pharyngonasal water bath; then drink a cup of cool water. Normal evacuation of the bowels may occur either before or after oral cleansing. Then take a bath.

2 Passive Invigoration. Assume accomplished posture (siddhasana) with the hands in the lap, palms up and the right on the left. Relax and be calm.

Now, think deeply that Guru, moon-white in colour, with his Power on his left side and red in colour, lies in the guru chakra. From them are flowing streams of death-conquering subtle substance of red colour by which you are bathed and you have become lifeful and powerful; you have no disease, no senility, no sorrow, but abundance of life and joy. All these should be done in deep thinking.

3 Active invigoration. Sit with the right leg extended forward, the perineum pressed with the left heel, and the hands placed on the right knee.

Now, inspire slowly and fully with both nostrils, and at the end of inspiration suspend the breath with chin-lock. Then bend the body forward and halfway downward, hold the toes of the right leg with both hands, and maintain this position until you are able to suspend the breath without much difficulty. Then bring the body to the original position and place the hands on the right knee as before, release the chin-lock and expire slowly and completely. Do it on the other side.

Contract the arms during inspiration and maintain the contraction during the suspension. Retract the abdomen during expiration, and at the end of expiration relax the arms and the abdomen.

Thereafter, place the right foot on the left one, with the hands in the lap, palms upward, and the right hand on the left. Now, inspire slowly and fully with both nostrils, and at the same time contract the anus, and then press gently the lower part of the abdomen near the genital region with the sides of the hands. At the end of inspiration, suspend the breath with chin-lock and at the same time make an inward abdominal pressure to a moderate degree, maintaining anal contraction. Suspend as long as you can without much difficulty. Then raise the head and expire slowly and fully and at the same time make abdominal retraction. At the end of expiration, relax the anus and the abdomen.

Finally, staying in the same position, inspire with anal contraction; then suspend the breath with chin-lock and make abdominal retraction, and then make sideward hip movements; then stop hip movements and expire and relax the anus and the abdomen.

4 Kapalabhati (abdominal short-quick) breathing. Assume the lotus posture (padmasana). First, expire quickly through both nostrils with the slight retraction of the front abdominal wall. Expiration should be immediately followed by a quick and passive inspiration through both nostrils with the relaxation of the abdomen. In this manner, quick expirations and inspirations should continue until the desired number is reached. The effective rate of expulsion is from 100 to 300 times a minute. Do 200 to 300 expulsions.

5 Hangsah (breath-reduction) breathing. Assume the accomplished posture (siddhasana). Now reduce the normal breathing rate to 4–3–2 a minute by relaxation and passivity of the body and tranquilization of the mind. It may take from 15 to 20 minutes or more. However, time will be shortened by regular practice. At a certain point the externalization of the mind will stop. This is the moment to start with bhutashuddhi proper.

6 Thought-concentration on Kundalini. The first part of bhutashuddhi is the thought-concentration on Kundalini in the muladhara. Sitting in the accomplished posture with the hands in your lap, think deeply that within the shining deep-red triangle in the muladhara is Swayambhu-linga as a shining deep red or black line, around which lies Kundalini in 3½ coils. Kundalini is supremely subtle, that is, it is extremely difficult to produce an impression of Kundalini in thought. Therefore, it is advisable to think of Kundalini as lightning-like splendorous, and appearing around the Swayambhu-linga line. The line should be gradually reduced to a point by deeper thought. At this stage

thought is centralized to the extent that it becomes possible to image Kundalini in thought as lightning-like splendorous conscious power.

Then, (7) thought-concentration on Jiwatman (being with I-principle). Think deeply that your being-consciousness as 'I' is like a motionless flame of a lamp, situated in the pericarp of the anahata chakra. Then bring the 'I' to the muladhara and unite it with Kundalini by thinking.

Then, (8) Kundalini-rousing. Inspire slowly and fully through the left nostril and at the same time think deeply of the mantra 'Yang' during the whole time of inspiration. At the end of inspiration, expire through the left nostril slowly and completely, and at the same time think deeply that kandarpa-energy is stimulated and concentrated in the muladhara triangle by the power of the mantra 'Yang', and the concentrated energy is knocking at Kundalini.

Then, inspire through the right nostril and at the same time think deeply of the mantra 'Rang'. At the end of inspiration expire through the right nostril and at the same time think that subtle fire from the mantra 'Rang' has been kindled in the muladhara triangle and that both kandarpa-energy and fire are focussed on Kundalini.

Then, inspire through both nostrils and at the same time think deeply that the combined apana and fire actions have produced so much heat that Kundalini is heated and agitated by it. Then, suspend breath with chin-lock, and at the same time contract the anus and mentally say the power-mantra 'Hung' and think deeply that Kundalini has been roused by the combined actions of apana, fire and the mantra 'Hung'.

Thereafter think that the 'earth'-principle ('earth'-mahabhuta and smell-tanmatra), the Deity Brahma, Power Dakini, and smell-principle—all have been absorbed into Kundalini.

Then, (9) Kundalini Conduction. Then, bring Kundalini from the muladhara to the swadhishthana by saying mentally the mantra 'Hangsah' in deep thinking. Then think that the 'water'-principle ('water'-mahabhuta and taste-tanmatra), the Deity Wishnu, Power Rakini and taste-principle are absorbed into Kundalini.

Then, bring Kundalini to the manipura by the

mantra 'Hangsah' in deep thinking. Here, the 'fire'-principle ('fire'-mahabhuta and sight-tanmatra), the Deity Rudra, Power Lakini, and sight-principle are absorbed into Kundalini by deep thinking.

Then, Kundalini is brought to the anahata in a similar manner, and the 'air'-principle ('air'-mahabhuta and touch-tanmatra), the Deity Isha, Power Kakini, and touch-principle are caused to be absorbed here by deep thinking.

Then, Kundalini is brought to the wishuddha where the 'void' (akasha)-principle ('void'-mahabhuta and sound-tanmatra), the Deity Sadashiwa, Power Shakini, and sound-principle are absorbed into Kundalini by deep thinking.

At this stage try to feel that you are at a point where the senses are no longer operating; think that you are without senses, and are in Kundalini.

Then, bring Kundalini to the talu chakra and rest there for some time, thinking that you are immersed in nectarous (having only life) fluid. Then, (10) Kundalini in Ajña System. Bring Kundalini to the ajña chakra where Power Hakini is absorbed into Kundalini by thinking.

Then, bring Kundalini to the manas chakra, and get chitta (sense-consciousness) absorbed into her; and then bring her to the indu chakra and get the Deity Parashiwa, Power Siddhakali, and buddhi (intellective mind) absorbed into Kundalini by deep thinking.

Then, bring Kundalini to the nirwana chakra. Here think deeply of Kundalini as the sole object, and that there is nothing but Kundalini.

Then, (11) Kundalini in Sahasrara. Bring Kundalini to the ama-kala point in the sahasrara and try to think of Kundalini as deep as possible. Then, at the nirwana-kala point get dhi (concentrative mind) and ahang (I-ness) absorbed into Kundalini; and then 'feel' by deep thinking that there is no mind-consciousness in any form, but only Kundalini remains. Now, Kundalini as Nirwana Shakti—the all absorbing power—remains alone.

Then, (12) Kundalini beyond Sahasrara. Now, Kundalini as supreme power is in $3\frac{1}{2}$ coils: the first coil at Supreme Bindu, the second coil at Supreme Nada, the third coil at the Shakti principle, and the half coil at Sakala Shiwa.

Then Kundalini begins to uncoil step by step, and absorbs Bindu, Nada, Shakti and Sakala Shiwa. Now, Kundalini is in her supreme aspect and only being. Then she becomes united with Parama Shiwa and fully absorbed into him, and becomes one and the same with him, in very deep thinking. Then think that you have become all life by the nectarous flow arising from the Shiwa-Shakti union in absorptive thought.

Then, (13) Pranayamic Purification. This purificatory process is to purify the subtle body (pranic and mental) as well as the physical body. The process consists of sahita breathing, mantras and thoughts. The relative measure of the breathing is 16–64–32.

Inspire slowly through the left nostril for 16 counts which are made by saying mentally the mantra 'Yang'; during inspiration say mentally 'Yang' 16 times, and at the same time think that 'Yang' is smoke-coloured and has the drying power. At the end of inspiration, suspend the breath with chin-lock for 64 counts by saying mentally the mantra 'Yang', and at the same time think that the body is being dried by the power of the mantra. Then expire slowly through right nostril by saying mentally the mantra 'Yang' 32 times, and at the same time think that the body has been dried.

Then, without stopping, inspire slowly through the right nostril by saying mentally the mantra 'Rang' 16 times, and at the same time think that 'Rang' is deep red in colour and has burning power. At the end of inspiration, suspend the breath with chin-lock by saying mentally the mantra 'Rang' 64 times, and at the same time think that the impurities of the body have been completely burnt by the power of 'Rang'. Then expire slowly through the left nostril by saying mentally 'Rang' 32 times and at the same time think that the impurities in the form of ashes are being eliminated from the body.

Then, without stopping, inspire slowly through the left nostril by saying mentally the mantra 'Thang' 16 times, and at the same time think that 'Thang' is moon-white in colour and by the power of the mantra, nectarous fluid is flowing from the moon-sphere in the indu chakra. At the end of inspiration, suspend the breath with chin-lock for 64 counts by saying mentally the mantra 'Wang' 64 times, and at the same time think that 'Wang' is white in colour, and by its power the nectarous life-substance is utilized in reconstructing the body as a new lifeful body. Then expire slowly through the right nostril by saying mentally the mantra 'Lang' 32 times, and at the same time think that 'Lang' is yellow in colour, and by its power the newly made body becomes strong and adamantine.

14 A Special Practice. This practice is especially meant for those practitioners who have been initiated and given the basic mantra (mulamantra).

After pranayamic purification, transform into Ishtadewata, by deep thinking and using the basic mantra, Shiwa-Shakti, that is, Parama Shiwa and Kundalini in union as one. Ishtadewata is the divine form of infinite Shiwa-Shakti roused by the power of the basic mantra. It can simply be said that Ishtadewata is the mantra-form of formless Shiwa-Shakti. The mantra is first made living, and then it is utilized for rousing Ishtadewata. So long as it is not possible to impart life to the mantra, it should be done by deep thinking.

Bring Ishtadewata to the sahasrara and think deeply of her (or his) form. Then open the hrit chakra by thinking. This chakra has eight golden petals where eight forms of superpower are situated. In its pericarp, there is a circular region as bright as the sun. Inside the sun-circle lies the moon-circle which is cool and calm. Inside the moon-circle is situated the fire-circle, where fire is burning and consuming everything except the gemmed seat which is there. This seat is your inner 'heart', the seat of deep feelings and inner power. Bring your Ishtadewata to the hrit chakra and place her (or him) on the heart-seat. Think that you are in the fire-circle, and everything—all your thoughts, feelings and desires—are being burnt by the fire. In this way being purified, you are in front of your Ishtadewata. Now, think deeply, without being deviated, but by focussing the whole thought, on Ishtadewata. This thought in time will lead to real concentration. This deep thinking may be done partly in conjunction with the mental use of the basic mantra. The thought should be saturated with the mantra

and centralized in Ishtadewata.

Thereafter, worship your Ishtadewata mentally by offering in the following manner:

Offer to Ishtadewata your body; then offer the 'earth'-principle, smell sense, enjoyment-action, and apana-force; then offer the 'water'-principle, taste-sense, organic actions, wyana-force; offer the 'fire'-principle, sight sense, locomotion, samana-force; offer the 'air'-principle, touch-sense, prehension, prana-force; offer the 'void'(akasha)-principle, sound-sense, speech, udana-force; offer sense-mind, intellective mind, I-ness.

Now, you can make japa of the basic mantra for 1008 times, or 508, or 108 times. Then bring Ishtadewata back to the sahasrara and from there to the infinite region by making her (or him) again transformed into Shiwa-Shakti.

15 Bringing back Kundalini to muladhara. Now think that Kundalini has emerged from Parama Shiwa and passes in a reversed way first to the sahasrara where samadhi consciousness is restored; then to the nirwana chakra where concentrative mind (dhi) is restored; then to the indu chakra where the Deity Parashiwa, Power Siddhakali, and intellective mind (buddhi) are restored; then to the manas chakra where sense-consciousness (chitta) is restored; then to the ajña chakra where Power Hakini is restored; then through the talu chakra to the wishuddha chakra where the 'void' (akasha)-principle, the Deity Sadashiwa, Power Shakini, and sound-principle are restored; then to the anahata chakra where the 'air'-principle, the Deity Isha, Power Kakini, and touch-principle are restored; then to the manipura chakra where 'fire'-principle, the Deity Rudra, Power Lakini, and sight-principle are restored; then to the swadhishthana chakra where the 'water'-principle, the Deity Wishnu, Power Rakini, and taste principle are restored; then to the muladhara chakra where the 'earth'-principle, the Deity Brahma, Power Dakini, and smell-principle are restored; and, finally, Kundalini encircles Swayambhu-linga in three and a half coils and becomes static. Thereafter, bring back I-ness (jiwatman) in the form of a still lamp flame from Kundalini to the anahata chakra. The bringing down of Kundalini and the restoration

of different principles, deities and powers are accomplished by deep thinking.

Bhutashuddhi ends here. At the end of the process, remain calm for some time.

Kundaliniyoga

In kundaliniyoga, Kundalini is actually roused and passes through all the chakras and becomes united with Parama Shiwa as one entity in supreme yoga, that is asamprajñata samadhi. Events that occur at different stages of the yoga are as follows:

First, rouse Kundalini by the mantra process of 'Yang'-'Rang'-'Hung' with yonimudra. The roused Kundalini manifests her great absorbing power, when she passes through the different chakras, which works in the consciousness of the practitioner, and as a result he (or she) is in a state of absorptive concentration which develops step by step as Kundalini passes through the chakras.

Roused Kundalini in the muladhara chakra absorbs the 'earth'-principle, the Deity Brahma, Power Dakini, and smell-principle. Because of this absorption, the practitioner's consciousness is being withdrawn from the smell impression. This is the first stage of absorptive concentration, occurring at the muladhara level.

Then Kundalini passes into the swadhishthana chakra and absorbs the 'water'-principle, the Deity Wishnu, Power Rakini, and taste-principle. This is the second stage of absorptive concentration in which the taste impression has been neutralized.

Then Kundalini passes into the manipura chakra and absorbs the 'fire'-principle, the Deity Rudra, Power Lakini, and sight-principle. This is the third stage of absorptive concentration in which consciousness is free from the sight impression as well as from smell and taste impressions.

Then Kundalini passes into the anahata chakra and absorbs the 'air'-principle, the Deity Isha, Power Kakini, and touch-principle. This is the fourth stage of absorptive concentration in which consciousness remains unaffected by touch, smell, taste, and sight impressions.

Then Kundalini passes into the wishuddha chakra and absorbs the 'void'-(akasha)-principle, the Deity Sadashiwa, Power Shakini, and sound-principle. This is the fifth stage of absorptive concentration in which the sound impression is neutralized. At this stage, the senses do not produce any impressions on consciousness, which is in absorptive concentration. So, there is an automatic pratyahara (sense-withdrawal).

Then Kundalini passes through the talu chakra into the ajña chakra and absorbs Power Hakini. Then Kundalini passes into the manas chakra and absorbs sense-consciousness (chitta); and then Kundalini passes into the indu chakra and absorbs Deity Parashiwa, Power Siddhakali, and intellective mind (buddhi). This is the sixth stage of absorptive concentration in which the perceptual and intellective functions of the mind cease. This means that mental consciousness is now actually elevated from the perceptive and intellective levels to the supramental level.

Then Kundalini passes into the nirwana chakra. Here, at first, automatic dharana occurs. Kundalini is held in consciousness so firmly and completely that there is no interruption, and so it continues. The uninterrupted continuation of the holding of Kundalini in consciousness at a certain point develops into very deep concentration, characterized by the uninterrupted, continuous deep flow of Kundalini-consciousness. This is dhyana. Now, the absorptive concentration is very deep, in which consciousness has been established in single-objectiveness. At this stage, the only object of consciousness is Kundalini; Kundalini fills the whole of consciousness; and Kundalini is held in consciousness so firmly that it is never without Kundalini, and so consciousness is wholly Kundalini.

When dhyana reaches a certain point, Kundalini passes into the sahasrara. Here, dhyana is transformed into samprajñata samadhi (superconscious concentration) in which consciousness is concentrated to a bindu (extremely concentrated point) which is all Kundalini, and without the feeling of I-ness. In this deepest concentration, there remains only Kundalini in her splendorous aspect. This is the seventh stage of absorptive concentration.

Thereafter, Kundalini absorbs samadhi consciousness and finally prakriti (the primary principle of mind and matter), and then there is nothing but Kundalini who, step by step, absorbs Supreme Bindu, Supreme Nada and Shakti, and ultimately becomes absorbed into Parama Shiwa in supreme yoga—asamprajñata samadhi.

This is kundaliniyoga, and bhutashuddhi is the foremost practice for its acquirement. At a certain point of its depth bhawana (thought) begins to be transformed into dharana and then dhyana. When the thought of Kundalini becomes intensely deep the image of the chakras appears automatically in consciousness. It is the sign that the time of the real rousing of Kundalini is near. When Kundalini is roused, bhutashuddhi is transformed into kundaliniyoga.

Note on the Pronunciation of Sanskrit Words and Mantras

The following is a key to the pronunciation of transliterated Sanskrit words and mantras (based on the Goswami method).

a	has the sound of o		in box
a	,, ,,	a	,, father
i	,, ,,	i	,, Italia (Italian) or almost as in 'bit' (English)
i	,, ,,	ee	,, see
u	,, ,,	u	,, Hund (German) or almost as in 'full' (English)
u	,, ,,	u	,, gut (German) or almost as 'oo' in 'moon' (English)
ri	,, ,,	ri	,, rivoluzione (Italian) or almost as in 'river' (English)
e	,, ,,	e	,, mehr (German) or as 'ay' in 'day' (Scottish pronunciation)
ai	,, ,,	oi	,, oil
o	,, ,,	o	,, hoch (German) or as 'oa' in 'coat' (Scottish pronunciation)
ou			is a diphthong, where the first part is pronounced as 'o' above, and the last part as 'u' in 'full'
k	,, ,,	k	,, sink
kh	,, ,,	kh	,, inkhorn
g	,, ,,	g	,, dog
gh	,, ,,	gh	,, log hut

ṅ	has the sound of ng		in king
ch	,, ,,	ch	,, catch
ch	,, ,,	chh	,, churchhill
j	,, ,,	j	,, job
jh	,, ,,	dgeh	,, hedgehog
ñ	,, ,,	ny	,, canyon
t	,, ,,	t	,, tie
th	,, ,,	th	,, anthill
d	,, ,,	d	,, dog
dh	,, ,,	dh	,, red-haired
n	,, ,,	rn	,, barn
t	,, ,,	t	,, vite (French) aspirated 't'
th			
d	,, ,,	d	,, dent (French) aspirated 'd'
dh			
n	,, ,,	n	,, noire (French)
p	,, ,,	p	,, map
ph	,, ,,	ph	,, haphasard
b	,, ,,	b	,, big
bh	,, ,,	bh	,, abhore
m	,, ,,	m	,, mother
y	,, ,,	y	,, yes
r	,, ,,	r	,, Roma (Italian) or Perth (Scottish pronunciation)
l	,, ,,	l	,, lettre (French) or almost as in 'letter' (English)
w	,, ,,	w	,, walk
sh	,, ,,	sh	,, shade
sh	,, ,,	sch	,, Schade (German)
s	,, ,,	s	,, see
h	,, ,,	h	,, hot
h	,, ,,	h	,, almost as in 'hot'
ng	,, ,,	ng	,, king
ng			gives a nasal tone to the preceding vowel

Glossary

Abalalaya The triangle situated in the pericarp of the guru chakra and formed by the three lines named A-line, Ka-line and Tha-line. In this triangle lies Kundalini.

Abhimana I-feeling.

Adhara The perineum.

Adhara-Shakti The power residing in the muladhara, that is, Kundalini.

Adhyatma-yoga Spiritual yoga.

Aditi Infinite Supreme Power as Supreme Consciousness, endowed with the specific power called prana.

Agarbha (or *Wigarbha*) Pranayama done without mantra and concentration (cf. Sagarbha).

Agni The catabolic principle of the body.

Ahang I-ness.

Ahara The Tantrika term for inspiration.

Ahingsa Love for all; harmlessness.

Akasha mahabhuta Void metamatter.

Amakala The power which maintains mental consciousness in a state of superconscious concentration (samprajñata samadhi).

Amrita Life-substance.

Amrita-warshana Shower of life-substance.

Ananda samadhi Superlove-concentration; superconcentration-in-divine-love.

Ananyabhakti Single-pointed, concentrated flow of love for God.

Antahkarana Mind in its entirety.

Antah-kumbhaka Inspiratory breath-suspension (cf. Bahya-kumbhaka).

Antahmanas Mind in its entirety.

Antaryaga Mental worship; specifically: the Tantrika process of concentration on Kundalini.

Ap mahabhuta Water metamatter.

Apana (or *Apanana*) Oupanishada terms for inspiration.

Apanana The centrifugal vital force-motion.

Apanayama A special form of pranayama for the control of apana-force.

Apasara The Tantrika term for expiration.

Arupa-dhyana Deep concentration without form.

Asamprajñata samadhi Non-mens concentration.

Asamprajñata yoga Non-mens supreme concentration.

Asana A posture in which the body is maintained motionless, which is necessary for the practice of pranayama and concentration; posture exercise in which the body undergoes various posture movements for physical development and control (especially prescribed in hathayoga). It constitutes the third stage of the eightfold yoga (ashtangayoga).

Ashabda Non-sound.

Ashtangayoga The eightfold yoga, consisting of eight main parts, viz.: yama, niyama, asana, pranayama, pratyahara, dharana, dhyana and samprajñata samadhi.

Awadhana Attention.

Bahyabhyantara-madhyama-kriya Externo-interno-median process, that is, the process of senso-mental control.

Bahya-kumbhaka Expiratory breath-suspension (cf. Antah-kumbhaka).

Bandha Control.

Bandhana Control.

Bhakti Spiritualized intense love; divine love.

Bhastra kumbhaka Thoracico-short-quick breath-control with suspension.

Bhastri Thoracico-short-quick breath-control.

Bhawa Feeling.

Bhawana Thought-concentration; thought.

Bhutashuddhi A process of deep thinking on those facts which actually happen in kundaliniyoga.

Bija Sound-specificity; sound-specificity-point.

Bija-mantra A highly concentrated power in sound-form, created by a particular combination of matrika-units.

Bindu   Immense Potential; supremely concentrated conscious power; consciousness-point; conscious form, as a deity.

Bindu-chakra   Sahasrara.

Bodha   Notion.

Brahma   Supreme Consciousness, manifesting creativity; God as creator.

Brahma nadi   See Brahmarandhra

Brahmacharya   Sexual control.

Brahmarandhra   The brahma nadi or brahmarandhra (nadi) inside the chitrini nadi; the terminal part of the brahma nadi where the sushumna nadi ends (in the cerebrum); the terminal part of sushumna; passage to the sahasrara centre; the brahmarandhra chakra, also termed the nirwana chakra.

Buddhi   Intellective mind.

Chakra   A subtle circular organization, containing mahabhuta, tanmatra, prana wayu and sensory principle, and situated within the body, not as a part of the material body but as a supra-material power-centre, only 'seen' in thought-concentration.

Chandra pranayama   Left-nostril inspiratory breath-control.

Chandra-danda   Brahma nadi.

Chandra-mandala   Indu chakra.

Charana   A system of skeletal muscular contraction and control; muscular control.

Chikirsha   Volition.

Chitrini   The third inner force-motion-line within the sushumna, in which the chakras are strung.

Chitta   Sense-consciousness; perceptive mind.

Chittakshaya   Absorption of sense-consciousness.

Dahana   Burning.

Daiwa manas   Supernormal mind.

Daiwa prana   Supernormal life-force.

Dewata   Supreme Consciousness-Power in form; deity.

Dharana   Holding-concentration, constituting the 6th stage of the eight-fold yoga (ashtangayoga); the Tantrika term for breath-suspension.

Dhatu   A basic constituent of the body.

Dhi   Concentrative mind; superconsciousness.

Dhyana   Deep concentration, constituting the seventh stage of the eight-fold yoga (ashtangayoga).

Drishti   Insight; intellective vision.

Dwadashantabrahmarandhra   Nirwana chakra.

Ekadhanawarodhana   Bio-energy control.

Ekatanata   Unchanging and uninterrupted, deeply concentrated consciousness.

Gunas   The three primary attributes.

Hridaya   The nonconscious aspect of mind, where post-conscious impressions are stored.

Hridayañjali mudra   A mode of aligning hands and fingers to make them hollow.

Ida and Pingala   The two vital force-motion lines or directions, situated on the left and right side of the vertebral column respectively.

Indriya aharana   Pratyahara; sense-withdrawal; sensory control.

Indriya manas   Sense-mind.

Indriya sangharana   The same as Indriya aharana.

Indriya sanniwesha   The same as Indriya aharana.

Indriya-yama   The same as Indriya aharana.

Ishtadewata   A divine form linked to a particular mantra. When the mantra is made living by japa and concentration, that divine form appears and is 'seen' in concentration. Also: the thought-form of Shiwa-shakti as an object of concentration.

Ishwara   The Supreme Consciousness in whom both yoga-power and pranic energy are in harmony, but who has full control over prana and has power to transform prana into mind-body.

Jalandhara   Chin-lock.

Japa   Mantra-practice, that is, the repetition of a mantra (a particular sound-form), verbally, in a low voice or mentally.

Jiwa   The embodied being.

Jñanatman   Sense-consciousness and intellect; perceptive mind; perceptive consciousness; chitta.

Jñanendriyas   Senses.

Kala   Time principle.

Kala   Life principle.

Kama   Desire.

Kamakala   Coiled creative omnipotency in sound-form; the principle of the actualization of the power as sound in a triangular process; an aspect of the supremely concentrated prana as bindu power, endowed with the capacity of transforming pranic force into pranawa, which releases fifty mantra-sound units as matrika and from which the universe of mind-matter comes into being.

Kama-wayu   Desire-radiating power.

Kañchupas   The powers of limitation which arise from maya.

Kanda-mula (or kanda)   Force-concentration centre from which all nadis originate; an oval-shaped, subtle, central nadi-root from which all nadis originate and which is situated inside the coccyx, just below the muladhara.

Kanda-sthana   An oval-shaped subtle space in the perineal region having a twelve-petalled centre.

Karana-samaharana Pratyahara; sense-withdrawal; sensory control.

Karmendriyas Conative faculties.

Kewala Non-inspiratory-non-expiratory suspension.

Kewala kumbhaka Automatic breath-suspension caused by pranayamic breathing and deep concentration; non-inspiratory-non-expiratory suspension.

Khechari mudra An advanced control exercise, by which a latent form of existence is achieved.

Kratu Conative impulse.

Kriti Conation.

Kula Kundalini; the muladhara chakra.

Kulakundalini Kundalini, when in the muladhara centre.

Kumbhaka Breath-suspension.

Kundalini Power-Consciousness dormant at the senso-intellective levels of consciousness, but realizable at the superconscious level.

Kundalini-kapata Door of Kundalini, that is, the entrance to sushumna.

Kundalirandhra-kanda Wajra nadi.

Kundali-sthana The seat of Kundalini in latent form, that is, in the muladhara centre.

Laya Deep absorptive concentration.

Layakriya Absorption process; absorptive concentration.

Linga-form A form which is thicker at its base and gradually tapers to become a point at its apex. Concentration starts at the base and gradually, as it becomes deeper, it automatically passes towards the apex, where concentration is the deepest. So the linga-form is an appropriate form for the development of concentration.

Madhyama Subliminal.

Mahabhuta Metamatter. It is that aspect of matter which lies beyond the boundary of elementary particles and anu-point.

Mahakulakundalini Mahakundalini, when residing in the muladhara centre as Kulakundalini.

Mahakundali Mahakundalini.

Mahakundalini Supreme Power in its supreme spiritual aspect.

Mahalaya Supreme absorptive concentration, leading to asamprajñata samadhi.

Mahan I-less supervast consciousness.

Mahan Manas Superconscious mind.

Mahanada-wayu Pranic force, exercising great control, which effects natural breath-suspension; suspensive power of great control.

Mahayoga Supreme yoga; the original yoga, consisting of eight fundamental practices, termed ashtangayoga; asamprajñata samadhi.

Manana Intellection.

Manas Will-mind; sense-mind; the sixth sense; subconscious mind; also mind as a whole—usually termed antahmanas or antahkarana—of which manas as sense-mind is a part.

Manas mandala Manas chakra.

Manas tattwa Principle of mind; mind as a whole.

Manas-nirodhana Sense-mind control.

Manasa-radiation Subconscious radiation.

Manasyana Will

Manasyana manas Will-mind.

Manisha Higher intellection; deeper thought-intellection; superintellect.

Mantra-chaitanya The process of life-impartation to a waikhari-mantra.

Mati Thought.

Matrika All the fifty particularized sound-forms together.

Matrika-unit A particular sound-form, which constitutes a lettered mantra and is used as a unit.

Matrika-warna Sound-units.

Maya The specific power of Supreme Power as negato-positivity, by which it is possible to manifest a limited phenomenon, such as the universe, in the unlimited sphere of Supreme Consciousness; negato-positivity.

Medha Retentive power.

Mitahara Moderation in eating.

Mudra Control exercise.

Mulabandha Anal-lock.

Mulamantra A special mantra given by the guru directly to a disciple in initiation; the basic mantra.

Nabhichakra A hen's-eggs-shaped plexus-like subtle centre from which all nadis originate and ramify in all directions.

Nada Causal or unmanifest sound; sound-radiating energy-point; sound-power.

Nadi That which is motional or in motion; a subtle line of direction along which the wayus move, that is, a pranic force-radiation-line. The nadis are no physical channels, neither nerves nor blood-vessels.

Nadi-chakra The nadi-system, i.e. the system formed by the subtle nadis, which originate from the nabhi-chakra and are distributed all over the body; force-motion field; force-field.

Nadi-kanda The subtle central aspect of the nadi-system.

Nadi-shodhana Pranic purification.

Nadi-shuddhi The purification of the subtle wayu (vital)-force operating as nadis, that is, force-motion lines.

Narayana   Supreme Consciousness, beyond creation; God in his supreme aspect.

Nigraha   Control.

Nirguna-dhyana   Deep concentration without any form.

Nirodha   Control.

Nirodhika   The power of supreme control.

Nirodhika-wahni   The power of supreme control exhibited by Kundalini.

Nirwana Shakti   All-absorbing Kundali-power.

Nirwanakala   The coiled power which is an aspect of Kundalini, exhibiting absorption-power.

Nirwikalpa samadhi   A synonym of asamprajñata samadhi, that is, non-mens concentration.

Nishkala   Having no manifestation of Shakti-Power; power absorbed in Shiwa.

Niyama   Observance—the second stage of control or discipline in the eightfold yoga (ashtangayoga).

Niyati   Regulatory principle.

Nyasa   A special method of purification by placing hands on certain parts of the body with appropriate mantras.

Ojas   The basic life-force. It is derived from prana as life-dynamism and, being infused into matter, transforms it into protoplasm.

Pañcha-dharana   Concentration, in conjunction with breath-suspension, on the earth, water, fire, air and void principles in stages, with their bija-mantras, in their appropriate centres.

Para   Supreme.

Parakundali   Supreme Power in its spiritual aspect; Supreme Kundali.

Parama kala   Supreme Kundalini.

Parama Shiwa   Supreme, infinite and whole Consciousness.

Parasharirawesha   A yogic process of entering into another's dead body to make it alive and functioning.

Pashchima-Linga   Swayambhu-Linga in the triangle of the muladhara centre. It is Supreme Consciousness in a specific form which shows the process of concentration.

Pashyanti   Radiant.

Pinda   Basic force of the body.

Pingala   See Ida.

Pitha-shakti   The holding, i.e. the holding-concentration power.

Plawana   Irradiation.

Prajñana   Superconcentratedness; superconsciousness.

Prakriti   The primary principle of force, mind and matter; primus.

Prana, Pranana   Oupanishada terms for expiration.

Prana-apana sangyama   Pranayama; breath-control.

Prana-mantra   Mantra in a vitalized form; a living mantra.

Pranana   The central vital force-motion; metabolism.

Pranawa-nada   The sound of the first mantra, Ong.

Prana-wayu(s)   The basic vital force exhibiting functions or motions; different forms of bio-energy.

Pranayama   A system of bio-energy control through short-quick and long-slow breathing and breath-suspension exercises.

Prithiwi mahabhuta   Earth metamatter.

Puraka   Inspiration.

Purusha   Primary consciousness principle.

Raga   Pleasure principle; love.

Ragatmika-bhakti   All-love.

Rajas   The primary energy-principle.

Rasa   The water content of the body, including intracellular fluid, interstitial fluid, lymph, plasma water, and fluids in the cartilage and bone.

Rechaka   Expiration.

Rodha   Control.

Ruchira   Oupanishada term for breath-suspension.

Rudra   Supreme Consciousness, manifesting the power of absorbing the creation; God who absorbs the universe.

Sagarbha   That form of pranayama in which mantra and concentration form parts.

Saguna-dhyana   Deep concentration on a form.

Sahaja state   Samadhi; superconcentration.

Sahita   Inspiratory-expiratory suspension.

Sakala Shiwa   Aroused power, remaining as the being of Shiwa.

Samadhi   Superconcentration.

Samanana   The equilibratory vital force-motion.

Samanya spanda   Basic infinitesimal motion, almost uniform in character.

Samata or Aikya   A state of oneness when the embodied spirit is absorbed into the Supreme Spirit to become one and the same with it.

Samprajñata samadhi   Superconscious concentration.

Samprajñata yoga   Superconscious concentration.

Sangjñana   Consciousness evoked by sensory impulses; the quality of chitta; sense-knowledge.

Sangskaras   Post-conscious and unconscious impressions.

Sangyama   Supercontrol.

Sangyoga   Superunion.

Saraswati-chalana   A process of muscular motion,

consisting of rolling movements of the rectus abdominis muscle from right to left and left to right repeatedly, while assuming the lotus posture and doing sahita suspension with chin-lock and anal-contraction. It is specially done for rousing Kundalini.

Sarupa-dhyana   Deep concentration on form.

Sarwabhawatmabhawana   Multiform consciousness.

Sarwa chitta   Multiform consciousness.

Sattwa   The primary sentience-principle.

Shabda tanmatra   Sound tanon.

Shabdabrahman   Kundalini as the source of sound.

Shakti-chakra   Power field.

Shaktichalana   A control process, consisting of the execution of anal-lock and abdomino-retraction in conjunction with the thoracico-short-quick breathing, while assuming the accomplished or adamantine posture. It helps in rousing Kundalini.

Shambhawa sthana   Indu chakra.

Shambhawi   A process of concentration by which the external seeing is transformed into an internal gazing.

Shankhini   Supreme Kundalini in the spiral form, lying above the sahasrara.

Shitali   Lingual breath-control.

Shiwa   Supreme Consciousness.

Shiwa-Shakti   A stage of non-mens concentration in which Shakti as yoga-power, lying in the being of Shiwa, is experienced.

Shoshana   Drying.

Shoucha   Cleanliness, consisting of external baths and internal lavage.

Shukra   The sexual energy which activates the sexual glands of the female and male to produce sexual secretions, both external and internal.

Siddha mantra   A mantra which is living and fully powerful and can accomplish the desired purpose.

Soma   The anabolic principle of the body.

Sthulakriya   A muscular control process.

Sukshmakriya   A breath-control process.

Supreme Bindu   Supreme power-concentration.

Surya kumbhaka   Right-nostril inspiratory breath-control.

Surya pranayama   Right-nostril inspiratory breath-control.

Suryabheda   Right-nostril breath-control.

Surya-mandala   Manas chakra.

Sushumnadhyanayoga   Concentration-on-centres-in-sushumna.

Sushumnadwara   The entrance to the sushumna nadi in the muladhara centre.

Sushumna-Kundali   The chitrini as power which

creates the inner-most void, termed brahma-randhra, through which Kundalini passes.

Swanana   Germ-mantra. Its abbreviated form is swanon.

Tamas   The primary inertia-principle.

Tanmatras   Concentrated sense forces, termed tanons.

Tanons   Tanmatras.

Tantrika   Relating to the Tantras; Tantric.

Tantrika yoga   An exposition by Shiwa (or Parwati) of Waidika yoga, in which various processes have been clearly explained and new ones incorporated, and which has been collected in the Tantras.

Tapas (or Tapasya)   Energizing process; static posture exercise to develop vital endurance and will power; ascesis; vigorous disciplining of body and mind.

Tejas mahabhuta   Fire metamatter.

Thought-concentration   Bhawana yoga.

Trikonashakti   Kundalini, when in the muladhara centre.

Trirasra   A triangle.

Udanana   The centripetal vital force-motion.

Uddiyana   Abdomino-retraction.

Udyana   The process of adamantine control and suction-power. (Also termed Udriyana.)

Ujjayi   Both-nostrils breath-control.

Unmani   Concentrated consciousness.

Wachaka-power of mantra   Kundalini in sound-form which appears as dewata by japa and concentration.

Wachya-power of Mantra   Mahakundalini as Supreme Consciousness, realized when con-centration on Kundalini as dewata is transformed into superconcentration.

Waidhi-bhakti   Ritualistic or devotional divine love.

Waidika   Relating to the Wedas; Vedic.

Waidika yoga   The original form of yoga, concealed in the Weda-mantras of the Sanghitas of the Weda in a contracted and highly technical Shrouta language, and explained and elaborated in the Upanishads.

Waikhari   Acoustic.

Waikhari-mantra   A mantra which is audible.

Wajra-kumbhaka   Adamantine suspension—a special form of breath-suspension for the conduc-tion of the roused Kundalini.

Wajroli   The adamantine control process of sex energy.

Warna   The specific power-line created by the operation of the force of a matrika-unit.

Wasana   The latent impression of feeling.

Wayu   That which exhibits constant motion; the motional or active state of pranic force.

Widya   Knowledge.

Wijñana   Intellection.

Wisarga   (1) The power-bridge, connecting the brahmarandhra with the guru chakra, through which Kundalini passes.
(2) That which separates sahasrara proper from Supreme Bindu.

Wishesha spanda   A particularized motion releasing a particularized sound.

Wishnu   Supreme Consciousness, manifesting the power of sustaining the creation; God as sustainer.

Writti   Mentimultiformity; an imaged consciousness; a knowledge-form; also a nonconscious form; an objective image.

Wyana, wyanana   Oupanishada terms for breath-suspension.

Wyanana   The diffused vital force-motion.

Wyayama   A controlled movement system to develop the body; physical education; muscular exercise.

Yajñastoma   The germ of power-manifestation which in Tantrika terms consists of Supreme Nada and Bindu.

Yama   Control; abstention—the first stage of control or discipline in the eightfold yoga (ashtangayoga).

Yoga-nidra   The state of non-mens supreme concentration; asamprajñata samadhi.

Yogasana   A posture in yoga; concentration posture.

Yoga-wibhuti   Omnipotency; great yoga-power.

Yojana   Union.

Yoni   The perineum; a triangle; a triangular-shaped region. (Also called kamakhya, kamarupa, kama and yonisthana.)

Bibliography

Weda

Rigwedasanghita

Upanishad

Adhyatmopanishad
Adwayatarakopanishad
Aitareyopanishad
Akshyupanishad
Amritanadopanishad
Annapurnopanishad
Atharwashikopanishad
Atmaprabodhopanishad
Brahmabindupanishad
Brahmawidyopanishad
Brahmopanishad
Brihadaranyakopanishad
Brihajjabalopanishad
Chandogyopanishad
Darshanopanishad
Dwayopanishad
Ganapatyupanishad
Gopalatapinyupanishad
Hangsopanishad
Ishopanishad
Kaiwalyopanishad·
Kathopanishad
Kenopanishad
Koushitakyupanishad
Kundikopanishad
Mahopanishad
Maitreyyupanishad
Mandalabrahmanopanishad

Mandukyopanishad
Muktikopanishad
Mundakopanishad
Nadabindupanishad
Narayanopanishad
Nirwanopanishad
Nrisinghatapanyupanishad
Paingalopanishad
Parabrahmopanishad
Pashupatabrahmopanishad
Prashnopanishad
Ramatapaniyopanishad
Sannyasopanishad
Shandilyopanishad
Shwetashwataropanishad
Sitopanishad
Soubhagyalakshmyupanishad
Subalopanishad
Taittiriya Aranyaka
Taittiriyopanishad
Tripadwibhutimahanarayanopanishad
Tripuratapinyupanishad
Trishikhibrahmanopanishad
Warahopanishad
Yogachudamanyupanishad
Yogakundalyupanishad
Yogarajopanishad
Yogashikhopanishad
Yogatattwopanishad

Tantra

Bhutashuddhitantra
Brihannilatantra
Dattatreyasanghita

Bibliography

Gandharwatantra
Gayatritantra
Goutamiyatantra
Grahayamala
Guptasadhanatantra
Jamala
Jñanachudamani
Jñanasankalinitantra
Jñanarnawa
Kamadhenutantra
Kankalamalinitantra
Koulawalitantra
Kubjikatantra
Kularnawa
Mahamuktitantra
Mahanirwanatantra
Mantramaharnawa
Mantramahodhadhi
Matrikabhedatantra
Mayatantra
Mridanitantra
Mundamalatantra
Nigamalata
Nilatantra
Niruttaratantra
Nirwanatantra
Padukapañchaka (MS; in possession of the
    author's guru)
Paranandasutra
Phetkarinitantra
Pranatoshanitantra
Prapañchasaratantra
Premayogatarangini
Purashcharanarasollasa
Purashcharyarnawa
Radhatantra
Rahasya Shadamnaya Nigama Sandarbha Tantra
Rudrayamala
Sammohanatantra
Sanatkumaratantra
Sarwollasatantra
Satwatatantra
Shadamnayatantra
Shaktakrama
Shaktanandatarangini
Shaktisangamatantra
Shaligramanighantubhushana
Sharadatilakatantra
Shatchakranirupana
Shatchakrawiwriti
Shiwasanghita
Shyamarahasya
Tantragandharwa
Tantrarajatantra

Tantrasara
Tantrabhaktisudharnawa
Tararahasya
Todalatantra
Tripurasarasamuchchaya
Tripurasaratantra
Wishwasaratantra
Yamala
Yogaswarodaya
Yoginihridaya

Purana

Agnipurana
Bhagawata
Brahmandapurana
Brahmapurana
Brahmawaiwartapurana
Dewibhagawata
Garudapurana
Kalikapurana
Kurmapurana
Lingapurana
Matsyapurana
Padmapurana
Shiwapurana
Skandapurana
Sourapurana
Wamanapurana
Warahapurana

Itihasa

Mahabharata

Darshana

Daiwimimangsadarshana

Yoga

Amarasanggraha (MS)
Brahmasiddhantapaddhati (MS)
Gherandasanghita
Hathadipika
Hathasanketachandrika (MS)

Tattwayogabindu (MS)
Yogakalpalatika (MS)
Yogaswarodaya
Yogawashishtha-Ramayana

Dictionaries

Apte's *The Practical Sanskrit-English Dictionary*
Bijabhidhana
Matrikanighantu
Monier-Williams, Sir Monier, *A Sanskrit-English Dictionary*, Oxford, 1899.
Shabdakalpadrumah
Tantrabhidhana
Wachaspatyam
Waidyakashabdasindhu
Warnabijakosha

Other Selected Works

Adhyatma Wiweka
American College of Chest Physicians, *Clinical Cardiopulmonary Physiology*, Grune & Stratton, New York, 1957.
Atma-tattwa-darshana, ed. Jaganmohana Tarkalankara, collected and published by Nilmani Mukhopadhyaya.
Bard, Philip, *Medical Physiology*, The C.V. Mosby Company, St Louis, 1961.
Campbell, E.J. Maran, *The Respiratory Muscles and the Mechanics of Breathing*, Lloyd-Luke (Medical Books) London, 1958.
Comroe, Jr, Julius H., *Physiology of Respiration*, Year Book Medical Publishers, Chicago, 1965.
Comroe, Jr, Julius H., Forster, II, Robert E., Dubois, Arthur B., Briscoe, William A., and Carlsen, Elizabeth, *The Lung*, Year Book Medical Publishers, Chicago, 1963.
Crosby, Elizabeth C., Humphrey, Tryphena, and Lauer, Edward W., eds, *Correlative Anatomy of the Nervous System*, Macmillan, New York, 1962.
Cunningham's Manual of Practical Anatomy, volume III, *Head and Neck and Brain*, revised by Romanes, G.J., 13th edn, Oxford University Press, London, New York & Bombay, 1967.
Cunningham's Textbook of Anatomy, ed. Romanes,

G.J., 10th edn, Oxford University Press, London, New York & Toronto, 1964.
Dorland's Illustrated Medical Dictionary, 24th edn, W.B. Saunders, Philadelphia & London, 1965.
Drinker, Cecil K., *The Clinical Physiology of the Lungs*, Charles C. Thomas, Springfield, Illinois, 1954.
Fenn, Wallace O., and Rahn, Hermann (section eds), *Respiration* (Section 3), vol. I (1964) and vol. II (1965), American Physiological Society, Washington, D.C.
Gitasara.
Gray's Anatomy, ed. Johnston, T.B., and Whillis, J., 30th edn, Longmans, Green, London, New York & Toronto, 1949.
Ganong, William F., *Review of Medical Physiology*, Lange Medical Publications, Los Altos, California, 1963.
Guyton, Arthur C., *Textbook of Medical Physiology*, W.B. Saunders, Philadelphia and London, 1966.
Houssay, Bernardo A., *Human Physiology*, Mcgraw-Hill, New York, Toronto & London, 1955.
Jackson, C.M., *The Effects of Inanition and Malnutrition upon Growth and Structure*, J. & A. Churchill, London, 1925.
Keele, Cyril A., and Neil, Eric, *Samson Wright's Applied Physiology*, Oxford University Press, London, 1961.
MacNalty, Sir Arthur Salusbury, ed. *The British Medical Dictionary*, 1st edn, The Caxton Publishing Company, London, 1961.
Margulis, Sergius, *Fasting and Undernutrition*, E.P. Dutton, New York, 1923.
Miller, William Snow, *The Lung*, Charles C. Thomas Publisher, Springfield, Illinois, 1947.
Parwati — Parameshwara — sangwada.
Ruch, Theodore C., and Patton, Harry D., *Physiology and Biophysics*, W.B. Saunders, Philadelphia and London, 1965.
Sachchidananda Saraswati, Swami, *Pujapradipa*.
Sachchidananda Saraswati, Swami, *Gitapradipa*.
Sachchidananda Saraswati Swami, *Gurupradipa*.
Sachchidananda Saraswati, Swami, *Jñanapradipa*.
Shrikramasanghita.
Sobotta, Dr Med. Johannes, trans. Uhlenhuth, Eduard, *Atlas of Descriptive Human Anatomy*, 7th english edn, vol 1-3, Habner Publishing Company, New York, 1957.
Waidika Sandhya-widhi.
Wishnusanghita.
Youmans, W.B., *Fundamentals of Human Physiology*, Year Book Medical Publishers, Chicago, 1962.

Index

BOOKS OF RELATED INTEREST

Chakras
Energy Centers of Transformation
by Harish Johari

Microchakras
InnerTuning for Psychological Well-being
by Sri Shyamji Bhatnagar and David Isaacs, Ph.D

Secret Power of Tantrik Breathing
Techniques for Attaining Health, Harmony, and Liberation
by Swami Sivapriyananda

The Yoga-Sūtra of Patañjali
A New Translation and Commentary
by Georg Feuerstein, Ph.D.

Yoga Spandakarika
The Sacred Texts at the Origins of Tantra
by Daniel Odier

Breath, Mind, and Consciousness
by Harish Johari

The Yoga of the Nine Emotions
The Tantric Practice of Rasa Sadhana
by Peter Marchand

The Yoga of Power
Tantra, Shakti, and the Secret Way
by Julius Evola

Inner Traditions • Bear & Company
P.O. Box 388
Rochester, VT 05767
1-800-246-8648
www.InnerTraditions.com

Or contact your local bookseller